Medical and Surgical Management of the Diabetic Foot

Medical and Surgical Management of the Diabetic Foot

Stephen J. Kominsky, D.P.M., D.A.B.P.S., F.A.C.F.S.
Director, Podiatric Medical Education
Washington Hospital Center
Clinical Instructor, Department of Medicine,
  Division of Endocrinology
George Washington University Medical Center
Clinical Instructor, Department of Orthopedic
  Surgery
George Washington University Medical Center
Partner, Diabetic Foot Centers
Washington, D.C.

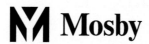 Mosby

St. Louis Baltimore Boston Chicago London Madrid Philadelphia Sydney Toronto

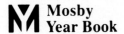

Mosby
Year Book

Dedicated to Publishing Excellence

Publisher: George Stamathis
Editor: James F. Shanahan
Developmental Editor: Jennifer Roche
Editorial Assistant: Anne J. Gleason
Assistant Director/Production, Editing, Design:
Frances M. Perveiler
Project Manager: Nancy C. Baker
Project Supervisor: Carol A. Reynolds
Proofroom Manager: Barbara M. Kelly
Designer: Carol A. Reynolds
Manufacturing Supervisor: John Babrick

Printed in the United States of America
Composition by Graphic World
Printing/binding by Maple–Vail

Mosby–Year Book, Inc.
11830 Westline Industrial Drive
St. Louis, Missouri 63146

Library of Congress Cataloging in
Publication Data
Medical & surgical management of the diabetic
foot / [edited by]
    Stephen Kominsky.
        p.   cm.
    Includes bibliographical references and index.
    ISBN 0-8016-6485-3
    1. Foot—Diseases.   2. Foot—Surgery.
    3. Diabetes—Complications.
  I. Kominsky, Stephen.
    [DNLM: 1. Diabetes Mellitus—
complications.   2. Foot Diseases—
therapy.   3. Foot Diseases—etiology.
WK 835 W489 1993]
RD563.M43 1993
617.5′85—dc20
DNLM/DLC
for Library of Congress   93-33481
                                            CIP

1 2 3 4 5 6 7 8 9 0 98 97 96 95 94

To my beautiful daughter
Danielle;
To Brian, the greatest son a dad
could ever have;
To my beautiful wife Karen, the
glue that keeps it all together;
Thank you for giving up "our
time" to provide me the
opportunity to make this book
happen.

I marvel that society would pay a surgeon a large sum of money to remove a patient's leg—but nothing to save it.

George Bernard Shaw

.   .   .

It has been forced upon me that diabetic gangrene is not heaven sent, but rather, earth borne.

E. P. Joslin (1934)

.   .   .

If you ignore your feet, they'll go away.

Anonymous

Over the last several years, I have often thought about the "dedication" for this textbook. Many circumstances that have an impact on the project arise during the course of the research and manuscript preparation for a project of this magnitude.

The plight of the diabetic patient, with respect to the foot, traditionally has been frought with frustration and anxiety. As we all know too well, the complications of the diabetic foot have been poorly understood, and mistreated for many years. As a result, the amputation rate has been unnecessarily high, and secondarily, mortality in the diabetic population is high.

Historically, these patients travel from physician to physician, looking for treatment for their foot problem(s), only to meet with no success. This compounds their anxiety and frustration as the search continues for the "diabetic foot doctor."

As anyone who treats these patients knows, there is a tremendous sense of reward and gratification with the successful healing of a chronic foot problem in this patient population. That patient truly becomes a patient for life. The look on that patient's face when he or she realizes that a lesion that wouldn't heal *has* healed is tremendously rewarding.

Therefore, this book is dedicated to that ever-growing population of diabetic patients who are susceptible to foot problems. Have the courage and conviction to hang in there and not give up, even in the face of adversity. Extremity amputation should be the absolute last resort, not a "quick fix" of the problem.

This text is also dedicated to those physicians with the interest and sensitivity needed in treating these patients. These pages are filled with stories of frustration as well as triumph. I hope they stimulate the reader to continue through the book and develop the skills needed to reduce the morbidity and mortality too often associated with the diabetic foot.

Stephen J. Kominsky, D.P.M.

CONTRIBUTORS

Christopher E. Attinger, M.D.
Assistant Professor, Plastic Surgery,
  Orthopedic Surgery, Otolaryngology
Georgetown University
Georgetown University Hospital
Washington, D.C.

Alan S. Banks, D.P.M.
Director of Residency Training
Northlake Regional Medical Center
Tucker, Georgia

James A. Birke, Ph.D., P.T.
Clinical Instructor, School of Allied Health
Louisiana State University
Director, Physical Therapy Department
Gillis W. Long Hansen's Disease Center
Carville, Louisiana

Paul W. Brand, M.D., B.S., F.R.C.S.
Clinical Professor Emeritus
Department of Orthopedics
University of Washington at Seattle
Seattle, Washington

Peter R. Cavanagh, Ph.D.
Distinguished Professor of Locomotion
  Studies, Biobehavioral Health and
  Medicine
Pennsylvania State University
University Park, Pennsylvania
Director of Research
Diabetes Foot Clinic, The Milton S. Hershey
  Medical Center
Hershey, Pennsylvania

James S. Chrzan, D.P.M.
Clinical Instructor in Surgery
Harvard Medical School
Division of Podiatry
New England Deaconess Hospital
Boston, Massachusetts

**Jeffrey M. Cohen, D.P.M.,
F.A.C.F.A.S.**
Adjunct Clinical Faculty-Barry University,
  School of Podiatric Medicine
Miami Shores, Florida
New York College of Podiatry
New York, New York
Director, Podiatric Residency Program,
  Englewood Hospital
Englewood Hospital & Medical Center,
  Podiatry Section
Englewood, New Jersey
Holy Name Hospital
Teaneck, New Jersey

William C. Coleman, D.P.M.
Ochsner Clinic
New Orleans, Louisiana

**Sandra Frankenheim, R.N., B.A.,
C.D.E.**
Private Practice
Washington, D.C.

**Robert G. Frykberg, D.P.M.,
F.A.C.F.S.**
Attending Podiatrist
New England Deaconess Hospital
Boston, Massachusetts

Joseph M. Giordano, M.D.
Professor and Chairman, Department of
  Surgery
George Washington University
Chairman, Department of Surgery
George Washington University
Washington, D.C.

John M. Giurini, D.P.M.
Clinical Instructor in Surgery
Harvard Medical School
New England Deaconess Hospital, Division
  of Podiatry
Boston, Massachusetts

Jean S. Gordon, M.D.
Assistant Director of Medical Education
Coastal Emergency Services
Attending Physician
Broward General Medical Center
Ft. Lauderdale, Florida

Geoffrey M. Habershaw, D.P.M.
Clinical Instructor in Surgery
Harvard Medical School
New England Deaconess Hospital, Division
  of Podiatry
Boston, Massachusetts

Yadollah Harati, M.D., F.A.C.P.
Professor of Neurology
Baylor College of Medicine
Chief, Neurology Service
Veterans Affair Medical Center
Houston, Texas

Patricia Herrera, M.D.
Attending Physician, Division of Infectious
  Diseases
Rush Medical College
Attending Physician, Department of
  Medicine, Division of Infectious Disease
Cook County Hospital
Chicago, Illinois

J. Phillip A. Hinton, M.D., F.A.C.S.
Medical Director, California Vascular
  Institute
Community Hospitals of Central California
Fresno, California

**Richard Martin Jay, D.P.M.,
F.A.C.F.A.S.**
Professor, Pediatric Foot and Ankle
  Orthopedics
Director of Pediatrics
Pennsylvania College of Podiatric Medicine
Director, Foot and Ankle Surgical Residency
  Program
The Graduate Hospital
President, American College of Foot and
  Ankle Pediatrics
Philadelphia, Pennsylvania

James S. Jelinek, M.D.
Assistant Professor Radiology, Uniformed
  Services University of Health Sciences
Bethesda, Maryland
Visiting Professor, Radiologic Pathology,
  Armed Forces Institute of Pathology
Diagnostic Radiologist, Chief
  Musculoskeletal Radiology
Washington Hospital Center
Washington, D.C.

Youssef M. Kabbani, D.P.M.
Visiting Professor
Department of Foot and Ankle Surgery/
  Medicine
Podiatrist
Department of Foot and Ankle Surgery
North Philadelphia Health Systems (St.
  Joseph's Division)
Philadelphia, Pennsylvania

**David R. Knighton, M.D., F.A.C.S.,
F.A.C.A.**
Clinical Associate Professor
University of Minnesota, Department of
  Surgery
University of Minnesota Hospital and Clinic
Minneapolis, Minnesota

**Stephen J. Kominsky, D.P.M.,
D.A.B.P.S., F.A.C.F.S.**
Director, Podiatric Medical Education
Washington Hospital Center
Clinical Instructor, Department of Medicine,
  Division of Endocrinology
George Washington University Medical
  Center
Clinical Instructor, Department of
  Orthopedic Surgery
George Washington University Medical
  Center
Partner, Diabetic Foot Centers
Washington, D.C.

Roy O. Kroeker, D.P.M.
Director of Podiatric Medicine
President, Diabetic Foot Center
Diplomat, National Board of Podiatric
  Medicine
Senior Podiatric Surgeon
Sierra Hospital
St. Agnes Medical Center
Fresno Community Hospital
Fresno, California

Stephen D. Lasday, D.P.M.
Grand Lake Foot and Ankle Specialists
Assistant Director Grand Lake Foot and
  Ankle Surgical Residency Program
Joint Township District Memorial Hospital
Associate Staff, Graduate Hospital, Foot and
  Ankle Surgical Residency
St. Mary's, Ohio

**Mark S. Lenes, B.S., M.S.Ed.,
R.Ph., P.D.**
Executive Vice President
NorthWest HealthCare
Columbia, Maryland

Elliot B. Levy, M.D.
Chief, Interventional Radiology Section
Southern Maryland Hospital
Clinton, Maryland

Frank W. LoGerfo, M.D., F.A.C.S.
Professor of Surgery
Harvard Medical School
Chief, Division of Vascular Surgery
New England Deaconess Hospital
Boston, Massachusetts

David P. Mayer, M.D.
Clinical Associate Professor
Department of Diagnostic Imaging, Temple
 University School of Medicine
Director, Graduate Hospital Imaging Center
The Graduate Hospital
Philadelphia, Pennsylvania

**Daniel J. McCarthy, M.R.E., M.A.,
Ph.D., D.P.M.**
Adjunct Clinical Professor
Ohio, Pennsylvania, New York, Des Moines
 Colleges of Podiatric Medicine
Chief, Podiatric Section, Surgical Service
VA Medical Centers of Baltimore; Fort
 Howard; Perry Point
Baltimore; Fort Howard; Perry Point;
 Maryland

John B. Nelson, M.D., F.A.C.C.
Director of Research
California Vascular Institute
Fresno Community Hospital
Fresno, California

Richard F. Neville, M.D.
Assistant Professor of Surgery
Georgetown University
Vascular Surgery
VA and Georgetown University Medical
 Centers
Washington, D.C.

J. Paul O'Keefe, M.D.
Professor of Medicine
Loyola University Stritch School of Medicine
Director, Division of Infectious Diseases
Foster G. McGaw Hospital
Maywood, Illinois
Hines VA Hospital
Hines, Illinois

**Maureen Smith Plombon, M.S., R.D.,
F.A.C.S.M.**
President
Integrated Health Consultants, Inc.
Oakton, Virginia

Robert E. Ratner, M.D., F.A.C.P.
Associate Professor of Medicine
George Washington School of Medicine
Director, Section of Endocrinology
Washington Hospital Center
Washington, D.C.

Barry I. Rosenbloom, D.P.M.
Clinical Instructor in Surgery
Harvard Medical School
New England Deaconess Hospital, Division
 of Podiatry
Boston, Massachusetts

Ronald A. Sage, D.P.M.
Associate Professor-Orthopaedic Surgery
Loyola University Stritch School of Medicine
Chief-Section of Podiatry
Loyola University Medical Center
Maywood, Illinois
Hines VA Hospital
Hines, Illinois

**Linda Selemba Schultz, R.N., M.S.N.,
A.N.P., C.D.E.**
Nurse Practitioner
Washington Hospital Center
Washington, D.C.

Anton N. Sidawy, M.D., F.A.C.S.
Associate Professor of Surgery
George Washington University
Chief, Vascular Surgery
VA Medical Center
Washington, D.C.

Herb S. Steb, C.PED., M.B.A.
Consultant and Pedorthic Faculty Member
Orthotic Prosthetic Division (Pedorthic
 Management)
Northwestern University Medical School
Chicago, Illinois
Director of Pedorthics
Diabetic Foot Centers of America
Washington, D.C.
President
Walk-Well Professional Fitters
Summit, New Jersey

**Jeffrey L. Tredwell, D.P.M.,
F.A.C.F.S., Diplomate A.P.B.S.**
President/Founder
Diabetic Foot Centers of America
Washington Hospital Center
Washington, D.C.

Jan S. Ulbrecht, M.D.
Associate Professor of Biobehavioral Health
Pennsylvania State University
Adjunct Associate Professor of Medicine,
   Dept. of Medicine
College of Medicine at the Penn State
   University
Hershey Medical Center
Hershey, Pennsylvania
Centre Community Hospital
State College, Pennsylvania

Sharon M. Wollman, R.N.
Director of Clinical Services
NorthWest HealthCare
Columbia, Maryland
Clinical Associate of American Academy of
   Pain Management (national)

FOREWORD

It is a real pleasure to congratulate Dr. Stephen Kominsky for recognizing the need for a comprehensive book such as this, and for gathering such a distinguished group of contributors so that we can now have on our shelves one of the first truly authoritative textbooks on every aspect of the management of the diabetic foot. Up until now, anyone seeking reliable information on this subject either had to read single chapters on the diabetic foot in large textbooks devoted to the disease of diabetes itself, or they had to find single chapters devoted to diabetic feet in textbooks of orthopaedic surgery, general surgery, or podiatric medicine.

I am personally gratified to see amongst the authors of the various chapters some of my own colleagues and others whom I have taught. From my armchair of partial retirement it is good to look back and see some of the developments which started during the study of the insensitive feet of leprosy patients in the 1940s and 1950s, and then widened and gained momentum as they were applied to meet the similar problems of diabetic patients whose feet were in danger of breaking down or being amputated.

The foot of a diabetic patient is a problem mainly because it becomes insensitive. Tissues break down with seemingly trivial stress, but not because they are fragile. Wounds fail to heal, but not because they lack growth factors. It is their lack of sensation that exposes them to constant minor trauma, the control of which

is usually enough to promote normal healing. Even those cases which have significant vascular problems seldom break down unless and until they lose their sensitivity to pain.

A second observation which is dealt with in several chapters of the book is that the breakdown and ulceration is almost always due to mechanical stress. This may be a single application of high stress at just one blow, or oft-repeated moderate stress thousands of times in succession (as in walking) or really quite low stress maintained continuously, resulting in aeschemia. Recognition of these factors should result in our concentrating on mechanical forces and modifying them so that the wound may heal and not recur. This book has good sections dealing with shoes and with plaster casts which deal with control of mechanical stress.

Finally, there is an important mental and psychological aspect to diabetic feet and this also is directly the result of the loss of sensation. Once a patient can no longer feel his foot and no longer has an interchange of information and control between his foot and his brain, there is a subtle but profound change in body image. To the patient, the foot feels dead. It is no longer part of him. So long as it remains attached to his leg, it may be used for walking on, but it will surely fall off or be amputated one day.

I sometimes feel that this mental rejection of a diabetic foot should have as much or more attention than all the other factors, because if once a person can change his or her subconscious mental image, and recognize that his foot is really alive and valuable and capable of carrying him for years to come, then he'll begin to take care of himself and assume responsibility for everything that happens to it. All of the other chapters in this book become futile if the patient loses interest in his foot. Conversely, if he can learn to accept responsibility on a day-to-day basis and inspect his foot regularly to pick up possible early signs of damage (temperature hot spots, for example) so that he can modify his behavior before real trouble starts, then the battle for foot survival has been won.

Too often we think of the patients as stupid, because they neglect our advice, and walk on their infected feet. Most of them are not stupid. You and I do not use intelligence in caring for our feet. We are equipped with pain, and that forces us to behave sensibly. We must give time and use patience and repetition to help our pain-free patients to understand the reality they cannot feel. This is referred to in the book. I just feel the need to add a little passion and extra emphasis to the things that nobody should miss. Now read on, and enjoy the feast.

Paul Brand, M.D.
Clinical Professor Emeritus
Department of Orthopaedics
University of Washington in Seattle
Seattle, Washington

PREFACE

My interest in the diabetic foot began years ago in a general podiatry practice. My partners and I began noticing that our diabetic patients were "being treated" for major complications by physicians outside of our practice, and were returning to us with amputated limbs. After awhile this became very disconcerting to us, and we decided to embark on something that would change our lives in a very positive way.

Over the years since that time, the role of the physician treating the diabetic foot has changed dramatically. Emphasis has been placed on the importance of saving limbs and reducing the morbidity and mortality once associated with this disease.

Statistics show that each year more than $6 billion are spent in the United States on direct medical costs associated with diabetic foot disease. The average duration of stay in the hospital nationwide for a diabetic patient with a foot infection is approximately 19½ days. The average diagnosis related group (DRG) payment/duration of stay is approximately 5 days. Therefore, one can quickly see that these patients cost the system a lot of money. In this era of "health care reform" these are important numbers.

In setting out to plan, and ultimately produce, this textbook, I believed that the material should be presented almost like telling a story. The first part sets the scene, that is, the basic science of the pathologic process. The first several chapters discuss diabetes itself; the disease and the physiologic complications that it causes. These include the vascular component, and the neurologic component. In addition, early in the text is a chapter on examination of the patient to better evaluate these systems.

The next group of chapters discusses diagnostic testing of the extremity to reach the appropriate diagnosis. Discussions on imaging, noninvasive vascular testing, and magnetic resonance imaging are included in these chapters.

The third group of chapters deals with treatment of the various problems as they develop. Some of these chapters include outpatient management of complications, surgical management of infections, and soft tissue reconstruction, to name just a few.

Finally, the last group of chapters discusses some controversial topics such as the use of hyperbaric oxygen in the treatment of ulcers. This section also includes aspects of nutrition, education, and home care from the perspective of the diabetic patient with a foot problem.

Certainly this text can be used as a reference for researching one particular component (e.g., complications, surgery, infections), but to really grasp the "whole story," it is recommended that you read the entire book.

This book is built on the frustrations and successes with all of our patients from each and every one of the fine contributing authors in this text.

Stephen J. Kominsky, D.P.M.

ACKNOWLEDGMENTS

A project of this magnitude requires the assistance of many people. It is my pleasure to take this opportunity to give credit to those who helped me realize my dream in producing this book.

I thank my partner, Jeffrey Tredwell, D.P.M., and former partner, Stuart Tessler, D.P.M., for providing me the opportunity within our practice, and inspiration in making this project a reality.

A special thank you to Annik Adamson, D.P.M., and Cassandra Darroch, D.P.M., for assisting me with all of the preliminary research.

Thank you to Bob Ratner, M.D., for professional guidance; and to Rick Jay, D.P.M., for being a friend and for pushing me to get started with this project.

Last, I thank all of my friends at Mosby who have made this book a reality; without any of them it would not have happened. Jim Shanahan and Anne Gleason, thank you so very much.

Stephen J. Kominsky, D.P.M.

CONTENTS

1 Overview of the Diabetic Foot

Robert E. Ratner, M.D.

DEMOGRAPHICS, EPIDEMIOLOGY AND HEALTH CARE COSTS

The importance of diabetes mellitus as a cause of lower-extremity disease was recognized well before the discovery of insulin. The surgical literature of the 19th century admonished that "gangrene occurring from trivial causes in persons presenting the appearance of usual health and in whom no evidence of atheromatous degeneration of the arteries can be detected should awaken the suspicion of the existence of diabetes and no time should be lost in making a careful examination of the urine."[1] In 1988, the last year for which complete data are available, 55,000 lower-extremity amputations were performed in individuals with diabetes mellitus.[2] Based upon previous data, diabetes accounts for 45% of all lower-extremity amputations and the individual with diabetes has a fifteenfold higher risk of requiring an amputation as compared to their age- and sex-matched nondiabetic control.[3] Perhaps of greatest concern, however, is the dramatic increase in incidence of lower-extremity amputations over the last decade (Fig 1–1). The Centers for Disease Control (CDC) has reported a 60% increase in the incidence of lower-extremity amputations in the diabetic population from 1980 through 1988.[2, 4] As with the prevalence of the diabetes itself, the burden of diabetes-related lower-extremity disease in the United States falls disproportionately on those in our society least able to deal with it. As compared to the white population, African Americans have twice the prevalence, Mexican Americans three times, and Native Americans five times the prevalence of diabetes. In addition, the incidence of diabetes mellitus increases with age so that 18% of the U.S. population over the age of 65 is affected.[5] Complications within these groups are markedly increased with the risk of amputation 2.3 times greater for African Americans[3] (Fig 1–2) and 3.7 times greater in certain Native American populations.[6] Sixty percent of all lower-extremity amputations among the diabetic population occur in individuals over the age of 65[2] (Fig 1–3).

Diabetic foot disease results in hospitalization more often than any other diabetic complication,[7] with 16% of all hospital admissions and 23% of total hospital days attributable to diabetic foot pathology.[8] The average hospital length of stay ranges from 18 to 21 days at a cost of $20,000 to $25,000, and diabetic foot disease accounts for approximately 10% of all direct costs related to diabetes care.[9]

These direct costs are only a small fraction of total societal costs related to diabetic foot pathology. Economic costs related to absenteeism, permanent disability, and mortality must also be factored in. Absenteeism in diabetic subjects with

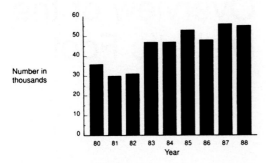

Number in thousands

FIG 1–1.
Nontraumatic lower extremity amputations related to diabetes, United States. (From Centers for Disease Control, U.S. Department of Health and Human Services, 1992.)

complications is 11-fold higher than that of an age-matched nondiabetic control population, accounting for 44 days per year at a cost of $365,000 per patient.[10] In this study, diabetes ranked third behind neurotic disorders and cardiac ischemia as the leading cause of permanent disability. As a result, early retirement resulted in 11 years of lost productivity due to diabetes-related permanent disability. Of course, the greatest societal loss is related to the overall mortality associated with lower-extremity disease. Acute mortality is difficult to quantify because death cer-

tificates seldom use diabetic foot ulcers as a cause of death. Rather, the subsequent occurrence of sepsis, myocardial infarction, and shock related to the foot disease predominate on official records. The prognosis for those individuals undergoing a lower-limb amputation remains dismal with a 3-year survival rate of 50%.[11]

Standards of Care

Despite the undisputed importance of diabetic foot pathology as a cause of significant morbidity and mortality, the overall level of medical care directed toward the foot remains woefully inadequate. Foot examinations by physicians at the time of routine medical visits for diabetes care occur in a disappointing 12% of visits. In addition, 73% of all foot examinations were performed by only 23% of the physicians included in the study, with only 49% of patients describing a foot examination by a health-care professional within the preceding year.[12] Utilization of foot care specialists in a consultative capacity was a disappointing 18%. This pattern of practice falls far short of the Standards of Foot Care adopted by the

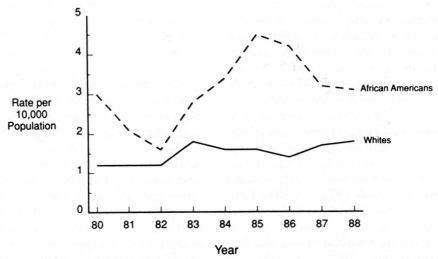

FIG 1–2.
Nontraumatic lower extremity amputations by race related to diabetes, United States. (From Centers for Disease Control, U.S. Department of Health and Human Services, 1992.)

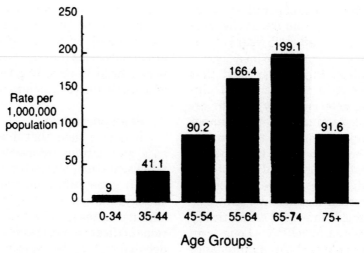

FIG 1–3.

Nontraumatic lower extremity amputations by age, related to diabetes, 1988. (From Centers for Disease Control, U.S. Department of Health and Human Services, 1992.)

American Diabetes Association.[13] Meeting these Standards of Foot Care and reducing risk factors for amputation have been projected to reduce by 50% the number of amputations within the diabetic population.[14]

Instituting a specialized foot clinic using the diverse skills of various health-care professionals is the most efficient means of both meeting the standards of care and successfully preventing lower-extremity amputations. In a prospective study, a dedicated foot clinic was able to reduce the incidence of major amputations by 50% and minor operations by 40% in the 3 years following its institution.[15] It remains an unfortunate truism that recognition of diabetic foot disease and appropriate intervention for its treatment is impossible unless patients and their health-care provider remove the shoes and examine the feet.

Glycemic Control and Complications

The etiology of diabetic foot disease is multifactorial. Multiple studies have examined the risk factors associated with diabetic foot ulcers and subsequent lower-limb amputations. As previously discussed, the risk of foot pathology increases with age and appears to be higher in minority populations with diabetes. In addition, there is clear evidence that men have foot ulcerations more commonly than women do. In the Pima Indians, duration of diabetes and the level of fasting and 2-hour postprandial glucose were significant factors for predicting amputation.[6] The role of glycemic control in causing chronic diabetic complications, however, has long been debated. From an epidemiologic standpoint, foot lesions, including gangrene, were twofold more frequent in those individuals with high glucose levels as compared with better controlled individuals with diabetes.[16] There also appears to be a relationship between glycemic control and the level of severity of peripheral vascular disease in age- and duration-matched patients with diabetes.[17]

Because of the multifactorial pathogenesis of diabetic foot disease, it is useful to examine the available data on the effect of glycemic control in general on the occurrence of diabetic complications. In his landmark personal observations, Pirart reported the prevalence of peripheral neuropathy progressing from 8% at the time of diagnosis to 50% after 25 years' duration of diabetes.[18] Using loose measures of glycemic control, Pirart suggested that those individuals with lower blood glucose levels (as determined by 24-hour urine glucose determinations, the number of insulin injections, and the number of hypoglycemic reactions) had less severe neuropathic signs and symptoms. In short-term studies, nerve conduction velocity increased significantly and perception thresholds improved dramatically with glycemic control.[19, 20] Long-term studies have confirmed the maintenance of improved nerve conduction velocity involving the nerves of the lower extremities after 3 years of intensive insulin therapy.[21]

Although atherosclerotic peripheral vascular disease has multiple risk factors, with diabetes being only one, it is now clear that diabetes coexists in higher instance with other atherosclerotic risk factors.[22] Diabetes alters existing lipids to render them more atherogenic,[23] and systemic hyperinsulinemia may be atherogenic in and of itself.[24]

Multiple studies have endeavored to show the relationship between glycemic control and progression of microvascular diabetic complications. In the Kroc, Steno Memorial Hospital, and Oslo studies, intensive glycemic control with multiple daily insulin injections or insulin pump therapy demonstrated reduced progression of diabetic complications.[25, 26, 27] These studies have been criticized for their short duration, small patient populations, and their failure to examine primary prevention. The Diabetes Control and Complications Trial is a prospective, randomized, controlled trial of intensive glucose control and its effects on diabetes complications in 1,441 patients followed for over 9,000 patient-years. By achieving average daily blood glucose levels of 155 mg%, the risk of new-onset clinically significant

neuropathy was reduced by 70%, while progression of pre-existant neuropathy was reduced by 58%.[28] There is now a broad consensus that near normoglycemia is beneficial in retarding the progression of diabetic microvascular complications.

Pathophysiology

It is now clear that diabetic foot disease stems from interaction among altered sensation, biomechanical abnormalities, trauma, infection, and impaired tissue oxygenation resulting from peripheral vascular disease. The relative contributions of these various factors has long been debated and can be examined in a variety of different ways. In one study,[15] 62% of foot ulcers were classified as neuropathic while 38% were considered to be ischemic in origin. Even so, the majority of those in the ischemic group had the presence of neuropathy as well. The absence of vibratory perception in the lower extremity increases the relative risk of amputation 15.5 fold, while a history of peripheral vascular disease increases the amputation risk ninefold.[29] This is further aggravated by the presence of biomechanical abnormalities resulting from either neuromuscular abnormalities or surgical procedures.[30] These factors predispose to tissue breakdown. When this is compounded by the presence of peripheral vascular disease resulting in $TcPO_2 < 20$ mm Hg the odds ratio of amputation rises to 161 times control. The presence of a chronic nonhealing ulcer then provides a portal of entry for infectious processes. In the study of Reiber et al,[29] infection was found in 68% of all amputated limbs.

In yet another analysis, it appears that isolated neuropathy or vascular insufficiency were insufficient alone to require amputation. Seventy-five percent of all diabetic limb amputations result from the sequence of events including minor trauma in the setting of peripheral neuropathy, subsequent skin ulceration, and faulty wound healing.[31]

The involvement of each individual component in this pathway will be covered in greater detail in subsequent chapters in this book. An understanding of the interaction of diabetic complications resulting in lower extremity disease provides an avenue for appropriate intervention for the ultimate prevention of ulceration and the subsequent need for amputation. This has been delineated as a major public health goal by the Department of Health and Human Services with a target reduction of amputations due to diabetic foot disease of 40% by the year 2000.[32]

REFERENCES

1. Senn N: *Principles of surgery,* Philadelphia, 1890, FA Davis, p 193.
2. *Diabetes in the United States: a strategy for prevention,* 1992, U.S. Department of Health and Human Services, National Center for Chronic Disease Prevention and Health Promotion, Division of Diabetes Translation.
3. Most RS, Sinnock P: The epidemiology of lower extremity amputations in diabetic individuals, *Diabetes Care* 6:87–91, 1983.
4. Wetterhall SF et al: Trends in diabetes and diabetic complications, *Diabetes Care* 15:960–967, 1992.
5. Harris MI et al: Prevalence of diabetes and impaired glucose tolerance and plasma glucose levels in the U.S. populations age 20–74 years, *Diabetes* 36:523–534, 1987.
6. Nelson RG et al: Lower extremity amputations in NIDDM: 12-year follow-up study in Pima Indians, *Diabetes Care* 11:8–16, 1988.
7. Gibbons Smith G, Eliopolos G: Infection of the diabetic foot. In Kozak G et al, editors: *Management of diabetic foot problems,* Philadelphia, 1984, Saunders, pp 97–102.
8. Smith D, Weinberger M, Katz B: A controlled trial to increase office visits and reduce hospitalizations of diabetic patients, *J Gen Int Med* 2:232–238, 1987.
9. Reiber GE: Diabetic foot care financial implications and practical guidelines, *Diabetes Care* 15(suppl 1):29–31, 1992.
10. Olivera EM, Perez-Duhalde E, Gagliardino JJ: Cost of temporary and permanent disability induced by diabetes, *Diabetes Care* 14:593–596, 1991.
11. Palumbo PJ, Melton LJ: Peripheral vascular disease and diabetes. In *Diabetes in America,* NIH Publication No 85-1468, Washington, DC, 1985, U.S. Government Printing Office, pp 1–21.
12. Bailey TS, Yu HM, Rayfield EJ: Patterns of foot examination in the diabetes clinic, *Am J Med* 78:371–374, 1985.
13. American Diabetes Association: Foot care in patients with diabetes mellitus, *Diabetes Care* 14(suppl 2):18–19, 1991.
14. National Diabetes Advisory Board: *The prevention and treatment of five complications of diabetes: a guide for primary care practitioners,* HHS Publication No 83-8392, Atlanta, 1983, Centers for Disease Control.
15. Edmonds ME et al: Improved survival of the diabetic foot: the role of the specialized foot clinic, *Q J Med* 232:763–771, 1986.
16. West KM: *Epidemiology of diabetes and its vascular lesions,* New York, 1978, Elsevier, North-Holland, pp 84–126.
17. Keen H, Jarrett R, editors: *Complications of diabetes,* London, 1975, Edward Arnold, pp 179–203.
18. Pirart J: Diabetes mellitus and its degenerative complications: a prospective study of 4,400 patients observed between 1947 and 1973, *Diabetes Care* 1:168–188, 1978.
19. Pietri A, Ehle AL, Raskin P: Changes in nerve conduction velocity after six weeks of glucose regulation with portable insulin infusion pumps, *Diabetes* 29:668–671, 1980.
20. Service FJ et al: Near normo glycemia improved nerve conduction and vibration sensation in diabetic neuropathy, *Diabetologia* 28:722–727, 1985.
21. Reichard P et al: Metabolic control and complications over three years in patients with insulin dependent diabetes: The Stockholm Diabetes Intervention Study, *J Int Med* 280:511–517, 1990.
22. Reaven GM: Role of insulin resistance of

human disease, *Diabetes* 37:1595–1607, 1988.

23. Garber AJ, Vinik AI, Crespin SR: Detection and management of lipid disorders in diabetic patients: a commentary for clinicians, *Diabetes Care* 15:1068–1074, 1992.

24. Durrington PN: Is insulin atherogenic?, *Diabetic Med* 9:597–600, 1992.

25. Kroc Collaborative Study Group: Blood glucose control and evolution of diabetic retinopathy and albuminuria, *N Engl J Med* 311:365–372, 1984.

26. Lauritzen T et al: The Steno Study Group: Two-year experience with continuous subcutaneous insulin infusion in relation to retinopathy and neuropathy, *Diabetes* 34(suppl 3):74–79, 1985.

27. Dahl-Jorgensen K et al: Effect of near-normo glycemia for two years on progression of early diabetic retinopathy, nephropathy, and neuropathy: The Oslo Study, *Br Med J* 293:1195–1199, 1986.

28. Diabetes Control and Complications Trial, *N Engl J Med,* in press.

29. Reiber GE, Pecoraro RE, Koepsell TD: Risk factors for amputation in patients with diabetes mellitus: a case control study, *Ann Intern Med* 117:97–105, 1992.

30. Bild DE et al: Lower extremity amputation in people with diabetes, *Diabetes Care* 12:24–31, 1989.

31. Pecoraro RE, Reiber GE, Burgess EM: Pathways to diabetic limb amputation, *Diabetes Care* 13:513–521, 1990.

32. Department of Health and Human Services: Healthy people 2000. In *National health promotion and disease prevention objections,* DHHS Publication No PHS 91-50212, Washington, DC, 1992, U.S. Government Printing Office.

2

The Initial Foot Examination of the Patient With Diabetes

William C. Coleman, D.P.M., D.A.B.P.O.

James A. Birke, M.S. P.T.

Several studies published during the past 20 years have concluded that the preferred form of clinical management for the patient with diabetes is the multidisciplinary team.[1-3] A specialist team should be able to differentiate a symptom attributable to diabetes from symptoms of other causes. For maximum efficiency and ideal patient care, each member of the team should be aware of the findings of the other specialists. Each should be capable of contributing a unique, essential component to the diagnosis and treatment of the patient's pathologic condition. Three questions should dominate the thought process of every member of the team:

1. Are the feet of the patient currently injured?
2. Is the patient at more risk of injury because his or her diabetes is compromising circulation or innervation?
3. Is the patient appropriately aware of the possible damage that could realistically develop on the foot if he or she does not maintain appropriate behavior consistent with the degree of risk?

If the team intends to treat large numbers of patients with diabetes, each member's examination must efficiently and effectively detect a present pathologic condition. Each finding must be included in a larger body of knowledge. These data must be readily available at the time decisions are being made for the definitive management of the patient. In larger clinics and hospitals this information can be difficult to extract from the record of patients who frequently have large charts because of a history of multiple diseases. For this reason not only should the information be included in this chart but a separate record of data relevant to the feet of a diabetic patient should be maintained. Standardized forms should be used in this specific record to make the information easily accessible for current clinical and historical purposes.

Though preferable, a team does not require face-to-face communication of information between team members. In many situations it is not practical for the members of the team to be in the same building or even belong to the same organization. Individual practitioners can establish a team with local professionals to coordinate care. In the interest of the diabetic population, in small communities this team must be accessible to every concerned caregiver.

The team approach works well only if the team members maintain communication with each other. Physicians who treat patients with diabetes routinely know that a high percentage of their patients do not adhere to recommended diet, exercise, or medical management protocols. This is true for foot care and shoe advice as well. Assal[4] has studied this problem for several years and has concluded the fault can be attributed to traditional education techniques in medical schools. He believes chronic diseases such as diabetes require a more holistic approach incorporating psychologic and sociologic management in addition to the biomedical perspective that dominates current medical practice.

Chronic disease in particular alters the patient psychologically in ways that are well defined in psychologic literature. Psychologic stages in chronic diseases have been compared to the psychologic phases of mourning.[5] Without going too far into psychology, the work of Assal et al.[6] in Geneva has been given much more credence because their techniques have resulted in an 85% reduction of lower-extremity amputations.

For purposes of consistency and to facilitate communication, the team should adopt history and physical forms containing the most relevant information for patient management. The history and physical forms in this chapter are included to serve as a starting point.

PATIENT HISTORY

This history form (Fig 2–1) was designed to include the information we consider to be most useful to help each patient minimize the possibility of catastrophic foot problems. Over the past few years a determined effort has been made to minimize useless information. Each element of the form should result in a comprehensive picture of the patient's problem and contribute to the design of an individualized patient education and treatment program.

Age, obesity, race, sex, and duration of having diabetes have been identified as factors that categorize patients as being in groups with higher risk of developing the secondary complications of neuropathy and peripheral vascular disease.[7] The incidence of peripheral vascular disease in patients with diabetes increased with age and duration of diabetes and is higher in men than in women.[8, 9] In Rochester, Minnesota, 8% of peripheral vascular disease at the time of the diagnosis of diabetes, 15% 10 years after diagnosis, 45% 20 years after diagnosis of diabetes.[9] Peripheral neuropathy was found in 8% of patients at the time of diagnosis of diabetes, 50% at 25 years with diabetes.[10] Risk of amputation in people with diabetes is greater in the black population than the white. The greater incidence of smoking and hypertension among blacks is probably a contributing factor.[11, 12] These factors are recorded at the top of the history form for quick reference and to emphasize the importance to the foot care team members. The patient's control of blood glucose levels are recorded by both the most recent fasting blood glucose level, or the patient's own home glucose monitor, and the glycosylated hemoglobin A_{1c} level.

For easy reference current medications are listed in the upper right-hand corner. Patients with multiple systemic diseases often forget specific terminology for them. In addition to the clinician's obvious need to know the list of medications for possible adverse interactions or contribution to current symptoms, the medication list aids in the identification of other chronic or acute diseases. Many patients and many physicians do not adhere to the principles of continuity of care. In such an environment, a complete list of the current medications may reveal a conflict in the patient management. If no primary physician can be identified by the patient, the physician who manages the patient's diabetes is recommended to fill this role. If the physician is not a member of the management team, he or she is telephoned to be advised of problems.

The presence of systemic diseases that have been identified as major contributing

OCHSNER FOOT CARE PROGRAM
DIABETIC PATIENT - FOOT HISTORY

NAME_____ CURRENT MEDICATIONS:

PATIENT NUMBER _____AGE_____ DATE_____

HEIGHT_____

WEIGHT(lbs.)_____

RACE_____

SEX ____

TIME w/ DIABETES: TYPE I_____ TYPE II _____

LAST BLOOD SUGAR_____ date _____ Gly Hemo A1c_____ date _____

CURRENT DIABETES PHYSICIAN _____

SYSTEMIC DISEASES:CAD ____ PVD____ Nephropathy ____ Retinopathy ____ Dialysis ____
    CVA ____ CHF ____ HTN ____ Hyperlipidemia _____

SOCIAL HISTORY: Smoking _____ pkg/yr EtOH _____ Occupation _____

HOME LOCATION _____

PAIN: Rest pain ____ claudication ____ > w/ walking ____ numbness/tingling ____ burning/sharp ____

PREVIOUS FRACTURES IN FEET _____

PREVIOUS VASCULAR SURGERY _____

PREVIOUS FOOT SURGERY _____

PREVIOUS FOOT ULCERATION _____

CHIEF FOOT COMPLAINT _____

HISTORY:

CURRENTLY WALKING ON UNPROTECTED WOUND: Y ___ N ___

CURRENT WOUND CARE _____

FOOT CARE PROVIDER _____

CURRENT PREFERRED FOOTWEAR: Pumps ____ slippers ____ loafers ____ oxfords ____
    boots ____ steel toes ____ sports ____ sandals ____

Material: plastic ____ leather ____ cloth ____ Heels: high ____ med ____ low ____

HISTORY OF PRESCRIBED FOOTWEAR _____

NAME OF SHOE FITTER _____

FIG 2–1.
Foot history form.

factors in the development or aggravation of the secondary complications affecting the lower extremities can be recorded by checking appropriate blanks. Hypertension increases the risk of intermittent claudication 2.5 times for men and 4 times for women.[13] Nephropathy and retinopathy are particularly ominous for the degree and rate of the advancement of diabetic complications. Hyperlipidemia is a risk factor for peripheral vascular disease.[13] Efforts to control these contributing pathologic precursors should reduce the patients risk of amputation.[3]

Smoking probably contributes to the development and rate of progression of peripheral vascular disease. The effects on blood components and vessels is well documented. (For example, atherosclerotic development is accelerated by smoking.) Smoking doubled the risk of intermittent claudication in both sexes in the Framingham study.[13] Direct correlations to the process of diabetic peripheral vascular disease, however, are still in contention.[13]

Alcoholism aggravates diabetes control but also is a potential source of neuropathy. If it can be extracted by history, the possibility of alcohol contributing to neuropathic symptoms has to be included.

Environmental factors also provide essential information to differentiate the neuropathic symptoms of diabetes from other occupational or neighborhood toxins.

Painful Neuropathy

There are several types of pain syndromes in diabetes. Though diabetes often results in segmental demyelination and axon loss as a result of metabolic abnormalities, the actual mechanism leading to damage is not yet conclusively defined. A high blood glucose level is a high-risk factor for peripheral neuropathy.[14, 15] Though there is a later chapter on neuropathy, here we will focus on the symptoms.

Diabetic mononeuropathies can involve a focal lesion of the lumbosacral plexus or a few nerve roots. The symptoms are usually asymmetric with sudden onset and may resolve quickly with only reassurance of the patient. These symptoms are far more prevalent among the elderly. Often it occurs with sensations of numbness or tingling in the feet. In the lower extremity it is primarily a motor neuropathy.

Polyradiculopathy often accompanies distal polyneuropathy. It begins unilaterally with pain, followed by weakness. The elderly are those usually affected. They recover substantially in 1 to 2 years. Amyotrophy effects L2, L3, and L4 nerve roots.[16] It manifests itself as adductor muscle weakness.

Diabetic amyotrophy leads to asymmetric severe pain, quadriceps wasting, and absent patellar reflexes. It is more common in men and usually resolves after several months.

Patients with neuropathic cachexia experience symmetric severe pain, weakness and wasting of muscles, weight loss, impotence, and depression. The clinical course is one of gradual improvement. Recovery ultimately occurs in about 1 year.[17]

Painful polyneuropathy is the most common form of the symptomatic neuropathies. Sensory symptoms in a stocking or glove pattern predominate, and objective findings may be minimal despite complaints of intense pain. The pain varies in character and intensity. Pain and paresthesias are more intense at night. The involved areas may be extremely sensitive to touch. Even hair follicles may be very sensitive. Onset of symptoms may follow the initiation of insulin or sulfonylurea therapy, injury, or infection.

It has been suggested that the progressive increase of pain may represent a sprouting of new nerve fibers with poorly developed function interpreted as pain.[18] In another form painful neuropathy comes many years after the onset of the disease. This pain can be persistent, debilitating, and progressive. Tobacco and alcohol have been implicated in the pathogenesis. In the past these symptoms have led to narcotic abuse. Depression with anorexia seems to be an integral part of painful neuropathies. The alert clinician will often recognize the desperate anxiety that often accompanies these symptoms leading to feelings of futility and an inabiltiy to cope with activities of daily living. Distal symmetric polyneuropathy is the most common form of neuropathy in individuals with diabetes.[14, 19] It may involve sensory, motor, and autonomic nerve fibers, as well as reduced pain sensation, numbness, and painful paresthesias.[18]

Rest pain is an indication for angiography and evaluation for vascular surgery. It usually indicates a series of at least two arterial blockages. The pain is thought to be caused by nerve ischemia. It is persistent with peaks of intensity that are worse at night. The pain decreases with limb dependency and increases with heat, limb elevation, and exercise.

Intermittent claudication is often used as a symptom of significant peripheral vascular disease.[13] The relative risk of intermittent claudication in the Framingham study was four to five times higher in individuals with diabetes when compared with nondiabetic subjects.[13]

In our clinical practice, the decision making is facilitated when the previously mentioned information is available when the history of the chief foot complaint is being obtained. The interrogation of the patient can be more focused on the differentiation of symptoms that may be related to diabetes.

Insensitivity

Insensitivity is the most common path toward lower-extremity amputation among patients with diabetes. A patient who has minimal or no symptoms while walking on an open foot wound should immediately create, in the mind of the cli-

nician, a clinical perspective to prevent further damage to the foot. To emphasize this need the reminder to record this information is placed as a yes or no responsive at the bottom of the history portion that occupies the middle of the form. It is there as a reminder to the whole team that this patient immediately requires the unique management techniques of insensate foot care.

Footwear is the primary, physical means of protecting insensate feet from injury. The patient's present footwear can be a source of injury. Many female patients are sensitive to a foot specialist's concern over pointed-toe, pump-style shoes and can be defensive or evasive about these shoes.

PHYSICAL EXAMINATION

The physical examination (Fig 2–2) form has evolved from a similar form originally designed to help evaluate patients with leprosy at the Gillis W. Long Hansen's Disease Center in Carville, Louisiana. It has been organized into sections. The general appearance of the foot is described at the top. This is followed by skeletal and muscle evaluations. A graphical representation of feet allows the examiner to draw or label specific findings. Sensory and vascular findings are recorded at the bottom. The footwear evaluation is not the least of the factors to be considered but it is at the bottom so as to be fresh in the mind of the clinician when treatment plans are formulated.

The foot type would be described in a word or short phrase such as rectus, forefoot adductus, rocker bottom, cavus, and planus. Color may be described as pale, cyanotic, rubrous, dependent rubor, erythematous, and so forth.

For the purpose of the initial physical examination of the foot, a specific note of a nail feature that poses a threat is all that is needed. In this area the examiner

OCHSNER FOOT CARE PROGRAM
DIABETIC PATIENT - PHYSICAL EXAM

DATE_____

NAME_____ PATIENT NUMBER _____

PHYSICAL APPEARANCE: Foot type_____ Color_____

Nails_____

Plantarflexed 1st Ray R___ L___   Plantarflexed lesser metatarsal R_____ L _____

LIMITATION OF ANKLE DORSIFLEXION: knee ext. R=____ L=____ knee flex. R=____ L=____
SUBTALAR JOINT ROM: R _____   L _____
REARFOOT: _____   FOREFOOT: _____

Manual Muscle Test:

Anterior Tibial	R____	L____	Drop Foot R_____ L _____
Extensor Hallucis Longus	R____	L____	
Flexor Hallucis Longus	R____	L____	Intrinsics R____ L _____
Posterior Tibial	R____	L____	
Peroneus Longus	R____	L____	
Gastoc/Soleus	R____	L____	

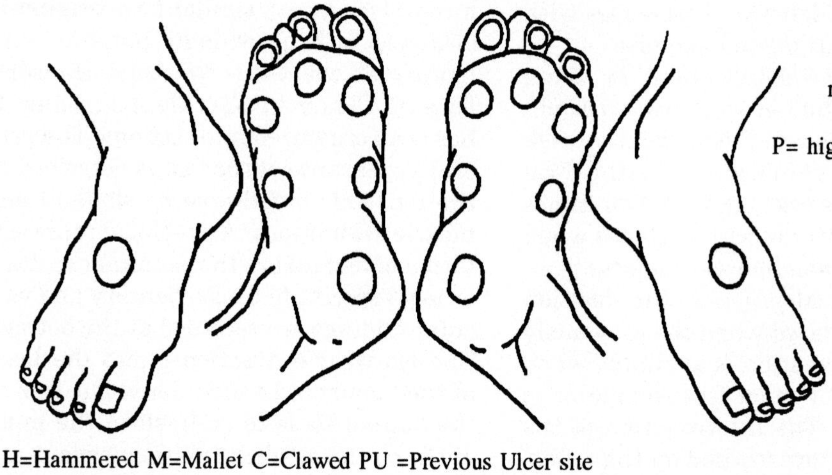

D= dryness
S= swelling
R= redness
n = temp. deg. C
callous
P= high pressure point

H=Hammered M=Mallet C=Clawed PU =Previous Ulcer site

Sensory Test (Semmes-Weinstein): 1=1 gram 2=10 grams 3=75 grams 4= No perception 75 grams
        Toes L ___ R ___ Forefoot L___ R ___ Heel L ___ R ___ Ankle L ___ R ___
Biothesiometer: R _____   L _____

PEDAL PULSES: Right: DP ____ PT ____   Left: DP ____ PT ____
Ankle/brachial Index: R _____ L _____ After one minute exercise: R _____ L _____
Footwear: Describe _____

FIG 2–2.
Physical examination form.

may note an ingrown nail, significant thickening, fungus, elongated, or other nail deformity.

Plantarflexed metatarsals are recorded because of the pressures generated at these points while the patient is walking. The first metatarsal is considered to be plantarflexed if the major portion of the total range of dorsiflexion to plantarflexion is plantar relative to the plane of the lesser metatarsal heads.[20] This is tested clinically while the subject is in a supine position. The lesser metatarsal heads are lifted into dorsiflexion by the tester's thumb with equal pressure under all heads. The other hand is used to grasp the first metatarsal head. The head is then dorsiflexed and plantarflexed, and the relative motion to the lesser metatarsal head plane is evaluated.

Equinus is defined as an inability to dorsiflex the foot at the ankle to a position representing a 90-degree angle to the leg. Functional equinus is present when the individual is unable to dorsiflex the foot to a position 10 degrees above the 90-degree position when the knee is extended. This dorsiflexion is considered necessary to minimize excessive pressure under the metatarsal heads as a person walks.

Limited joint range of motion may be a secondary effect of diabetes. It is thought to be a manifestation of diffuse collagen abnormalities.[21] Limited joint range of motion has been correlated to increased pressure under the foot of persons with peripheral neuropathy.[22] This is evaluated with the patient prone. The calcaneus and the lower third of the leg are bisected with straight lines. The angle between full inversion and full eversion in the frontal plane is then recorded. The highest pressures were found under feet where a limited subtalar joint range of motion and neuropathy were present.[23] Subtalar joint range of motion in normal individuals is generally about 30 degrees. Limited subtalar range of motion is around 20 degrees.[23]

Rearfoot alignment to the leg in the frontal plane is recorded below the total range of motion of the subtalar joint. This would be recorded as a description of the position of the calcaneus when the subtalar joint is in neutral position (Fig 2–3). It would be recorded as varus, valgus, or perpendicular. The evaluation is done while the patient is in the prone position to measure total subtalar joint range of motion.

Also, while the patient is prone, the forefoot alignment as represented by the plantar plane of the metatarsal heads in the frontal plane, is described by the relative position to the previously drawn bisection of the calcaneus (Fig 2–4). This relationship of the forefoot to the calcaneal bisection is done with the subtalar joint in neutral position and the forefoot dorsiflexed by pressure under the fifth metatarsal neck. The examiner while looking at the foot from the posterior side records the relative alignment as being in varus, valgus, or perpendicular.

These rearfoot and forefoot alignments effect pressures under the foot in gait. A more detailed justification for recording this information is beyond the scope of this chapter but is available in the increasingly more frequent studies on the biomechanical function of the foot.

Manual muscle testing as described in definitive texts[24] is more relevant to assessing the effects of trauma or disease.[25] A more relevant measurement for muscles for most clinics treating diabetic foot problems are the three levels of strong, weak, and absent. Intrinsic muscles are measured by having the patient spread the toes or extend the toes. These are recorded as present or absent.

Advanced motor neuropathy can result in drop foot. Though this is a relatively rare finding, manual muscle testing is done specifically to extract the presence of such weakness or paralysis. A drop foot may be in an early stage of development. If weakness of the anterior muscle group

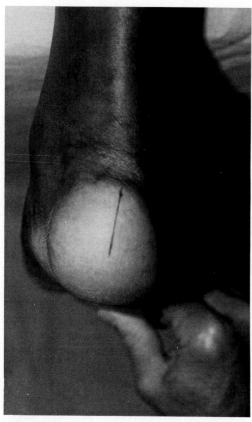

FIG 2–3.
A line is drawn on the skin of the posterior heel to represent a bisection of the calcaneus. The line can then be used to determine the position of the calcaneus when the subtalar joint is in neutral position. The total range of subtalar joint, frontal plane motion can also be determined while the patient is in this position.

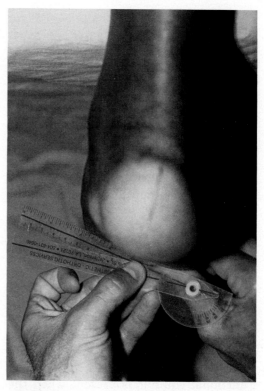

FIG 2–4.
The total range of frontal plane motion of the front of the foot changes with the position of the subtalar joint. Therefore, the alignment of the forefoot is measured relative to the bisection of the calcaneus.

Thermometry

Thermometry can be used to monitor the effects of stress on soft tissues by quantifying the degree of surface skin temperature elevation that comes with an inflammatory response.[28, 29] Temperature should be measured after a patient has been resting, with feet elevated for at least 20 minutes with shoes and socks removed. This will allow temperatures resulting from local reactive hyperemia to subside and leave focal areas of inflammation that remain warm.

Temperatures should be quantified by an accurate device for measuring skin temperature. If only occasional surface temperature measurements are taken a contact thermistor probe would suffice. For practitioners who do many evalua-

is found, the examiner should question the patient about a possible history of tripping, falling, or other gait problems.

Motor neuropathy leads to intrinsic muscle paralysis. This is noticed most often involving the lumbricales. The resultant imbalance between the flexors and extensors leads to the characteristic intrinsic minus foot with clawing of the toes and prominent metatarsal heads.[26]

Identification of areas where callous is present is important because higher pressures are present in these locations during gait. Removal of these callouses can reduce these pressures.[27]

tions of diabetic feet, an infrared thermometer is essential for rapid accuracy (Fig 2–5). The temperature is recorded as the only numbers on the drawings of the foot.

For clinical purposes it is not the absolute temperature that is most relevant unless the whole foot is close to core body temperature (37°C). The important feature of surface skin temperature on insensate feet is that it can reveal focal areas of elevated temperature, indicating inflammation from underlying injury. This is an invaluable tool for use on patients whose symptoms are masked or diminished by sensory neuropathy. In our clinical practice a focal area of increased temperature 2°C greater than the same location on the contralateral foot or greater than the ambient temperature of the same foot is regarded as significant injury. Even with no corroborating radiograph, bone scan, or other test results, the foot is treated to prevent further injury.

Foot Pressures

Neuropathy alone does not result in injury of the tissues of the foot. An external force

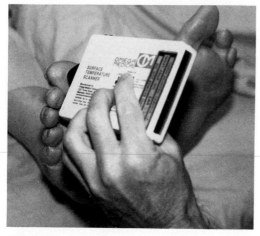

FIG 2–5.
An infrared thermometer is a quick, accurate method of quantifying surface skin temperature. The unit shown here displays a numerical reading of the temperature with a resolution to 0.1°C.

or excessive thermal cause must also be present. Damage of this sort is not unique to persons with diabetes but is shared with all diseases that lead to neuropathy. Forefoot pressures are greater under insensate walkers than under feet with normal sensation. Ulcerated sites correlate well with regions under the foot that are subjected to the highest pressure.

A British study has shown that 51% of neuropathic feet in diabetic patients have abnormally high pressures under metatarsal heads. This compares with 17% of diabetic patients without neuropathy and 7% among nondiabetics. Foot pressure studies may be used as a predictive or management aid in determining risk areas for possible ulceration (Figs 2–6 to 2–9). Pressures under the foot do not significantly increase under the feet of obese individuals. The foot seems able to adapt to increased weight.[30] This testing is recommended for individuals with neuropathy.[31] Measurement of pressures under the foot, as a person walks over a measurement device, seems to be most relevant for predicting areas of potential ulceration.[32] In virtually all cases, locations of previous ulceration show increased pressure on laboratory tests. Static measurements of pressure have not been as reliable.[32] The areas of high pressure as found by pressure assessment by pedobarograph or electrical sensors are not recorded as pressure units but with the letter P.

Proper fit of footwear should be determined by a professional shoe fitter, but the clinician can perform some simple evaluations to identify high-risk footwear. Footwear should be the size and shape appropriate for the patient's foot. The shoe should be ½ to ⅝ in. longer than the longest toe while the patient is standing.[33] To minimize metatarsal head pressures, heel heights should be less than 2 in.[34] Pointed-toe shoes should be avoided.

On the graphical representation of feet the letters designating toe deformi-

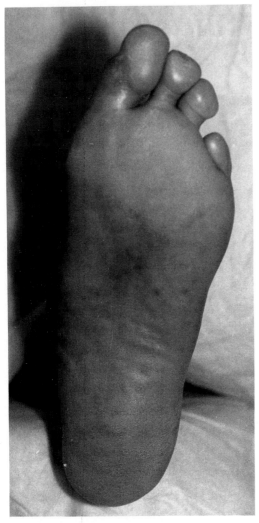

FIG 2–6.
The foot shown has a history of ulceration under the great toe. Callous is present under the second metatarsal head.

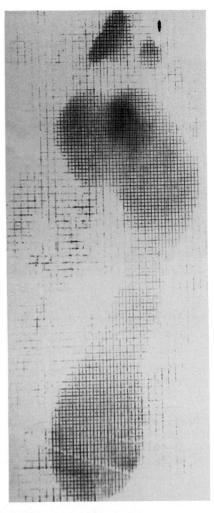

FIG 2–7.
After the patient whose foot is pictured in Figure 2–6 walked over a Harris mat, high pressures were found in the areas of callous and scar.

ties are usually written over the involved toe. Interdigital maceration is recorded as a U-shaped figure drawn around the involved interdigital area (Fig 2–10). Areas of involvement with callous, ulceration, scarring, gangrene, or amputation are drawn on the figures.

The circles are present on the foot for data collection purposes. Each circle can be assigned a number to facilitate recording findings in each portion of the foot.

Neurologic Examination

Peripheral neuropathy is the most important factor for the development of foot ulcers.[2, 35] Though the patient is more distressed with painful neuropathy, the clinician should be more concerned with polyneuropathy results in sensory loss. When retrospective surveys are conducted on the factors that have resulted in limb amputation among persons with diabetes, insensitivity is the most common initial

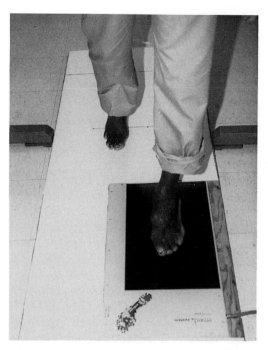

FIG 2–8.
The patient from Figures 2–6 and 2–7 then walked over an EMED system pressure platform.

sign. It has been noted that patients with chronic pain from neuropathy do not develop foot ulcers.[36] Most persons with neuropathic foot ulcers cannot recall a history of nerve pain.[37]

Frequently the development of insensitivity is not noticed by the patient. Symptoms they may relate include a nonspecific sensory change or a feeling that the feet are always covered by a sock. Distal development of motor neuropathy is often revealed by the presence of clawed toe deformities.

It is important for the clinical team to be aware of the loss of protective levels of sensation. For clinical purposes, protective sensation can be defined as sensory levels that are adequate to protect the patient from the common forms of injury attributable to insensitivity and enough sensation to produce appropriate levels of pain when an injured foot is used.

In the past clinicians have used a variety of sensory testing techniques. Few

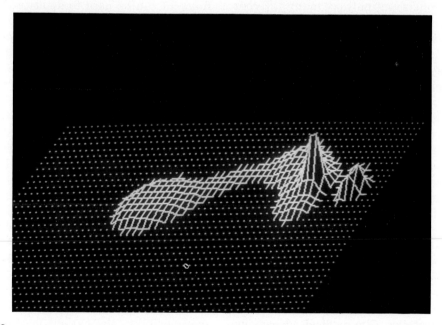

FIG 2–9.
The EMED system (see Fig 2–8) then produced a three-dimensional graphic representation of the levels of pressure generated under the foot in gait. This method provides quantification of the pressures in addition to location.

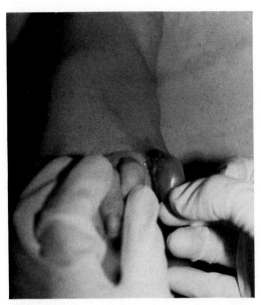

FIG 2–10.
Careful clinical examination should always include the interdigital areas. When neuropathy is present, the patient is usually unaware of the presence of an interdigital ulceration, as in this case.

professionals routinely use many different means of testing nerve function, and even fewer use the results of these tests to effect a change in their clinical decision-making.

Foot care for persons with diabetes has been evolving toward a focus on prevention rather than crisis management. To effectively anticipate problems, the clinical team must be able to concentrate their efforts on persons at the most risk of developing a pathologic condition. It is the reliable quantification of protective sensation that will allow us to differentiate varying degrees of patient risk. Recent publications seem to indicate that we are close to having a definitive clinical test to quantify protective sensation.

Of the techniques now available, the Semmes-Weinstein monofilaments, biothesiometer (Bio-medical, Newbury, Ohio), and the 128-Hz tuning fork have been clinically correlated to protective sensation. Myerson et al.[38] found that the use of Semmes-Weinstein monofilaments

for pedal sensory evaluation failed to reveal all patients with diabetes who would develop foot ulceration. This group concluded that using both the Semmes-Weinstein filaments and the biothesiometer would identify all patients with pedal sensory loss.

Semmes-Weinstein monofilaments are nylon fibers of various diameters. Each filament is attached to a handle. Thicker filaments require more force to bend them. When the tip of a filament is pressed against the skin, thicker filaments are easier to feel. Sets comprised of many filaments have been used to map subtle sensations over the entire body. On the feet, most people are unable to differentiate many of the filaments from each other. So, for pedal testing, only three-filament thicknesses have been routinely used. When the patient is unable to feel the filament that bends with a linear force of 10 g on their foot, protective sensation is considered lost (Fig 2–11).[39, 40] A 1-g filament can be used to detect early sensory loss. A 75-g filament is used to test for even greater deficit of sensation.

A biothesiometer is used by measuring the vibration threshold while the vibrating tip of the device is placed against the hallux (Fig 2–12). The rate of vibration rate is varied. A scale of 0 to 50 is displayed on the unit. As the vibration rate of the tip increases, the readings on the scale increase. Using the biothesiometer, persons who did not feel the vibration at less than 25 had a tenfold increased risk of having ulcerations when compared with those who would feel feel vibrations. If the reading was more than 43, there was a 30 times increase in risk of ulceration.[35] The average vibratory perception threshold was 40 in those with ulceration and was 23.5 in those with no ulceration.[35] For reproducibility the patient is prone with the top of the feet resting on an elevated pad. The bottom of the feet are toward the ceiling. The biothesiometer is rested on the toe. The weight of the handpiece is the

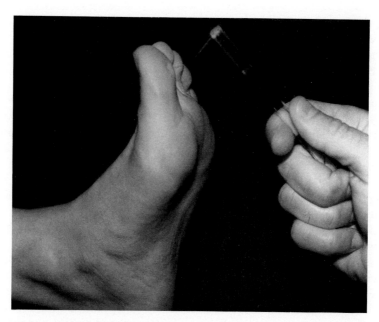

FIG 2–11.

A Semmes-Weinstein monofilament is used for sensory testing by placing one end of the filament against the surface of the skin. Force is then applied to the other end of the filament until the filament bends. The patient states whether or not he or she perceives the touch as the end of the filament. More force is required to bend thicker filaments.

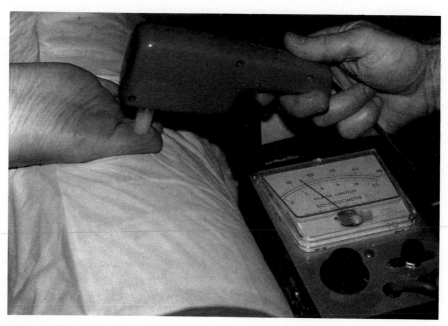

FIG 2–12.

The biothesiometer is used to quantify a patient's perception of vibration. The vibrating tip of the handle is rested against the skin using only the weight of the instrument to improve intertest reliability. Readings are in voltage units from 0 to 50.

only force on the toe. The rate of vibration at the tip is varied during three separate tests on each hallux. The recorded value is the mean results on each hallux.[23]

Patients who are unable to perceive a 128-Hz tuning fork on the hallux should be regarded as being at risk.[35] This study also showed that this vibration perception threshold most closely correlated with the presence of foot ulceration.[41]

Autonomic neuropathy on the feet is usually diagnosed by the absence of sweating. This can result in cracking of the skin, which can lead to ulceration or dry scaling, which can lead to injury when the person tears the skin by pulling off the larger scales (Fig 2–13). Autonomic neuropathy can result in atrophy of the smooth muscles that regulate small vessel flow. This has been suggested to result in arteriovenous shunting.[42, 43] When the flow is diverted through these shunts, blood supply to the smaller distal vessels can be reduced.[44] Cardiovascular reflexes

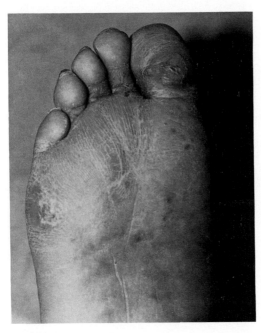

FIG 2–13.
Autonomic neuropathy results in the loss of sweating in the effected areas. Dry skin cracks and the brittle nature of anhidrotic skin can lead to ulceration.

can be used to test for autonomic neuropathy.[37]

Vascular Examination

Peripheral vascular disease is 20 times more common in persons with diabetes than in the nondiabetic population. The development of macroangiopathy is relatively unrelated to the length of time since diabetes was diagnosed and may even be detected before the diagnosis of diabetes. Peripheral vascular disease tends to involve arteries between the knee and ankle.[45, 46]

The absence of dorsalis pedis and posterior tibial pulses can be a significant clinical sign. It has been reported that as many as one third of diabetics may have small areas of digital gangrene even with palpable pedal pulses. If pedal pulses are present because of collateral circulation, the foot will become pale, and the pulses will disappear after a brisk walk. The possibility of having two independent testers record absent pedal pulses is not much greater than chance.[47, 48]

Pallor with limb elevation, prolonged venous filling time (>15 seconds), and dependent rubor are hallmarks of significant lower extremity vascular disease. About 75% of diabetic patients with significant arterial occlusive disease in their legs have no intermittent claudication. The blockage tends to be found more distally in persons with diabetes and can therefore be present beyond the branching of calf muscle vessels. Neuropathy can also mask claudication symptoms.

Many clinics use the ankle-brachial index (ABI) developed at Rancho los Amigos, in Los Angeles in the 1960s. The index is a value created when the systolic pressure measured by Doppler at the ankle is divided by the systolic pressure in the arm (Fig 2–14).[49, 50] The ABI will show decrease after the artery is greater than 50% occluded.[51] It is very reproducible and easy to perform clinically. The postexer-

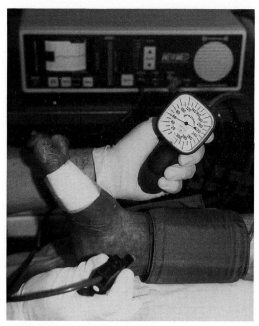

FIG 2–14.
A pneumatic tourniquet is used around the ankle to occlude the arteries. Then a Doppler is used to record the ankle systolic pressure as the pressure in the cuff is slowly released.

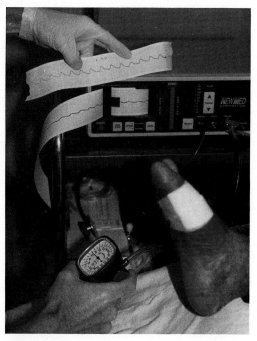

FIG 2–15.
A pulse volume recorder is used to show the amplitude of flow through an artery. The strip being held above the recorder represents the proximal flow for this patient. The recording in the machine shows the diminished amplitude at the ankle.

cise ABI was recommended by a committee of the American Heart Association as the method of choice for field studies.[17] A normal index would fall in the range between 0.95 and 1.25. An index greater than 1.31 comes as the result of medial calcification of the arteries, making the vessels more difficult or impossible to compress. Sclerotic or calcified noncompressible arteries in the lower extremities occur more frequently in individuals with diabetes than among nondiabetic individuals.[52, 53] A value of 0.89 or less indicates occlusive disease.

Pulse volume recorders are used in many clinics. In occlusive disease, arterial waveforms show decreased amplitude and a loss of diastolic forward flow (Fig 2–15). Arterial stiffening is demonstrated by an increase in pulse wave velocity.

Nondiabetic patients with peripheral occlusive disease are more likely to have occlusion in vessels in the foot than peripheral vascular disease patients with diabetes.[54] Presently many vascular specialists do not consider microangiopathy to be a significant factor in diabetic foot lesions.[45] Arteries of the foot are most often spared. Infection can lead to thrombosis of digital vessels. Digital skin infarcts are caused by thrombi, microthrombi, or microemboli from more proximal atheromatous plaques. Emboli can cause blue toe syndrome, a sudden onset of pain and cyanosis in one or more digits. These blockages often result in a sharp demarcation between well-perfused and poorly perfused tissues and can come as the result of anticoagulant therapy.

Open Ulceration

The foot must be closely examined for open wounds. Interdigital ulcers and ul-

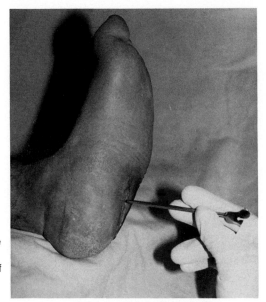

FIG 2–16.
A nasal sinus probe can be used clinically to locate the presence of sinus tracts within an ulcer. These openings are often not apparent during gross examination of the wound. Probing every wound will reveal these frequently missed complications.

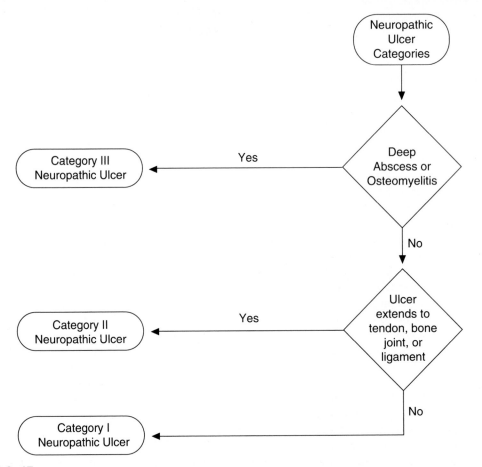

FIG 2–17.
This small algorithm graphically represents the need to examine every foot wound for signs of more serious complications first and rule them out to classify the wound as being less complicated. Categories 4 and 5 are for gangrene but have been excluded to simplify the algorithm.

cers posterior to the heel or ankle are frequently missed by clinicians. Once the wound is found, the size and depth should be recorded. Many clinics now use a piece of exposed, sterile, x-ray film to draw the perimeter of the ulcer for their records and to monitor healing rates.

A blunt tipped nasal probe should be used to complete the examination of any ulcer on an insensate foot (Fig 2–16). Many of these ulcers have deeper involvement even when they appear superficial. Frequently sinus tracts to necrotic tissue or a joint are found in these ulcers. Also deeper abscess can be revealed in this way.

The Wagner classification of ulcers is still the most commonly accepted means of determining the severity of an ulcer.[55] Figure 2–17 is a small algorithm depicting this classification system.

The categories for gangrene have been excluded to simplify the decision making hierarchy for open wounds. Wounds should be examined by expecting the worst problem and working back to simpler forms so as not to miss deeper complications. Wounds are covered in depth in later chapters.

Neuropathic Fractures

There are several systems described in medical publications to classify neuropathic (Charcot's) fractures. Figure 2–18

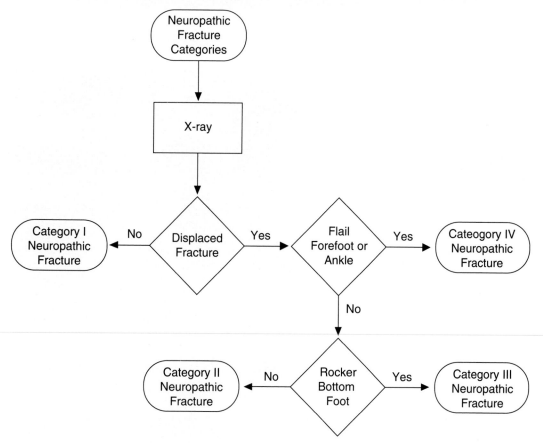

FIG 2–18.
This simple algorithm illustrates a system of classifying neuropathic fractures according to their difficulty in management.

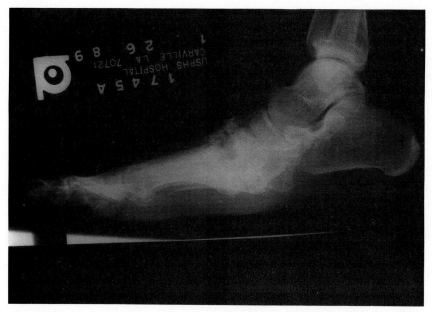

FIG 2–19.
A neuropathic fracture at the first metatarsal-cuneiform joint resulted in collapse of the medial arch.

FIG 2–20.
The fracture represented in Figure 2–19 resulted in a large plantar prominence that will pose a very difficult design problem for the construction of definitive footwear.

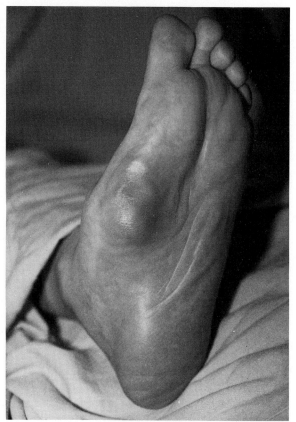

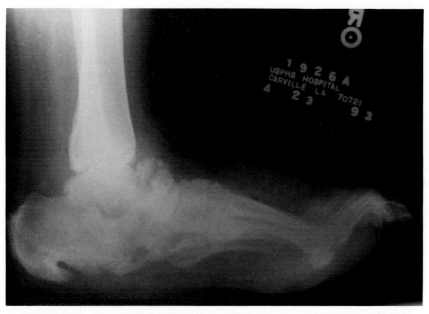

FIG 2–21.
Fractures at the head of the talus usually in collapse of the entire midfoot region.

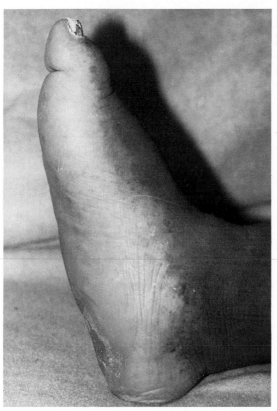

FIG 2–22.
The fracture in Figure 2–21 healed into a rocker-bottom foot. Conventional depth footwear and standard commercial footwear are rarely effective in the prevention of ulcers under this high-pressure area.

TABLE 2–1.

Risk Categories for Diabetic Feet

Risk category 0
  These patients have diabetes, but they have protective sensation, have never had a foot ulcer, and may have a foot deformity.
Risk category 1
  These patients have diabetes but have lost protective sensation. They have no history of foot ulceration and do not have a foot deformity.
Risk category 2
  These patients not only have diabetes and sensory loss but also have a foot deformity. They have never had a foot ulcer.
Risk category 3
  These patients have diabetes and have sensory loss. In addition, either they have had a foot ulceration in the past or vascular testing proves the presence of significant vascular disease.

---

is another small algorithm depicting how we classify these fractures according to management difficulty.

Nondisplaced neuropathic fractures are usually found in our clinics by thermographic evaluation. We refer to them as category 1 because they have the best prognosis and are the easiest to manage.

Category 2 fractures are minimally displaced at the fracture site. Decisions on their management are more complicated.

Fractures that are displaced so as to create a rocker-bottom foot are potentially far more serious and are category 3 (Figs 2–19 and 2–20). The plantar exostosis becomes a high-pressure point for possible ulceration (Figs 2–21 and 2–22). Footwear is more complex in design to protect this foot.

Category 4 fractures are flail at the ankle or midfoot. These unstable components are extremely difficult to manage, and large orthoses or amputation is often required for long-term management.

Risk Determination

After the feet have been examined and before the final treatment plan is formulated, we recommend assigning a degree of risk to every patient who is not currently injured. This will facilitate the patient's management and aid in the design of an education program. Table 2–1 represents the system originally conceived by Joseph Reed, R.P.T., and modified by clinical practice with leprosy patients.

The patients true risk can be ascertained only by a complete history and physical examination. Forms, such as the ones in this chapter, can help ensure a consistent, comprehensive initial patient evaluation. It is easy for health care providers who treat patients with diabetes regularly to be frustrated with frequent periods of burnout. Persons with diabetes can engender feelings of apathy or hostility on the part of the clinical team because of noncompliance. But with a determination to be thorough, the clinical team will be successful far more often than they fail.

REFERENCES

1. Davidson JK, Alonga M, Goldsmith M et al: Assessment of program effectiveness at Grady Memorial Hospital-Atlanta. In Steiner G, Lawrence PA, editors: *Educating Diabetic Patients,* New York, 1981, Springer-Verlag New York.
2. Edmonds ME, Blundell, MP, Morris HE et al: The diabetic foot: Impact of a foot clinic, *Q J Med* 232:763, 1986.
3. Bild DE, Selby JV, Sinnock P, et al: Lower-extremity amputation in people with diabetes, *Diabetes Care* 12:24, 1989.
4. Assal J-P: A global integrated approach to diabetes: A challenge for more efficient therapy. In Davidson JK, editor: *Clinical diabetes mellitus: A problem-oriented approach,* New York, 1991, Thieme Medical Publishers.
5. Kübler-Ross E: *On death and dying,* New York, 1969, Macmillan.
6. Assal JP, Muhlhauser I, Pernat A et al: Patient education as a basis for diabetic foot care in clinical practice, *Diabetologia* 28:602, 1985.
7. Most RS, Sinnock P: The epidemiology of

lower extremity amputations in diabetic individuals, *Diabetes Care* 6:87, 1983.

8. Beach KW, Strandress DE Jr: Arteriosclerosis obliterans and associated risk factors in insulin-dependent and noninsulin-dependent diabetes, *Diabetes* 29:822, 1980.

9. Melton LJ III, Macken KM, Palumbo PJ et al: Incidence and prevalence of clinical peripheral vascular disease in a population based cohort of diabetic patients, *Diabetes Care* 3:650, 1980.

10. Pirart J: Diabetes mellitus and its degenerative complications: A prospective study of 4,400 patients observed between 1947 and 1973, *Diabetes Care* 1:168, 1978.

11. Miller AD, Van Buskirk AH, Verhoek-Oftedabl W et al: Diabetes-related lower extremity amputation in New Jersey 1979–1981, *J Med Soc NJ* 82:723, 1985.

12. Ogbuawa B, Williams JT, Henry WL: Diabetic gangrene in black patients, *South Med J* 75:285, 1982.

13. Kammel WB, McGee DL: Update on some epidemiologic features of intermittent claudication: The Framingham study, *J Am Geriatr Soc* 33:13, 1985.

14. Harati Y: Diabetic peripheral neuropathies, *Ann Intern Med* 107:546, 1987.

15. Winegrad AI, Simmons DA, Martin DB: Has one diabetic complication been explained?, *N Engl J Med* 308:152, 1983.

16. Ellenberg M: Diabetic neuropathic cachexia, *Diabetes* 23:418, 1974.

17. American Heart Association Council on Epidemiology (Prineas RJ, Harland WR, Jonzon L, Kannel W): Recommendations for use of non-invasive methods to detect atherosclerotic peripheral arterial disease in population studies (AHA special report), *Circulation* 65:1561, 1982.

18. Levin ME: Pathogenesis and management of diabetic foot lesions. In Levin ME, O'Neal LW, Bowker JH, editors: *The diabetic foot,* ed 5, St Louis, 1993, Mosby–Year Book.

19. Guy RJC, Clark CA, Malcom PN et al: Evaluation of thermal and vibration sensation in diabetic neuropathy, *Diabetologica* 28:131, 1985.

20. Root ML, Orien WP, Weed JH: *Normal and abnormal function of the foot: Clinical biomechanics,* Vol 2, Los Angeles, 1977, Clinical Biomechanics Corporation.

21. Crisp AJ, Heathcoate JG: Connective tissue abnormalities in diabetes mellitus, *JR Coll Phys Lond* 18:132, 1984.

22. Delbridge L, Perry P, Marq S et al: Limited joint mobility in the diabetic foot: relationship to neuropathic ulceration, *Diabetic Med* 5:333, 1988.

23. Fernando DJS, Nasson EA, Veves A et al: Relationship of limited joint mobility to abnormal foot pressure and diabetic foot ulceration, *Diabetes Care* 14:8, 1991.

24. Kendall FP, McCreary EK: *Muscles: Testing and Function,* ed 3. Baltimore, 1983, Williams & Wilkins.

25. Cavanagh PR, Ulbrecht JS: Biomechanics of the diabetic foot: A quantitative approach to the assessment of neuropathy, deformity, and plantar pressure. In Jahas MH, editor: *Disorders of the foot and ankle: Medical and surgical management,* Philadelphia, 1991, WB Saunders.

26. Lippmann HI, McLellan GE, Klenerman L: The neuropathic foot of the diabetic, *Bull NY Acad Med* 52:1159, 1976.

27. Young MJ, Cavanagh PR, Thomas G et al: The effect of callus removal on dynamic plantar foot pressures in diabetic patients, *Diabetic Med* 9:55, 1992.

28. Bergtholdt HT, Brand PW: Temperature assessment and plantar inflammation, *Lepr Rev* 47:211, 1976.

29. Chan AW, MacFarlane IA, Bowsher DR: Contact Strenonography of painful diabetic neuropathic foot, *Diabetes Care* 14:918, 1991.

30. Cavanagh PR, Sims DS Jr, Sanders LJ: Body mass is a poor predictor of peak plantar pressure in diabetic men, *Diabetes Care* 14:750, 1991.

31. Veves A, Fernando DJS, Walewski P et al: A study of plantar pressures in a diabetic clinic population, *Foot* 1:89, 1991.

32. Duckworth T, Boulton AJM, Betts RP et al: Plantar pressure measurements and the prevention of ulceration in the diabetic foot, *J Bone Joint Surg* 67B:79, 1985.

33. Rossi WA, Tennant R: *Professional shoe fitting,* New York, 1984, National Shoe Retailers Association.

34. Snows RE, Williams KR, Holmes GB: The effects of wearing high heeled shoes on pedal pressure in women, *Foot Ankle* 13:85, 1992.

35. Boulton AJM, Kubrusly DB, Bowker JH et al: Impaired vibratory perception and diabetic foot ulceration, *Diabetic Med* 3:335, 1986.

36. Ward JD, Armstrong W, Preston E et al: Pain in the diabetic leg: A trial of aspirin and dipyridamole in diabetic neuropathy, *Pharmatherapeutica* 2:642, 1981.

37. Young RJ, Zhou YQ, Rodriquez E et al: Variable relationship between peripheral somatic and autonomic neuropathy in patients with different syndromes of diabetic polyneuropathy, *Diabetes* 35:192, 1986.

38. Myerson M, Papa J, Eaton K et al: The total contact cast for management of neuropathic plantar ulceration of the foot, *J Bone Joint Surg* 74A:261, 1992.

39. Birke JA, Sims DS: Plantar sensory threshold in the ulcerative foot, *Lepr Rev* 57:261, 1986.

40. Holwski JJ, Stess RM, Graf PM et al: Aesthesiometry: Quantification of cutaneous pressure sensation in diabetic peripheral neuropathy, *J Rehabil Res* 25:1, 1988.

41. Boulton AJM, Hardisty CA, Betta RP et al: Dyrsciruic foot pressure and other studies as diagnostic and management aids in diabetic neuropathy, *Diabetes Care* 6:26, 1983.

42. Borowski M: An experimental study on the role of arteriovenous anastomoses in the pathogenesis of trophic ulcer, *Arch Immunol Ther Exp* 21:363, 1973.

43. Edmonds ME: The neuropathic foot in diabetes, *Diabetic Med* 3:111, 1986.

44. Ward JD, Simms JM, Knight G et al: Venous distension in the diabetic neuropathic foot, *J Royal Soc Med* 76:1011, 1983.

45. LoGerfo FW, Coffman JD: Vascular and microvascular disease of the foot in diabetes, *N Engl J Med* 311:1615, 1984.

46. Janka HU, Standl E, Mehnert H: Peripheral vascular disease in diabetes mellitus and its relation to cardiovascular risk factors screening with Doppler ultrasonic technique, *Diabetes Care* 3:207, 1980.

47. Ludbrook J, Clarke AM, McKenzie JK: Significance of absent ankle pulse, *Br Med J* 1:1724, 1962.

48. Marinelli MR, Beach KW, Glass MJ et al: Noninvasive testing vs clinical evaluation of arterial disease: A prospective study, *JAMA* 241:2031, 1979.

49. Chamberlain J, Housley E, MacPherson AIS: The relationship between ultrasound assessment and angiography in occlusive arterial disease of the lower limb, *Br J Surg* 62:64, 1975.

50. Keoabtaki N, Lindfors O, Pekkola P: The ankle/arm systolic blood pressure ratio as a screening test for arterial insufficiency in the lower limb, *Ann Chir Gynecol* 72:57, 1983.

51. Carter SA: Clinical measurement of systolic pressures in limbs with arterial occlusive disease, *JAMA* 207:1869, 1969.

52. Emanuele MA, Buchanan BJ, Abraira C: Elevated leg systolic pressures and arterial calcification in diabetic occlusive vascular disease, *Diabetes Care* 4:289, 1981.

53. Neubauer B, Gundersen HJG: Calcifications, narrowing and rugosities of the leg arteries in diabetic patients, *Acta Radiol Diagn* 24:401, 1983.

54. Cantelmo NL, Snow JR, Menzoian JO et al: Successful vein bypass in patients with an ischemic limb and palpable popleteal pulse, *Arch Surg* 121:217, 1986.

55. Wagner FW Jr: A classification and treatment program for diabetic, neuropathic, and dysvascular foot problems, in AAOS instructional course lectures, vol 28, St Louis, 1979, Mosby–Year Book.

3

Plantar Pressure and Plantar Ulceration in the Neuropathic Diabetic Foot

Jan S. Ulbrecht

Arleen Norkitis

Peter R. Cavanagh, Ph.D.

The scope and the cost of the problems that can affect the lower extremities of persons with diabetes are large, both in personal and in public health terms.[1-4] Amputation is one of the most feared lower-extremity complications of diabetes: it is disfiguring, the rehabilitation process is often lengthy, and rehabilitation is not always complete. Thus, prevention of this irreversible complication of diabetes must be a priority for all involved in the care of these patients. Skin ulceration is a major risk factor for amputation; for instance, in a recently published study the path to amputation in patients with diabetes included a skin ulcer in 84% of the cases.[5] Furthermore, skin ulceration itself represents significant morbidity. Because healing will usually take many weeks, an ulcer will often prevent the patient from working. Medical care of an ulcer is labor-intensive and, therefore, costly.[6-8]

It is appropriate that a discussion of approaches to prevention of foot ulcer-ation in patients with diabetes forms a major part of any discussion of lower-extremity problems among these patients. Prevention of any disease becomes possible only when its pathogenesis is understood. Therefore, in this chapter we will first explore the relationship between mechanical conditions at the interface between the foot and its environment and ulceration. We will then examine the implications of this relationship for the screening and care of patients with diabetes.

THE ETIOLOGY OF FOOT ULCERS: AN OVERVIEW

Acute significant trauma can injure the skin in anyone. However, most of the foot ulcers seen in patients with diabetes occur as a consequence of relatively minor trauma that is repeated many times during foot contact in walking. As is discussed elsewhere in this book, patients with significant diabetic neuropathy are at risk for this classical diabetic foot ulcer (see Chapter 7). These patients are at risk because neuropathy (loss of protective sensation) is permissive to skin breakdown.[9–14] Ulceration occurs because patients with loss of protective sensation cannot perceive this repeated trauma to the skin.

On the dorsal surface of the foot and on the toes ulceration is most commonly a consequence of poorly fitting footwear.[15] Most of the ulcerations not involving the toes are, however, plantar,[15] and these appear to occur at areas of highest interface pressure between the plantar aspect of the foot and the supporting surface during gait.[9, 16–18] This association between high plantar pressure and ulceration has long been suspected, and Brand stands out as the investigator who has done the most over the years to advance this hypothesis.[19] Brand was also probably the first to measure pressure under the insensitive foot[20] and he has for many years encouraged clinicians to measure plantar pressure routinely, using the Harris mat, before prescribing footwear for patients at risk.[21]

PLANTAR ULCERATION AND PLANTAR PRESSURE

The first group to actually demonstrate the association between high plantar pressure and ulceration was Stokes et al.[16] A similar study with more sophisticated equipment was conducted by Ctercteko et al[17] a few years later (for a more detailed discussion of these studies see Cavanagh and Ulbrecht[13]). Barefoot pressures under the feet of a group of patients with diabetes and plantar ulceration were compared to those of a group with diabetes but without ulceration and to a nondiabetic control group. In both studies, the patients with ulcers tended to have higher pressures than subjects in the other

groups and the site of the ulceration appeared to correlate well with the site of the highest pressure. Both of these studies were cross-sectional, as was another extensive study to confirm these same findings.[9] Boulton and his associates[18] were also the first investigators to extend these findings prospectively. In this most recent study they followed several groups of patients for 30 months on average. The neuropathic group comprised 86 patients and, of these, 14 (16%) developed plantar ulcers during the follow-up. All of the patients who ulcerated were noted to have "abnormally high" plantar pressures at baseline. Of the 86 subjects, 43 (50%) did not have elevated pressures at the baseline evaluation and none of these patients developed plantar ulcers.

PLANTAR PRESSURE ULCERATION THRESHOLD

The obvious question to ask next is: At what level of plantar pressure does a person become at risk for ulceration? Before proceeding, it must be pointed out that plantar pressure results obtained from the same person will be different when different types of pressure platforms are used (this will be discussed in further detail later). Thus, the apparent normal values for plantar pressure found in healthy populations obtained on different pressure-measuring platforms differ. Boulton and his associates have defined the upper limit of normal plantar pressure as the mean peak pressure anywhere under the foot in a healthy population plus one standard deviation. They found this value to be 1,207 kPa using the optical pedobarograph.[22] We have reported values of mean plus two standard deviations almost 30% less using a piezo-electric platform built in our laboratory (881 kPa at the hallux).[13] Perry[23] found a mean plus two standard deviations of 815 kPa in nondiabetic subjects using the EMED SF pressure platform. Future research may show that age-adjusted norms would be more appropriate to define normal ranges. It may also be more reasonable to use a one-tailed probability to define the statistical confidence limits (where the 95% confidence limits would be 1.64 standard deviations from the mean). Such an approach would result in adjusted thresholds of 1458 kPa, 814 kPa, and 767 kPa, respectively, for Veves, Cavanagh and Ulbrecht, and Perry.

Based on a retrospective study of neuropathic diabetic patients who have ulcerated, Boulton et al[9] have suggested that the danger pressure threshold for ulceration is 1,080 kPa using the optical pedobarograph. This represented the lowest value found at the ulcer site in any patient. In striking contrast to this value, we have found that the lowest barefoot pressure using an EMED platform at a site of plantar ulceration in 52 ulcer patients was only 270 kPa. The wide discrepancy between these two values suggests that many additional factors need to be taken into account before a threshold can be determined.

Another method to define a threshold for injury is to examine peak pressure at the ulcer site after healing in neuropathic ulcer patients and to use the mean peak pressure (rather than the lowest value) obtained as the threshold. We have attempted such a procedure in 46 apparently nontraumatic lesions in 34 neuropathic patients.[24] The 20% of patients with the lowest pressure at the ulcer site were assumed to have ulcerated due to unreported trauma and were excluded from further analysis. The mean peak pressure at the ulcer site in the remaining patients was 450 kPa and we currently consider this value as our "working" danger threshold on the EMED SF platform. Note that this value is well within the normal ranges established using healthy subjects presented earlier.

Perhaps the most critical question with respect to the "normal" data described earlier is: Can the mean plus two standard deviations for a healthy population measured on a given platform be used as the danger threshold for the diabetic patient at risk? We believe that the answer to this question is an emphatic "no" and will now examine the rationale underlying this belief.

Persons without neuropathy remain free of ulceration not because their plantar pressures are low, but because they can perceive injury. They probably change the way they walk, or change shoes, or rest if their feet hurt; they do not usually just keep walking until skin breakdown occurs. (Occasionally people with intact sensation do continue through "pain barriers"—in sport for example—and a "blister" representing partial thickness skin breakdown occurs.) A reasonable definition of ulceration threshold is that pressure which, if repeatedly applied to the same location during prolonged walking, is just high enough such that plantar ulceration will occur. A pressure just a little lower than this "threshold" would be low enough so that skin breakdown would not occur regardless of the amount of activity the patient engaged in or the footwear used.

All discussions of plantar pressure thus far have referred to measurements between the bare foot and the floor, but skin breakdown occurs in the majority of patients while they are wearing shoes. As we will discuss in more detail later, it is now possible to measure pressure at the interface between the foot and the shoe insole. Does this imply that the risk status of a neuropathic patient should be defined in terms of in-shoe pressure? We suggest that barefoot measurement is the preferred method for the identification of feet "at risk" for ulceration and we will explain this point by a consideration of two hypothetical patients. In the first case, let us examine a foot with peak barefoot pressure under the first metatarsal head of 900 kPa. Let us make the assumption that the skin in this area of the patient's foot would break down if exposed to 800 kPa for 30 minutes of walking, 600 kPa for 2 hours, and 400 kPa for 4 hours of walking, but that ulceration would never occur during walking if the pressure could be reduced to 200 kPa. This hypothetical patient would not ulcerate in bed (an obvious but important point!), she could walk barefoot for less than 30 minutes, and she would do well for up to 4 hours in shoe A, which reduced the pressure in this region down to 400 kPa. In shoe B, which reduced the pressure down to 150 kPa, she would never ulcerate. If this patient came to the clinic in shoe B (and if the actual ulceration threshold of 200 kPa was known), measurement of in-shoe pressure would lead the clinician to conclude that the patient is not "at risk." But if she came in shoe A, she would be identified as being "at risk." The barefoot measurement would, however, immediately identify her as "at risk." Compare this with a second patient who in the same shoe B demonstrated peak pressure under his foot of 130 kPa, but in this same region had a pressure of only 290 kPa barefoot. This second patient could be considered as basically not at risk because he would need to walk barefoot for many hours before ulcerating. However, measurement of pressure in shoe B would not differentiate these two patients.

The concept of the true ulceration threshold has now been alluded to several times, and this is worth exploring further. This threshold was defined earlier as the plantar pressure below which ulceration will never occur regardless of the activity level. Actually, a better and more practical definition would be, "the pressure below which ulceration will not occur given that particular patient's activity level." It is probable that this threshold varies from patient to patient, and quite possibly from time to time and from site to site. In practice, we know that some patients do not

seem to ulcerate despite high plantar pressure, poor footwear, and footcare habits while other similar patients are very difficult to keep healed. These differences between patients may be due to any of the multiple variables that are thought to contribute to ulceration risk. For instance, it seems likely that the areas of the foot specialized for weight bearing—the heel and metatarsal head regions—may withstand higher pressures than the midfoot, which is not usually involved in weight bearing, although it can become very much involved in a foot with a Charcot fracture deformity.[25] If ischemia is part of the mechanism of tissue injury in an area of high pressure[19, 26] then the state of the circulation may be important. "Quality" of the plantar tissue may also be relevant; for instance, freshly healed plantar tissue is less compliant than healthy plantar tissue and will probably ulcerate more easily than healthy plantar tissue (described later in this chapter). Aging may also affect plantar tissue "quality" as may glycosylation of collagen occurring as a consequence of the diabetic state.[27, 28] Gait patterns have also been proposed as relevant.[29–31] It has been suggested that some patients may load different parts of the plantar surface with each step while others (possibly those with more severe neuropathy) may load the feet more consistently from step to step and, therefore, may expose a particular area to more repeated loading. These assertions remain to be demonstrated experimentally.

Although there is certain to be marked variability in the ulceration pressure threshold from case to case, knowledge of the range for this quantity would be extremely useful in footwear prescription. We have recently had the opportunity to obtain such a value for an individual patient using the Micro EMED pressure-measuring insole. The pressure at the ulcer site in a shoe in which the patient had repeatedly ulcerated was 215 kPa. At that same site in a new shoe, in which he remained ulcer free for several months, the pressure was 150 kPa.[14] Thus for this patient at this site and at this time the in-shoe ulceration threshold was somewhere between 150 and 215 kPa. It is likely that a set of upper and lower boundaries for the ulceration threshold in different groups of patients can be developed by similar repeated measurements. Such data would be extremely useful in footwear prescription in a setting where routine use of in-shoe pressure measurement was available before footwear was dispensed. This issue is discussed in more detail in Chapter 23.

CUMULATIVE PLANTAR PRESSURE AND SHEAR

Before leaving the topic of risk of ulceration, two other issues must be briefly discussed: the role of cumulative load and shear stress. In all previous studies in which the association between plantar pressure and ulceration has been demonstrated, the pressure measured was the peak normal (i.e., vertical) pressure reached at any point in the gait cycle. Loading at that pressure level may have occurred for just a small fraction of the gait cycle, or it may have been prolonged. Some measure of the interaction of pressure and time may in fact be a better predictor of ulceration, particularly if tissue ischemia is relevant to injury. In our clinic we routinely display the time integral of pressure, which we call "cumulative pressure".[13, 32] While these data have not yet been analyzed systematically, there appears to be a strong correlation between the peak and cumulative pressure measurements. However, differences do exist and such differences may be another reason why some patients with apparently high peak pressure do not ulcerate.

While pressure is a measure of the vertical loading experienced by the plantar surface, shear is a measure of load acting parallel to the plantar surface. Shear on the plantar surface of the foot cannot yet be usefully measured, though several laboratories are in the process of developing such shear-measuring devices. Several authors have suggested that shear stress may be involved in plantar tissue injury[20, 33–36] and in the development of callus, which is detrimental to plantar tissue function (see later). It is even possible that shear is the major injurious force involved in plantar ulceration and that the association of peak normal plantar pressure with ulceration occurs only because of an association between pressure and shear. Only simultaneous direct measurement of both normal and shear stress will answer these questions. Some interesting preliminary data addressing shear have been presented by Pollard et al.[35] In a study of 10 healthy subjects walking under a variety of conditions, Pollard et al. found marked reductions in shear stress in two commonly employed interventions: rocker bottom shoes and plaster casts. Clearly, this topic merits further study.

A THEORETICAL FRAMEWORK FOR PREDICTING RISK OF ULCERATION

A theoretical framework that summarizes the previous discussions on threshold for ulceration can be found in Figure 3–1. In this figure we follow a single hypothetical patient with sensory neuropathy (which is considered permissive for ulceration). The overall risk for ulceration can be determined from the combined influence of four groups of factors—all of which must be considered if a final determination of risk is to be made. These factors are as follows:

1. Structural factors that affect the peak pressure under the foot (such as prominent metatarsal heads, displaced fat pads, midfoot collapse).

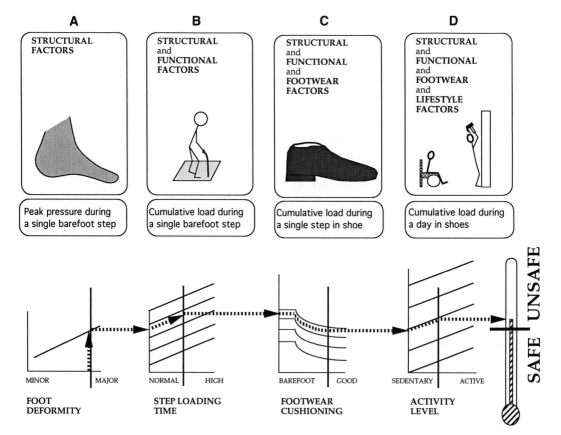

FIG 3-1.

A conceptual framework for the linkage between barefoot pressure measurement and the risk of ulceration in a single hypothetical neuropathic patient.

For each patient, a judgment is made about each of the previously mentioned factors and a vertical line is drawn at the appropriate place on each of the four horizontal axes. For example, the patient shown has major foot deformity, greater-than-average step loading time, well-cushioned shoes, and is rather inactive.

To determine this patient's risk of ulceration, a line through all four graphs must be followed. First, we move vertically up the deformity line until the sloping graph is met. Notice that greater deformity is predicted to result in higher pressure. We then move horizontally (dotted line) at a value representing the peak plantar pressure that results from a single barefoot step.

As soon as the Y axis of the step loading time graph is met, we move parallel to the contours on the graph until the vertical line representing this patient's step loading time is met. We now move horizontally to the footwear cushioning line at a level that indicates the combined effect of pressure and loading time in each single barefoot contact with the ground.

On meeting the axis of the footwear cushioning graph, we again move parallel to the contours until the vertical line representing this patient's shoes is met. Note that footwear, in general, has the tendency to move our line down (reducing the overall risk) because most footwear reduces peak pressure. However, this does not happen immediately (see the horizontal part of the contours) because some footwear, such as leather oxfords, have almost no beneficial effect on pressure reduction.[23] In this example the patient has

well-cushioned shoes, and on meeting the vertical line representing these shoes, we move horizontally at a level indicating the combined effect of deformity, step loading time, and footwear.

On the activity level graph, notice that any activity whatsoever, other than total bedrest, moves our line upward (increasing the risk level). This reflects the relatively few cycles of ground contact that may be required to raise the threshold above tissue injury level if the preceding factors (deformity, step loading time, and footwear) are sufficiently influential. Once the activity level line for this patient is intersected, we move horizontally and finally arrive at a thermometer display for cumulative load that this patient experiences in a complete day given his foot structure, gait pattern, footwear, and activity level.

In this case, despite the relatively good footwear, the combined effect of the patient's deformity, step loading time, and activity levels are sufficient to result in a daily cumulative load that puts him into the unsafe region of the final display, which indicates that tissue breakdown and ulceration are likely.

There are many simplifications and assumptions in this theoretical framework. For example, cumulative daily trauma may not be directly related to the risk of ulceration without a consideration of other important factors not shown in the figure. However, the framework is useful because it identifies the challenge for research in the future that must quantify the various unknowns in this theoretical model and identify factors not shown such that actual risk of ulceration can be predicted for a given patient.

2. Functional factors that may affect the duration of loading of a boney prominence under the foot during ground contact (such as aerobic capacity, joint pain, lower extremity strength, general debility).
3. Footwear factors that reflect the amount of cushioning the shoe provides (on a spectrum from barefoot to good cushioning).
4. Life-style factors that affect the total number of loading cycles the foot experiences during a day (on a scale from sedentary to extremely active).

In the example given in the figure, an individual with marked deformity, a longer-than-average loading time, well-cushioned shoes, and a low activity level is, nevertheless, above threshold for tissue damage. This example serves to indicate the need for consideration of all the structural, functional, footwear, and behavioral issues when assessing whether or not a patient is at risk for ulceration. There are many assumptions and many simplifications in this approach, but it does serve to identify the challenge for research in the future. There is a pressing need to quantify the various unknowns in this theoretical model such that the actual risk of ulceration can be predicted for a given patient.

IMPLICATIONS FOR ULCER HEALING

The obvious implication of the discussion so far is that patients who are at risk of plantar ulceration because of neuropathy and high plantar pressure can be protected from ulceration at a given activity level by footwear that adequately distributes plantar loading and, therefore, lowers plantar pressure below the ulceration threshold in key areas for that patient. This has been the premise of footwear design for the "at risk" neuropathic patient

for decades.[19, 33] However, healing of an ulcer almost certainly requires much greater unloading than prevention of ulceration. It is also likely that the prevention of reulceration after complete healing at the same site also requires greater unloading. We are unaware of any measurements to date of this healing pressure threshold, but based on clinical experience it is likely that this value is extremely low.

This statement is based on the observation of many patients in our clinic who were strongly advised to maintain non-weight-bearing on the ulcerated foot through the use of crutches, wheelchairs, etc. However, when questioned further, these patients reported that they may go to the bathroom at night barefoot without using crutches and that they may do the same twice a day to get a cup of coffee—and they do not heal. They may even use footwear that would probably be adequate to prevent ulceration, but healing does not take place. These patients usually heal rapidly when placed at bed rest or in a total contact cast.[6] In our clinic we use total contact casting as much as possible to heal plantar ulcers, but occasionally patients will decline casting. We could probably be described as extreme in instructing our patients who choose non-weight-bearing as a means of healing an ulcer to never put the affected foot on the ground. It is, therefore, likely that our patients may be more compliant with non-weight-bearing procedures than other patient groups might be. Yet the mean healing time of 60.6 days (± 33.7) that we have achieved for 32 plantar ulcers in casts is the same (59.3 days $\pm$ 41.3) as that for 34 ulcers with non-weight-bearing treatment despite the fact that the mean area of the ulcers treated by casting was over twice the area of those not cast. This comparison, in the same clinic where all other aspects of treatment were the same, is an enticing suggestion of the superiority of the total contact cast method although a statistically significant difference in healing rates was not demonstrated.

Intuitively it seems likely that shear forces must play a significant role in prevention of healing because the tissue of a healing or just healed ulcer is often adherent to deeper structures because of fibrous tissue. However, this statement is also simply a matter of speculation.

Based on these largely clinical and certainly uncontrolled observations, it seems prudent to recommend that clinicians who take care of patients with plantar ulcerations should ensure that such patients *never* bear weight on that foot without that foot being in a total contact cast (or possibly a Scotchcast boot.[7, 37]) It is also possible to heal a forefoot ulcer in a shoe that has no load bearing under the distal 50% of the foot.[38] Non-weight-bearing with the use of crutches, walkers, or wheelchairs is probably a viable treatment option, particularly when the expertise or personnel to provide total contact casting are not available or when the patient is not a candidate for casting. But the patient must understand what total non-weight-bearing means. We challenge clinicians who choose to prescribe anything less than total non-weight-bearing to show that healing is achieved reasonably rapidly under those circumstances.

SURGICAL APPROACH TO PLANTAR PRESSURE RELIEF

The topic of surgical alteration of the foot to relieve plantar pressure is discussed elsewhere in this book (see Chapter 22). Only a brief discussion of the topic will be conducted here. Essentially, all areas of high plantar pressure and therefore of ulceration are associated with a bony prominence. The most common are the metatarsal heads while less common are the base of the fifth metatarsal and prominences in the midfoot due to a Charcot fracture.[15] Ulceration under the heel is quite unusual, possibly because of the large amount of soft tissue usually found in this region. In the preceding section it has been stated that a logical approach to plantar ulcer prevention is to redistribute the forces acting on the plantar surface using footwear. However, an equally logical approach would be to alter the foot. The types of surgery performed for this purpose include metatarsal head osteotomy,[39, 40] metatarsal head resection,[41] removal of a bony fragment associated with a Charcot fracture,[42] surgical repair of a Charcot fracture,[43] and possibly even an amputation of a particularly deformed foot or part of a foot.[44]

There are no controlled studies comparing the short-term and the long-term results of altering footwear in prevention of plantar ulceration or reulceration versus altering the feet surgically. Some clinics are biased toward footwear intervention (for instance our clinic), while others are biased toward surgery.[39] Controlled studies with adequate long-term follow-up in clearly defined clinical situations must be performed before clear choices can be made, and before criteria for individual patients can be identified. In the meantime, those of us who favor footwear solutions are obliged to show that reulceration and future complications are at least as good as those achieved with prophylactic surgery. This will involve ensuring that we are able to find appropriate footwear solutions quickly, that the footwear is acceptable to the patient, that the patient has the resources (both financial and personal) to use the footwear consistently and correctly, and that the patient is functional in the footwear (footwear solutions can be bulky and cumbersome). Those who favor surgery must provide evidence that serious complications can be avoided consistently. This applies, in particular, to avoidance of nonhealing due to infection or due to unrecognized vascular disease and the need for further surgery such as revascularization or amputation. It should also be recognized that any surgical intervention in a neuropathic foot may be a risk factor for Charcot fracture. Follow-up studies using pressure distribution are needed to show that relief of plantar pressure and, therefore, of ulceration can be achieved consistently and that transfer lesions (ulceration at another site due to transfer of pressure to that site) do not occur frequently. Although there are studies of the outcome of a program that emphasizes footwear solutions,[45] and other studies of postprophylactic surgical complications,[40, 41, 46–48] none of these have been done in the same institutions with the same strict criteria for patients assignment and treatment. There are certainly no controlled studies available to show that such procedures as panmetatarsal head resection for the first forefoot ulcer have results superior to an aggressive footwear intervention.

HIGH PLANTAR PRESSURE AND DIABETES

As has been discussed earlier, plantar ulceration can occur at pressure levels that can be seen in healthy patients. However, diabetes, and in particular diabetes complicated by neuropathy, is associated with higher-than-normal plantar pressures. This was first demonstrated by Boulton et al[9] and has since been confirmed.[22, 49] In the early study, Boulton et al found that 51% of diabetic neuropathic feet had peak plantar pressures that were considered abnormal, while this was true of 17% of patients with diabetes but without neuropathy and of 7% of healthy controls. The logical inference from this cross-sectional data is that pressure under the feet of patients with diabetes, and particularly so with diabetic neuropathy, will increase over time. This prediction was confirmed in the most recent study of Veves et al.[18] They found that after 30 months of follow-up, on average, the peak plantar pressure

under the feet of a neuropathic diabetic group increased from 1,197 to 1,452 kPa; in the diabetic nonneuropathic group this change was from 1,099 to 1,324 kPa and in the healthy controls there was no change (755 to 775 kPa).

In most of the studies described above the average body weights of the groups being compared were very similar, so that the differences in peak plantar pressures observed between the groups could not be attributed to differences in body mass. In fact we have recently shown that body weight has little impact on plantar pressure.[50] In a study of 56 patients with diabetes and neuropathy we have found a statistically significant correlation between weight and peak plantar pressure, but this correlation was quite weak ($r = 0.37$; $r^2 = 0.14$).[50] A very similar correlation value ($r = 0.224$) relating peak plantar pressure to weight has been reported by Veves et al.[22] These studies imply that the anatomy of the plantar surface is much more important in the generation of focal plantar pressures than in the overall loading force.

Potential Causes of High Plantar Pressures in Diabetes

The commonly accepted causes of high plantar pressure in diabetes have been reviewed recently elsewhere and will be summarized here only briefly.[14, 51, 52] Some research addressing this issue has been carried out over the last few years, but much is yet to be learned. Further study of this field is important because a better understanding of how diabetes causes high pressure may lead to the future development of strategies to prevent these changes in the foot in diabetes.

Bony deformities are an obvious potential cause of increased plantar pressure. Such deformities could be a consequence of poorly healed traumatic fractures and especially of Charcot fractures.

In a random and blind radiographic study, evidence of traumatic fracture in the foot was found in 22% of patients who had a history of neuropathic ulcer. This was significantly greater than the prevalence seen in nondiabetic controls, age-matched diabetic patients without neuropathy, or in neuropathic patients without history of ulceration.[53] Most of the fractures in the ulcer patients had not been previously diagnosed, presumably because the patients had no pain as a result of neuropathy. In addition, a 16% prevalence of Charcot fractures was found in the neuropathic ulcer patients. Elevated plantar pressure could also be a consequence of more subtle bone trauma and remodeling, or it could be a reflection of changes in tarsal anatomy due to motor neuropathy. In a quantitative extension of the same x-ray study, we also examined the relationship between the bony architecture of the foot and plantar pressure.[54] A variety of angular and linear measurements was taken from standardized weight-bearing x-rays. Using stepwise multiple regression, the strongest predictors of pressure under the first metatarsal head were found to be the inclination of the first metatarsal in the sagittal plane, the frontal plane splay of the first and fifth metatarsals, and the soft tissue thickness under the metatarsal head. These observations do not in themselves explain why plantar pressure is higher in patients with diabetes, but they do offer a method for investigating this question further in terms of the bony architecture of the foot.

By identifying the soft tissue thickness under the first metatarsal head as relevant to plantar pressure, this work supports the long hypothesized and intuitively obvious key role of plantar soft tissue in cushioning the plantar surface. Plantar soft tissue abnormalities are therefore very likely to contribute to the high plantar pressures found in diabetes. One possible mechanism by which the plantar soft tissues could be altered in di-

abetes is related to clawing of the toes. Clawed toes are a frequent clinical finding among patients with diabetic neuropathy and this phenomenon has been ascribed to neuropathic atrophy of the intrinsic muscles that control the position of the proximal phallanges on the metatarsals.[55] Objectively this change can be measured as a reduction in plantar toe pressures in these patients.[49] In addition to increasing the likelihood of dorsal ulceration from footwear, it has been hypothesized that the soft tissue metatarsal cushions that are normally situated under the metatarsal heads are displaced anteriorly with the toe plantar flexor tendons as the toes become clawed.[56] This has been postulated to leave the condyles of the metatarsal heads covered with much less plantar soft tissue than normal. The only studies to examine plantar soft tissue thickness under the metatarsal heads have not, however, been conclusive.[57, 58]

Another possible alteration of plantar soft tissue in diabetes is glycosylation of collagen.[59] Glycosylation is the nonenzymatic, concentration-dependent attachment of glucose to protein. Almost all proteins so far examined have been found to be glycosylated in diabetes and both collagen and keratin have been found to become "stiffer" when glycosylated.[27, 59] This could alter the "cushioning" properties of the plantar soft tissues in diabetes, but this hypothesis has yet to be supported by any experimental data.

It is also still only a matter of hypothesis and clinical suspicion that diabetes predisposes patients to the production of excessive plantar callus.[60] However, if this association proves to be true, it will explain at least a part of the causation of higher plantar pressures in these patients. This assertion is based on the recent demonstration that removal of callus under bony prominences in the forefoot reduces plantar pressure by an average of 29%.[61] Excessive callus could form in the diabetic foot because of increased loading, normal or shear, thereby setting up a vicious cycle of pressure causing callus, which then itself contributes to even higher pressure. Callus could also form because of decreased sweating due to autonomic neuropathy, increased keratin glycosylation,[27] or for other reasons. The objective observation that callus reduction can markedly decrease plantar pressure confirms the critical importance of callus care in patients at risk for neuropathic ulceration. This point is true regardless of whether or not more callus develops because of diabetes, or whether or not the amount of callus in these patients is normal.

Another commonly accepted by-product of nonenzymatic glycosylation is the observed limitation in the range of movement in many joints of the body in patients with diabetes.[62] Limited joint mobility (LJM) has been observed in the joints of the foot and ankle,[63, 64] and decreased subtalar joint mobility has been associated with elevated plantar pressure.[63, 65] Presumably, a major means of keeping pressures within reasonable bounds is to use the adaptability afforded by motion of joints of the foot and ankle particularly the subtalar and metatarsophalangeal joints, and this mechanism is impaired by LJM.

TECHNICAL ASPECTS OF PLANTAR PRESSURE MEASUREMENT

The technical aspects of plantar pressure measurement have also been recently reviewed extensively elsewhere by ourselves and by others.[13, 14, 32, 66-69] From a clinical perspective it would be convenient if one could simply order the test, look at the results, and treat the patient. A similar approach would also be convenient in the research setting. However, the field of plantar pressure measurement is still new and the methodology is not yet fully developed or standardized. The user of the equipment must know how to use it and must know its limitations. Some key points and potential pitfalls related to plantar pressure measurement will therefore be reviewed in the next few paragraphs.

Hardware.—Several "mats" for barefoot plantar pressure measurement are currently commercially available and two "in-soles" for in-shoe pressure measurement have also been recently introduced commercially.[68] These are all matrix instruments (multiple individual pressure transducers arranged next to each other in a matrix). Individual sensors have been available much longer, but they have many disadvantages compared to the matrix devices.[68] Several different principles for measuring pressure are used in the different devices and there are many technical factors that affect accuracy and reproducibility.[13] The "garbage in, garbage out" principle is certainly true for plantar pressure measurement. If the hardware for measuring pressure is unreliable, it matters little (and may actually confuse) if the display of the results is spectacular or if the software that processes the data is sophisticated. It will benefit all users of plantar pressure-measuring instruments to be familiar with the hardware before looking too much at the software.

Specifically, key issues are the reliability of the transducers (site to site, walk to walk, and day to day), the usable pressure range of the device, and the accuracy at higher pressures, which are often the most important part of the measurement range. Effects of foot temperature and of other environmental factors may complicate data collection. Devices that ostensibly measure vertical pressure may also be sensitive to shear stress and bending—both of which are unavoidable in a typical measurement situation. Some method of calibration is extremely important and preferably this should calibrate all elements that are in the device rather than just taking an average of those that happen to be active in some contrived situation. The manufacturer should be consulted on how often calibration needs to be repeated—particularly when prospective studies are being conducted. Spatial resolution is a consequence of element size, and the effective element size has a major effect on the absolute values of pressure obtained. Generally speaking, the smaller the sensor, the larger the apparent pressure recorded in the same region of the same foot.[32] Thus as already discussed, normative data must be developed for each instrument used, and plantar pressure results obtained with one device simply *cannot* be directly compared to the results from another.

In-shoe applications are particularly demanding on durability and the measuring device can often be damaged either locally or more globally by attempting to measure pressure in a shoe that has ridges in the insole. Some insoles can also crease during normal use and this often results in a off-scale indication in a small local region. Care should be taken not to interpret this as a high pressure that has been generated by the foot-shoe interaction.

Software.—In many research paradigms, pressure values from each transducer at each point in the step cycle may need to be accessed and analyzed. However, for clinical applications and for most research purposes, some summary method of presenting the data is needed. The most popular graphic presentation of plantar pressure data is the contour plot, which can be either in color or black and white and in a two-dimensional or three-dimensional display. The peak pressure reached at any time during the step cycle can be shown in a summary plot, or the data can be presented as a series of "snapshots" taken throughout the contact phase, or indeed as a "movie" that replays the instantaneous pressures on all parts of the foot

in slow motion. Plots that present the "integral" of pressure over the ground contact time (see earlier) may also be useful.[13] In our work we most often also present average pressure results by region based on a standard computer generated division of the footprint.[13] Some of the commercial software packages allows for "masks" that divide the footprint into regions of interest to be developed for each subject. These masks can then be applied for multiple foot contacts. The choice of regions of interest can also be made in some systems on screen by using a mouse. Key to any software is that it should allow, if necessary, inspection of the raw data for each trial. Preferably, data at all points in the step cycle from each element should be available so that unusual results presented in an average plot can be checked.

Data collection.—Several aspects of the data-collection process will influence the results so that the protocol for plantar pressure measurement must be selected carefully and must be described when the results are presented. The subject related factors that will have an impact on the results include stride length and the speed of walking, both of which can be either natural or mandated. Hughes et al[70] have examined the day-to-day reliability of pressure measurement when such factors are controlled. For barefoot collection on a platform, the results will be somewhat dependent (particularly in the heel) on whether the first step from rest is analyzed or a middle step during a longer walk is measured. For patients with poor vision and an unsteady gait, we believe that first-step collection has significant advantages. In our clinic, we have also chosen not to standardize walking speed or stride length to make the steps as normal for the subject as possible on the day of testing. We recognize that some of the differences we may see from day to day are likely to be a consequence of changes in the gait rather than in the feet. However, this approach is justifiable clinically, because in the clinic we are interested in plantar pressure during the patient's "natural" gait on that day, and the patient's perception of what speed he or she can manage is a factor in the definition of "normal." In barefoot studies we average five "first steps" although, for in-shoe testing, averaging over many more steps is easily accomplished during full gait.

PLANTAR PRESSURE MEASUREMENT—THE PRESENT

As Brand has long postulated,[19] it has now been clearly established that most plantar ulcers occur in patients who are "at risk" because of loss of protective sensation in areas of high plantar pressure. Although ulceration can occur at sites where pressure is apparently still within normal limits (as defined by a healthy population), patients with diabetes tend to develop higher-than-normal plantar pressures— thereby increasing the risk. This happens for a variety of, as yet, poorly understood reasons that we have previously reviewed in this chapter.

Brand has long proposed that plantar pressure measurement be used routinely in all subjects "at risk" for plantar ulceration and the strong evidence relating ulceration to pressure that is now available leads us to agree with that recommendation. In particular the data linking ulceration to high pressure prospectively[67] provides clear impetus for screening patients at risk using pressure measurement before they ever ulcerate, and then intervening to prevent ulceration.[18] Brand many years ago, and more recently Boulton[18] have recommended the use of the Harris Mat in routine clinical work. We disagree with this recommendation because this device has poor performance characteristics compared with the newer instruments, although it is much less expensive. It does not provide quantitative

information and it saturates at a pressure value (470 kPa) well below barefoot pressures usually seen at ulcer sites.[71] Choices have to be made, but when possible we recommend the routine screening of patients with loss of protective sensation using one of the newer platform devices. Patients who are then identified as "at risk" should be prescribed footwear that is designed to protect them in the regions of high pressure that have been identified. This recommendation assumes that values that are close to "ulceration thresholds" will, in the near future, be identified for each device used. It must be recognized that, at present, plantar pressure measurement is a sensitive, but not particularly specific, method for predicting plantar ulceration. For example, in the study mentioned earlier[18] all patients who ulcerated had elevated pressures at baseline (100% sensitivity). However, 67% of the neuropathic patients with elevated plantar pressure at baseline did not ulcerate during the follow-up (60% specificity). A better understanding of the additional factors contributing to ulceration should improve specificity.

It is more difficult to recommend in-shoe pressure measurement routinely yet, because the technique is newer and its use is not yet well substantiated by research. Methodological issues also still loom large. We have, however, used in-shoe pressure testing on a case-by-case basis in our clinic and it has proven invaluable in several situations. In particular, we have used it when prescribing a new footwear iteration to a patient who has reulcerated in shoes we thought to be adequate. We have then measured pressure in the shoes that caused the ulcer and compared the pressure in the new footwear before dispensing the new shoes to the patient. We believe that this approach has saved our patients from further ulceration in footwear that was simply no better than the failed prescription. Use of in-shoe pressure measurement in specialized, research oriented diabetes foot clinics should probably soon be routine.

PLANTAR PRESSURE MEASUREMENT—THE FUTURE

What does the future hold? Treatment and, in particular, preventive care for the diabetic patient "at risk" for foot problems must improve[58] and plantar pressure measurement has the potential to play a major role in this improvement. In the near future, barefoot plantar measurement should be used much more routinely to identify patients at risk. Better danger thresholds using the barefoot measurement need to be, and will be, developed for each device used. We also need to learn why some patients with apparently the same degree of neuropathy, the same plantar pressure, the same activity level, the same footwear etc., do not ulcerate, while others do. This may be a consequence of patient attributes such as the degree of plantar tissue glycosylation or the state of the circulation—it should then become possible to measure these cofactors and develop a better risk profile for each patient. But the fact that all patients with high peak plantar pressure do not ulcerate may also be a function of what we measure—peak plantar pressure may not be the only injurious quantity, but rather cumulative pressure or shear may be responsible. This is an area that should be explored further. We should also explore further why diabetes causes high plantar pressure and develop strategies for preventing this process. For example, exercise programs to prevent the progression of foot deformity or LJM have not been well explored.

In-shoe pressure measurement is in its infancy, but the potential for clinical use in this area is almost beyond imagination. We must begin to learn what the true in-shoe threshold for ulceration is. This is likely to vary markedly from patient to patient (and we may need to look at shear rather than just at peak pressure). But this variability can also be addressed in terms of other patient-related risk factors. Thus it should be possible eventually to measure plantar pressure in shoes when they are prescribed and to know if the shoes are safe to enable the patient to live an active and ulcer-free life.

Acknowledgment

The work of Drs. Cavanagh and Ulbrecht on this chapter was supported in part by NIH grant 1-RO1-DK42912.

REFERENCES

1. Bild DE et al: Lower-extremity amputation in people with diabetes—epidemiology and prevention, *Diabetes Care* 12(1):24–31, 1989.
2. Reiber GE: Diabetic foot care. Financial implications and practice guidelines, *Diabetes Care* 15(Suppl 1):29–31, 1992.
3. Reiber GE, Pecoraro RE, Koepsell TD: Risk factors for amputation in patients with diabetes mellitus. A case-control study, *Ann Intern Med* 117:97–105, 1992.
4. Fylling CP, Knighton DR: Amputation in the diabetic population: incidence, causes, cost, treatment, and prevention, *J Enterostom Ther* 16:247–255, 1989.
5. Pecoraro RE, Reiber GE, Burgess EM: Pathways to diabetic limb amputation: basis for prevention, *Diabetes Care* 13:513–521, 1990.
6. Myerson MS et al: The total-contact cast for management of neuropathic plantar ulceration of the foot, *J Bone Joint Surg* 74A(2):261–269, 1992.
7. Jones GR: Walking casts: effective treatment for foot ulcers? *Pract Diabetes* 8:131–132, 1991.
8. Fylling CP: Wound healing: an update. Comprehensive wound management for prevention of amputation, *Diabetes Spectrum* 5(6):328–359, 1992.
9. Boulton AJM et al: Dynamic foot pressure and other studies as diagnostic and

management aids in diabetic neuropathy, *Diabetes Care* 6(1):26–33, 1983.

10. Holewski JJ et al: Aesthesiometry: quantification of cutaneous pressure sensation in diabetic peripheral neuropathy, *J Rehabil Res Dev* 25(2), 1988.

11. Sosenko JM et al: Comparison of quantitative sensory-threshold measures for their association with foot ulceration in diabetic patients, *Diabetes Care* 13(10):1057–1061, 1990.

12. Birke JA et al: A review of causes of foot ulceration in patients with diabetes mellitus, *J Prosthet Orthotics* 3:13–22, 1991.

13. Cavanagh PR, Ulbrecht JS: Biomechanics of the diabetic foot: a quantitative approach to the assessment of neuropathy, deformity, and plantar pressure. In Jahss MH, editor: *Disorders of the foot and ankle,* ed 2, Philadelphia, 1991, WB Saunders.

14. Cavanagh PR, Ulbrecht JS: Biomechanics of the foot in diabetes. In Levin ME, O'Neal LW, Bowker JH, editors: *The diabetic foot,* ed 5, St Louis, 1993, Mosby–Year Book.

15. Apelqvist J, Larsson J, Agardh CD: The influence of external precipitating factors and peripheral neuropathy on the development and outcome of diabetic foot ulcers, *J Diabetic Complications* 4:21–25, 1990.

16. Stokes IAF, Faris IB, Hutton WC: The neuropathic ulcer and loads on the foot in diabetic patients, *Acta Orthop Scand* 46:839–847, 1975.

17. Ctercteko GC et al: Vertical forces acting on the feet of diabetic patients with neuropathic ulceration, *Br J Surg* 68:608–614, 1981.

18. Veves A et al: The risk of foot ulceration in diabetic patients with high foot pressure: a prospective study, *Diabetologia* 35(7):660–663, 1992.

19. Brand PW, Coleman WC: The diabetic foot. In Rifkin H, Porte D Jr, editors: *Ellenberg and Rifkin's diabetes mellitus: theory and practice,* ed 4, New York, 1990, Elsevier Science.

20. Bauman JH, Brand PW: Measurement of pressure between foot and shoe, *Lancet* March:629–632, 1963.

21. Brand PW: Management of the insensitive limb, *Phys Ther* 59(1):8–12, 1979.

22. Veves A et al: A study of plantar pressures in a diabetic clinic population, *Foot* 2:89–92, 1991.

23. Perry JE: *The effect of running shoes and oxfords on plantar pressures in diabetic patients,* master's thesis, University Park, 1992, Pennsylvania State University.

24. Hsi WL et al: Plantar pressure threshold for ulceration, *Diabetes* (abstract) 42(suppl 1):103A, 1993.

25. Wolfe L, Stess RM, Graf PM: Dynamic pressure analysis of the diabetic Charcot foot, *J Am Podiatr Med Assoc* 81(6):281–287, 1991.

26. Brand PW: Repetitive stress in the development of diabetic foot ulcers. In Levin ME, O'Neal LW, editors: *The diabetic foot,* ed 4, St Louis, 1988, Mosby–Year Book.

27. Delbridge L, Ellis CS, Robertson K: Nonenzymatic glycosylation of keratin from the stratum corneum of the diabetic foot, *Br J Dermatol* 112:547–554, 1985.

28. Brownlee M, Cerami A, Vlassara H: Advanced glycosylation end products in tissue and the biochemical basis of diabetic complications, *N Engl J Med* 318:1315–1321, 1988.

29. Brand PW: The diabetic foot. In Ellenberg M, Rifkin H, editors: *Diabetes mellitus. Theory and practice,* ed 3, New Hyde Park, NY, 1983, Medical Examination Publishing.

30. Helm PA, Walker SC, Pullium G: Total contact casting in diabetic patients with neuropathic foot ulcerations, *Arch Phys Med Rehabil* 65(11):691–693, 1984.

31. Ward D: Footwear in leprosy, *Lepr Rev* 34:94–105, 1962.

32. Cavanagh PR, Ulbrecht JS: Plantar pressure in the diabetic foot. In Sammarco GJ, editor: *The diabetic foot,* Philadelphia, 1991, Lea & Febiger.

33. Brand PW, Ebner JD: Pressure sensitive devices for denervated hands and feet, *J Bone Joint Surg* 51A(1):109–116, 1969.

34. Coleman WC, Brand PW, Birke JA: The total contact cast: a therapy for plantar ulceration on insensitive feet. *J Am Podiatr Med Assoc* 74(11):548–552, 1984.

35. Pollard JP, Le Quesne LP, Tappin JW: Forces under the foot, *J Biomed Eng* 5:37–40, 1983.

36. Thompson DE: The effects of mechanical stress on soft tissue. In Levin ME and O'Neal LW, editors: *The diabetic foot,* ed 4, St Louis, 1988, Mosby–Year Book.

37. Burden AC et al: Use of a "Scotchcast Boot" in treating diabetic foot ulcers, *Br Med J* 286:1555–1557, 1983.

38. Ravina A: Management of plantar ulcers, *Diabetic Med* 7:465, 1990 (letter).

39. Griffiths GD, Wieman TJ: Metatarsal head resection for diabetic foot ulcers, *Arch Surg* 125(7):832–835, 1990.

40. Dannels EG: A preventive metatarsal osteotomy for healing pre-ulcers in American Indian diabetics, *J Am Podiatr Med Assoc* 76(1):33–37, 1986.

41. Jacobs RL: Hoffman procedure in the ulcerated diabetic neuropathic foot, *Foot Ankle* 3(3):142–149, 1982.

42. Sanders LJ, Frykberg RG: Diabetic neuropathic osteoarthropathy: the Charcot foot. In Frykberg RG, editor: *The high risk foot in diabetes mellitus,* New York, 1991, Churchill Livingstone.

43. Myerson MS, Papa J, Girard P: Arthrodesis for salvage of hindfoot and ankle neuroarthropathy, *J Bone Joint Surg* (in press).

44. Wagner FW Jr: Lower extremity amputations. In Frykberg RG, editor: *The high risk foot in diabetes mellitus,* New York, 1991, Churchill Livingstone.

45. Edmonds ME et al: The diabetic foot: impact of a foot clinic, *Q J Med* 232:763–771, 1986.

46. Gudas CJ: Prophylactic surgery in the diabetic foot. In Harkless LB, Dennis KJ, editors: *Clinics in podiatric medicine and surgery: the diabetic foot,* Philadelphia, 1987, WB Saunders.

47. Giurini JM et al: Sesamoidectomy for the treatment of chronic neuropathic ulcerations, *J Am Podiatr Med Assoc* 81(4):167–173, 1991.

48. Giacalone VF, Krych SM, Harkless LB: Our experience with foot surgery in diabetes: elective and infected foot surgery, *J Foot Surg,* (in press).

49. Boulton AJM et al: Abnormalities of foot pressure in early diabetic neuropathy, *Diabetic Med* 4:225–228, 1987.

50. Cavanagh PR, Sims DS, Sanders LJ: Body mass is a poor predictor of peak plantar pressure in diabetic men, *Diabetes Care* 14(8):750–755, 1991.

51. Boulton AJM, Veves A, Young MJ: Etiopathogenesis and management of abnormal foot pressures. In Levin ME, O'Neal LW, Bowker JH, editors: *The diabetic foot,* ed 5, St Louis, 1993, Mosby–Year Book.

52. Cavanagh PR, Simoneau GG, Ulbrecht JS: Ulceration, unsteadiness, and uncertainty: the biomechanical consequences of diabetes mellitus, *J Biomech* 26(suppl 1): 23–40, 1993.

53. Cavanagh PR et al: Radiographic abnormalities in the feet of patients with diabetic neuropathy, *Diabetes Care* (accepted for publication, 1993).

54. Cavanagh PR et al: Correlates of structure and function in neuropathic diabetic feet, *Diabetologia* 34(suppl 2):A39, 1991 (abstract).

55. Myerson MS, Shereff MJ: The pathological anatomy of claw and hammer toes, *J Bone Joint Surg* 71A(1):45–49, 1989.

56. Habershaw G, Donovan JC: Biomechanical considerations of the diabetic foot. In: Kozak GP et al, editors: *Management of diabetic foot problems,* Philadelphia, 1984, WB Saunders.

57. Gooding GAW et al: Heel pad thickness: determination by high-resolution ultrasonography, *J Ultrasound Med* 4:173–174, 1985.

58. Gooding GAW, Stess RM, Graf PM: Sonography of the sole of the foot: evidence for loss of foot pad thickness in diabetes and its relationship to ulceration of the foot, *Invest Radiol* 21:45–48, 1986.

59. Brownlee M, Vlassara H, Cerami A: Nonenzymatic glycosylation and the pathogenesis of diabetic complications, *Ann Intern Med* 101:527–537, 1984.

60. Sage RA: Diabetic ulcers: evaluation and management. In Harkless LB, Dennis KJ, editors: *Clinics in podiatric medicine and surgery: the diabetic foot,* Philadelphia, 1987, WB Saunders.

61. Young MJ et al: The effect of callus removal on dynamic plantar foot pressures in diabetic patients, *Diabetic Med* 9(1):55–57, 1992.

62. Rosenbloom AL et al: Limited joint mo-

bility in childhood diabetes mellitus indicates increased risk for microvascular disease, *N Engl J Med* 305:191–194, 1981.

63. Fernando DJS et al: Relationship of limited joint mobility to abnormal foot pressures and foot ulceration, *Diabetes Care* 14(1):8–11, 1991.

64. Birke JA, Cornwall MA, Jackson M: Relationship between hallux limitus and ulceration of the great toe, *J Orthop Sports Phys Ther* 10(5):172–176, 1988.

65. Cavanagh PR et al: Limited joint mobility (LJM) and loss of vibration sensation are predictors of elevated plantar pressure in diabetes, *Diabetes.* 40(suppl 1): 531A, 1991 (abstract).

66. Alexander IJ, Chao EYS, Johnson KA: The assessment of dynamic foot-to-ground contact forces and plantar pressure distribution: a review of the evolution of current techniques and clinical

applications, *Foot Ankle* 11(3):152–167, 1990.

67. Betts RP, Franks CI, Duckworth T: Foot pressure studies: normal and pathologic gait analyses. In Jahss MH, editor: *Disorders of the foot and ankle,* ed 2, Philadelphia, 1991, WB Saunders.

68. Cavanagh PR, Hewitt FG Jr, Perry JE: In-shoe plantar pressure measurement: a review, *Foot* 2(4):185–194, 1992.

69. Masson EA, Boulton AJMB: Pressure assessment methods in the foot. In Frykberg RG, editor: *The high risk foot in diabetes mellitus,* New York, 1991, Churchill Livingstone.

70. Hughes J et al: Reliability of pressure measurements: the EMED F system, *Clin Biomechan* 6:14–18, 1991.

71. Silvino N, Evanski PM, Waugh TR: The Harris and Beath footprinting mat: diagnostic validity and clinical use, *Clin Orthop* 151:265–269, 1980.

4

Vascular Disease in the Diabetic Lower Extremity

Frank W. LoGerfo, M.D.

Anton N. Sidawy, M.D.

The complex pathophysiology of diabetic foot lesions often involves the combination of ischemia, neuropathy, and infection. In recent years there have been considerable improvements in our understanding of the vascular disease leading to ischemia and improvements in surgical technique to restore blood flow to the foot. The well-perfused foot is more resistant to ulceration and has an improved capacity to heal following foot surgery and can recover better from infection. Thus a well-perfused foot opens up many therapeutic options in the long-term care of the diabetic foot. An understanding of the underlying vascular disease and its management is therefore an essential aspect of diabetic foot care.

Unfortunately, an appropriate understanding of the nature of vascular disease in the diabetic has been significantly hampered by some past misconceptions. The most prominent of these is the idea that patients with diabetes have an occlusive vascular disease involving the microcirculation. This misconception can be traced to an early observational study of the vasculature derived from histologic studies of amputation specimens. It was concluded that diabetics had an arteriolosclerosis and endothelial proliferation that was occluding the microvasculature. However, numerous subsequent prospective studies have failed to confirm the existence of such a lesion in association with diabetes.[1] In a prospective study of amputation specimens using blinded histology, Strandness[2] found no evidence of a microvascular occlusive lesion that was more common in diabetics than in nondiabetics. Similarly, Conrad[3] conducted a prospective study of amputation specimens using a sophisticated arterial casting technique that again demonstrated no evidence of an arteriolar occlusive lesion associated with diabetes. If patients with diabetes did indeed have arteriolosclerosis, they would be presumed to have a high fixed peripheral resistance in the lower extremity. Barner tested this hypothesis by measuring the flow rate in femoro-popliteal vein grafts before and after injecting papaverine to cause vasodilatation.[4] There was no difference in the capacity for vasodilatation between diabetics and nondiabetics with similar runoff. With the same reasoning, Irwin et al.[5] used noninvasive techniques to assess peripheral resistance in diabetics and nondiabetics presenting with foot ulceration and again demonstrated no evidence of higher resistance in the diabetic. Thus there have been many studies using various experimental approaches. All of these studies have been unable to confirm the existence of a microvascular occlusive lesion. If indeed a microvascular occlusive lesion did exist, it would connote a hopeless prognosis for patients with diabetic foot lesions. Thus an important step toward appropriate clinical management is rejecting the concept of a microvascular or small vessel occlusive disease associated with diabetes.

There are abnormalities in the microcirculation of the diabetic which are not occlusive but which may alter the physiology of the foot. Most prospective studies have confirmed the existence of a thickened capillary basement membrane.[6] Again, this is not associated with an occlusive lesion. In fact, the capillary lumen in the diabetic is actually slightly larger than that in the nondiabetic.[7, 8] The capillary basement membrane plays an important role in the exchange of nutrients, metabolic products, and cells between the capillary and the interstitium. It is therefore possible that the thickened capillary membrane interferes with these processes through, as yet, undefined mechanisms. The chemical structure of the basement membrane is altered as a result of glycosylation. This leads to greater crosslinking of proteins and a decreased number of highly charged sulfur groups.[9] This is one explanation for the established observation that highly charged molecules, such as albumin[10] and pentetic acid,[8] leak through the capillary basement membrane in the diabetic. There does not appear to be any impairment of oxygen diffusion to the extent that diabetics presenting with foot ulceration actually have a higher transcutaneous PO_2 than nondiabetics.[11]

Most studies have demonstrated a difference in the microanatomy of the capillaries. With diabetes, there are fewer of the simple "hair-pin loop" capillaries. There is an increased number of capillaries that take a tortuous path, appearing more as tufts than as simple loops. Following ischemia, there is less recruitment of new capillaries into the circulation although the overall number of existing capillaries per gram of tissue appears to be no different.[12] Following induction of ischemia it takes longer for the red cell velocity within the capillaries to reach peak velocity in the diabetic as compared with

the nondiabetic.[13] Thus there appears to be several abnormalities in the microcirculation that might contribute to an altered physiologic milieu in the diabetic. However, it is again important to note that none of these lesions are occlusive in nature, and thus do not represent an impediment to blood flow.

Atherosclerotic occlusive disease is the underlying cause for ischemia in the diabetic foot. Histologically, there is no difference in the atherosclerotic lesion when it occurs in association with diabetes.[14] However, the incidence of occlusive disease is higher, and the progression is more rapid among diabetics.[15] There is a very important difference in the pattern of atherosclerotic occlusive disease when it occurs with diabetes. The occlusion has a propensity to involve the infrageniculate arteries, i.e., the anterior tibial, posterior tibial, and peroneal arteries. Suprisingly, the arteries in the foot, especially the dorsalis pedis artery, are often spared. This pattern of occlusive disease with involvement of the infrageniculate arteries but with sparing of the foot arteries has been documented by histologic studies[2] and arterial casting studies.[3] In addition, using angiographic studies this pattern of atherosclerotic involvement in diabetic patients was further evaluated.[16] Arteriograms of diabetic and nondiabetic patients admitted for the evaluation of their symptomatic peripheral vascular disease were studied. A score was assigned to each of the plantar arch, anterior and posterior tibial, and the peroneal arteries; diabetic patients had significantly more disease in the tibial and peroneal arteries in the leg, however, the magnitude of plantar arch occlusive involvement was not significantly different.[16] In recent years, this observation has become critically important because it opens up the possibility of arterial reconstruction to the foot arteries. When arteriography is performed to assess the site of atherosclerotic occlusion, the status of the foot vessels must always be established even when the tibial and peroneal arteries are totally occluded. This can be accomplished by using digital subtraction arteriography or other angiographic techniques. In diabetics with pre-existing renal failure, there is always concern about contrast-induced renal failure as a complication of arteriography. The most important measure to prevent this is adequate hydration of the patient prior to the angiogram. When renal failure occurs, it is almost always reversible,[17] but it may delay the arterial reconstructive surgery for several days before the creatinine returns to baseline.

An important technical advance in the management of the ischemic diabetic foot is the excellent results achieved with bypass grafts to the pedal arteries (Fig 4–1).[18] The advantage of extreme distal bypass grafts is that they restore maximum arterial pressure to foot vessels. In the presence of neuropathy and/or infection, maximum perfusion is necessary to obtain and maintain healing of the foot.

Diabetic neuropathy is a key factor in the formation of foot ulcers in diabetic patients. Repetitive trauma, from wearing a tight-fitting shoe for example, leads to the formation of lesions in the insensate diabetic foot even in the presence of palpable foot pulses. This contributes to the misconception that diabetic patients have occlusive disease involving their microcirculation despite patent arterial system. Thus foot protection in diabetic patients suffering from neuropathy is very important to prevent foot lesions. The ease by which infection can develop in diabetics contributes to the complexity of diabetic foot problems. The addition of infection to even a simple lesion may lead to disastrous results; therefore, the immediate control of any infection is very important despite possible delay in revascularization.

The impact of our current understand-

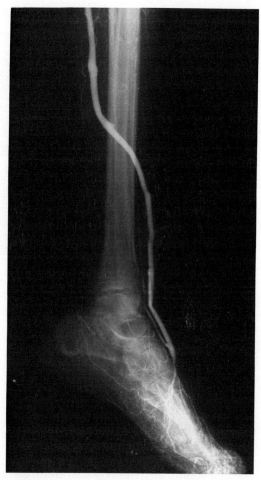

FIG 4–1.
An intraoperative arteriogram of a saphenous vein bypass to the dorsalis pedis artery. Note the excellent foot runoff.

ing of vascular disease and the use of extreme distal bypass grafting is illustrated in Fig 4–2.[19] Maximum benefit from revascularization can be achieved through an integrated interdisciplinary approach to the complex pathobiology of the diabetic foot. Thus it remains a priority to debride and drain abscesses or any contained infections prior to revascularization. Following revascularization, the wound can be managed with attention toward elimination of pressure points and deformities that are likely to lead to recurrent ulceration especially in the pres-

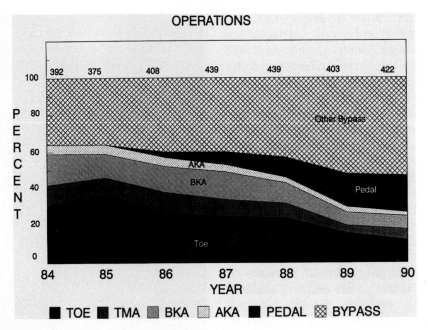

FIG 4–2.
Operative experience on patients with diabetes and foot lesions over a 7-year period comparing incidence of lower extremity bypass grafts with incidence of amputation. *Pedal* = bypass graft to the dorsalis pedis artery; *AKA* = above-knee amputation; *BKA* = below-knee amputation; *TMA* = transmetatarsal amputation; *toe* = toe amputation. Note that the incidence of all amputations has decreased in recent years. This decrease corresponds with the increasing use of vein bypass grafts to the dorsalis pedis artery.

ence of neuropathy. Our overall management plan may be summarized as follows:

1. Prompt intravenous antibiotic administration, drainage of abscesses, and debridement of necrotic tissue to control systemic sepsis.
2. Evaluation for ischemia.
3. Arteriography to demonstrate the arterial anatomy of the entire leg down to and including the foot. In particular, the status of the foot arteries must be determined even when the arteries in the leg are occluded.
4. Arterial reconstruction designed to restore maximum foot perfusion.
5. Reconstructive foot surgery to obtain tissue closure and to eliminate pressure points or deformities.
6. Foot protection using appropriate footwear to prevent further injury and tissue loss.

Clinical management of the diabetic foot is a demanding and complex task. This is best accomplished through an interdisciplinary team of vascular surgeons, podiatrists, orthopedic surgeons, plastic surgeons, infectious disease experts, diabetologists, physical therapists, etc. An understanding of the pathophysiology of ischemia and its management provides the foundation on which this care can be provided with the greatest degree of success.

REFERENCES

1. LoGerfo FW, Coffman JD: Vascular and microvascular disease of the foot in diabetes: implications for foot care, *N Engl J Med* 311:1615–1619, 1984.

2. Strandness DE Jr, Priest RE, Gibbons GE: Combined clinical and pathologic study of diabetic and nondiabetic peripheral arterial disease, *Diabetes* 13:366–372, 1964.

3. Conrad MC: Large and small artery occlusion in diabetics and nondiabetics with severe vascular disease, *Circulation* 36:83–91, 1967.

4. Barner HB, Kaiser GC, Willman VL: Blood flow in the diabetic leg, *Circulation* 43:391–394, 1971.

5. Irwin ST et al: Blood flow in diabetics with foot lesions due to "small vessel disease," *Br J Surg* 75:1201–1206, 1988.

6. Siperstein MD, Unger RH, Madison LL: Studies of muscle capillary basement membrane in normal subjects, diabetic and prediabetic patients. *J Clin Invest* 47:1973–1999, 1968.

7. Britland ST et al: Relationship of endoneural capillary abnormalities to type and severity of diabetic polyneuropathy, *Diabetes* 39:909–913, 1990.

8. Katz MA et al: Relationships between microvascular function and capillary structure in diabetic and nondiabetic human skin, *Diabetes* 38:1245–1250, 1989.

9. Brownlee M, Cerami A, Vlassara H: Advanced glycosylation end products in tissue and the biochemical basis of diabetic complications, *N Engl J Med* 318:1315–1321, 1988.

10. Parving HH, Rasmussen SM: Transcapillary escape rate of albumin and plasma volume in short- and long-term juvenile diabetes, *Scand J Clin Lab Invest* 32:81–87, 1973.

11. Wyss CR et al: Transcutaneous oxygen tension measurements on limbs of diabetic and nondiabetic vascular disease, *Diabetes* 13:366–372, 1964.

12. Katz MA, McNeill G: Defective vasodilation response to exercise in cutaneous precapillary vessels in diabetic humans. *Diabetes* 36:1386–1396, 1987.

13. Fargell B et al: Vital capillary microscopy for assessment of skin viability and microangiopathy in patients with diabetes mellitus, *Acta Med Scand* 687(suppl):25–28, 1989.

14. Ruderman NB, Haudenschild C: Diabetes as an atherogenic factor, *Prog Cardiovasc Dis* 26:373–382, 1984.

15. Beach KW et al: Progression of lower-extremity arterial occlusive disease in type II diabetes mellitus, *Diabetes Care* 11:464–472, 1988.

16. Menzoian JO et al: Symptomatology and anatomic patterns of peripheral vascular disease: differing impact of smoking and diabetes, *Ann Vasc Surg* 3:224–228, 1989.

17. Parfrey PS et al: Contrast material-induced renal failure in patients with diabetes mellitus, renal insufficiency, or both. A prospective controlled study, *N Engl J Med* 320:143, 1989.

18. Pomposelli FB Jr et al: A flexible approach to infra-popliteal vein grafts in patients with diabetes mellitus, *Arch Surg* 161:724–729, 1991.

19. LoGerfo FW et al: Trends in the care of the diabetic foot: expanded role for arterial reconstruction, *Arch Surg* 127:617–621, 1992.

5 _____ Noninvasive Vascular Testing

Joseph M. Giordano, M.D.

The diagnosis and treatment of vascular disease has depended on concurrent advances in medical technology including sophisticated arteriographic techniques, grafts for arterial bypass, and instrumentation used for diagnosis. These new diagnostic instruments stimulated development of peripheral vascular laboratories that have become essential components of the vascular evaluation, enhancing the impression of the physician and allowing the objective physiological measurements of the extent of vascular disease.

These vascular laboratories use Doppler, plethysmography, and ultrasound techniques to evaluate patients with cerebrovascular, peripheral arterial, and venous disease. The labs have become so effective that carotid arterial stenoses can be accurately diagnosed in 95% of cases. And duplex ultrasound scans have replaced venography as the gold standard for the diagnosis of deep venous thrombosis. In the lower extremities, these same techniques are used to evaluate patients with arterial vascular insufficiency and are particularly valuable in the diabetic patients who present with ischemic vascular disease of the feet.

This chapter discusses the role of the vascular laboratory in the diagnosis and management of diabetic patients with vascular disease in the lower extremity. I will explain the basic physiology that determines arterial blood flow to the foot, the tests available to diagnose peripheral arterial disease, and pathophysiological factors unique to the diabetic.

VASCULAR HEMODYNAMICS

The arterial side of the cardiovascular system is a closed circuit of conduits, i.e., blood vessels, with a central pump, the heart, that generates pressures to overcome peripheral resistance allowing for the flow of blood. Blood flow depends on the following relationships: Blood flow equals $\Delta P/R$ with the ΔP being the difference in arterial pressures between any two points in the vascular bed, and R being the resistance in the vascular bed to the flow of blood. Blood flow then depends not only on arterial pressures, but on the relationship between pressure and resistance. If the arterial pressure gradient is the same, then blood flow is inversely related to peripheral resistance so that lowering peripheral resistance increases blood flow, and an increase of resistance reduces blood flow. If resistance remains constant as in a fixed arterial plaque, then blood flow is directly related to the arterial pressure gradient between two points in the vascular bed.

The system of blood vessels is a closed circuit with one central pump. Therefore in an individual lying in a supine position, arterial pressures will be the same in any major artery. In the standing position, gravity influences pressure so that arterial pressure in the ankle will be higher than arterial pressure in the arm. If, however, there is a stenosis or occlusion of a major artery, the arterial pressure distal to the occlusion is reduced, affecting the flow of blood. Documentation of reduced arterial pressure in a particular vascular bed, such as the lower extremity, compared to the central aortic pressure, as measured in the upper arm, indicates an occlusion or critical stenosis in the major artery to the lower extremities.

VASCULAR LABORATORY TESTS

Arterial Pressure Measurements

Segmental arterial pressure measurements of the lower extremities is the most basic and useful test to detect peripheral vascular disease. The concept of the test is similar to the measurement of routine arm pressures. A blood pressure cuff placed on the leg is inflated to occlude arterial blood flow. Detecting blood flow distal to the cuff after deflation determines arterial pressure of the leg. Unlike arm pressures, acoustic signals in the lower extremity are unreliable, and a Doppler probe is used to detect the return of blood flow.

Segmental pressures are frequently, but not always, measured in five different levels of the lower extremity: upper thigh, lower thigh, below the knee, ankle, and toe. Blood pressure cuffs are applied to these segments. An arterial signal at the ankle is located with the Doppler. Starting at the thigh, each cuff is inflated to above systolic arterial pressure as measured by a pressure cuff. The cuff is then slowly deflated until a Doppler signal is heard at the ankle. The pressure of the occluding cuff that marks the return of the Doppler arterial flow at the ankle is the arterial pressure at that cuff level. For measuring toe pressures, a 2 cm cuff is placed on the proximal phalanx. The return of the arterial flow after deflation of the cuff is detected not by Doppler signals, but usually

by the reappearance of oscillations as detected by a photoplethysmography.

In theory, segmental pressures of the lower extremity should be the same as central aortic pressure measured by the brachial arm pressure. In practice, however, measuring lower extremity arterial pressures with pressure cuffs has pitfalls. If the width of the thigh cuff is less than 1.2 times the circumference of the thigh, then pressures higher than actual intra-arterial pressures are obtained.[1] With the arterial toe pressures, the small size of the cuff and toe make measurements difficult so that toe pressures in normal patients are frequently found to be less than systolic arterial pressures. The pressure in the cuff must be reliably transmitted to the artery to accurately reflect the intraarterial pressure. Large amounts of tissue, noncompliant skin, and calcified arteries may interfere with the transmission of cuff pressure needed to occlude the artery and distort the recorded values.

Ankle pressures are the most accurate and useful of the segmental leg pressures.[2] It is accurate because ankle circumference, which is consistent from patient to patient, has an optimal relationship to the width of a standard blood pressure cuff. In addition, the absence at the ankle of large amounts of muscle, fat, and subcutaneous tissue allow for a true transmission of pressure from the cuff to the arteries of the ankle so that the pressure measured is the actual intraarterial pressure.

Ankle pressures are expressed as the ankle/arm index. This index is represented by the systolic pressure at the ankle divided by the brachial systolic pressure. In normal patients, the pressure is usually 1 or slightly greater than 1. Values under 0.9 are clearly abnormal, indicating a degree of vascular insufficiency. Because central aortic pressure influences ankle pressure and frequently fluctuates in the same patient, the ankle/arm index compensates for these fluctuations and will accurately reflect the degree of arterial occlusive disease. A reduction in the ankle/arm index indicates worsening of arterial occlusive disease, not just change in the central aortic pressure. In the presence of calcification, the vessel walls may be noncompressible which would artificially inflate the index to greater than 1. However, absolute ankle pressures are useful to determine the potential for an ulcer to heal, to confirm the diagnosis of rest pain, and establish the viability of the lower extremity and foot.

Plethysmography

Plethysmography records volume changes in a limb, finger, or toe that qualitatively reflects the amount of pulsatile blood flow. Different types of plethysmography exist depending on the sensing mechanism used to record the volume changes. Devices that are water, air, and mercury filled, in addition to electrical impedance devices, and photoplethysmography have all been used and advocated. However, the air-filled plethysmograph and the photoplethysmograph are currently most commonly used. The air-filled plethysmograph uses a thin-walled cuff filled with air that is connected to a pressure transducer. The cuff is placed around the extremity, inflated to 65 cm Hg, and then opened to the pressure transducer. Changes in the cuff's volume with pulsatile blood flow causes pressure changes within the cuff that is sensed by the transducer and recorded as a tracing. Photoplethysmography uses a light source to illuminate a portion of tissue. Reflected light picked up by photoelectric sensor connected to a recorder is related to capillary blood volume. A pulsatile wave form is generated with characteristics similar to wave forms by other types of plethysmography. The device can be applied directly to the skin in an area without the need of a cuff surrounding the digit or extremity. Because photoplethysmography reflects the changes in skin perfusion, maintaining room temperature is important and a major problem with interpretation of this test.

Plethysmographic tracings are evaluated with both qualitative and quantitative techniques.[3] The normal contour of the recording, including a sharp upswing and downswing with a dicrotic notch, are indications of normal arterial inflow. In a properly calibrated instrument, the height of the wave form can be closely correlated with the degree of arterial occlusive disease. Tracings at the ankle

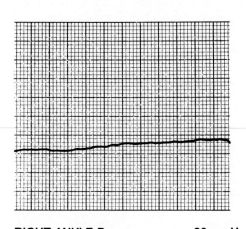

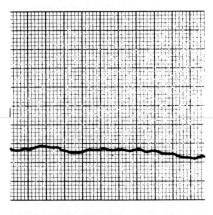

RIGHT ANKLE P sys   28 mmHg   **LEFT ANKLE P sys**   34 mmHg

FIG 5–1.
Flat tracings and low ankle pressure are diagnostic of severe peripheral arterial ischemia.

greater than 15 mm are normal while flat tracings indicate severe peripheral ischemia (Fig 5–1).

Plethysmographic tracings are usually consistent with ankle pressure. However, ankle pressures are misleading if the peripheral arteries are stiff from calcification and extensive atheroscleroses. The pressure in the calf needed to overcome wall stiffness to collapse the artery for measuring ankle pressure is much higher than the actual intraarterial pressure. In these circumstances, the recorded pressures are falsely elevated. Plethysmographic tracings are useful in this setting since the volume changes are more reflective of peripheral arterial blood flow (Fig 5–2).

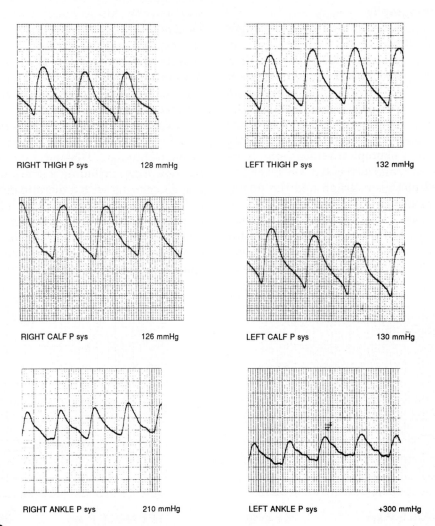

BRACHIAL BLOOD PRESSURE

RIGHT ARM 100/60   LEFT ARM 110/70

RESTING SEGMENTAL PLETHYSMOGRAPHY AND SYSTOLIC PRESSURES

RIGHT THIGH P sys 128 mmHg	LEFT THIGH P sys 132 mmHg
RIGHT CALF P sys 126 mmHg	LEFT CALF P sys 130 mmHg
RIGHT ANKLE P sys 210 mmHg	LEFT ANKLE P sys +300 mmHg

FIG 5–2.
Segmental pressures and tracings. Note high ankle pressures due to noncompressible calcified arteries. *Tracings* indicate adequate arterial blood flow.

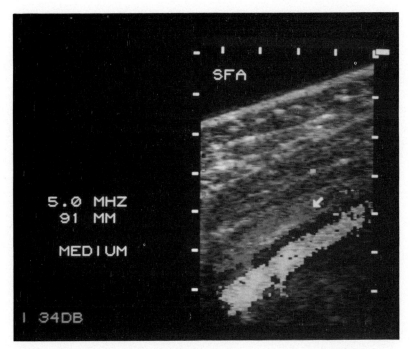

FIG 5–3.
Color coding allows easy distinction between femoral artery *(arrow)* and femoral vein.

Duplex Scan

Duplex scans have become the gold standard for the diagnosis of carotid arterial and peripheral venous disease and have been applied to the lower extremity arterial system.[4] It uses the combination of a real time B-mode scanner, along with a directional Doppler. Recently, the duplex scan was modified to become user friendly by adding a color flow technique. A Doppler probe is placed over the artery and vein (Fig 5–3). Because the directional Doppler can determine whether blood is flowing toward or away from the probe, flow is color coded depending on flow direction. Arterial and venous flow are always in the opposite directions, and therefore will be assigned different colors to allow easier distinction between the artery and vein. For diagnosing arterial disease, a duplex scan uses the images provided by the scan to identify the artery and determine the areas of plaque formation or narrowing that may be amenable to balloon dilata-

tion (Fig 5–4). More important, with the area of narrowing identified, the Doppler beam is placed in its center to determine the velocity of blood flow and the presence of flow turbulence. At any point of a branchless segment of an artery, flow defined as mL/minute is the same. This holds true even if there is a narrowing of an arterial segment. What changes, however, is the velocity of flow, i.e., how fast blood flow is moving is expressed as cm/sec. To understand this concept a useful analogy is to picture a quiet stream of water that narrows to become a dangerous rapids. The flow of water in mL/minute over any point of this stream or rapids must be the same. To maintain the same flow through the narrow part, the velocity of flow must greatly increase to produce the rapids. Dramatic increases in the velocity of flow indicates arterial stenosis. If both flow Doppler signal and color are absent, the artery is occluded.

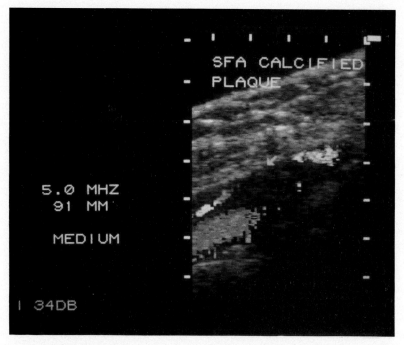

FIG 5–4.
Stenosis of the arterial lumen is obvious from the reduction in the color flow image.

Transcutaneous PO₂ Measurements

Transcutaneous (TC) PO_2 is the oxygen tension on the surface of the skin detected by an electrode. Usually PO_2 on the skin surface is almost zero. However, by increasing the local skin temperature, and thereby increasing skin blood flow, the TC PO_2 rises to measurable levels. Low TC PO_2 levels have been correlated with severe peripheral arterial disease. The test is not widely used in vascular laboratories due to difficulty in performing and interpreting the results. Factors that influence the skin PO_2 includes thickness of skin, diffusing capacity of skin, cardiac output, and degree of sympathetic stimulation.

THE DIABETIC PATIENT

Nondiabetic patients with ischemic foot problems usually have rest pain whereas diabetic patients are more likely to have foot ulcerations. These ulcerations may be ischemic, neurotrophic, or a combination of both. With ten million diabetics and the increased risk of atherosclerosis in diabetic patients, this clinical problem is indeed significant.

The diabetic patient with an ischemic foot has unique problems that make examination in the vascular laboratory more challenging. Medium-sized arteries from the superficial femoral artery to the tibial vessels at the ankle are frequently calcified and therefore noncompressible. Pressure cuffs used to determine ankle pressures cannot overcome the arterial wall stiffness unless high pressures are used. These high pressures are inaccurate because they reflect the intraarterial pressure at the level of the cuff and the pressure needed to overcome arterial wall stiffness. Thus the performance of ankle pressure in diabetic patients may not be accurate.

Nevertheless there are three clinical problems in the ischemic diabetic foot that are helped by an evaluation in the vascular laboratory. These are as follows:

1. Determination of the adequacy of blood flow to heal a foot ulcer.
2. Evaluation of foot pain.
3. Selection of an amputation site.

Ankle pressures are used to predict wound healing in nondiabetic patients. Most physicians would agree that minor foot ulcerations will not heal if the ankle pressure is under 65 mm Hg. In diabetic patients, however, a pressure greater than 90 mm Hg is necessary to heal foot ulcerations.[5] This difference may be due to the calcified arteries of a diabetic causing erroneously high values so that the diabetic patient with an ankle pressure of 90 mm Hg actually has an intraarterial pressure of 65 mm Hg. However, there may be other explanations. Wyss[6] suggests that for a given ankle pressure, a diabetic patient has less blood flow to the foot than a nondiabetic patient. It is tempting to suggest that this is due to the small vessel disease of diabetics. LoGerfo,[7] however, concluded that small vessel disease, defined as involvement of foot arteries, is no different in diabetics compared to the nondiabetic population. Perhaps the higher pressure necessary to heal a diabetic foot ulcer may reflect the increased need of diabetic patients for more blood flow because of decreased resistance to infection and the presence of neuropathy.

Other strategies in the evaluation of diabetic foot ulceration must be used. These include plethysmography and digital arterial pressure. Plethysmography is an accurate qualitative reflection of arterial blood flow to the foot. The test is not affected by calcification of peripheral arteries. Plethysmography can be used at the ankle, transmetatarsal, or digital level. As discussed previously, interpretation depends on evaluation of pulse contour and amplitude of the tracings. In diabetic patients, calcification does not usually involve digital arteries. Therefore, toe pressures with the use of a 2 cm cuff on the proximal toe and photoplethys-mography distally to determine the return of pulsations can be used to determine the adequacy of blood flow. It is generally accepted that a toe pressure of 30 to 40 mm Hg is the minimum needed to heal a toe ulcer in a diabetic patient.

Foot pain in the diabetic patient can be due to many causes. Because rest pain from ischemic vascular disease can be considered pregangrenous, it is important to accurately diagnose ischemic rest pain in the diabetic patient. In a nondiabetic patient, a good history plus the absence of pulses below the femoral are adequate to establish the diagnosis of ischemic rest pain. The diabetic patient frequently has palpable popliteal pulses and the presence of neuropathy that complicate the interpretation of foot pain. The performance of ankle pressures and tracings should be all that is necessary to diagnose ischemic rest pain. The presence of flat plethysmographic tracings with either low ankle pressures or high pressures due to noncompressible leg arteries establishes the diagnosis of ischemic rest pain.

Determining the optimal level for an amputation has been an elusive goal. Relying on clinical factors such as skin color and temperature, peripheral pulses, and bleeding at the time of incision have proven to be unreliable. Use of the vascular laboratory has not produced a standard test or battery of tests that can accurately predict the optimal level of amputation. Many authors have advocated various combinations of plethysmography and segmental pressures to predict the healing of an amputation site. However, if laboratory values to determine the site of amputation are placed too high, then, although patients with values above that level always heal from an amputation, many patients with values below that level still might heal but will be denied a more distal amputation site. Conversely, if the lab values are too low, then some amputations may not heal requiring a secondary operation.

Transcutaneous PO_2 values has recently been shown to be a promising new technique. Differences exist in the criteria used and further experience is necessary before definite recommendations can be made. One can clearly state that a patient with a TC PO_2 of 0 mm Hg will not heal from an amputation at that level. And likewise, all patients with values above 40 mm Hg will heal. Values between 0 to 40 mm have been problematic. Harwood, et al reports that if a TC PO_2 is below 10 mm Hg and a less than 10 mm Hg increase occurs after exposure to 100% oxygen, the amputation site will not heal.[8] Karanfilian also reports a low chance of successful healing of an amputation site if the TC PO_2 was less than 10 mm of mercury.[9] Clearly, more comprehensive studies are needed to define the absolute criteria necessary to heal or to predict healing of an amputation site.

SUMMARY

Most diabetic patients with ischemic foot disease can be evaluated in the vascular laboratory with simple ankle pressures and tracings. Toe tracings with a photoplethysmography would give helpful information for patients with toe ulcerations who have normal ankle pressure and tracings. These patients might have disease distal to the ankle that would be diagnosed with abnormal toe tracings. For patients with high ankle pressures from calcified arteries, attention should be focused on the pulse contours of the tracings. For routine evaluation, duplex scan of the lower leg arteries is unnecessary. However, in patients who may need intervention but are poor candidates for surgery, a duplex scan of the proximal lower extremity arteries could reveal areas of stenosis that are amenable to balloon dilatation.

One other new technique for determination of lower extremity healing potential is magnetic resonance flowmetry (see Chapter 6 for detailed discussion). Although quite new, and possibly controversial, this technique shows some promise.

REFERENCES

1. Alexander H, Cohen ML, Steinfeld L: Criteria in the choice of an occluding cuff for the indirect measurement of blood pressure, *Med Biol Eng Comput* 15:2, 1977.
2. Carter SA: Clinical measurement of systolic pressures in limbs with arterial occlusive disease, *JAMA* 207:1869, 1969.
3. Darling RG et al: Quantitative segmental pulse volume recorder: a clinical tool, *Surgery* 72:873, 1972.
4. Jager KA, Rickets HJ, Strandness DE Jr: Duplex scanning for the evaluation of lower limb arterial disease. In Bernstein EF, editor: *Noninvasive diagnostic techniques in vascular disease,* ed 2, St Louis, 1985, Mosby–Year Book.
5. Carter SA: The relationship of distal systolic pressure to healing of skin lesions in limbs with arterial occlusive disease with special reference to diabetes mellitus, *Scan J Clin Lab Invest* 31(suppl 128):239, 1973.
6. Wyss CR et al: Relationship between transcutaneous oxygen tension, ankle blood pressure and clinical outcome of vascular surgery in diabetic and nondiabetic patients, *Surgery* 101:56, 1987.
7. LoGerfo F, Coffman J: Vascular and microvascular disease of the foot in diabetes, *N Engl J Med* 311:1615, 1984.
8. Harwood T et al: Oxygen inhalation induced transcutaneous PO_2 changes as a prediction of amputation level, *J Vasc Surg* 2:220, 1985.
9. Karanfilian RG et al: The value of laser doppler velocimetry and transcutaneous oxygenation determination in predicting healing of ischemic forefoot ulcerations and amputations in diabetic and non-diabetic patients, *J Vasc Surg* 4:511, 1986.

6
Measuring Arterial Blood Flow by Nuclear Magnetic Resonance

J. Philip A. Hinton, M.D.

J. R. Nelson, M.D.

Roy Kroeker, D.P.M.

Nuclear magnetic resonance can be used to measure arterial blood flow in an extremity or in a single artery. This technology allows objective, direct measurement of arterial blood flow in an entirely noninvasive manner. It is unaffected by calcification or incompressibility of the arterial wall. Therefore, arterial blood flow can be accurately measured in even the most difficult circumstances, such as the diabetic patient with medial sclerosis of the arteries.

Measurement of arterial flow to an extremity is critical for decision making. In patients with foot ulceration, it is especially important to identify the presence of ischemia as a primary etiology of chronic nonhealing wounds.

Traditional noninvasive vascular laboratory studies have included Doppler-derived segmental blood pressures. The most commonly reported parameter is the ankle/brachial index, which compares systolic pressure at the ankle to systolic pressure at the arm. However, this technique is only an indirect measurement of leg hemodynamics. The diabetic presents a challenge in the application of pressure measurements because arterial wall calcification makes pressure measurements unreliable and results in erroneously elevated ankle pressures that are thus nondiagnostic.[1]

Many attempts have been made to correlate toe pressures with the ability to heal foot lesions.[2] However, cumulative data suggest that healing occurs when toe pressures exceed 30 mm Hg, but usually do not occur when pressure is less than 20 mm Hg. Sondgeroth et al found that the normal variability of toe pressures is 10 mm Hg.[3] It becomes obvious that minor changes in systemic pressure and the technique and skill of the technician can drastically alter the reliability of these studies. This variability makes accurate assessment of wound healing potential unpredictable. In addition, when flow to the lower limb is provided by extensive collaterals, toe pressures may be less than 20 mm Hg, even close to zero, because of the higher resistance of collaterals. This would account for the instances where toe pressures are significantly less than 20 mm Hg, and yet healing of the lesion occurs.

Bidirectional Doppler waveform analysis is useful to separate normal flow patterns (triphasic) from proximal obstruction patterns (monophasic). However, this analysis will not allow identification of the subgroup with limb threatening ischemia. Transcutaneous oxygen levels are used to predict ischemia, but are less reproducible and more prone to technician variance than are ankle brachial indices.[4]

Similarly, laser Doppler studies do not accurately detect ischemia.[5] Pulse volume recording (PVR) has the limitation that the line between abnormal and ischemic flow is not well defined.[6] Color flow duplex scanning measures velocity of flow and measures the diameter of a vessel at the point of use. If the entire length of an artery is scanned, stenoses and obstructions can be identified, at least to the popliteal level. Anatomic location and the degree of the disease's stenosis can be assessed, but again, no information is obtained to separate out an ischemic subgroup.[7]

Magnetic resonance angiography is gaining acceptance as a noninvasive modality to assess arterial anatomy, but hemodynamic quantification of arterial flow in the lower extremity is limited. Excellent information is obtained with contrast arteriograms, but adequacy of flow is not measured with arteriograms. The inability of these methods to accurately assess flow has prompted the development of new technology.

Although based on the same underlying physics, magnetic resonance flow (MRF) scanning differs technologically from magnetic resonance imaging (MRI).[8] MRI systems use intense pulses of radiofrequency (RF) and magnetic energy to create images of anatomic structures. MRF scanning requires weaker, continuous magnetic and RF fields to generate signals proportional to the volume of arterial blood flowing during each cardiac cycle. As blood moves through a steady magnetic field, nuclear magnetization is induced due to the alignment of hydrogen nuclei in the blood along the direction of the applied field. As this magnetization is carried into a constant RF field that is oscillating at the magnetic resonance frequency, the magnetization tips away from, and precesses about the direction of the steady magnetic field. The precessing magnetization induces a voltage in a receiver coil that is proportional to the volume flow rate of blood being swept into

the receiver coil with each cardiac cycle. The receiver coil completely encircles the limb being measured, so that all the flow in arterial lumens within that cross section, major and minor arteries as well as collaterals, contribute to the pulsatile flow signal.

By adding continuously rotating gradient fields to the steady magnetic field, the conditions for magnetic resonance can be limited to the vicinity of a selected individual artery. By this means, flow through individual arteries can be measured. There is a commercially available, FDA-approved MRF system that uses this technology to measure pulsatile arterial flow in a cross section of an extremity, or in an individual artery in that cross section (Metriflow AFM-100; Metriflow Corp., Milwaukee; Fig 6–1).

The Metriflow scanner consists of a 6000-lb permanent magnet with a movable patient exam bed, a computer workstation with printer, and radiofrequency detector electronics. Because it is a dedicated small-parts (arm or leg) scanner with a 0.1 tesla magnetic field, its cost is a small percentage of a magnetic resonance imager's cost. The low magnetic field also eliminates many of the hazards of the high-strength MRI units. Patients with stents and metal prostheses are routinely scanned in the Metriflow scanner. At present, patients with pacemakers are not scanned.

The patient lies supine on a movable table with one limb placed in the bore of the MRF scanner (Fig 6–2). Incremental measurements of flow are made at intervals in the extremity. Five sites are measured between the ankle and the knee, and two sites are measured in the thigh. By measuring the circumference of the extremity at each test site, and by determining the size of the foot (shoe size), the volume of tissue distal to each measurement site is determined. Two reports are generated from this data.

The Rapid Vascular Assessment

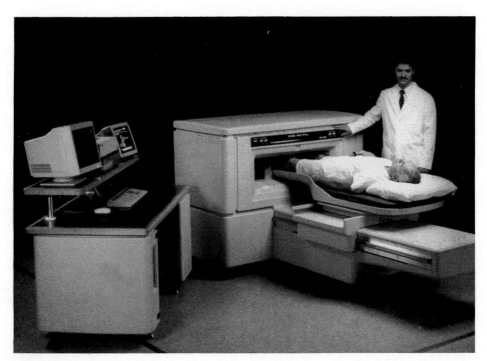

FIG 6–1.
Metriflow AFM-100 scanner.

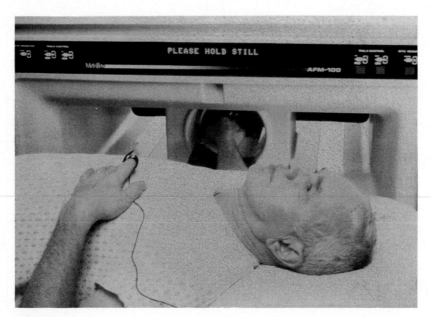

FIG 6–2.
Metriflow scanner with patient limb in the bore.

(RVA) lists the pulsatile arterial blood flow, in cc per minute, at each test site, with a corresponding arterial flow waveform displayed at each level. Figure 6–3 demonstrates a patient with the right side normal, and the left side abnormal secondary to stenosis of the left external iliac artery. The waveform morphology has proven to be useful, in addition to the flow number. Waveforms typical of normal arterial flow (Fig 6–4) demonstrate rapid systolic upstroke, tapering diastolic down-

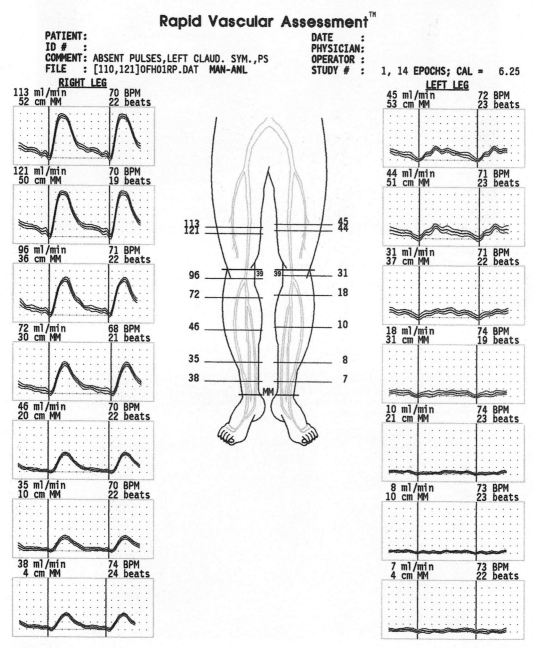

FIG 6–3.
Metriflow rapid vascular assessment *(RVA)* report-right side normal, left side abnormal.

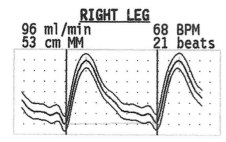

FIG 6–4.
Normal waveform, rapid vascular assessment *(RVA).*

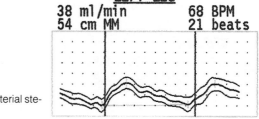

FIG 6–5.
Abnormal waveform secondary to proximal arterial stenosis, rapid vascular assessment *(RVA).*

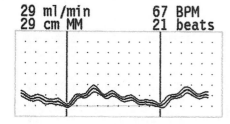

FIG 6–6.
Abnormal waveform demonstrating collateral flow, rapid vascular assessment *(RVA).*

stroke, and a width at half height equal to about 25% of the cardiac period. Stenosis of proximal arteries produces slow upstroke, and flattening of the waveform resulting in a width at half height 30% to 60% of the cardiac period (Fig 6–5). Functional collateral arterial flow is demonstrated by "jagged" waveforms, as the peak flow of systole arrives a few milliseconds later in smaller collaterals.[9] Figure 6–6 demonstrates the waveform in a patient with total occlusion of the superficial femoral artery in its mid portion with reconstitution via collateral vessels at the adductor hiatus. The blunted upstroke with "jagged" waveform is typical for such disease.

The Perfusion Analysis (PA) correlates the arterial flow at each level with the amount of distal tissue which that flow supplies. This is reported as milliliters per minute per 100 cubic centimeters of distal tissue (mL/min/100 cc distal tissue). Figure 6–7 demonstrates a patient with occlusion on the left side of the superficial femoral artery. The limb perfusion values on the left demonstrate the decrease in flow that is secondary to this pathology. This removes the variable of limb size from the study, and allows creation of a nomogram (Fig 6–8). This nomogram when used together with waveform morphology, reliably separates normal flow from abnormal and separates ischemic levels from claudication levels of flow.[10]

With this information, it is possible to determine the adequacy of arterial perfusion for wound healing.[10] This assessment of limb perfusion is especially important in the diabetic. First, the presence of vascular occlusive disease must be detected. Second, it must be established if

PERFUSION ANALYSIS

PATIENT:
ID # :
COMMENT: PS, LEFT LEG CLAUD. SYM., AB PULSES
FILE : [110,107]07700RP.DAT AUTO-ANL

DATE :
PHYSICIAN:
OPERATOR :
STUDY # : 0, 14 EPOCHS; CAL = 6.80

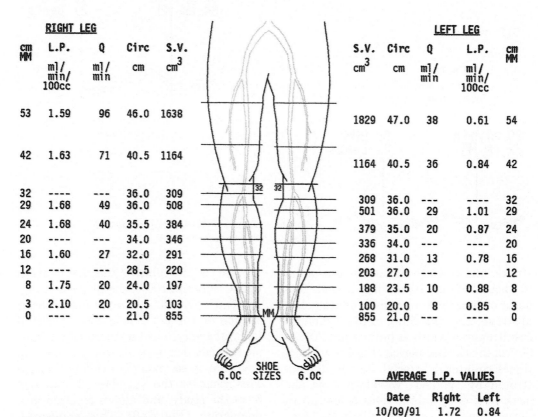

RIGHT LEG

cm MM	L.P. ml/min/100cc	Q ml/min	Circ cm	S.V. cm³
53	1.59	96	46.0	1638
42	1.63	71	40.5	1164
32	----	---	36.0	309
29	1.68	49	36.0	508
24	1.68	40	35.5	384
20	----	---	34.0	346
16	1.60	27	32.0	291
12	----	---	28.5	220
8	1.75	20	24.0	197
3	2.10	20	20.5	103
0	----	---	21.0	855

LEFT LEG

S.V. cm³	Circ cm	Q ml/min	L.P. ml/min/100cc	cm MM
1829	47.0	38	0.61	54
1164	40.5	36	0.84	42
309	36.0	---	----	32
501	36.0	29	1.01	29
379	35.0	20	0.87	24
336	34.0	---	----	20
268	31.0	13	0.78	16
203	27.0	---	----	12
188	23.5	10	0.88	8
100	20.0	8	0.85	3
855	21.0	---	----	0

SHOE SIZES
6.0C   6.0C

AVERAGE L.P. VALUES

Date	Right	Left
10/09/91	1.72	0.84

Circ : Circumference of the LEG at cm MM

L.P. : Limb Perfusion (perfusion to total tissue volume distal to cm MM)

Q. : Volume flow measured with AFM-100 at cm MM

S.V. : Segmental Volume (volume of the segment based on circumferential data)

FIG 6–7.
Perfusion analysis *(PA)* demonstrating normal right side and abnormal left side secondary to superficial femoral artery occlusion.

LIMB PERFUSION NOMOGRAM FOR THE LEG

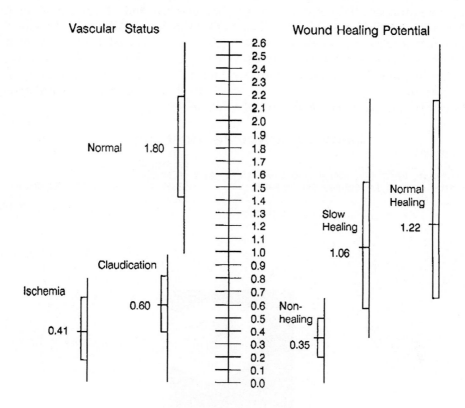

Perfusion Ranges and Means (+/- 1 Standard Deviation) in the Leg
as Related to Vascular Status and Wound Healing

AFM-100 Measured Resting Blood Flows, ml/min/100cc of distal tissue

November 1991

FIG 6–8.
Nomogram for perfusion analysis *(PA)*.[10]

there is adequate arterial flow to allow healing. Often, even when significant arterial occlusive disease is present, perfusion is adequate to heal wounds. Of greatest importance, however, is identifying a patient with ischemia. C. Daniel Proctor et al. recently found that diabetic lesions with perfusions of less than 0.70 mL/min/100 cc of distal tissue did not heal. Thus, the Metriflow scanner reliably stratifies diabetic foot lesions into healing versus nonhealing categories. PA accurately assesses the functional significance of arterial occlusion.

In addition to cross-sectional arterial volume flow measurements, flow can be measured in individual arteries. Using flow sensitive voxels of varying sizes to scan the extremity, arteries are located and the flow in each artery is measured individually. This is then compared to the total blood flow in the extremity at that level, expressed as a percentage of the total arterial flow. This Individual Artery Performance (IAP) report demonstrates the position of each artery and the flow in each artery. Figure 6–9 demonstrates a normal superficial femoral artery. Figure 6–10 shows superficial femoral artery obstruction.

Individual Artery Performance™

```
PATIENT:                                    DATE    :
ID #   :                                    PHYSICIAN:
COMMENT: RIGHT SFA, NORMAL FEMALE VOLUNTEER, 24 Y  OPERATOR :
FILE   : [110,133]09ROORP.DAT   MAN-ANL     STUDY # :   0,  2 EPOCHS; CAL =   6.57
```

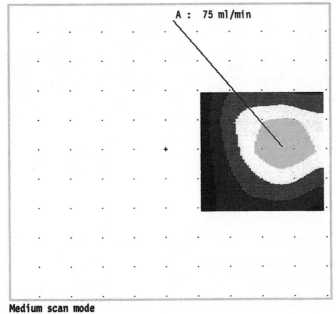

A : 75 ml/min

Medium scan mode

75 ml/min (77%) A 86,49

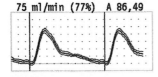

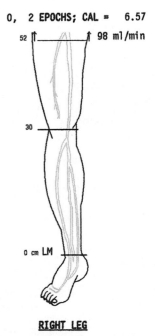

52 ⇧   ⇧ 98 ml/min

30

0 cm LM

RIGHT LEG
52 cm LM

WHOLE LIMB
98 ml/min   51 BPM

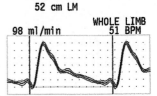

FIG 6–9.
Individual artery report *(IAP)*, normal right superficial femoral artery.

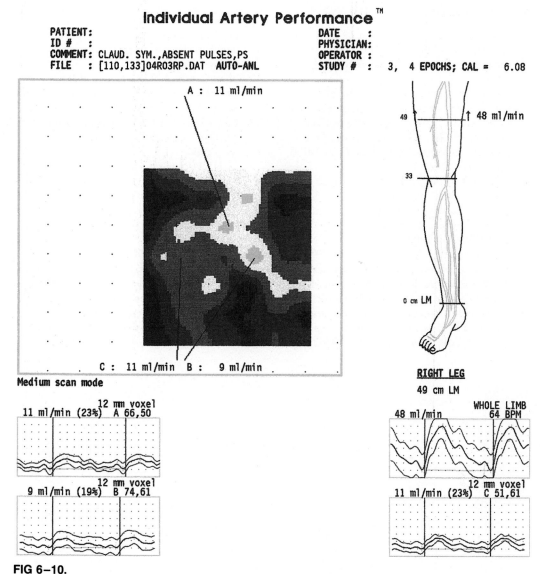

FIG 6–10.
Individual artery report *(IAP)*, with obstruction of the right superficial femoral artery.

The IAP is useful to follow the results of interventions such as bypass grafts and endovascular reconstructions. Restenosis of the artery or graft becomes apparent by progressive deterioration of flow volume. In addition, stenosis of the superficial femoral artery can be reliably determined.

In summary, magnetic resonance flow studies yield diagnostic information of great clinical use. Vascular assessment in diabetics is particularly useful because of the unreliability of cuff-pressure measurement in this group. Prediction of wound healing, determination of the functional significance of arterial occlusions, follow-up of arterial reconstructions, and screening of patients with claudication-like symptoms are all excellent uses of this technology.

REFERENCES

1. Hobbs JT et al: A limitation of the Doppler ultrasound method of measuring ankle systolic pressure, *Vasa* 3:160-162, 1974.
2. Towne JB: Complications of the diabetic foot. In *Complications of vascular surgery*, Philadelphia, 1985, Grune & Stratton.
3. Sondgeroth TR et al: Variability of toe pressure measurements, *BRUITVI*:14-16, September 1982.
4. Backrach JM et al: Predictive value of transcutaneous oxygen pressure and amputation success by use of supine and elevated measurements, *J Vasc Surg* 15(3):558-563, 1992.
5. Karanfilian RG, Lynch TG, Zirul VT: The value of laser Doppler velocimetry and transcutaneous oxygen tension determination in predicting healing of ischemic forefoot ulcerations and amputations in diabetic and nondiabetic patients, *J Vasc Surg* 4:511-517, 1986.
6. Raines JK et al: Vascular laboratory criteria for the management of peripheral vascular disease of the lower extremities, *Surgery* 79:21-29, 1976.
7. Moneta GL et al: Accuracy of lower extremity arterial duplex scanning, *J Vasc Surg* 15(2):275-284, 1992.
8. Battocletti J: Blood flow measurement by NMR, *Crit Rev Biomed Eng* 13(4):311-367, 1986.
9. Rice KL, Naslund TC, Procter CD: Magnetic resonance flowmetry for evaluation of peripheral arteries in diabetic patients. Proceedings of the sixth San Diego Symposium on Vascular Diagnosis, January 1992.
10. Procter CD et al: Comparison of ankle-brachial indices and magnetic resonance flowmetry in prediction outcome in diabetic patients. Proceedings of the sixteenth annual meeting of the Southern Association for Vascular Surgery, January 1992.

7 _____ Diabetic Peripheral Neuropathy

Yadollah Harati, M.D.

A feature of diabetes mellitus is its propensity to cause certain complications, including vascular disease, nephropathy, retinopathy, and peripheral neuropathies. In addition to hyperglycemia and insulin deficiency, multiple other metabolic, genetic, and environmental factors play a role in the development of these syndromes. Because of the diversity of these causative and contributing factors, no single satisfactory pathogenetic explanation or therapy for any of these complications has been forthcoming. To understand the pathogenesis of diabetic neuropathy, one must not only know why many diabetics develop this complication but also understand why many others do not, even after many years of disease. A full understanding of the pathogenesis and treatment of diabetic complications may well await the discovery of the exact cause of diabetes itself.

In this chapter, I will address the present understanding of diabetic peripheral neuropathies and their relation to foot complications of diabetes mellitus.

DEFINITION

Although the definitions of cranial neuropathies, limb mononeuropathies, multiple mononeuropathies, and thoracoabdominal neuropathies are relatively straightforward, there is a general lack of agreement among neurologists and diabetologists regarding a standard definition for *diabetic polyneuropathy*. It is this form of neuropathy that often contributes to the foot complications of diabetes. To some physicians, minor paresthesias in the feet constitute neuropathy; to others, more rigid criteria must be met to establish such a diagnosis. Some physicians may diagnose neuropathy only when clinical symptoms or signs appear, whereas others consider it to be present when slowed motor and sensory nerve conduction, elevated sensory perception threshold, or abnormal autonomic function tests are documented, even in the absence of symptoms. Subclinical electrophysiologic changes will ultimately lead to the development of symptoms in a significant number of patients reexamined years later.

The character of symptoms and signs of diabetic peripheral neuropathy depends on a number of factors, including:

1. Type of nerve affected (motor, sensory, autonomic, or mixed).
2. Class and level of axons affected (large vs. small, proximal vs. distal).
3. Specific pathologic process (axonal degeneration, segmental demyelination, or both).
4. Course and severity of pathologic process.
5. Degree of nerve regeneration.
6. Ectoptic impulse regeneration.
7. Age at onset.
8. Other complications (e.g., arthropathy, angiopathy).

Varying combinations of these factors lead to varying patterns of symptoms. Nerve dysfunction may give rise to positive symptoms, negative symptoms, or both. Positive symptoms include pain, cramping, spasm, neuromyotonia, and sensations of prickling, tightness or crawling in the distribution of affected nerves. Negative symptoms include weakness, fatigability, hypesthesia or anesthesia, and unsteadiness in gait. Positive or negative autonomic symptoms (e.g., hypohidrosis or orthostatic hypotension) may also be present. Positive sensory symptoms tend to be worse at night. By far the most frequent form of diabetic peripheral nerve disorder is a length-dependent sensory polyneuropathy of insidious onset. Involvement of distal upper limbs usually evolves when the leg symptoms have extended to the upper third of the foreleg. Some patients with untreated diabetes without neuropathy after an episode of ketotic coma complain of positive symptoms in the feet that rapidly subside after glycemic control. Whether these transient symptoms herald the future development of a progressive neuropathy is not known.

In summary, the presently accepted definition of diabetic neuropathy is that of a demonstrable (clinical or subclinical) disorder of somatic or autonomic parts of the peripheral nervous system ocurring in the setting of diabetes mellitus. Because diabetes is a common disorder and may coincide with other conditions causing peripheral neuropathy, the mere association of neuropathic symptoms with diabetes mellitus is not sufficient for a diagnosis of diabetic neuropathy, and other causes of peripheral neuropathy must be excluded.

EPIDEMIOLOGY

Elucidating the epidemiology of diabetic neuropathy has been hampered by the lack of a standard definition for diabetic polyneuropathy, intraobserver and interobserver differences in eliciting symptoms and signs, and the lack of reliable, sensitive, reproducible tests. Although methods of assessing peripheral nerve function are improving, no one test is indicative of nerve disease, and there are still wide variations in the coefficient of variation of many estimations. Based on these considerations, The San Antonio Conference of Diabetic Neuropathy[2] recommend obtaining at least one measure from each of the following categories to better define and classify diabetic neuropathy: clinical symptoms, clinical examination, electrodiagnostic studies, quantitative sensory testing, and autonomic function testing. Unfortunately, methodologies vary between different laboratories and investigators and comparison of data is usually not possible. Standardization of these methods, however, is feasible and must be encouraged. When the neurologic examination is standardized and quantified, there is substantial correlation with the observed nerve pathology.[3]

There is virtually no reliable information on prevalence, incidence, severity, morbidity, mortality, natural history, or public health costs of diabetic neuropathy. Estimates for clinical and subclinical neuropathy have varied between 5% and nearly 60% and even 100% if patients with asymptomatic abnormalities of nerve conduction are included. This tremendous variability is due to the use of different tests, neuropathic end-point evaluations, and patient cohorts, and the lack of standard criteria for the diagnosis of neuropathy. The most frequently cited reference on the prevalence of diabetic neuropathy is that of Pirart,[4] who prospectively studied 4,400 patients (primarily elderly non-insulin-dependent diabetics) between 1947 and 1973, 7.5% of whom had clinical neuropathy at the time of diagnosis of diabetes mellitus. This rate increased linearly to 50% after 25 years. Another study by Mincu[5] shows an overall prevalence of neuropathy of 11.6% in newly diagnosed diabetics, 19% in those with symptoms for 15 months before diagnosis, and only 4% in those with symptoms for less than 5 months before diagnosis. The Rochester Diabetic Neuropathy Study, a population-based study of neuropathy in noninsulin-dependent diabetes mellitus (NIDDM), yielded a cumulative incidence of distal symmetric polyneuropathy of 4% after 5 years and 15% after 20 years of diabetes, with a median time of 9 years to development of neuropathy after diagnosis.[6] This ongoing study includes approximately 38% of all Rochester Minnesota diabetics and provides a reasonable cohort on which conclusions about the cause and natural history of diabetic neuropathy may be based.[7] In this prospective study, patients are evaluated at periodic preset-dates, tests, and risk factors are predetermined, and comprehensive criteria for abnormality are well defined. Population-based studies are valuable because they provide represenative information about a given population that may then be compared with and extrapolated to a more general population.

A recent surveillance program of 1,150 diabetics compared with 480 age- and sex-matched nondiabetics reveal a prevalence rate of 7.4% of past or present foot ulcerations among diabetics but only 2.5% in controls. Of the ulcers found on examination, 39.4% were mixed, suggesting the important role of neuropathy in their pathogenesis. The predictors of the presence of ulcers were duration of diabetes, absent light touch, impaired pain perception, absent dorsalis pedis pulse, and the presence of retinopathy.[8]

Information on the prevalence of diabetic autonomic neuropathy is minimal. Four percent of patients with insulin-dependent diabetes mellitus (IDDM) studied by Canal et al.[9] had autonomic symptoms within the first year, rising to 28% after 5 years. Fernandez-Castaner et al.[10] found that 53% of an unselected series of dia-

betics had symptoms suggestive of autonomic dysfunction. Nearly all diabetics with autonomic neuropathy have an associated somatic neuropathy[11] that precedes abnormalities of autonomic function.[12]

Early studies[13, 14] and the general experience of pediatricians suggest that neuropathy occurs infrequently in children with diabetes. Among diabetic teenagers, symptoms of autonomic neuropathy are very rare.[15] More systematic and prospective studies of diabetic children, using quantitative electrophysiologic, sensory threshold studies, and autonomic tests, are required to better understand the epidemiology of neuropathy in children.

Despite the fundamental difference in the pathogenesis of IDDM and NIDDM, the prevalence of diabetic neuropathy is similar.[41] Diabetic neuropathy also occurs in secondary forms of diabetes (e.g., pancreatectomy, nonalcoholic pancreatitis, and hemochromatosis).[16] There are no large series of patients with secondary diabetic neuropathies, and no epidemiologic conclusions can be derived from available reports.

Notwithstanding the discrepancies previously discussed, the following conclusions regarding diabetic neuropathy are generally accepted: it is an extremely common medical problem because of the high incidence of diabetes; manifestations are usually not revealed at the time of diagnosis of diabetes and may take years to develop; prevalence increases with the duration of diabetes; it occurs in IDDM, NIDDM, and secondary forms of diabetes, ultimately affecting up to 50% of patients with long-standing diabetes; and it is usually associated with other complications such as retinopathy and nephropathy.[7]

PATHOGENESIS

The exact pathogenesis of diabetic neuropathy has remained elusive to investigators. Many hypotheses supported by experimental and clinical studies have been proposed (see Table 7–3), but none has gained general acceptance. Research in the pathogenesis of diabetic neuropathy has been complicated by the clinical heterogeneity of neuropathy, its occurrence in IDDM and NIDDM with different causes, and lack of a single animal model to sufficiently reproduce the human disease. Most of the hypotheses and debates surrounding the cause of diabetic neuropathy have focused on metabolic and vascular factors and their interaction. There are several lines of experimental and clincial evidence to suggest the pivotal role of long-term hyperglycemia in the pathogenesis of diabetic neuropathy. Experimentally, hyperglycemia results in changes in polyols, myo-inositols, sodium-potassium-ATPase, and nonenzymatic glycosylation; reduction of axonal transport, diameter and nerve conduction, and axoglial dysjunction, microangiopathy, endoneurial hypoxia, and demyelination.[34] The earliest effects of hyperglycemia are generally metabolic; electrophysiologic and morphologic changes are considered to be late occurrences. The early metabolic effect is thought to result from direct exposure of nerve structures to glucose, where, unlike other tissues, its uptake and transfer do not require insulin.

The most popular metabolic hypothesis involves myo-inositol depletion, a consequence of increased polyol pathway flux. Myo-inositol depletion results in reduced synthesis and turnover of phosphoinositides, required for the production of diacylglycerol, a second messenger for stimulation of sodium-potassium-ATPase activity.[35] Reduced sodium-potassium-ATPase activity may then cause a series of abnormalities, to include reduced nerve conduction velocity, paranodal swelling, axoglial dysjunction, and subsequent axonal degeneration or demyelination.[34]

Despite strong evidence in favor of increased polyol pathway activity and de-

creased nerve myo-inositol in diabetic peripheral nerves, long-term trials with dietary myo-inositol supplementation have failed to show improvement in nerve function in human beings,[36] and the therapeutic effect of several aldose reductase inhibitors has been modest. This and other recent experimental evidence[37, 38] cast doubt on the role of myo-inositol in the pathogenesis of diabetic neuropathy. It is possible, however, that increased polyol activity and sorbitol accumulation exert their pathogenic role in some way not yet fully understood. One possibility is that the increased water content of nerve and edema lead to ischemia and nerve damage. Griffey et al.,[39] using magnetic resonance spectroscopy, showed increased sural nerve water content in more than half of patients with symptomatic diabetic neuropathy but not in those being treated with aldose reductase inhibitors. This finding may provide a link between metabolic and vascular theories for the pathogenesis of diabetic neuropathy.

Many studies suggest vascular abnormalities in diabetic peripheral nerves. Evidence for endoneurial microvascular abnormalities in human diabetic nerves includes basement membrane thickening and duplication, endothelial cell swelling and proliferation, occlusive platelet thrombi,[40–42] multifocal-ischemic proximal nerve lesions[42, 43] and increased numbers of closed capillaries in the sural nerve.[44] These abnormalities are thought to cause multifocal nerve ischemia-hypoxia, resulting in polyneuropathy. The initiating factor for microvascular pathology may be the formation of advanced glycosylated end products (AGEs) resulting from hyperglycemia and their effect on the rigidity of plasma membranes.[45] This, along with increased blood viscosity and decreased erythrocyte deformability observed in the peripheral capillaries of diabetics, is conductive to the formation of free radicals.[46] The free radicals may damage endothelial cells, disrupt blood-nerve barriers, and inhibit prostacyclin activity. Reduced prostacyclin activity results in an imbalance in the epidemiology of neuropathy in children.

CLASSIFICATION OF DIABETIC NEUROPATHIES

A rigid classification of diabetic neuropathies is difficult to establish because mixed syndromes are frequently seen. The most accepted and practical classification is one that divides the neuropathies into symmetric polyneuropathies and focal and multifocal neuropathies.[17] Each category is then divided into several subtypes (Table 7–1).

The issue of selective nerve fiber damage (small-fiber vs. large-fiber) in diabetic polyneuropathy is still unsettled, and classification into small-fiber or large-fiber neuropathy is presently not justified.[18] Small myelinated nerve fibers with slower conduction convey pain and temperature sensation, whereas the fast-conducting and larger myelinated fibers carry vibratory and position sense and unmyelinated nerves fiber the autonomic impulses. A varying degree of small-fiber involvement is seen in all diabetic polyneuropathies and can be determined by detailed autonomic and sensory threshold testing in some patients.[19] Whether there is a pure

TABLE 7–1.

Classification of Diabetic Neuropathies*

Symmetric polyneuropathies
    Sensory or sensorimotor polyneuropathy
    Symmetry proximal lower limb motor neuropathy
    Acute or subacute distal motor neuropathy
    Autonomic neuropathy
Focal and multifocal neuropathies
    Cranial neuropathy
    Trunk and limb mononeuropathy
    Asymmetric lower limb motor neuropathy
Mixed forms

*From Thomas PK: *JR Coll Physicians Lond* 7:154, 1973. Used by permission.

diabetic autonomic neuropathy remains controversial. In nearly all patients with diabetic autonomic neuropathy, some degree of involvement of the somatic afferent nerve fibers is usually detected with careful testing. Autonomic neuropathy remains a major complication of diabetes, often causing impotence, gastric stasis, diarrhea, postural hypotension, impaired counterregulatory responses to hypoglycemia, and possibly sudden death by cardiac arrest.[20, 21] The salient manifestations of diabetic autonomic neuropathy are listed in Table 7–2. Of these, the sudomotor and vasomotor abnormalities are of particular importance in the development of diabetic foot complications. Disturbances of skin microcirculatory blood flow regulation, paradoxical vasoconstriction in response to skin heating, increased arteriovenous shunting, neuropathic edema, hypohidrosis, and hyperthyrosis-resulting from peripheral autonomic denervation are major contributing factors to the development of foot ulcerations. In fact, when tests for peripheral autonomic denervation such as the acetylcholine sweat spot test are performed, it is universally abnormal in patients with diabetic neuropathic foot ulceration.[22]

In painless foot ulceration there is universal severe dysfunction of all nerve populations, determined by nerve conduction studies, vibration, cooling and warming thresholds, heart rate–dependent cardiac autonomic reflexes (parasympathetic system), orthostatic blood pressure determination, and plasma norepinephrine level (sympathetic system). By contrast, in painful neuropathy the small nerve fibers are uniformly abnormal, whereas other modalities may be normal or only minimally affected. The cause of pain, however, is not known. Involvement of both small and large fibers, axonal atrophy, ectopic nerve impulse generation at the dorsal root ganglion, or precipitation of nociceptive impulse generation by blood glucose are among several widely quoted

TABLE 7–2.

Manifestations of Diabetic Autonomic Neuropathies*

Cardiovascular
  Postural hypotension
  Resting tachycardia
  Painless myocardial infarction
  Sudden death (with or without association with
    general anesthesia)
Gastrointestinal
  Esophageal motor incoordination
  Gastric dysrhythmia, hypomotility (gastroparesis
    diabeticorum)
  Pylorospasm
  Uncoordinated intestinal motility ("diabetic diar-
    rhea," spasm)
  Intestinal hypomotility (constipation)
  Gallbladder hypocontraction (diabetic cholecystop-
    athy)
  Anorectal dysfunction (fecal incontinence)
Genitourinary
  Diabetic cystopathy (atonic bladder, postmicturi-
    tion dribbling)
  Male impotence
  Ejaculatory disorders
  Reduced vaginal lubrication, dyspareunia
Respiratory
  Impaired breathing control (?)
  Sleep apnea (?)
  Decreased bronchial response to methacholine or
    cold air
Thermoregulatory
  Sudomotor (diminished, excessive, or gustatory
    sweating)
  Vasomotor (vasoconstriction, vasodilatation, neu-
    ropathic edema)
Pupillary
  Miosis
  Disturbance of dilatation
  "Algyll-Robertson"-like pupils
Neuroendocrine
  Reduced pancreatic polypeptide release
  Reduced somatostatin release
  Reduced motilin and gastric inhibitory peptide re-
    lease
  Enhanced gastrin release
  Reduced norepinephrine release (orthostatic, ex-
    ercise, and hypoglycemic induced)
  Reduced parathyroid hormone secretion (hypocal-
    cemic induced)
  Elevated immunoreactive atrial natriuretic hormone
  Impaired glucose counterregulation (hypoglycemia
    unawareness) (?)

*From Harati Y, Low PA: Autonomic peripheral neuropathies:
Diagnosis and clinical presentation. In Appel SH, editor: *Cur-
rent neurology.* St Louis, 1990, Mosby–Year Book, p 105.
Used by permission.

hypotheses. Development of foot ulcers is related primarily to tissue damage of which the patient is unaware because of loss of pain and temperature sensation. The presence of neuropathy even in its earliest stage may itself disturb the posture of the foot and predispose it to local increases in pressure at the sites of high mechanical pressure, resulting in ulceration.

RISK FACTORS FOR DEVELOPMENT OF DIABETIC NEUROPATHIES

There is a clear relationship between the duration of diabetes and the development of diabetic neuropathy.[23] Males[23] and tall individuals[24] are at greater risk to develop neuropathy, and elderly diabetics, regardless of the duration of diabetes, tend to develop neuropathy more frequently.[23] It is possible that younger individuals have a relative resistance to the development of neuropathy, as has been demonstrated for retinopathy. Females with anorexia nervosa and diabetes[25] and patients with a recent episode of ketosis or after the establishment of tight glycemic control may have a precipitated acute painful neuropathy.[26] No familial tendency for the development of neuropathy has been suggested, and earlier claims that there may be a genetic predisposition for diabetic neuropathy were not confirmed by Boulton et al.[27] One recent study, however, suggested that there may be an underlying genetic predisposition for the development of autonomic neuropathy in the families of subjects with type I diabetes. This study demonstrated a greater incidence of serum complement–fixing antibodies against the adrenal medulla, sympathetic ganglia, and the vagus nerve, as well as subclinical autonomic dysfunction among the family members of patients with type I diabetes.[28] The prevalence of symptomatic peripheral neuropathy is significantly higher among diabetics who consume excessive alcohol.[29] Tobacco use may also predispose to earlier development and more severe symptoms of diabetic neuropathy, presumably by inducing vasoconstriction and nerve ischemia. One recent report suggests that diabetics with lower limb ischemia caused by peripheral vascular disease have a more severe neuropathy than diabetics without limb ischemia.[30] It is therefore prudent that patients with diabetic neuropathy and its foot complications abstain from alcohol and tobacco and that improvement of limb perfusion be attempted for those with vascular insufficiency.

Further elucidation of risk factors for the occurrence of diabetic neuropathies is clearly important for prevention and therapy.

ANIMAL MODELS

Diabetic animal models have been invaluable for exploring morphologic, functional, and metabolic abnormalities under strict experimental conditions.[31] Most animal studies using chemical agents cytotoxic to pancreatic beta cells have used the rat as the preferred species. Alloxan, a pyrimidine derivative with structural similarities to uric acid and glucose, is diabetogenic not only in rats but also in rabbits, dogs, cats, monkeys, and mice. Guinea pigs are completely insensitive to alloxan. Alloxan has been supplanted in modern times by streptozocin (STZ), an antibiotic. STZ has diabetogenic action thought to be similar to that of alloxan. STZ, however, is more specific for beta cells than is alloxan. Intravenous injection of STZ causes diabetes in rats, mice, guinea pigs, monkeys, and dogs but not rabbits. Despite the extensive use of these two agents to induce experimental diabetes, their mechanisms of action are

only partially understood. Both agents provide a relatively permanent diabetes, allowing for the study of long-term complications, such as neuropathy. Alloxan- or STZ-induced diabetes simulate IDDM in human beings with respect to pancreatic beta cell destruction. Diabetes induced by both agents results in biochemical, electrophysiologic, and morphologic nerve changes that may be improved by insulin treatment. The major problem encountered with animal models has been the unpredictability of the severity of chemically induced diabetes, thus hampering the reproducibility of results and comparison of data among investigators.

In 1974, a genetically susceptible rat (BB rat) with spontaneous diabetes was identified and has served as a model for human IDDM. The basis for the development of diabetes in both genetic and immunologic, resulting in an autoimmune-mediated destruction of the beta cells. The onset of diabetes is abrupt and severe, resulting in the death of many animals, not treated with insulin. The BB rats also develop a genetic thyrotoxicosis, complicating some aspects of diabetes. The primary pathologic changes in peripheral nerve of diabetic BB rats occur at the node of Ranvier, causing axoglial dysjunction.[32]

There is also a genetically diabetic mouse strain that is insulin resistant and generally reflects features of NIDDM. The pattern of hyperglycemia in this model is complex, covering the spectrum from an insulin-resistant state to an insulin-deficient state, making it difficult to compare data obtained at different stages of hyperglycemia among various studies. Some of the motor disabilities exhibited by these animals may be attributed to their gross obesity rather than to neuropathy. However, there are some nerve electrophysiologic and pathologic changes to suggest the development of neuropathy, although these changes do not always invariably correspond to those observed in other animal models or in humans.[33]

One species of Chinese hamster demonstrates a diabetic mutation in approximately 30% of animals. There is substantial variation in the onset and severity of diabetes among various sublines of the diabetic Chinese hamsters.[34] Slowed motor nerve conduction velocity has been demonstrated, but conflicting reports exist on the morphologic changes of the nerves. Pathologic changes observed in the autonomic nervous system, however, are more pronounced than in other species.[33]

Spontaneous diabetes also occurs in dogs. Although the long life span of dogs provides important possibilities for the study of the long-term complications of diabetes, there are no systematic studies of neuromuscular disorder in this model. There is, however, a significant reduction in motor and sensory nerve conduction velocity and a decrease in amplitude of evoked compound muscle action potential in dogs without clinical evidence of neuropathy.[33]

There is no one ideal animal model for diabetic neuropathy. The inherent between prostacyclin and thromboxane A,[47] thereby promoting vasoconstriction and platelet aggregation. Endoneurial ischemia induced by vasoconstriction and reinforced by hemorrheologic abnormalities, nonenzymatic glycosylation of capillary structures and the free radical cascade will ultimately result in microvascular pathology and nerve fiber loss as previously described.[48] Ischemia, when induced by a proximal arteriovenous shunt in rats, results in 50% to 75% reduction of endoneurial blood flow within the sciatic nerve associated with a 25% to 30% reduction in nerve conduction velocity. This reduced nerve conduction velocity was thought to be secondary to morphologically observed alterations in the node of Ranvier with increased nodal capacitance and slowing of saltatory conduction.[49] The presence of endoneurial hyp-

oxia by direct in vivo measurement has been demonstrated in the sural nerve of diabetic patients.[50] Moreover, unlike in normal individuals, nerve conduction velocity fails to increase after exercise in patients with diabetic neuropathy, suggesting poor blood flow.[51] Diabetics with lower-limb vascular insufficiency develop a more severe neuropathy.[30] Another study evaluating the occurrence of neuropathy in patients with chronic obstructive airway disease shows a mild neuropathy in more than 40% of patients, some showing pathologic changes in sural nerve biopsy specimens.[52] This study lends additional support to the concept that hypoxia plays a role in the pathogenesis of neuropathy.

The role of nonenzymatic glycosylation of proteins in the development of diabetic complications has received substantial attention in recent years. Glycosylation of proteins occur by the attachment of glucose to amino groups. In addition to their effect on the capillary basement membranes, AGEs also affect other proteins such as skin collagen, extracellular matrix components, and peripheral[53] and central nervous system proteins.[54, 55] The most affected proteins of nerve structures are the tubulins of microtubules, essential structures for axonal transport. This may, in part, explain previous reports of the defective, slow axonal transport of diabetic nerves.[56] Vitamin C, by a competitive mechanism, may inhibit glycosylation of short-lived proteins in nondiabetic subjects.[57] Further studies in diabetic patients are required before vitamin C is used therapeutically to delay or prevent the chronic complications of diabetes. Also, aminoguanidine-HCl, a nucleophilic hydraxine, has been shown to inhibit the accumulation of AGEs on peripheral nerve and to ameliorate the functional and structural impairments of peripheral nerves of rats with streptozotocin-induced diabetes.[58] Similar effects have been observed in rats' kidneys[59] and retinas.[60–62] Aminoguanidine may also reverse nerve ischemia and more gradually improve nerve electrophysiology by an action on nerve microvessels.[63] The exact mechanism by which aminoguanidine inhibits the formation of AGEs has not been determined.[64] Daily long-term administration of another nucleophilic compound, diaminoguanidine, to normoglycemic and alloxan-induced diabetic rats not only inhibits AGE production in eye lenses but also inhibits aldose reductase activity and sorbitol accumulation.[65] This suggests a link between abnormal glycation and the polyol pathway or, alternatively, an independent effect of this compound on these two systems.

In addition to metabolic and vascular abnormalities, other explanations for diabetic neuropathy have been proposed (Table 7–3). One such theory implicates the reduction of endogenous concentrations of nerve growth factors (NGF),[66, 67] which shares several molecular, structural, and physiologic properties with insulin. NGF levels are decreased in patients with diabetic neuropathy, and such levels correlate with the severity of the neuropathy.[66, 68] Insulin itself also acts as a trophic factor, and NGF-responsive cells respond in a similar way to high concentrations of insulin[69]; therefore, it is plausible that the combined deficiency of NGF and insulin is deleterious to nerve cells.

TABLE 7–3.

Abnormalities Implicated in the Pathogenesis of Diabetic Peripheral Neuropathy

Abnormalities suggestive of a vascular etiology
    Basement membrane thickening
    Endothelial cell swelling and proliferation
    Occlusive platelet thrombi
    "Closed" capillaries
    Multifocal "ischemic" proximal nerve lesions
    Epineurial vessel atherosclerosis
    Decreased erythrocyte deformability
    Nerve hypoxia
Abnormalities suggestive of a metabolic etiology
    Accumulation of sorbitol
    Reduction in the rate of synthesis and transport of intra-axonal proteins
    Reduction in nerve sodium-potassium-ATPase
    Alterations in protein kinase C
    Reduced amino acid incorporation into dorsal root ganglion
    Reduced incorporation into myelin of glycolipids and amino acids
    Abnormal inositol lipid metabolism
    Excessive glycogen accumulation
    Increased nonenzymatic peripheral nerve protein glycosylation
    Nerve hypoxia
Other abnormalities
    Increased nerve edema
    Increased blood-nerve permeability
    Reduced endogenous NGF
    Insulin deficiency

PATHOLOGY OF HUMAN DIABETIC NEUROPATHY

There is substantial evidence that distally accentuated axonal loss of myelinated and unmyelinated nerve fibers is the salient pathologic change in diabetic polyneuropathy. The loss appears to be multifocal and is present in both elderly and young patients.[70, 71] The diffuse distal fiber loss is thought to result from more proximal ischemic multifocal lesions, presumably caused by vascular abnormalities.[40] Although segmental and paranodal demyelination can occur (Fig 7–1), it is seldom a striking feature of distal nerve pathology in more advanced diabetes. It is not clear if the demyelination is of the primary[72] or secondary type.[18] As suggested by Vlassara et al.,[73] demyelination may result from the removal of glycosylated myelin protein recognized by macrophages. Because of the preponderance of axonal degeneration, inclusion of diabetic neuropathy in the differential diagnosis of demyelinating neuropathies is not justified. Axonal regeneration (multiple regeneration clusters or axonal sprouts) is prominent in nerve biopsy specimen of patients with chronic sensory motor neuropathy.[18] Patients with painful neuropathy and an associated severe autonomic neuropathy have more profound

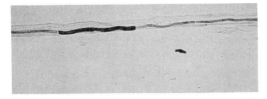

FIG 7–1.
A single teased nerve fiber showing three demyelinated segments and one intact myelinated segment.

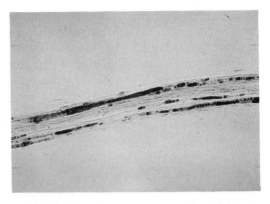

FIG 7–2.
Teased nerve fiber preparation showing several nerve fibers undergoing axonal degeneration and breakdown of myelin into ovoids and balls.

sural nerve fiber loss than do patients with painful neuropathy alone.[18] As discussed earlier, the nerve fiber loss involves both small- and large-diameter fibers; therefore, selective vulnerability based on fiber diameter does not appear likely.[18, 70] In cases of acute painful diabetic neuropathy, extensive active fiber breakdown is evident in teased nerve fiber preparations (Fig 7–2). The presence of spontaneous pain is, in general, related to small nerve fiber damage. Whether ectopic impulses arising from regenerating small myelinated and unmyelinated fibers also play a role in pain generation remains controversial.[18, 47, 75]

TREATMENT

There is presently no effective treatment for diabetic peripheral neuropathy. The following therapeutic approaches, however, have been more frequently studied in the recent years.

Glycemic Control

Although an unequivocal answer to the question regarding the role of glycemic control in the cause of diabetic neuropathies and other complications cannot be provided, the attainment and maintenance of normal blood glucose and lipids, in conjunction with ideal body weight, remains the cornerstone of treatment of diabetes. Based on imperfect, retrospective studies,[4, 76] a relationship between the duration of diabetes and the development of

neuropathies before treatment, and the improved motor nerve conduction and resistance to ischemic conduction block after therapy is now fairly well established.[36, 77–82] The improvement may not be evident until after 6 months of treatment, however.[82] Therefore, the absence of improved nerve conduction after short periods of treatment appears irrelevant. As shown by Service et al., measurement of neurologic function and nerve conduction after continuous subcutaneous insulin infusion compared with conventional insulin treatment shows no apparent difference at 4 months but significant differences in nerve conduction velocity and vibratory thresholds at 8 months, favoring the former therapeutic regimen.[83] There remain several questions in respect to the effect of glycemic control on peripheral neuropathy: Are the reported improvements a reflection of structural nerve recovery or simply a result of alteration in axon caliber related to fluid and electrolyte shifts after control of plasma and tissue osmolality? Can an improvement in electrophysiologic measures be translated into a noticeable clinical response? Do all aspects of neuropathies, both somatic and autonomic, respond to the same degree of glycemic control? Is improvement in the painful diabetic neuropathies after institution of glycemic control related to reduced levels of glucose as a pain-producing substance or to structural changes of nerve? Multicenter studies are currently underway to determine precisely the degree of glycemic control required to reduce late complications. The ongoing large-scale Diabetes Control and Complication Trial is designed to look at the differences between conventional and excellent control during the course of diabetes. In very tightly controlled diabetes, however, there is a risk for repeated iatrogenic hypoglycemic reactions that may aggravate the underlying neuropathy.

Pancreas transplantation in diabetic patients may have the potential to halt or reverse the complication of diabetes by reinstitution of normal glycemic state. A recent study by Kennedy et al.[84] described a trend toward improved motor and sensory function and stable autonomic function 42 months after pancreas transplantation. Other long-term studies from Europe have also reported a slight improvement or stabilization of different aspects of neuropathy after pancreas transplantation. The major problem in assessing the effect of pancreas transplant on diabetic neuropathy is the more advanced nature of neuropathy among these patients, the presence of renal failure, frequent hypoglycemic reactions, and severe orthostatic hypotension, all of which adversely affect the course and prognosis of neuropathy.

Aldose Reductase Inhibitors

As discussed in the previous sections, accumulation of sorbitol in tissues is dependent on the enzymatic reduction of glucose to sorbitol by aldose reductase. Although the physiologic role of aldose reductase in nerves, if any, remains unknown, inhibition of this enzyme by aldose reductase inhibitors results in reduced levels of tissue sorbitol. Despite their effect on nerve function and structure in both animal and

human diabetes, clinical trials using a variety of aldose reductase inhibitors with different potencies, half-lifes and side effects have generally failed to produce clear-cut evidence of efficacy. Many of these trials have been hindered by insufficient knowledge of the natural history of diabetic neuropathy, small or heterogeneous patient populations, unreliable end points, and ineffective drug dosage.

The first orally absorbed aldose reductase inhibitor, alrestatin, resulted in conflicting claims as to its efficacy and proved to have substantial hepatotoxicity.[85] In a Japanese trial, ONO-2235 (epalrestat) given for 1 month produced small subjective improvement in pain.[86] Sorbinil, when administered for less than 6 months, resulted in mild improvement in symptoms of pain and paresthesia and an improvement in nerve conduction velocity of less than 2 m/sec.[87] The relevance of such a modest improvement in nerve conduction velocity to clinical symptoms has been questioned. Based on cross-sectional epidemiologic data, a minimum improvement of 2.9 m/sec for ulnar motor nerve and 2.2 m/sec for peroneal nerve is needed to be considered clinically meaningful. The corresponding changes of amplitude are 1.2 and 0.7 mV, respectively.[88] The results of other trials with sorbinil have been relatively uniform in their findings. Many of these small studies varied in their patient selection and efficacy end points. A more recent multicenter study involving 202 patients but of short duration showed statistically significant improvement in maximum and overall pain.[89] Another multicenter study of 12 months' duration also showed modest improvement in several symptoms of neuropathy.[90] When the same sural nerve of a subgroup of patients who received sorbinil for 12 months had to have a second biopsy performed on it at a more proximal level, a 25% increase in nerve fiber density, a fourfold increase in nerve fiber regeneration, and a decrease in abnormality index was seen. This correlated with improvement in the amplitude of sural nerve sensory action potentials.[33] Unfortunately, in 10% of patients receiving sorbinil, severe hypersensitivity reactions developed, which resulted in discontinuation of all human trials. This side effect was thought to be caused by the hydantoin structure of sorbinil. Tolrestat, a nonhydantoin drug with minimal side effects, administered to 550 patients in a U.S. multicenter, dose-ranging, randomized, double-blind, placebo-controlled trial of 12 months' duration produced a small increase in motor nerve conduction velocity but not of median or sural nerve sensory conduction.[91] This effect was observed only with the highest dose of 200 mg/day. Withdrawal of therapy from some of the patients treated for 4 years resulted in electrophysiologic and morphologic deterioration of nerve.[92] Encouraged by these modest results, a multicenter, double-blind, placebo-controlled trial of tolrestat involving 300 patients is currently under way in the United States and Canada. This study will assess clinical, electrophysiologic, and sural nerve biopsy parameters over an 18-month period. A recent placebo-controlled 24-week study of 44 patients in England showed no clinical or electrophysiologic benefit from ponalrestat, another aldose reductase inhibitor.[93]

The two major problems encountered in previous multicenter studies were poor standardization for both symptom assessment (pain and paresthesias) and electrophysiologic testing. Because of the differences in training and experience of electromyographs and the lack of standardization of techniques and equipment, the results were subject to considerable variability. The modest improvement in conduction velocities seen in all aldose reductase inhibitor trials, however, may also be partially explained by the predominant involvement of slower-conducting (small myelinated) fibers, at least in some

patients. In contrast to the large-diameter fibers, the smaller myelinated fibers' participation in compound nerve conduction velocity is minimal. Therefore, their improved function clinically is not expected to result in electrophysiologic improvement as reflected by compound nerve conduction velocity. None of the aldose reductase inhibitors is currently approved for clinical use in the United States.

Gangliosides

Because of the recent publication regarding the recovery of motor function after spinal cord injury after GM-I ganglioside therapy,[94] there has been a resurgence of interest in exogenous gangliosides in treating diabetic neuropathy. Gangliosides are complex sialoglycolipids particularly concentrated in nerve cell membranes of nerve terminals and nerve growth cones.[95–99] There is increasing evidence that systemic administration of gangliosides results in some degree of recovery after nerve injury. This effect may be attributed to one or several of the following mechanisms: stimulation of sprouting mechanisms,[100–102] incorporation of ganglioside at the neuronal membrane level,[100] activation of certain enzyme activity (including sodium-potassium-ATPase),[98, 102] or promotion of the production of NGF by Schwann cells.[103] (For a comprehensive review of gangliosides see Rodden et al.[104] and Samson[105].)

Several European[41] and two U.S. studies[106, 107] of the effect on diabetic neuropathy of a mixed ganglioside preparation (cronassial), containing 21% GM-I, report modest improvement. Crepaldi's study involved 140 patients in a double-blind, cross-over trial using 20 mg/day of cronassial for 6 weeks. Although there were some statistically significant improvements in electrophysiologic variables and symptoms, functional changes were minimum.[41] The two double-blind, placebo-controlled trials in the United

States involved 28 and 37 patients, respectively, and used 40 mg intramuscularly daily of cronassial and found no improvement in quantitative features, including electrophysiology. The study with the smaller number of patients, however, showed a statistically significant improvement in lower-limb sensation. The paucity of well-designed studies using a large number of patients and standardized, sensitive, quantitative sensory and electrophysiologic techniques has recently prompted the initiation of a large-scale, multicenter, placebo-controlled study in the United States using a pure form of GM-I. Despite recent concern about the development of Guillain-Barré syndrome in a few patients after injection of cronassial,[108] epidemiologic studies have shown no causal relationship.[109] Other side effects of gangliosides include mild transient pain at the injection site, psychomotor agitation, vertigo, and dryness of the mouth.[104]

Pain Management

Approximately 10% of diabetics have pain associated with diabetic neuropathy.[6] The mechanisms of this neuropathic pain are multiple and complex. Management of pain is often difficult and disappointing. It is important to inform the patient who has severe pain that a spontaneous resolution of pain may occur, but it may take several months. Such simple reassurance that the pain will not be permanent is usually sufficient to obtain patients' cooperation in coping with the pain. Simple analgesics may be tried for milder cases but are usually of little value when pain is severe. Some patients gain substantial relief by soaking their feet in ice-cold water. However, frequent and prolonged soaking should be discouraged because extreme cold itself may aggravate the neuropathy. A double-blind trial of the tricyclic antidepressant,[110] amitriptyline has clearly demonstrated significant benefits in re-

ducing burning, aching, sharp, throbbing, and stinging pain. This dose-dependent effect is independent of mood elevation.[110] The use of amitriptyline in patients with heart block, urinary tract obstruction, orthostatic hypotension, or narrow angle glaucoma is contraindicated. The drug should be started at a low dose (10–20 mg every night) and increased gradually (once or twice weekly) until pain control is achieved or limiting side effect occur. Achievement of pain relief may require as high as 150 mg of the drug per day for 3 to 6 weeks. Patients who show slight or no relief of pain may have low serum levels of amitriptyline requiring an increase in dosage. Withdrawal from amitriptyline, however, must be gradual to prevent rebound insomnia. The use of amitriptyline in patients with autonomic neuropathy is complicated because many of its side effects tend to be more severe in these patients. These include orthostatic hypotension, urinary retention, bowel hypomotility, and dryness of the mouth. In such cases, if the patient appears to have responded to amitriptyline, a trial of nortriptyline, which is a major metabolite of amitriptyline with a lesser propensity to cause orthostatic hypotension, may be worthwhile. The combined use of fluphenazine and amitriptyline is not recommended because of an excessive sedating effect and the possibility of tardive dyskinesia. In a 12-week controlled cross-over study, Max et al.[111] show that desipramine, an antidepressant with selective noradrenergic action at a mean dose of 201 mg/day, caused significant relief of pain after 5 weeks of treatment. Although pain relief was greater in depressed patients, reduction in pain was also seen in patients who were not depressed. Despriamine's anticholinergic and sedative side effects are less than those of amitriptyline, but this drug may also cause severe orthostatic hypotension and heart block.

If treatment with amitriptyline is not

successful, anticonvulsants may be used. Phenytoins commonly used in the treatment of painful neuropathy[112] are shown in a double-blind cross-over study to be of no significant value.[113] My experience also suggests that response to phenytoin is rarely satisfactory. In addition, because of phenytoin's inhibitory effect on insulin secretion, its use is best avoided in diabetics, especially in those with unstable disease. In three controlled, double-blind studies,[114-116] carbamazepine was shown to be of value in painful diabetic neuropathy, but because of potential toxicity of the drug, its use should be limited to those who failed tricyclic antidepressant therapy. The usual effective dose of carbamazepine is 400 to 1,200 mg/day in divided doses, with an initial dose of 100 mg twice daily. Clonazepam has been reported to be more effective than carbamazepine and phenytoins for lancinating pains[117] and may be tried in patients experiencing brief, shooting pains.

Baclofen, a γ-aminobutyric analog, may be used for pain that is aggravated by spasm. There has been no systematic, controlled study of its use in painful diabetic neuropathy. Clonidin, an α_2-adrenergic agonist, relieved nocturnal neuropathic leg pain and cramping in three patients immediately after its use.[118] This is in agreement with the reported benefit of this drug in postherpeutic neuralgia.[119] The mechanism of action of clonidin may involve inhibition of the firing of dorsal horn nociceptors[120] or generalized inhibition of efferent sympathetic activity.

The anesthetic agent lidocaine used intravenously at a dose of 5 mg/kg over 30 minutes results in the relief of pain associated with diabetic neuropathy and lasted up to 2 weeks after the infusion in some patients.[121] Lidocaine is not available in an oral form, but mexiletine is shown, in a controlled study, to relieve both lancinating and chronic dysesthetic pains in 16 diabetics.[122] The effective dose is 10 mg/kg daily. The dosage should be gradually increased over the first week to minimize gastrointestinal upset and dizziness, the two most prominent side effects of mexiletine. Patients with suspected or proved cardiac arrhythmias may have worsening of their arrhythmia with this drug. My experience with lidocaine for painful diabetic neuropathy has not been as satisfactory as that reported here.

Topical use of capsaicin-containing creams in the treatment of painful diabetic neuropathy has received considerable attention in the past 2 years. Capsaicin is contained in a variety of capsicum hot pepper species, and its topical application has been reported to relieve diabetic dysesthetic pain and painful paresthesias by as yet incompletely understood mechanisms.[123] Its topical and systemic application results in depletion of substance P, a principal neurotransmitter of polymodal nociceptive afferent fibers.[124-128] Depletion is selective from primary nociceptive afferent fibers and type C fiber terminals. In experimental animals, capsaicin also causes loss of unmyelinated fibers and degeneration of primary sensory ganglion neurons containing substance P, cholecystokinin, somatostatin, and vasoactive-intestinal polypeptide. The mechanism of substance P depletion appears to be secondary to the release of substance P from nerve terminals, diminished axonal transport of substance P to replenish it in the nerve terminals, and inhibition of its synthesis.[126-128] The initial release of substance P results in a lower threshold of thermal, chemical, and mechanical nociceptors, presumably from direct stimulation of receptors. This results in local erythema, burning, warmth, and spontaneous pain, as is experienced by many patients. After repeated and continued application, desensitization and elevation of thresholds occur, resulting in pain relief.

Although the use of capsiacin-containing ointments in painful diabetic neuropathy and other neuropathies has been widely promoted, personal experience and that of others suggests that most patients find the initial irritation after topical application too unpleasant and discomforting to warrant its further use. The reported controlled studies suggest that benefits of drug application become evident only after 4 weeks of use, when a significant number of patients find it necessary to discontinue treatment because of the burning sensation after application. In fact, in the large randomized, double-blind, vehicle-controlled study using 0.075% topical capsiacin ointment four times daily in 277 patients with diabetic neuropathy,[129] local pain was reported four times as often by patients who used capsiacin as by those who used a placebo. This, along with neuropathic pain relief reported by patients receiving a placebo (53.4% vs. 69.5% receiving capsiacin) has resulted in skepticism about the efficacy of this drug. In addition, the burning caused by local application of capsaicin, and the sneezing and coughing resulting from inhalation of airborne ointment, makes it difficult to accept this study as a true double-blind study.

PROGNOSIS OF DIFFERENT FORMS OF DIABETIC PERIPHERAL NEUROPATHY

The diverse syndromes resulting from diabetic mononeuropathies and multiple mononeuropathies are usually reversible. The recovery period for diabetic third cranial nerve palsy is usually 3 to 6 months.[130] The syndrome of unilateral or bilateral painful diabetic thoracoabdominal neuropathy,[131, 132] usually associated with rapid weight loss and depression, is reversible but occasionally recurs. The recovery period may last up to 30 months but is usually complete within 6 months.[131] The acute painful diabetic neuropathy[74] is a self-limited syndrome associated with profound weight loss and

depression, resembling diabetic neuropathic cachexia.[133] These syndromes are more prevalent in males and may occur at any time during the course of both type I and type II diabetes. Some patients exhibit no other features of neuropathy. Recovery from severe pain is always associated with restitution of normal body weight and is usually complete in less than 12 months. When pain is less severe or other neuropathic features are also evident, the pain may persist for many years.[134]

Diabetic proximal motor neuropathy (femoral neuropathy, diabetic amyotrophy, Bruns-Garland syndrome) with severe unilateral or bilateral anterior thigh pain, followed by wasting and weakness of quadriceps muscles and loss of knee reflex, is more common in middle aged or elderly patients with NIDDM and usually carries a good prognosis.[135] A spontaneous and near-complete recovery often occurs from within a few months to up to 3 years. Recurrent episodes may occur in up to 20% of patients.[136] It appears that institution of insulin therapy after the onset of symptoms does not influence the rate of recovery.[136]

The prognosis for the slowly progressive symmetric sensory motor polyneuropathy is difficult to assess because of the slow rate of progression, variable involvement of different nerve fibers, and high coefficients of variations in methods of nerve function measurement. If patients are followed for 2 years, no observable change or very small deterioration may be detected.[76, 83, 137, 138] Observation for 5 years by Bishoff,[139] however, suggests deterioration of motor nerve conduction velocity, whereas a 10-year follow-up by van der Vliet et al.[140] shows no deterioration. These conflicting results indicate that the final answer to the question of prognosis of diabetic polyneuropathy must await the result of the ongoing large-scale Diabetic Control and Complication Trial.

The presence of diabetic neuropathy

increases mortality risks in diabetics. Ewing et al.[141] showed that when patients with diabetic autonomic neuropathy are followed prospectively, the calculated mortality may reach 53% after 5 years. About half of the deaths result from renal failure. O'Brien et al.,[142] studying 506 randomly selected patients with IDDM, screened for autonomic neuropathy with a series of cardiac autonomic function tests and found the cumulative 5-year mortality rate five times greater in diabetics with autonomic dysfunction than in those without autonomic dysfunction. The increased mortality rate was reported to be from renal failure. Whether the autonomic neuropathy is directly or indirectly responsible for death is not known. Sampson et al.[143] studied the evolution of autonomic symptoms in young insulin-dependent diabetics, first identified as having abnormal autonomic function 10 to 15 years earlier. Symptoms of autonomic neuropathy, especially gastrointestinal symptoms, were intermittent occurring at varying intervals and rarely worsened or remitted over 10 to 15 years. The severity of orthostatic hypotension was also variable with no tendency to deterioration.

Acknowledgments

I gratefully appreciate the support of Andrea and Claud Walker from Taylor, Louisiana. I thank Ms. Stacie Liuzzo for typing the manuscript.

REFERENCES

1. Young RJ, MacKintyre CCA, Martyn CN, et al: Progression of subclinical polyneuropathy in young patients with type 1 (insulin-dependent) diabetes: Associations with glycaemic control and microangiopathy (microvascular complications), *Diabetologia* 29:156, 1986.
2. Report and recommendations of the San Antonio conference on diabetic neuropathy, *Neurology* 38:1161, 1988.
3. Dyck PJ, Karnes JL, Daube J, et al: Clinical and neuropathological criteria for the diagnosis and staging of diabetic polyneuropathy, *Brain* 108:861, 1985.
4. Pirart J: Diabetes mellitus and its degenerative complications: A prospective study of 4,400 patients observed between 1947 and 1973, *Diabetes Care* 1:168, 1978.
5. Mincu I: Micro- and macroangiopathies and other chronic degenerative complications in newly detected diabetes mellitus, *Rev Roum Med Int* 18:155, 1980.
6. Melton H, Dyck PJ: Epidemiology. In Dyck PJ, Thomas PK, Asbury AK, et al, editors: *Diabetic neuropathy,* Philadelphia, 1987, WB Saunders, p 27.
7. Dyck PJ, Kratz KM, Lehman KA, et al: The Rochester diabetic neuropathy study, *Neurology* 4:799, 1991.
8. Walters DP, Gatling W, Mullee MA, et al: The distribution and severity of diabetic foot disease: A community study with comparison to a non-diabetic group, *Diabetic Med* 9:354–358, 1992.
9. Canal N, Comi G, Saibene V, et al: The relationship between peripheral and autonomic neuropathy in insulin dependent diabetes: A clinical and instrumental evaluation. In Canal N, Pozza G, editors: *Peripheral neuropathies,* New York, 1978, Elsevier North-Holland, p 247.
10. Fernandez-Castaner M, Mendola G, Levy I, et al: The prevalence and clinical aspects of the cardiovascular autonomic neuropathy in diabetic patients, *Med Clin (Barc)* 84:215, 1985.
11. Tackmann W, Kaeser HE, Berger W, et al: Autonomic disturbances in relation to sensorimotor peripheral neuropathy in diabetes mellitus, *J Neurol* 224:273, 1981.
12. Peretti A, Nucciotti I, Francica D, et al: Autonomic and sensory-motor neuropathy in diabetes mellitus: Intercorrelation and relationship with metabolic control and disease duration, *Electroencephalogr Clin Neurophysiol* 61:519, 1985.
13. Hoffman J: Peripheral neuropathy in children with diabetes mellitus, *Acta Neurol Scand* 40(suppl 8):1, 1964.

14. Lawrence DG, Locke S: Neuropathy in children with diabetes mellitus, *BMJ* 1:784, 1963.
15. Young RJ, Ewing DJ, Clarke BF: Nerve function and metabolic control in teenage diabetics, *Diabetes* 32:142, 1983.
16. Osuntokun BO: The neurology of non-alcoholic pancreatic diabetes mellitus in Nigerians, *J Neurol Sci* 11:17, 1970.
17. Thomas PK: Metabolic neuropathy, *J R Coll Physicians Lond* 7:154, 1973.
18. Llewelyn JG, Gilbey SG, Thomas PK, et al: Sural nerve morphometry in diabetic autonomic and painful sensory neuropathy, *Brain* 114:867, 1991.
19. Young RJ, Zhou YQ, Rodriguez E, et al: Variable relationship between peripheral somatic and autonomic neuropathy in patients with different syndromes of diabetic polyneuropathy, *Diabetes* 35:192, 1986.
20. Harati Y, Low PA: Autonomic peripheral neuropathies: Diagnosis and clinical presentation. In Appel SH, editor: *Current neurology*. St Louis, 1990, Mosby–Year Book, p 105.
21. Niakan E, Harati Y, Comstock JP: Diabetic autonomic neuropathy, *Metabolism* 35:224, 1986.
22. Ryder REJ, Kennedy RL, Newrick PG, et al: Autonomic denervation may be a prerequisite of diabetic neuropathic foot ulceration, *Diabetic Med* 7:726–730, 1990.
23. DCCT Research Group: Factors in development of diabetic neuropathy. Baseline analysis of neuropathy in feasibility phase of diabetes control and complications trial (DCCT), *Diabetologia* 37:476, 1988.
24. Sosenko JM, Gadia MT, Fournier AM, et al: Body stature as a risk factor for diabetic sensory neuropathy, *Am J Med* 80:11031, 1986.
25. Steele JM, Young RJ, Lloyd GG, et al: Clinically apparent eating disorders in young diabetic women: Associations with painful neuropathy and other complications, *BMJ* 294:859, 1987.
26. Llewelyn JG, Thomas PK, Fonseca V, et al: Acute painful diabetic neuropathy precipitated by strict glycaemic control. *Acta Neuropathol* (Berl) 72:157, 1986.

27. Boulton AIM, Hardisty CA, Worth RC, et al: Metabolic and genetic factors in diabetic neuropathy, *Diabetologia* 23:157, 1982.
28. Brown FM, Watts M, Rabinowe SL: Aggregation of subclinical autonomic nervous system dysfunction and autoantibodies in families with type I diabetes, *Diabetes* 40:1611, 1991.
29. McCulloch DK, Campbell IW, Prescott RJ, et al: Effects of alcohol intake on symptomatic peripheral neuropathy in diabetic men, *Diabetes Care* 3:245, 1980.
30. Ram Z, Sadeh M, Walden R, et al: Vascular insufficiency quantitatively aggravates diabetic neuropathy, *Arch Neurol* 48:1239, 1991.
31. Sharma AK, Thomas PK: Animal Models: pathology and pathophysiology. In Dyck PJ, et al, editors: *Diabetic neuropathy*. Philadelphia, 1987, WB Saunders, p 237.
32. Sima AA, Lattimer SA, Yagihashi S, et al: Axo-glial dysjunction. A novel structural lesion that accounts for poorly reversible slowing of nerve conduction in the spontaneously diabetic bio-breeding rat, *J Clin Invest* 77:474, 1986.
33. Sima AAF, Bril V, Nathanial V, et al: Regeneration and repair of myelinated fibers in sural nerve biopsies from patients with diabetic neuropathy treated with sorbinil, an investigational aldose reductase inhibitor, *N Engl J Med* 319:548, 1988.
34. Greene DA, Lattimer-Greene S, Sima AF: Pathogenesis of diabetic neuropathy: Role of altered phosphoinositide metabolism, *Crit Rev Neurobiol* 5:143, 1989.
35. Tomlinson DR: Polyols and myoinositol in diabetic neuropathy—of mice and men, *Mayo Clin Proc* 64:1030, 1989.
36. Gregersen G: Variations in motor conduction velocity produced by acute changes in the metabolic state in diabetic patients, *Diabetologia* 4:273, 1968.
37. Calcutt NA, Tomlinson DR, Biswas S: Co-existence of nerve conduction deficit with increased Na^+/K^+-AThase activity in galactose-fed mice, *Diabetes* 39:663, 1990.

38. Carrington AL, Ettlinger CB, Calcutt NA, et al: Aldose reductase inhibition with imirestat—effects on impulse conduction and insulin stimulation of Na$^+$/K$^+$-adenosine triphosphatase activity in sciatic nerves of streptozotocin-diabetic rats, *Diabetologia* 34:397, 1991.

39. Griffey RH, Eaton RP, Sibbitt RR, et al: Diabetic neuropathy: structural analysis of nerve hydration by magnetic resonance spectroscopy, *JAMA* 260:2872, 1988.

40. Dyck PJ, Karnes JL, O'Brien P, et al: The spatial distribution of fiber loss in diabetic polyneuropathy suggests ischemia, *Ann Neurol* 19:440, 1986.

41. Crepaldi G, Fedele D, Tiengo A, et al: Ganglioside treatment in diabetic peripheral neuropathy: A multicenter trial, *Acta Diabetol Lat* 10:265, 1983.

42. Johnson PC, Doll SC, Cromey DW: Pathogenesis of diabetic neuropathy, *Ann Neurol* 19:450, 1986.

43. Sugimura K, Dyck PJ: Multifocal fiber loss in proximal sciatic nerve in symmetric distal diabetic neuropathy, *J Neurol Sci* 53:501, 1982.

44. Dyck PJ, Hansen S, Karnes J, et al: Capillary number and percentage closed in human diabetic sural nerve, *Proc Natl Acad Sci USA* 82:2513, 1985.

45. Brownlee M: Glycosylation products as toxic-mediators of diabetic complications, *Annu Rev Med* 42:159, 1991.

46. Low PA, Nickander KK: Oxygen free radical effects in sciatic nerve in experimental diabetes, *Diabetes* 40:873, 1991.

47. Asbury AK, Fields HL: Pain due to peripheral nerve damage: An hypothesis, *Neurology* 34:1587, 1983.

48. Low PA, Langerlund TD, McManis PG: Nerve blood flow and oxygen delivery in normal diabetic and ischemic neuropathy, *Int Rev Neurobiol* 31:355, 1989.

49. Sladky JT, Tschoepe RL, Greenberg JH, et al: Peripheral neuropathy after chronic endoneurial ischemia, *Ann Neurol* 29:272, 1991.

50. Newrick PG, Wilson AI, Jakubowski J, et al: Sural nerve oxygen tension in diabetes, *BMJ* 293:1053, 1986.

51. Tesfaye S, Harris N, Wilson RM, et al: Exercise induced conduction velocity increment: a marker of impaired peripheral blood flow in diabetic neuropathy, *Diabetologia* (in press).

52. Malik RA, Masson EA, Sharma AK, et al: Hypoxic neuropathy: Relevance to human diabetic neuropathy, *Diabetologia* 33:311, 1990.

53. Cullum NA, Mahon J, Stringer K, et al: Glycation of rat sciatic nerve tubulin in experimental diabetes mellitus, *Diabetologia* 34:387, 1991.

54. Vlassara H, Brownlee M, Cerami A; Nonenzymatic glycosylation of peripheral nerve protein in diabetes mellitus, *Proc Natl Acad Sci USA* 78:5190, 1981.

55. Williams SK, Howarth NL, Devenny JJ, et al: Structural and functional consequences of increased tubulin glycosylation in diabetes mellitus, *Proc Natl Acad Sci USA* 79:6546, 1982.

56. Tomlinson DR, Mayer JH: Defects of axonal transport in diabetes mellitus—a possible contribution to the etiology of diabetic neuropathy, *J Auton Pharmacol* 4:59, 1984.

57. Davie SJ, Gould BJ, Yudkin JS: Effect of vitamin c on glycosylation of proteins, *Diabetes* 41:167, 1992.

58. Yagihashi S, Kamijo M, Baba M, et al: Effect of aminoguanidine on functional and structural abnormalities in peripheral nerve of STZ-induced diabetic rats, *Diabetes* 41:47, 1992.

59. Soulis-Liparata T, Cooper M, Papazogloud, et al: Retardation by aminoguanidine of development of albuminuria, mesanglial expansion, and tissue fluorescence in streptozocin-induced diabetic rat, *Diabetes* 40:1328, 1991.

60. Ellis EN, Bowen W: Aminoguanidine ameliorates glomerular basement membrane (GBM) thickening in experimental diabetes [abstract], *Diabetes* 39(suppl 1):71A, 1990.

61. Hammes H-P, Martin S, Federlin K, et al: Aminoguanidine treatment inhibits the development of experimental diabetic retinopathy [abstract], *Diabetes* 39(suppl 1):62A, 1990.

62. Nicholls K, Mandel TE: Advanced glycosylation end-products in experimental

murine diabetic neuropathy: Effect of islet isografting and of noguanidine, *Lab Invest* 60:486, 1989.

63. Kihara M, Schmelzer JD, Podulso JF, et al: Aminoguanidine effects on nerve blood flow, vascular permeability, electrophysiology and oxygen free radicals, *Proc Natl Acad Sci USA* 88:6107, 1991.

64. Edelstein D, Brownlee M: Mechanistic studies of advanced glycosylation end product inhibition by aminoguanidine, *Diabetes* 41:26, 1991.

65. Kumari K, Uhar S, Bansal V, et al: Inhibition of diabetes-associated complications by nucleophilic compounds, *Diabetes* 40:1079, 1991.

66. Faradji V, Sotelo J: Low serum levels of nerve growth factor in diabetic neuropathy, *Acta Neurol Scand* 81:402, 1990.

67. Hellweg R, Hartung HD: Endogenous levels of nerve growth factor are altered in experimental diabetes mellitus: A possible role for NGF in the pathogenesis of diabetic neuropathy, *J Neurosci Res* 26:258, 1990.

68. Sotelo VF: Low serum levels of nerve growth factor in diabetic neuropathy, *Acta Neurol Scand* 81:402, 1990.

69. Frazier WA, Hogue-Angeletti R, Bradshaw RA: Nerve growth factor and insulin, structural similarities indicate an evolutionary relationship reflected by physiological action, *Science* 76:482, 1972.

70. Dyck PJ, Lais A, Karnes JL, et al: Fiber loss is primary and multifocal in sural nerves in diabetic polyneuropathy, *Ann Neurol* 19:425, 1986.

71. Llewelyn JG, Thomas PK, Gilbey SG, et al: Pattern of myelinated fiber loss in the sural nerve in neuropathy related to type 1 (insulin-dependent) diabetes, *Diabetologia* 31:162, 1988.

72. Said G, Slama G, Selva J: Progressive centripetal degeneration of axons in small fiber diabetic polyneuropathy. A clinical and pathological study, *Brain* 106:791, 1983.

73. Vlassara H, Brownlee M, Cerami A: Recognition and uptake of human diabetic peripheral nerve myelin by macrophages, *Diabetes* 34:533, 1985.

74. Archer AG, Watkins PJ, Thomas PK, et al: The natural history of acute painful neuropathy in diabetes mellitus, *J Neurol Neurosurg Psychiatry* 46:491, 1983.

75. Britland ST, Young RJ, Sharma AK, et al: Association of painful and painless diabetic polyneuropathy with different patterns of nerve fiber degeneration and regeneration, *Diabetes* 39:898, 1990.

76. Lauritzen T, Frost-Larsen K, Larsen HW, et al: Two-year experience with continuous subcutaneous insulin infusion in relation to retinopathy and neuropathy, *Diabetes* 34:74, 1985.

77. Daube JR: Electrophysiologic testing in diabetic neuropathy. In Dyck PJ, Thomas PK, Asbury AK, et al, editors: *Diabetic neuropathy,* Philadelphia, 1987, WB Saunders, p 162.

78. Fraser DM, Campbell IW, Ewing DJ, et al: Peripheral and autonomic nerve function in newly diagnosed diabetes mellitus, *Diabetes* 26:546, 1977.

79. Horowitz SH, Ginsberg-Fellner F. Ischemia and sensory nerve conduction in diabetes mellitus, *Neurology* 29:695, 1979.

80. Pietri A, Ehle AL, Raskin P: Changes in nerve conduction velocity after six weeks of glucose regulation with portable insulin infusion pumps, *Diabetes* 29:668, 1980.

81. Terkildsen AB, Christensen NJ: Reversible nervous abnormalities in juvenile diabetics with a recently diagnosed diabetes, *Diabetologia* 7:113, 1971.

82. Ward JD, Barnes CG, Fisher DJ, et al: Improvement in nerve conduction following treatment in newly diagnosed diabetics, *Lancet* 1:428, 1971.

83. Service FJ, Rizza RA, Daube JR, et al: Near normoglycaemia: Improved nerve conduction and vibration sensation in diabetic neuropathy, *Diabetologia* 28:722, 1985.

84. Kennedy WR, Navarro X, Goetz FC, et al: Effects of pancreatic transplantation on diabetic neuropathy, *N Engl J Med* 322:1031, 1990.

85. Harati Y: Diabetic peripheral neuropathies, *Ann Intern Med* 107:546, 1987.

86. Goto Y, Oikawa N, Akanuma Y, et al: Clinical study of a new aldose reductase inhibitor (ONO-2235) on diabetic neuropathy—a multicenter study, *J Jpn Diabetes Soc* 28:89, 1985.

87. Judzewitsch RG, Jaspan JB, Polonsky KS, et al: Aldose reductase inhibition improves nerve conduction velocity in diabetic patients, *N Engl J Med* 308:119, 1983.

88. Dyck PJ, O'Brien PC: Meaningful degrees of prevention or improvement of nerve conduction in controlled clinical trials of diabetic neuropathy, *Diabetes Care* 12:649, 1989.

89. Jaspan J, Malone J, Nikolai T, et al: Clinical response to sorbinil in painful diabetic neuropathy, *Diabetes* 38:14A, 1989.

90. Sorbinil Neuropathy Study Group: Clinical response to sorbinil treatment in diabetic neuropathy, *Diabetes* 38:14A, 1989.

91. Boulton AIM, Levin S, Comstock J: A multicentre trial of the aldose reductase inhibitor tolrestat in patients with symptomatic neuropathy, *Diabetologia* 33:431, 1990.

92. Gonen B, Bochenek W, Beg M, et al: The effect of withdrawal of tolrestat, an aldose-reductase inhibitor, on signs, symptoms and nerve function in diabetic neuropathy, *Diabetologia* 34(suppl 2):A153, 1991.

93. Florkowski CM, Rowe BR, Nightingale S, et al: Clinical and neurophysiological studies of aldose reductase inhibitor ponalrestat in chronic symptomatic diabetic peripheral neuropathy, *Diabetes* 40:129, 1991.

94. Geisler FH, Dorsey FC, Coleman WP: Recovery of motor function after spinal-cord injury—a randomized placebo-controlled trial with GM-I ganglioside, *N Engl J Med* 324:1829, 1991.

95. Hannsson HA, Holmgran J, Svennerholm L: Ultrastructural localization of cell membrane GMI ganglioside by cholera toxin, *Proc Natl Acad Sci USA* 74:3782, 1977.

96. Ledeen RW, Skrivanek JA, Tirri LJ, et al: Gangliosides of the neuron: localization and origin, *Adv Exp Med Biol* 71:83, 1976.

97. Morgan IG, Tattamani G, Gombos C: Biochemical evidence on the role of gangliosides in nerve endings, *Adv Exp Med Biol* 71:137, 1976.

98. Marini P, Vitadello M, Binachi R, et al: Impaired axonal transport of acetylcholinesterase in sciatic nerve of alloxan-diabetic rats: Effect of ganglioside treatment, *Diabetologia* 29:254, 1986.

99. Sebille A: Nerve regeneration in exogenous cerebral ganglioside-treated rats, *Muscle Nerve* 7:278, 1984.

100. Gorio A, Carmignoto G, Facci L, et al: Motor nerve sprouting induced by gangliosides: possible implications for gangliosides on neuronal growth, *Brain Res* 197:236, 1980.

101. Gorio A, Marini P, Zanoni R: Muscle reinnervation: III. Motorneuron sprouting capacity, enhancement by exogenous gangliosides, *Neuroscience* 8:417, 1983.

102. Leon A, Facci G, Toffano S, et al: Activation on (NA^+K^+) AThase by nanomolar concentrations of GMI ganglioside, *J Neurochem* 37:350, 1981.

103. Ohi T, Farukawa S, Hayashi K, et al: Ganglioside stimulation of nerve growth factor synthesis in cultured rat Schwann cells, *Biochem Int* 20:739, 1990.

104. Rodden FA, Wiegandt H, Bauer BL: Gangliosides: The relevance of current research to neurosurgery, *J Neurosurg* 74:606, 1991.

105. Samson JC: GM1 ganglioside treatment of central nervous system injury: clinical evidence for improved recovery, *Drug Develop Res* 19:209, 1990.

106. Hallett M, Flood T, Slater N, et al: Trial of ganglioside therapy for diabetic neuropathy, *Muscle Nerve* 10:822, 1987.

107. Horowitz SH: Ganglioside therapy in diabetic neuropathy, *Muscle Nerve* 9:531, 1986.

108. Schonhofer PS: GM-I ganglioside for spinal cord injury, *N Engl J Med* 326:493, 1992.

109. Granieri E, Casetta I, Govoni V, et al: Gangliosides therapy and Guillain-Barre syndrome, *Neuroepidemiology* 10:161, 1991.

110. Max MB, Culnane M, Schafer SC, et al: Amitriptyline relieves diabetic neuropa-

thy pain in patients with normal or depressed mood, *Neurology* 37:589, 1987.

111. Max MB, Kishor-Kumar R, Schafer SC, et al: Efficacy of desipramine in painful diabetic neuropathy: A placebo-controlled trial, *Pain* 54:3, 1991.

112. Ellenberg M: Treatment of diabetic neuropathy with diphenylhydantoin, *NY State Med J* 68:2653, 1968.

113. Saudek CD, Werns S, Reidenberg MM: Phenytoin in the treatment of lancinating pain. A comparison, *Anaesthesia* 36:1129, 1981.

114. Chakrabarti AK, Samantary SK: Diabetic peripheral neuropathy: Nerve conduction studies before, during and after carbamazepine therapy, *Australia NZ Med* 6:565, 1976.

115. Rull JA, Quibrera R, Gonzalez-Millan H, et al: Symptomatic treatment of peripheral diabetic neuropathy with carbamazepine (tegretol): Double-blind crossover trial, *Diabetologia* 5:215, 1969.

116. Wilton TD: Tegretol in the treatment of diabetic neuropathy, *S Afr Med J* 48:869, 1974.

117. Swerdlow M: Review: Anticonvulsant drugs and chronic pain, *Clin Neuropharmacol* 7:51, 1984.

118. Tan Y-M, Croese J: Clonidine and diabetic patients with leg pains, *Ann Intern Med* 105:633, 1986.

119. Max MB, Schafer SC, Culnane M, et al: Association of pain relief with drug side-effects in post-herpetic neuralgia: A single-dose study of clonidine, codeine, ibuprofen, and placebo, *Clin Pharmacol Ther* 43:363, 1988.

120. Fleetwood-Walker S, Mitchell R, Hope PJ, et al: An a2 receptor mediates the selective inhibition by noradrenaline of nociceptive responses of identified dorsal horn neurones, *Brain Res* 334:243, 1985.

121. Kastrup J, Angelo HR, Petersen P, et al: Treatment of chronic painful diabetic neuropathy with intravenous lidocaine infusion, *BMJ* 292:173, 1986.

122. Dejgard A, Petersen P, Kastrup J: Mexiletine for treatment of chronic painful diabetic neuropathy, *Lancet* 1:9, 1988.

123. Tandan R, Lewis GA, Krusinski PB: Topical capsaicin in painful diabetic neuropathy, *Diabetes Care* 15:8, 1992.

124. Bernstein JE: Capsaicin in the treatment of dermatologic disease, *Cutis* 39:352, 1987.

125. Bernstein JE, Bickers DR, Dahl MV, et al: Treatment of chronic postherpetic neuralgia with topical capsaicin: A preliminary study, *J Am Acad Dermatol* 17:93, 1987.

126. Buck SH, Burks TF: The neuropharmacology of capsaicin: Review of some recent observations, *Pharmacol Rev* 38:179, 1986.

127. Go VLW, Yaksh TL: Release of substance P in the cat spinal cord, *J Physiol (Lond)* 391:141, 1987.

128. Lembeck F, Donnerer J, Calpaert FC: Increase of substance P in primary afferent nerves during chronic pain, *Neuropeptides* 1:175, 1981.

129. Capsaicin Study Group: Effect of treatment with capsaicin on daily activities of patients with painful diabetic neuropathy, *Diabetes Care* 15:159, 1992.

130. Watkins PJ: Natural history of the diabetic neuropathies, *Q J Med* 284:1209, 1990.

131. Harati Y, Niakan E: Diabetic thoracoabdominal neuropathy: A cause for chests and abdominal pain, *Arch Intern Med* 146:1493, 1986.

132. Stewart JD: Diabetic truncal neuropathy: Topography of the sensory deficit, *Ann Neurol* 25:233, 1989.

133. Ellenberg M: Diabetic neuropathic cachexia, *Diabetes* 23:418, 1974.

134. Boulton AIM, Armstrong WD, Scarpello JHB, et al: The natural history of painful diabetic neuropathy, *Postgrad Med J* 59:556, 1983.

135. Barohn RJ, Sahenk Z, Warmolts JR, et al: The Bruns-Garland syndrome (diabetic amyotrophy), *Arch Neurol* 48:1130, 1990.

136. Coppack SW, Watkins PJ: The natural history of diabetic amyotrophy, *Q J Med* 79:307, 1991.

137. Dahl-Jorgensen K, Brinchmann-Hansen O, Hanssen KF, et al: Effect of near normoglycaemia for two years on progression of early diabetic retinopathy, nephropathy and neuropathy: The Oslo Study, *BMJ* 293:1195, 1986.

138. Jakobsen J, Christiansen JS, Kristoffersen I, et al: Autonomic and somato-

sensory nerve function after 2 years of continuous subcutaneous insulin infusion in type I diabetes, *Diabetes* 37:452, 1988.

139. Bischoff A: The natural course of diabetic neuropathy: A follow-up, *Hormone Metab Res* 9(suppl):98, 1980.

140. van der Vliet JA, Navarro X, Kennety WR, et al: Long-term follow-up polyneuropathy in diabetic kidney transplant recipients, *Diabetes* 37:1247, 1988.

141. Ewing DJ, Campbell IW, Clarke BF: The natural history of diabetic autonomic neuropathy, *Q J Med* 193:95, 1980.

142. O'Brien IA, McFadden JP, Corral RJM: The influence of autonomic neuropathy on mortality in insulin dependent diabetes, *Q J Med* 79:495, 1991.

143. Sampson MJ, Wilson S, Karagiannis P, et al: Progression of diabetic autonomic neuropathy over a decade in insulin-dependent diabetes, *Q J Med* 75:635, 1990.

8

Pathophysiology of Tissue Breakdown in the Diabetic Foot

Jeffrey L. Tredwell, D.P.M.

It is well known that diabetes can be devastating to the feet. Global statistics from organizations such as the American Diabetes Association, the Centers for Disease Control, and the American Association of Diabetes Educators reveal that the medical and podiatric communities in general have not successfully focused their energies and vast academic resources on treatment programs that can significantly reduce the great morbidity associated with lower-extremity problems that result from diabetes.

According to various studies, there are approximately 14 million diabetics, diagnosed and undiagnosed, in the United States and many millions more worldwide. In the United States alone, there are approximately 600,000 newly diagnosed diabetics entering the health-care system each year. Of the more than 100,000 major amputations that occur each year, of the nontraumatic ones, five of six occur in the diabetic population. This does not include relatively minor procedures such as metatarsal head resections, toe amputations, and other forefoot surgery secondary to soft tissue and bone infection. It has been estimated that diabetics are 17 times more likely to develop gangrene. From clinical observation, we know that if a major or minor amputation occurs, within a relatively short period of time more surgery and more amputation will follow until the patient can no longer be independently mobile. We have observed that most patients who develop a foot complication will have recurrence of the same complication in a relatively short period of time.[1-7] This sad predicament causes further impact on disability insurance payments, rehabilitation, home nursing, and custodial costs.

It is clear, based on these alarming statistics, that from both a clinical and economic point of view, it is of paramount importance that a program of early recognition be developed in the physician's office that allows the physician to address the devastating forces of diabetes that lead to lower-extremity complications. By successfully addressing the clinical importance, the potential for maintaining the independence of the diabetic patient will further enhance the potential for a better quality of life, and will allow him to continue his contribution to his family, employer, and community.

There is a tremendous void in medicine when it comes to dealing with the diabetic foot. The general medical community, who holds millions of diabetics under their care, too many times takes a watchful, waiting approach until an overt complication occurs. Once the complication becomes too serious to care for on a local treatment basis, the primary physician refers the patient for a major surgery or amputation. The patient is then referred back to the primary physician who takes a watchful, waiting approach until the next complication. Unfortunately, the patient is caught in this vicious cycle of repetitive treatment.

Probably the most difficult task that a physician who treats the diabetic foot has is to accurately assess where the patient falls in the natural evolution of the complication. This is because unlike other disease entities, and with the exception of obstruction that leads to gangrene, the physician is treating a patient who does not complain of pain. Consequently, the patient is at risk for a major problem. Therefore a diabetic patient is a patient for life. And whether or not the patient has a very minor problem with good intact skin and good pulses, or whether or not the patient has a very major problem that will ultimately lead to amputation, he is forever our patient who we will continue to see to ensure that a complication does not develop or reoccur.

A common misconception among many physicians is that if a foot complication in the diabetic occurs, ultimately the foot will have to be removed. And this misconception has caused undue hardships on patients and families. Therefore doctors who treat the diabetic foot must understand the mechanisms of injury that lead to the destruction. In so doing, the catastrophic effects of diabetes on the lower extremities can be demonstratively and dramatically reduced.

To successfully implement a program to treat the effects of diabetes on the foot, the practitioner must first understand the different factors caused by diabetes that in turn cause the destruction of the diabetic foot. The key is in recognizing, identifying, and comprehending the mechanisms of injury that lead to the destruction. Once these mechanisms are understood, a treatment program can be followed that has been designed to allow the doctor to predict and prevent complications before they develop. Where the overt complication has already developed, such as a plantar ulcer or acute Charcot joint, the treatment program should be followed to allow the doctor to reverse the mechanism of injury before major surgery

and amputation are necessary. The treatment program then should allow a continued ongoing effort to ensure that the destructive mechanism of injury remains dormant so as to control any recurrences of the complication.

COMPLICATIONS OF DIABETES LEADING TO DESTRUCTION OF THE FOOT

There are two general complications of diabetes that in turn lead to complications of the foot. It is important for the practitioner to be able to immediately differentiate between these two in order to initiate appropriate treatment. One complication leads to peripheral vascular disease, which in turn leads to obstruction and gangrene. The other leads to peripheral neuropathy, which in turn leads to ulcers and Charcot joints.

Complications of diabetes lead to:
1. Peripheral Vascular Disease
   a. obstruction
   b. gangrene
2. Peripheral Neuropathy
   a. ulcers
   b. Charcot joints

Lesions that are caused by the effects of peripheral neuropathy will not be helped by vascular reconstructive procedures, unless there is also an underlying vascular obstruction preventing enough blood to the area for healing to occur. Conversely, one cannot apply techniques used for reversing neuropathic lesions if vascular disease is the cause for the lesion. A combination of treatments used by the peripheral vascular surgeon, who treats obstruction, and the podiatric specialist who treats lesions resulting from the neuropathy, works best when the lesion is secondary to the effects of neuropathy, but there is inadequate blood flow to heal that lesion. Successful vascular reconstructive surgery to ensure adequate blood flow followed by biomechanical stress-corrective techniques to close plantar ulcers generally is quite successful.

An individual whose feet are totally intact, but whose vascular status is minimal, can be kept ambulating even though the perfusion is inadequate to fight infection, as long as the skin remains intact. To successfully understand and implement a complete patient care program for the diabetic, one must understand the vascular component. Experts in the field of vascular surgery have written in other chapters in this text regarding this subject. However, a familiarity with their work is mandatory if one is to evaluate and treat diabetic foot patients.

Logerfo and Coffman, in researching the subject of vascular and microvascular disease of the feet in diabetes state that in particular, there is a wide-spread misconception that patients with diabetes mellitus have arteriolar occlusive disease, which can cause ischemic lesions even in the presence of normal pedal pulses. This view often leads to inappropriate care of the patient and a hopeless attitude on the part of the physician.[8]

When atherosclerosis occurs in diabetics in the lower extremity, it is most common in the femoral popliteal segment, the same as nondiabetics.[9, 10] There is, however, a very common signature occlusive lesion of the arteries of the lower leg in the tibial and peroneal arteries. The tibial lesion does not generally extend into the foot, and so the arterial system in the foot is less frequently involved with atherosclerosis in diabetics than in nondiabetic patients.[10] This knowledge allows the diabetic foot specialist to work with peripheral vascular surgeons who look for open vessels in the feet of diabetic patients to do reconstructive bypass surgeries with the goal of saving a limb instead of deciding to amputate because of an inappropriate diagnosis (Figs 8–1 and 8–2).

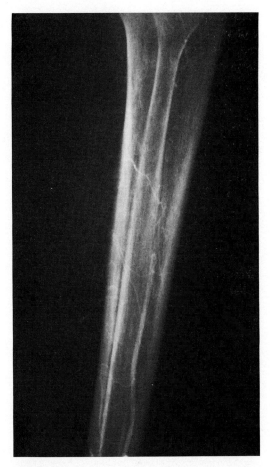

FIG 8–1.
Arteriogram of 80-year-old diabetic with vessel obstruction and plantar ulcer. No palpable pulses in the foot, but with a strong popliteal pulse.

Although the vascular component is extremely important, the reason for most complications that most physicians see in the feet of diabetic patients is due to peripheral neuropathy, the inability of patients to feel to protect themselves from injury. Understanding the effects of neuropathy on the lower extremity is a prerequisite to successful treatment of diabetic foot lesions. Understanding the psychological effects of the loss of the pain-protective mechanism can only come with seeing and experiencing dozens of patients who have large draining ulcers, or hot swollen feet with multiple fractures, and their condition has been present for

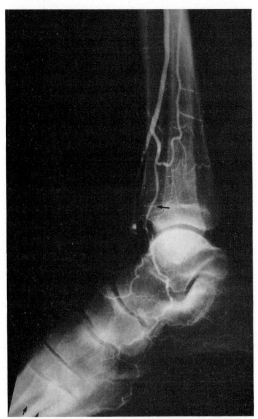

FIG 8–2.
Patient underwent a successful distal bypass surgery and eventual closure of ulcer by stress-corrective techniques. (Courtesy Anton Sidawy, MD, Veteran's Administration Hospital, Washington, DC.)

many months, even years, and have gone untreated or undetected.

This combination of the inability to feel pain to protect oneself from injury and the psychological denial process of visually observing a problem on one's own foot, but disassociating that part from the rest of the body, is a challenge for the physician. That is, the physician who treats these problems must also be compassionate, understanding, and very patient. Only then can the doctor successfully treat the complication.

Although motor neuropathy causes a weakening of the muscles of the foot and contractures that result in hammer toes, cavus feet, and other deformities, it is the sensory peripheral neuropathy that is the major cause of most complications that we see in our offices today.

MECHANISMS OF INJURY THAT LEAD TO DESTRUCTION OF THE DIABETIC FOOT

In the presence of insensitivity, where the pain-protective mechanism is no longer intact, there are four mechanisms of injury by which the diabetic foot is destroyed. Each is different and distinct from the other (Table 8–1).[11]

The first way in which the foot is destroyed is through direct mechanical disruption of tissue.[11] The second is through a small amount of pressure that is sustained over time that leads to ischemia.[11] The third is through a moderate amount of force that is repeated over and over again that leads to inflammation.[11] This inflammation causes an enzymatic autolysis of tissue from within. Finally if one of these three mechanisms of injury occurs, then an ulcer develops.[11] Through that hole in the skin, bacteria enters and is driven deeper, and eventually the fourth mechanism of injury, spreading cellulitis and osteomyelitis, develops. However, this ulcer cannot develop, unless one of the first three mechanisms occur first. Therefore one of the main missions that the specialist who treats the diabetic foot has, is to make sure that the skin does not break down. If we can accomplish this, and just this alone, then we can eliminate many of the amputations and partial amputations that are currently being performed today.

The first mechanism in which the foot is destroyed is through *direct mechanical disruption of tissue.* It takes several hundred pounds of force per square inch to penetrate the skin, which can lead to this first mechanism of destruction. An example of this would be a diabetic with loss of the pain-protective mechanism who walks barefoot and steps on an object such as a nail, a tack, or a piece of glass that penetrates the skin (see Fig 8–3). The open skin barrier allows bacteria to enter and to be driven into the deeper tissues as the diabetic walks without noticing the trauma. Because there is no warning sign of pain, the cycle continues until overt infection occurs.

This first way in which the diabetic foot is destroyed can be virtually eliminated if patients always protect their feet. If they always wear shoes or slippers and never go barefoot, then the disruption of tissue should not occur.

The importance of patient education cannot be overstated. A strong educational program designed to teach the patient not only what to do, but *why,* has been very effective in helping to eliminate this first mechanism of injury.

The second mechanism of injury that leads to the destruction of the diabetic foot results from a *small amount of pressure that is sustained over a period of time that leads to ischemia.* Whereas it takes several hundred pounds per square inch to penetrate the skin and cause the first mechanism of injury, it only takes a couple of pounds per square inch that is sustained that leads to ischemia and breakdown. In the first mechanism of injury, the skin barrier is abruptly broken. This second mechanism relies on pressure without a

TABLE 8–1.

Mechanisms of Injury That Destroy the Foot

Mechanisms of Injury	Example
Direct mechanical disruption of tissue	Patient steps on nail while walking barefoot abruptly breaking the skin barrier (see Fig 8-3)
Small amount of force that is sustained over time that leads to ischemia	1. Foot on footrest of wheel chair may lead to mid-foot ulcer (see Fig 8-4) 2. Patient at bed rest in hospital may lead to decubitus ulcer of heel (see Fig 8-4) 3. Tight shoe may lead to breakdown of bunion site (see Fig 8-7)
Moderate amount of force that is repeated over and over leads to inflammation and enzymatic autolysis of tissue	Plantar metatarsal ulceration (see Fig 8-5)
Infection	1. Development of pus foot (see Fig 8-6)

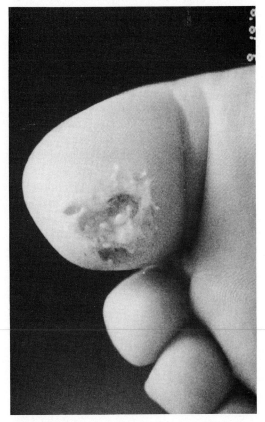

FIG 8–3.
Result of great toe stepping on nail. This is an example of the first mechanism of injury.

break in the integrity of the skin. The pressures are so low that they are generally not noticed until damage has occurred. Capillary blood flow may be obstructed by these extremely small pressures. Actual ischemic gangrene takes several hours to occur and is due to deprivation of oxygen to the tissue. For this reason a person with normal sensation will be warned that damage is taking place and will take measures to reduce the constant irritation at low pressures that is causing the pain. The warning sign will take place prior to damage occurring. Ischemic gangrene that occurs on the foot is rarely due to the pressures of ambulatory weight-bearing, which are usually intermittent. It is almost always due to the pressure of a shoe that is too tight, or a foot resting against something.[11]

Experiments at the National Hansen's Disease Center in Carville, Louisiana, by Dr. Paul Brand using pressure pads on the backs of pigs demonstrated that small amounts of pressure exerted over 5 to 7 hours, just the pressure of a tight shoe, was enough to destroy the fat pad beneath the skin. He observed that although the greatest pressure was at the central portion, it was at the periphery of the pressure pads, where pressure and nonpressure met, that sheer stress occurred. These twisting forces were found to be most damaging to tissue, much more so than even direct pressure. He found that comparisons of just a couple of pounds per square inch difference on a foot in a shoe was enough to cause this second mechanism of injury.[11]

This second mechanism of injury is unfortunately seen in both ambulatory and nonambulatory patient populations. Examples of the second mechanism of injury in a nonambulatory patient would be a patient who is confined to a wheelchair and is constantly resting his or her feet on the foot rest, or in a patient who is bed

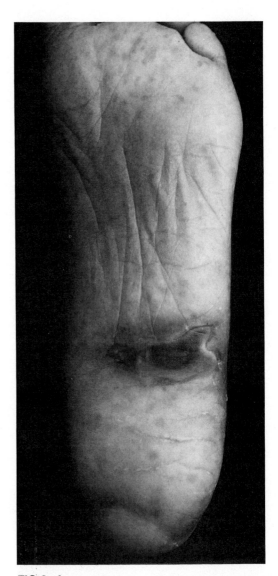

FIG 8–4.
Patient who was wheelchair-bound and developed ischemia from the second mechanism of injury at the midfoot area. The same patient also developed a decubitus ulcer because of lack of heel protection while at bed rest.

ridden and develops decubitus ulcers of his or her heels (Fig 8–4). Recognizing the reasons for the very serious problems of heel ulcers from bed rest that occur in hospitals, nursing homes, and among dialysis patients dictates that prevention should take an aggressive approach. Temperatures around the heel area of potential breakdown will always be elevated, and atrophy of the heel fat pad can generally be palpated. Reversing this mechanism of injury does not work as well as eliminating it in the nonambulatory patient. In this regard, any diabetic with neuropathy who is placed in a position at rest with the heels accepting even a minimal amount of force per square inch, which can be seen as nothing more than a blanching of the skin, is too much pressure. Appropriate protocols should be followed that allow the heels to float in appropriate heel protective devices so that there is no greater than zero pounds per square inch of pressure exerted. Following this protocol will greatly reduce, and hopefully eliminate, most of the lesions caused by the second mechanism of injury in the nonambulatory patient.

In an ambulatory patient, we should never see the results of this second mechanism of injury. The sad fact is that we too often do, and it is commonly the fault of the health-care worker. It may be the pedorthist who places a bulky orthotic in a shoe, or the nurse practitioner who applies a bulky bandage on the foot and then requires the patient to get into a shoe, or the physician who places a thick unna boot on a foot and then allows the patient to put that foot into his shoe. In these instances, the well-fitting shoe now becomes a tight-fitting shoe. That extra 1 or 2 pounds per square inch that is exerted on the foot is just enough to cause the ischemia and breakdown secondary to low

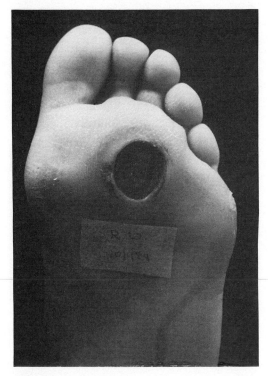

FIG 8–5.
Plantar ulceration representing the result of the third mechanism of injury.

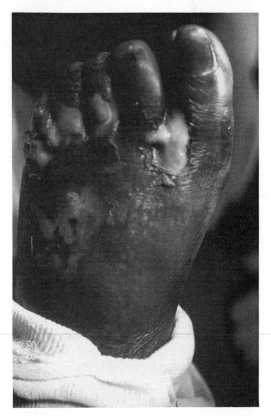

FIG 8–6.
This foot represents the fourth mechanism of injury, spreading cellulitis and osteomyelitis and death by bacterial toxicity.

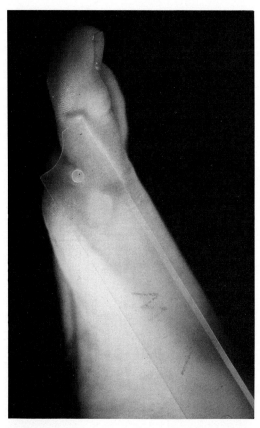

FIG 8–7.
Just two pounds per square inch, is enough to cause the second mechanism of injury. Note the blanching of the skin beneath the tractograph.

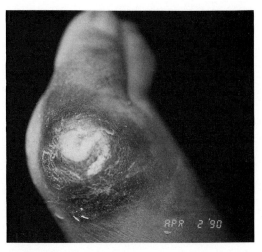

FIG 8–8.
The pressure of a tight shoe is enough to cause breakdown by the second mechanism of injury. Note the ulceration on the bunion.

grade pressure that is sustained over several hours (Figs 8–7 and 8–8).

Doctors who deal with treating the diabetic foot must understand and appreciate this second way in which the foot is destroyed. Tight-fitting shoes are the major cause of ulcers on the medial and lateral aspects of the forefoot and on dorsal bony prominences such as hammer toe deformities. The reason for this occurrence can be explained by the formula that states *tension produces pressure exactly in inverse proportion to the radius of the curvature of the curve.* To understand this, think of an oval such as an egg. If a string is tied around that egg, every point on that string will have identical tension. But the pressure produced by that tension will be greatest around the curvature. Correlate this to the transverse section of a shoe as it cuts through the metatarsal heads. There is a gentle slope of the dorsum of the foot so there will be very little pressure produced by the tension of the shoe on top of the foot and no breakdown will occur. The plantar surface of the foot is flat or slightly concave, so there will be very little pressure produced by the ten-

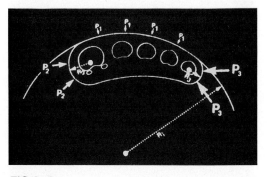

FIG 8–9.
A cross section of a shoe and foot at the metatarsal heads. Ulcers from tight shoes occur on the medial and lateral borders of the foot because pressure produced by the tension of the shoe is greatest at these points. (From Brand PW: The insensitive foot [including leprosy]. Seminars and Lecture Series on the Insensitive Foot, U.S. Public Health Service Hospital, Carville, La.)

sion of the shoe on the bottom of the foot. If an ulcer develops because of a tight shoe, it commonly develops on the medial and lateral aspects of the foot where the radius of curvature is smaller (Fig 8–9).[11] This formula leads to the academic rationale for prophylactic surgical procedures in diabetics with insensitivity and adequate circulation. The idea is to eliminate the bony prominences, such as bunion deformities, and therefore increase the radius of the curve that in turn decreases the pressure produced by the tension of the shoe at that point. This concept is discussed in detail in this text, in the chapter on prophylactic surgery.

In summary then, this second mechanism of injury can be addressed and greatly reduced in nonambulatory patients by supporting their feet and reducing all pressure from the heel areas and the plantar surface areas. In ambulatory patients, it is very important to ensure that a shoe is not too tight to the point where medial and lateral aspects will have ischemia from increased small constant pressure. It is important to note that the patient who experiences insensitivity will almost always try to "feel" the shoe pressure because of a greater feeling of security. If the patient can feel the snugness of shoe pressure, most of the time the shoe is too tight on the sides. It is therefore important that a specially educated and trained certified pedorthist who appreciates the effects of neuropathy on the foot help in the shoe fitting and fabrication of orthotics. This member of the team is extremely valuable in helping to prevent initial problems and recurrences of problems.

The best ways to eliminate the second mechanism of injury in an ambulatory patient are to make absolutely certain that the shoes are fitted properly and checked periodically by a pedorthist well versed in the effects of neuropathy on the foot. Next, convince the patient to change shoes at least two times per day. By doing this,

even if the shoe is too tight, he won't wear it long enough to do permanent damage.

The third mechanism of injury by which the diabetic foot can be destroyed is through a *moderate amount of pressure that is repeated, which leads to inflammation and breakdown* into plantar ulcers (see Fig 8–5) or multiple fractures and dislocations of the joints (Charcot joints). This is the reason for the vast majority of foot complications in diabetic patients. Understanding and appreciating this mechanism of injury has allowed us to design a set of treatment protocols where we can:

1. Predict and prevent complications before they develop.
2. Reverse the mechanism of injury to prevent major surgery and amputation.
3. Greatly reduce the recurrence rate of complications that is usually seen in the diabetic foot.

Whereas it takes several hundred pounds to penetrate the skin and cause the first mechanism of injury, and it takes only a couple of pounds per square inch to initiate the second mechanism of injury, the next question of the researchers was how and why tissue breaks down in an ambulatory population that is insensate. Two classic experiments were performed by Brand at the National Hansen's Disease Center. The first demonstrates how repetitive stress at moderate pressure, just the stress of walking, leads to inflammation and an enzymatic autolysis of tissue. The second, using thermography studies in a normal, healthy runner, demonstrates the difference between the intact and absent pain-protective mechanism, and how this robs individuals of the ability to protect themselves from the outside forces of trauma. In the first instance, an experiment was created and a machine designed that would repetitively stress the foot pad of a rat at 10,000 times a day at 20 pounds per square inch (psi). Brand found that a progressive inflammation developed in soft tissues and that by the third day inflammation was literally concentrating pressure to itself. By the eighth day necrosis of tissue had developed and the epidermis was destroyed. This experiment shows that the overt ulcer develops from strictly mechanical stress. *The stress remained constant throughout, but the tissue changed as inflammation was concentrated with even more inflammation* (Plates 1 to 5).

This experiment shows the essence of what really occurs in the diabetic foot that leads to plantar ulcers and destruction. It is not that the diabetic patient with insensitivity breaks down any faster than the normally sensate patient, or even any easier. But the patient with insensitivity is robbed of the memory of inflammation and pain to protect himself from injury. Normally sensate individuals may limp, or take off their shoe and rest, or do anything they can to prevent walking on the inflamed area because pain is so great. However, diabetics with insensitivity who have excessive inflammation will continue to apply the stress of weight bearing to the inflamed area. This is because they cannot feel the pain and therefore can't protect themselves from the injury. As a result, ulcers will develop.

The second experiment involves a normal, healthy, sensate individual who was asked to run in his stocking feet. He ran for a total of 8 miles in 2-mile segments. After each segment, thermograms were done of his feet. He was not allowed to see any of the thermography films and after the 8th mile he was asked how he felt. He stated that he wasn't sure but he thought in the 7th or possibly the 8th mile his great toe was starting to hurt him. This was correct. Thermography studies showed that by the end of the 8th mile the second toe was even hotter, more inflamed, than the great toe ever was. Without consciously realizing it, the runner was su-

pinating his foot to take pressure off of the great toe. Subconsciously, the great toe was sending a message through the pain-protective mechanism that said "roll off me, I'm hurting" and so the second toe began accepting the greater forces of the big toe. The smaller area of the second toe required a greater energy necessary to do the job of the great toe, and therefore a greater temperature resulted. If the runner was a diabetic with insensitivity, he would not have gotten the message to supinate, and eventually inflammation would have led to a reduced damage threshold and ulceration (Plates 6 to 11).

Although the pathophysiology is different in the acute Charcot joint syndrome, the mechanism of injury for development of this serious problem falls into the category of the third mechanism of injury. The Charcot joint is discussed in great detail elsewhere in this text, but it

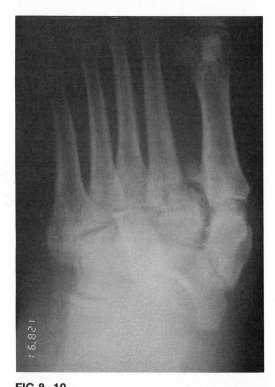

FIG 8–10.
AP view of Charcot joint syndrome. Note displacement and subluxation at Lisfranc's joint area.

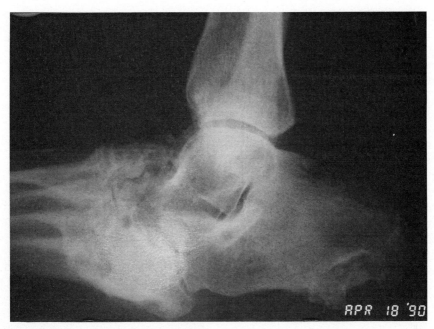

FIG 8–11.

Lateral view of Charcot joint. Note the rocker bottom appearance of the foot with prominent plantarly dis- placed cuboid and destruction of the midtarsus area. Note the head of the talus is plantigrade.

is important to mention here because the treatment goal, controlling, and then reversing inflammation once the mechanism of injury is understood, will allow healing and consolidation of the joints to take place. Even minimal trauma to the foot, a seemingly benign stress fracture, or a minor strain may be enough to initiate the Charcot joint. Whereas initial trauma will be too painful to allow continued weight-bearing in a normal sensate individual, the insensate individual will continue to apply weight. This in turn causes capsular and ligamentous stretching, joints exceeding their maximum range of motion, grinding of bones and joints against each other (which results in fracturing), and a hyperemic response. Continued weight-bearing makes this traumatic cycle continue, resulting in even more blood flow to the area. Ultimately, the hyperemic response becomes so great that the normal ground substance of bone is washed away. In accepting continued weight-bearing, the softened

bones and joints collapse, resulting in the Charcot joint, most commonly seen at Lisfranc's joint and the metatarsal phalangeal joints (Figs 8–10 to 8–11).

Strategy for treatment is similar in both the plantar ulcer and the acute Charcot joint. First control, then reverse inflammation until healing takes place. In the case of a plantar ulcer, allow healing to take place by using stress-corrective techniques, then continue using stress-corrective techniques to ensure that recurrence does not take place.

In the case of a Charcot joint, reverse the hyperemic response through stress-reduction, then continue stress-reduction until consolidation occurs. In all cases, remember that the insensitivity is present. *This is the constant, and is not reversible.* Frequent monitoring by the physician, scheduled at set periods of time, and by the patient daily, will help decrease the great morbidity that we see throughout the diabetic population.

To reverse the third mechanism of injury and relieve the inflammation and control its devastating effects, weight-bearing must be significantly reduced. This goal is met through a mechanical stress-reduction plan. This may take the form of complete bed rest, which takes all weight-bearing off of the feet, but introduces a potential second mechanism of injury. It may also cause other medical problems associated with a nonambulatory diabetic patient. Or it may take the form of a healing sandal that allows the foot to gently roll over the concentrated point of inflammation or shoes and orthotics that significantly reduce the point of contact where inflammation is concentrated.

The cornerstone of treatment, and this author's most effective treatment for both plantar ulcers and Charcot joints is the ambulatory total contact cast (Fig 8–12).[12–15] This method of treatment is described in detail elsewhere in this text. Applying the ambulatory total contact cast should be evaluated and applied as carefully as you would plan for a surgical procedure. The beauty of the ambulatory total contact cast is that it reduces pressure on the plantar surface of the foot to less than 5 pounds per square inch (psi). This allows ambulation, reversibility of inflammation, and healing to occur concurrently. It is the most effective way to close ulcers that occur from the third mechanism of injury. In my experience, grade II ulcers can close on average of about 7 weeks from initiation of treatment with total contact casting, regardless of how long the lesion has been present.[16]

Regarding acute Charcot joints, it takes an average of 4 months to reduce the hyperemic response as measured by temperature and another 4 months for consolidation of joints to occur.[16] Prevention of actual gross deformity during this time has not always been successful, and in some cases, a combination of total contact casting and non-weight-bearing may be more effective in the initial stages of the hyperemic response.

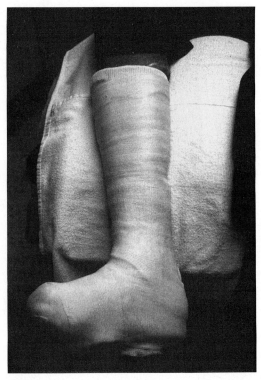

FIG 8–12.
Ambulatory total contact cast. This is a very effective modality in reducing weight-bearing strategy. The cast reduces pressure to less than 5 pounds per square inch.

Successful treatment requires that inflammation in the presence of neuropathy and repetitive stress be recognized as causing the complication. Insensitivity is the constant. Removing repetitive stress will decrease inflammation and allow healing to occur. In the worse-case scenario, the patient goes on to develop a plantar ulcer, the break in the skin barrier and repetitive weight-bearing allows infection to be driven into deeper tissues. This sets up the fourth mechanism of injury, *spreading cellulitis and eventual osteomyelitis.* Appropriate treatment including hospitalization, debridement, and antibiotics must be accomplished. Once acute infection is under control, the patient may again begin to ambulate and be treated on an outpatient basis with appropriate stress-reduction techniques.

SUMMATION OF EVALUATION AND TREATMENT

In summary, prevention of the ulcer can be accomplished if the physician recognizes and evaluates the patient for the first three mechanisms of injury. The philosophy of treatment should include evaluating all diabetics for insensitivity. If insensate points are found, evaluation of these points for bony prominences and abnormal weight distribution should then be performed. Temperature probes should be used to determine if inflammation is present. Stress-correction techniques should follow to reduce or prevent the specific mechanism of injury.

Appropriate treatment of the complication should be established once the mechanism of injury is known. If plantar ulcers are present, reverse the inflammation with stress-reduction techniques. Once the ulcers are closed, continue stress-reduction techniques to prevent recurrence. If Charcot joints develop, a physician must use ambulatory total contact casting to reduce hyperemia and initiate healing and consolidation. Once joints are consolidated, particularly if gross deformity occurs, protection of new bony prominences is necessary by stress-reduction, which may also include surgical procedures.

Evaluation and treatment of the diabetic foot is extremely complex. The physician must have full knowledge of the effects of neuropathy on the foot. With this knowledge, prediction and prevention of further complications as well as reversing the mechanisms leading to destruction can be accomplished. A knowledge of the denial process in general and appreciating the significance of the loss of pain-protective mechanisms all further enhance the potential for the success of treatment. Patient education of the various ways by which the foot is destroyed will also help accomplish a successful patient care program. Patients will comply with instruc-

tions much easier and will begin to take responsibility for themselves if they understand the underlying causes.

Three cases illustrate examples of how understanding mechanisms of injury allow for a strategy of treatment. The first case predicts and then prevents the overt problem from occurring. Cases two and three first reverse, then heal, and finally control the forces that lead to breakdown.

CASE #1

Presentation.—A 37-year-old woman recently diagnosed as having type II diabetes was referred by her primary physician for a diabetic podiatric evaluation. The patient offered no complaints.

Assessment.—Pedal pulses were palpable both at the anterior tibial and posterior tibial arteries bilaterally. No history of rest pain or claudication was noted. Both feet were totally intact. Biomechanical observation showed a small callus beneath the third metatarsal head on the left foot, which was prominent in relation to the adjacent metatarsal heads. A Semmes-Weinstein sensory evaluation measured at 5.07 at all plantar points bilaterally with the exception of the third metatarsal on the left foot, which measured at 6.10. Temperature gradients were symmetrical and in the mid-80s at all plantar points bilaterally with the exception of the third metatarsal on the left foot, which measured at 91° versus 85° at the contralateral point.

Intervention.—Shoes were modified and orthotics fabricated to allow pressure to be reduced from the third metatarsal head on the left foot.

Outcome.—Continued follow-up has helped keep the foot intact with no occurrence of ulceration.

Discussion.—The mechanism of injury causing plantar ulcers in diabetics is most typically abnormal pressure leading to inflammation in the presence of neuropathy.

A Semmes-Weinstein evaluation quantitatively determines the level of loss of sensation.[16-19] Measurement at 6.10 indicated insensitivity at the third metatarsal area, and that the pain-protective mechanism was no longer intact. Temperature probes indicated inflammation was present, but due to the insensitivity, the patient could not feel the pain of the inflammation.

Modified shoes and orthotics substantially decreased a concentration of pressure and subsequently the inflammation, thus preventing an ulcer from developing beneath the third metatarsal head, left foot.

CASE #2 (Figs 8–13 to 8–17)

Presentation.—A 55-year-old man presented with a diabetic ulceration beneath the right first metatarsal head, duration 13 months.

History.—Previous complications included hospitalization for a plantar ulceration of the second metatarsal head 2 years prior to his initial visit to the diabetic foot center. Metatarsal head resection due to osteomyelitis and 6 weeks of in-patient IV antibiotic therapy followed. Three months after surgery, an ulcer beneath the third metatarsal head developed with the patient experiencing a similar treatment and hospital course.

The patient was hospitalized twice for the ulcer, once by a surgeon who suggested

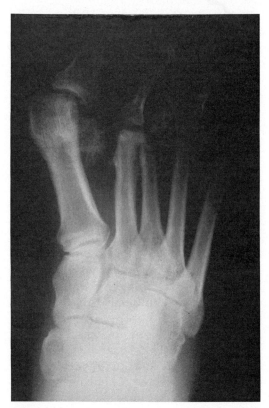

FIG 8–14.
Patient was subsequently hospitalized because of third metatarsal ulceration that developed after resection of the second metatarsal head. The patient followed a similar hospital course and third metatarsal head was removed. X-ray demonstrates resection of second and third metatarsal heads. Note hallux valgus deformity.

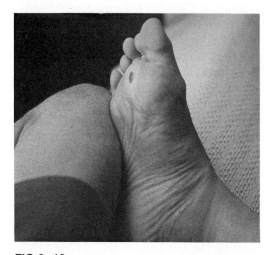

FIG 8–13.
Plantar ulceration beneath the second metatarsal head, right foot. Patient was hospitalized for 6 weeks on IV antibiotics. Second metatarsal head had to be resected because of osteomyelitis.

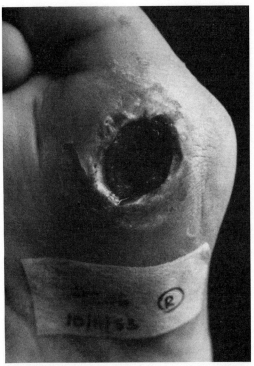

FIG 8–15.
Presenting plantar ulceration beneath the first metatarsal head had been present for 13 months. Patient was hospitalized twice for this ulceration, once by a surgeon who suggested BK amputation and once by a plastic surgeon who unsuccessfully attempted a skin graft.

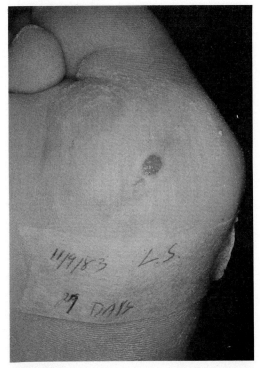

FIG 8–16.
Using ambulatory total contact casting on an out-patient basis, ulcer showed dramatic decrease in size at 29 days.

a BK amputation due to recurrent ulcers, which was rejected by the patient, and subsequently by a plastic surgeon who attempted a skin graft that was unsuccessful once ambulation began. Total medical expenses that year were nearly $100,000.

Assessment.—Examination revealed pedal pulses to be palpable bilaterally. A Semmes-Weinstein evaluation measured at 6.10 at all plantar points indicating insensitivity and complete loss of the pain-protective mechanism. Temperatures were elevated at the ulcer site and measured 8° higher than the contralateral point. Radiographic evaluation was negative for bone infection.

Intervention.—Application of ambulatory total contact cast technique with weekly changes done on an out-patient basis.

Outcome.—The ulcer closed in 41 days. Modified shoes and orthotics to reduce pressure, and the third mechanism of injury, over the forefoot prevented any further recurrences.

Discussion.—Patients who present with a plantar ulcer will heal in the presence of adequate circulation if the mechanism of injury can be reversed. In this case, a Semmes-Weinstein evaluation indicated neuropathy with complete loss of the pain-protective mechanism.

Abnormal pressure beneath the first metatarsal head was present due to previous resection of the second and third

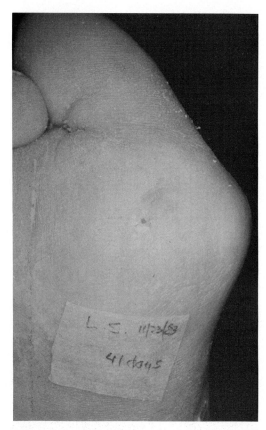

FIG 8–17.
Using total contact casting, ulcer was closed in 41 days.

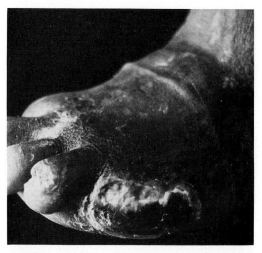

FIG 8–18.
Lateral aspect of the foot following 5th toe amputation. The tight shoe at the small radius of curvature caused this second mechanism of injury to occur.

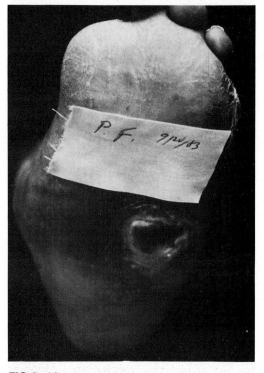

FIG 8–19.
Patient had undergone previous amputation of his great toe due to the second mechanism of injury. Note the rocker bottom appearance of the foot, which is classic in a Charcot joint syndrome.

metatarsal heads. This abnormal pressure over the first metatarsal head in the presence of insensitivity led to the inflammation that ultimately caused the ulcer.

Reducing pressure beneath the first metatarsal head, and thus reducing inflammation, allowed the ulcer to close. The ambulatory total contact cast allowed reduction of pressure and reversal of inflammation. It also allowed the patient, who would otherwise have been bed-ridden to ambulate and heal at the same time.

Recognizing that recurrence of the mechanism of injury is a strong possibility, frequent assessment for increased temperatures, and protection of the foot with stress-corrective devices, such as modified shoes and orthotics, protected the foot against further breakdown.

CASE #3 (Figs 8–18 to 8–26)

Presentation.—A 45-year-old insulin-dependent diabetic man presented with fresh amputation site at the fifth toe area, plantar ulceration at the cuboid area, and acute Charcot joint syndrome. The patient had been hospitalized at bed rest for 3 months prior to his assessment. He was scheduled for an above-the-knee amputation. The plantar ulceration had been present for about 1 year.

History.—Previous hospitalizations had been necessary for a plantar ulceration of the right toe that had developed into osteomyelitis and subsequent amputation of the great toe. The patient was in end-stage renal disease. An arteriogram was not performed because of a possibility of complete renal shut down.

Assessment.—Examination revealed pedal pulses to be minimally palpable at the anterior tibial and posterior tibial areas. A Semmes-Weinstein evaluation measured at 6.10 at all plantar points, indicating insensitivity and complete loss of the pain-protective mechanism. Temperatures were elevated to 93° at the area of Lisfranc's joint and was 7°

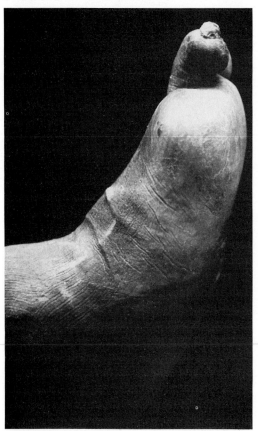

FIG 8–20.
Ulceration is noted beneath prominent cuboid, which has shifted during destructive phase at midtarsus area.

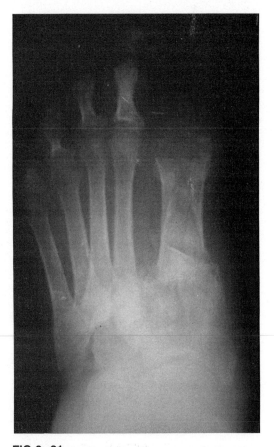

FIG 8–21.
AP of the foot showing complete destruction at Lisfranc's joint.

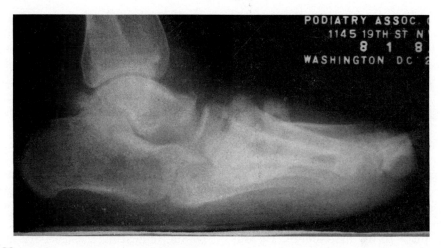

FIG 8–22.

Lateral view of the acute Charcot joint showing devastating results. Note the rocker bottom appearance of the foot at the midtarsus area. Also note the dorsal protrusion of the metatarsal bases.

higher than the contralateral side. Radiographic evaluation revealed Charcot joint disease with complete destruction of the midtarsus. A plantar ulceration was noted secondary to the cuboid prominence. The ulcer was at a grade II stage. No sinus tracts were noted. It was believed that osteomyelitis was not present because the ulceration did not penetrate to deeper tissues. The lateral aspect of the foot showed a fresh incision site from the amputation of the fifth toe.

Intervention.—The patient was discharged 2 days following consultation and was placed into an ambulatory total contact cast with weekly changes on an outpatient basis.

Outcome.—The plantar ulceration closed in about 5 months. The lateral amputation site closed in 7 months. Complete consolidation and revascularization of the midtarsus occurred in 8 months. Modified shoes with tridensity orthotics and bracing to reduce pressure, and the third mechanism of injury, over the entire foot have prevented further complications.

Discussion.—In patients who present with acute Charcot joint syndrome, a successful treatment program using total contact casting can be obtained in about 8 months. It generally takes about 4 months for the hyperemic response to be reversed, and another 4 months for consolidation to occur. In the absence of radiographic findings for bone infection, if the plantar ulceration has not penetrated to deeper tissues, using the total contact cast is an acceptable first step. If however the ulceration has penetrated to deeper tissues, a biopsy of the underlying bony prominence may be appropriate.

Once consolidation has occurred, a graded return to weight-bearing is necessary. Atrophy of the leg muscles is very common and a transition device from the cast to the modified shoe with brace is suggested. Bracing can be removed between 6 months and 1 year when the leg muscles are strong enough to support body weight.

Using temperature probes at the area of the Charcot joint is the best way to monitor the hyperemic response and to determine if the acute stage of this process and a reversal of the mechanism of injury are occurring.

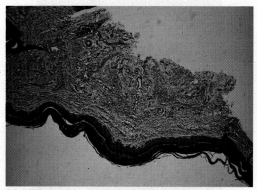

PLATE 1.
Intact epidermal layer of skin. No break in the stratum corneum.

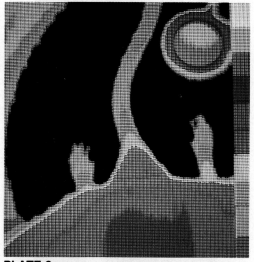

PLATE 2.
Thermography of the foot pad of the rat prior to the experiment beginning. Note that the foot is cool.

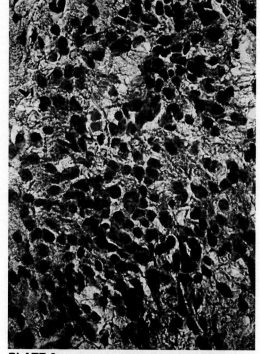

PLATE 3.
On third day of experiment, acute inflammatory cells present. Inflammation is concentrating pressure to itself.

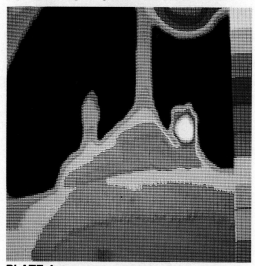

PLATE 4.
Thermography reading on 3rd day. Note that one foot pad is about 10° hotter than the opposite side. This demonstrates the effects of the repetitive stress leading to inflammation.

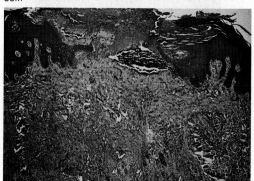

PLATE 5.
On the 8th day of the experiment, continued repetitive stress caused an ulcer to develop. Note the disruption of the stratum corneum.

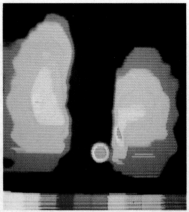

PLATE 6.
Thermogram of the feet of runner prior to experiment.
Toes are in the dark areas and are not shown.

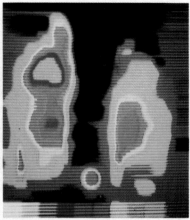

PLATE 7.
After 2 miles, inflammation is noted at the midmeta-tarsal head areas.

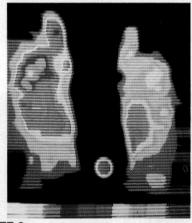

PLATE 8.
At 4 miles the metatarsal heads are hotter.

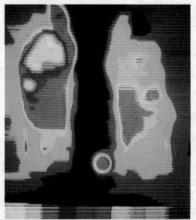

PLATE 9.
At 6 miles the metatarsal heads are hotter and the fifth
metatarsal head comes into view.

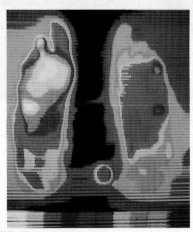

PLATE 10.
After 8 miles, the second toe is hotter than the hallux.
This demonstrates an intact pain-protective mecha-nism in a healthy individual. Subconsciously, the run-ner began to supinate the foot to take pressure off of
the great toe. (Plates 1–10 courtesy of Paul Brand,
M.D., Seattle, Washington.)

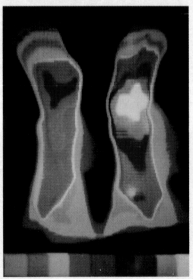

PLATE 11.
Thermography showing increased hyperemia in a pa-tient with acute Charcot joint syndrome.

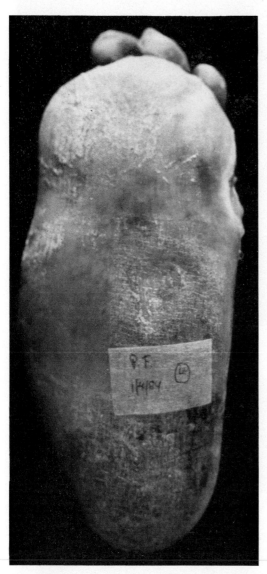

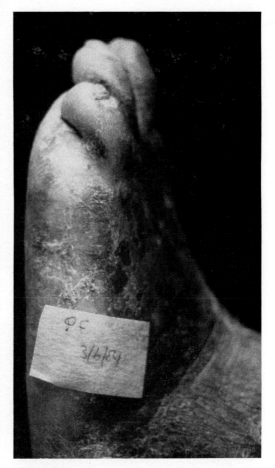

FIG 8–24.
Lateral amputation site closed in 7 months using total contact casting.

FIG 8–23.
Ulcer was closed in 5 months using ambulatory total contact casting on an out-patient basis.

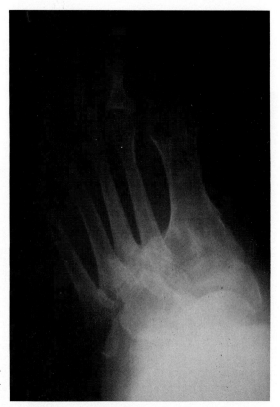

FIG 8-25.
AP view showing complete consolidation and revascularization after 8 months using ambulatory total contact casting.

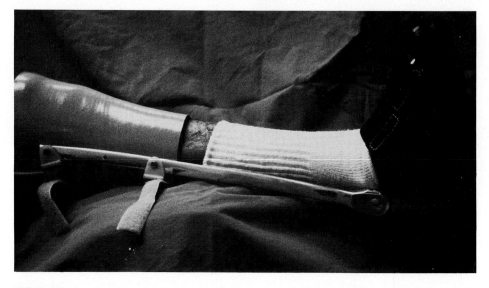

FIG 8-26.
Molded shoe with tridensity inserts and bracing to lock foot in place and allow body weight to gently roll over foot during ambulation.

Once consolidation has taken place and the patient is in a specially molded shoe to accommodate the deformity, new bony prominences must be monitored closely. If stress corrective techniques do not maintain the integrity of the skin, then surgical procedures are appropriate to reduce the bony prominence and therefore reduce the potential for further breakdown.

Acknowledgment

The author wishes to thank William Coleman, D.P.M., Former Chief of Podiatry, National Hanson's Disease Center in Carville, Louisiana, for numerous informal conversations during the decade of the 1980s.

REFERENCES

1. Most RS, Sinnock P: The epidemiology of lower extremity amputations in diabetic individuals, *Diabetes Care* 6, 1983.
2. Bild DE et al: Lower extremity amputation in people with diabetes epidemiology and prevention, *Diabetes Care* 12:1, 1989.
3. Polumbo PJ, Melton LJ: Peripheral vascular disease and diabetes. Diabetes in America, NIH Publication No 85, Washington, DC, 1984, US Government Printing Office.
4. Levin ME, O'Neil LW: *The diabetic foot: pathophysiology, evaluation and treatment,* ed 4, St Louis, 1988, Mosby-Year Book.
5. Ecker LM, Jacobs BS: Lower extremity amputations and diabetic patients, *Diabetes* 19:189, 1970.
6. McCullough NC et al: Bilateral BKA in patients over 50 years of age, *J Bone Joint Surg* 54A:1217, 1972.
7. Bodily KC, Burgess EM: Contralateral limb and patient survival after leg amputation, *Am J Surg* 146:280, 1983.
8. LoGerfo FW, Coffman JD: Vascular and microvascular disease of the foot in dia-
betes, *N Engl J Med* 311:1615–1619, 1984.
9. Strandness DE Jr, Priest RE, Gibbons GE: Combined clinical and pathologic study of diabetic and nondiabetic peripheral arterial disease, *Diabetes* 13:366–372, 1964.
10. Conrad NC: Large and small artery occlusion in diabetics and nondiabetics with severe vascular disease, *Circulation* 36:83–91, 1967.
11. Brand PW: The insensitive foot (including leprosy). Seminars and Lecture Series on the Insensitive Foot, U.S. Public Health Service Hospital, Carville, La.
12. Brand PW: personal correspondence with author, 1983.
13. Ellenberg M, Rifkin H: *Diabetes mellitus, theory and practice,* ed 3.
14. Jahss NH: *Disorders of the foot.* vol 2, p 1280.
15. Lowe SV, Ruderman RJ, Goldner JL: The management of intractable ulcerations in the neurologically impaired and the dysvascular foot, *Orthop Transact J* 6:185, 1982.
16. Tredwell JL: Treatment of complications of the diabetic foot, *J Foot Surg* 26:555–556, 1987.
17. Bell-Krotoski J, Tomancik E: The repeatability of testing with Semmes-Weinstein monofilaments, *J Hand Surg* 12A:155–161, 1987.
18. Bell JA: Semmes-Weinstein monofilament testing for determining cutaneous light touch/deep pressure sensation, *The Star* November/December 1984.
19. Birke JA, Sims DS: Plantar sensory threshold in the ulcerative foot, *Lepr Rev* 57:261–267, 1986.

BIBLIOGRAPHY

Boulton AJM et al: Dynamic foot pressure and other studies as diagnostic and management aids in diabetic neuropathy, *Diabetes Care* 6:1, 1983.
Duckworth T et al: Plantar pressure measurements and the prevention of ulceration in the diabetic foot, *J Bone Joint Surg* 167B:, 1985.

Helm TA, Walker SC: Total contact casting
in diabetic patients with neuropathic foot
ulcerations, *Arch Phys Med Rehabil*
65:691–693, 1984.

Kosiak M: Etiology and pathology of ischemic ulcers, *Arch Phys Med Rehabil* 40:62,
1959.

Omer GE Jr, Spinner M: *Management of peripheral nerve problems,* Philadelphia, WB
Saunders.

Pollard JP, Le-Quesne LP: Method of healing
diabetic forefoot ulcers, *Br Med J*
286:1236–1237, 1983.

9 A Clinical Guide to the Charcot Foot

Alan S. Banks, D.P.M.

Charcot foot is a progressive condition that affects multiple tissues in the lower extremity. The process has classically been characterized by pathologic fractures and/or dislocations resulting in variable degrees of deformity, dysfunction, and additional complications. Due to the obvious radiographic changes, many physicians have used the term "neuroarthropathy" to denote the condition. However, more than just the osseous structures are affected, and therefore, the term Charcot foot is preferred.

For a Charcot foot to develop, there must be some underlying neurologic deficit. In the past, Charcot foot was associated with tabes dorsalis. Today, diabetes mellitus is the most common disease state related with this condition. The exact prevalence of Charcot foot within the diabetic population is not certain. A prevalence ranging from 0.16%[1] to 2.4%[2] has been reported. These studies are somewhat dated, however, and one might expect that there would be an increase in the number of limbs affected as management techniques for treating diabetes improve. It is feasible that as these individuals live longer they may begin to sustain more of the complications related to diabetes such as Charcot foot.

There are a large number of conditions other than diabetes that may lead to a Charcot foot (Table 9–1). Furthermore, not all diabetics will have a Charcot foot. The clinical manifestations of neuropathy are dependent on the magnitude and duration of the injury as well as the types of nerve fibers that are affected. Although the emphasis of this book is on diabetes, the principles are applicable to any patient with a Charcot foot regardless of the underlying disease.

DISTAL SYMMETRICAL POLYNEUROPATHY

In some circles the diabetic foot has become known as the insensitive foot because many of these patients develop sensory deficits as a result of the peripheral neuropathy. However, there is also the implication that the only neurologic aberrations are sensory. Patients with Charcot foot have both autonomic and motor nerve fibers affected, usually to an equal degree. Distal symmetrical diabetic polyneuropathy is believed to involve all three fiber types in approximately 70% of the patients.[3] The motor and autonomic components of the neuropathy, however, have been largely ignored despite their profound influence on the lower extremity. A basic knowledge of these features of the neuropathy is essential to understand the Charcot process and for optimal care.

Sensory Neuropathy

The role of sensory deficits in the pathogenesis of diabetic foot problems has been

TABLE 9–1.

Outline of Diseases and Processes Resulting in a
Neuropathic Foot*

> I. Neuropathy associated with systemic disease
>   Diabetes mellitus
>   Uremia
>   Amyloidosis
> II. Neuropathy associated with nutritional distur-
>   bances
>   Alcoholism
>   Pernicious anemia
> III. Neuropathy associated with infectious diseases
>   Leprosy
>   Syphilis
>   Poliomyelitis
> IV. Neuropathy on a vascular basis
>   Cerebral vascular accident
>   Spinal cord infarction
>   Diabetic mononeuropathy
>   Arteritis
>   Peripheral vascular disease
> V. Hereditary motor and sensory neuropathy
>   (HMSN)
>   Roussy-Lévy syndrome
>   Charcot-Marie-Tooth disease
> VI. Hereditary sensory and autonomic neuropathy
>   (HSAN)
>   Hereditary sensory neuropathy
>   Congenital sensory neuropathy
>   Dysautonomia (Riley-Day syndrome)
> VII. Cerebellar degeneration
>   Friedreich's ataxia
> VIII. Motor neuron disease
>   Amyotrophic lateral sclerosis
> IX. Diseases of the spinal cord
>   Spina bifida
>   Syringomyelia
> X. Trauma
>   Spinal cord injury
>   Peripheral nerve injury
>   Spinal root trauma
> XI. Compressive neuropathy
>   Spinal cord tumor
>   Peripheral nerve compression
> XII. Toxic Neuropathy
>   Lead poisoning
> XIII. Other
>   Cerebral palsy

*From Heatherington VJ: The neuropathic foot. In McGlamry
ED, Banks AS, Downey MS, editors: *Comprehensive textbook
of foot surgery,* ed 2, Baltimore, 1992, Williams & Wilkins,
p 1352.

appropriately emphasized in recent years. Insensitivity places the extremity at risk regardless of the cause of neuropathy. However, loss of sensation is not the primary component involved in the development of a Charcot foot, as evidenced by the large number of patients with sensory neuropathy, yet the relatively small number of these individuals with Charcot foot.

Autonomic Neuropathy

Within the lower extremity, the functions of the autonomic nervous system are provided by the sympathetic fibers. The primary function of the sympathetic nerves is to effect vasodilation and vasoconstriction of the small arterioles. When the autonomic nerves are impaired, these vessels lose their constrictive tone and the arterioles remain dilated. Consequently, there is an increase in the vascular perfusion to the extremity. A clinical examination will reveal a warm foot with diffuse swelling and distention in the venous tree. This has been termed "neuropathic edema." The integument will be dry due to associated aberrations in sweat gland function, although the xerosis may presumptively be attributed to tinea pedis. To compensate, the patient may sweat profusely over the trunk and upper extremities.

In more recent years a greater understanding of the vascular implications of diabetes has been derived, particularly in relation to autonomic neuropathy. Previous studies[4] that indicated an increase in blood flow to the lower extremities of diabetic patients have led to the finding that the venous PO_2 of those with neuropathy is much higher than that of control subjects.[5] In some patients, the PO_2 in the veins is comparable to that of the arteries.[6] Increased arteriovenous shunting is postulated as the cause for this phenomena, which in turn could be attributed to autonomic neuropathy.[5] The administration of ephedrine, a sympathomimetic agent, is noted to reduce the neuropathic edema and create a more normal triphasic vascular pattern via Doppler evaluation, confirming the role of the sympathetic fibers in this process.[7]

In addition to neuropathic edema, patients are noted to possess resting skin temperatures as much as 5° C to 8° C higher than nondiabetics or diabetics without neuropathy. Skin blood flow is increased at both the hallux and midfoot levels on average five times greater than controls.[8] When technetium scans are performed in diabetics with neuropathy, a greater perfusion of the isotope is demonstrated in all three phases, again representative of the relative hypervascularity to the foot.[9]

Increased rigidity of the vessels, increased blood flow velocities, and medial arterial wall calcification are noted in diabetics with peripheral neuropathy. Radiographic evidence of vascular calcification is noted in a large number of diabetics and is not related to the age, severity, or duration of the disease, but to the degree of neuropathy. This prompted Edmonds et al. to report that this phenomena is a specific complication of diabetes and is associated with neuropathy.[12]

In reviewing two large studies of Charcot foot, 78% and 90% of the patients, respectively, demonstrate radiographic evidence of vascular calcification.[1, 13] This same vascular calcification in the foot is noted in both diabetics and nondiabetics several years after undergoing surgical sympathectomy.[14] Experimental findings demonstrate that once sympathetic tone is interrupted the muscles within the media of the arterioles atrophy, then secondarily calcify.[15] Furthermore, patients with medial arterial calcification demonstrate normal transcutaneous oxygen levels both at rest[10] and with exercise.[11] Therefore, radiographic evidence of vascular calcification should not be interpreted as representative of occlusive vascular disease, but as representative of autonomic neuropathy.

Vascular calcification may prevent the clinician from palpating the pedal pulses. The stiff arterial wall also makes occlusion of the vessel more difficult, which falsely elevates the ankle arm index.[12] Therefore, other noninvasive tests may prove more accurate in assessing peripheral arterial flow.

The peripheral hyperemia that ensues with autonomic neuropathy does not selectively affect the soft tissues. Several investigators have shown that the bones are highly innervated by sympathetic nerves and that sympathectomy results in an increase in bone blood flow between 10% to 115%.[16–19] This creates an osteopenia that may weaken the skeleton. Diabetic patients with neuropathy have been noted to have a significantly lower bone mass in both the hands and feet, although the greater osteopenia was found in the feet.[20] Therefore, the degree of osteopenia correlates with the distribution of the sympathetic fibers.

Several authors have specifically noted evidence of autonomic neuropathy in their studies of Charcot feet.[1, 21, 22] However, in most instances the method used to diagnose sympathetic dysfunction has been to correlate information regarding autonomic integrity in more proximal areas (i.e., cardiac function, gastrointestinal symptoms) and extrapolate this to the lower extremity. Obviously, this is not specific or accurate. It is reasonable to presume that these small nerve fibers are affected early in the disease process, certainly prior to more proximal involvement.[8, 23, 24, 25]

The scientific advances that demonstrate hyperemia within the neuropathic foot only confirm what some physicians have known for years: that many diabetics possess adequate circulation for healing, contrary to standard medical dogma. Although there is a large volume of data that demonstrate that diabetics have macrovascular disease, to date there is still no objective evidence that diabetics have a greater incidence of occlusive peripheral microvascular disease. This concern is still cited, however, as the reason for inadequate foot care in many patients.[26] Furthermore, studies indicate that capillary ischemia is not a feature of diabetic neuropathy under resting conditions.[27]

Motor Neuropathy

Impairment of motor nerves in the lower extremity may create muscular imbalances that predispose the foot to more acute complications. The intrinsic muscles of the foot are usually affected initially. In fact, Lippman has referred to the diabetic foot as the "intrinsic minus" foot.[2] Losing intrinsic muscle function will permit the development of digital contractures. This may occur as a result of swing phase (extensor substitution) or stance phase (flexor stabilization) imbalance. Either condition may be present as a consequence of a deformity that was present prior to the onset of neuropathy. Flexor stabilization may develop as a consequence of insensitivity as the patient actively grasps with the toes in an attempt to compensate for the loss of proprioception. A rocker-bottom Charcot foot may also lead to the development of hammertoes because the intrinsic muscles will usually atrophy significantly following tarsal collapse.

Regardless of the specific factors involved, once the digit is contracted it is now susceptible to irritation at the dorsal aspect of the proximal interphalangeal joint and the distal pulp. The nail will begin to thicken as the toe bears weight on the distal tip. This should not be errantly dismissed as onychomycosis. Contracture usually progresses to involve the metatarsophalangeal joint so that the vectors of force about that level are significantly altered. The retrograde force against the metatarsal head is now directed plantarly, which increases weight-bearing pressure in the ball of the foot. This pressure increases the risk of hyperkeratosis or ulceration.

Muscle imbalance does not necessarily limit itself to the foot. Quite often the anterior leg muscles, or extensors, will become weakened. At times this is profound enough to create a drop foot. In other less remarkable cases, there is enough weakness to result in a loss of the normal muscle antagonism. Therefore, the posterior musculature, particularly the gastrosoleal complex, gains a mechanical advantage and an ankle equinus deformity develops.

Equinus creates several unfavorable circumstances in the neuropathic foot including the exacerbation of digital deformity. In an attempt to achieve adequate dorsiflexion, the extensor muscles will fire prematurely, creating an extensor substitution. This either assists in the creation or progression of digital and metatarsal contractures. Additionally, the tight heel cord will independently increase plantar weight-bearing and shearing forces in the forefoot as the patient propels in gait. This will also help the development of calluses and tissue compromise.

An ankle equinus results in excessive stress being applied to other areas of the foot. As the patient enters the propulsive phase of gait, 10° of dorsiflexion will be required for normal function.[28] If this motion is not available at the ankle, then the patient will usually create the necessary motion through excessive pronation and by breeches within the joints of the foot. This most often affects the midtarsal or tarsometatarsal articulations. The stress that is applied may lead to hyperostosis or an acute Charcot collapse. Once present, plantar prominences at the midfoot are subjected to greater stress, encouraging ulceration. Probably one of the most common sources of failure for conservative care measures in the Charcot foot is the failure of the physician to appreciate and treat the coexisting ankle equinus deformity (Fig 9–1).

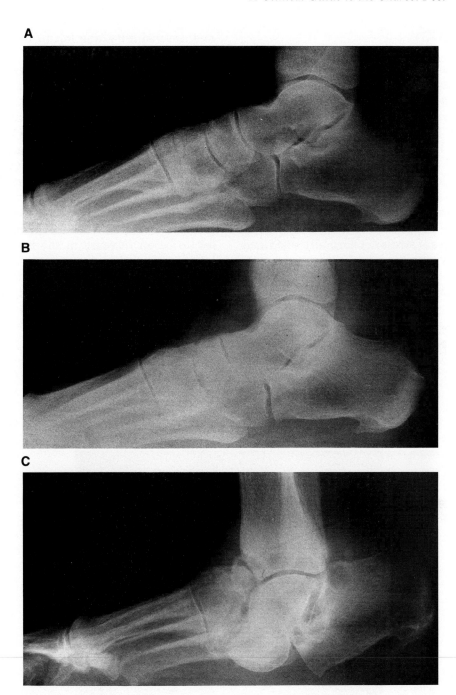

FIG 9–1.
A, B, lateral radiographs of a 62-year-old diabetic female. Note the increased joint space at the calcaneocuboid joint of the left foot. This patient possesses a significant gastrosoleal equinus. **C,** the same patient 1 year later following an acute Charcot collapse. The equinus deformity was not addressed previously, thereby creating unnecessary bending forces within the foot in compensation for the lack of ankle motion. This picture clearly depicts how the tight achilles will use the calcaneus as a long lever arm and create a potentially disruptive force at the weakest areas of the foot.

ETIOLOGY

Theories regarding the etiology of Charcot foot have not always been consistent. In part, this has been due to the two different radiographic appearances of neuroarthropathy. The variant most commonly noted is the hypertrophic form that is characterized by deformity and a proliferative or fairly dense osseous reaction with healing (Fig 9–2). For years it was proposed that the loss of sensation to the affected part allowed the patient to subject the joint to extremes of stress not normally sustained, thereby resulting in fractures. An exuberant repair process then followed. This was termed the neurotraumatic theory

and, insensitivity was felt to be the primary factor in the development.

Another less common variety of Charcot joint was also noted in some individuals. Conversely, one witnessed a resorption of bone from the affected area, sometimes termed diabetic osteolysis (Fig 9–3). The classic rationale for this presentation was that a hyperemic response within the limb created a resorption of bone prior to or as opposed to healing. This was termed the hypervascular theory and the primary factor in the development was felt to be an increase in the local circulation.

Experimental confirmation of the neurotraumatic theory was said to have

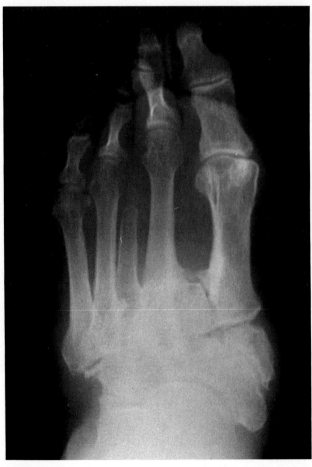

FIG 9–2.
Hypertrophic form of neuroarthropathy with dense bone formation.

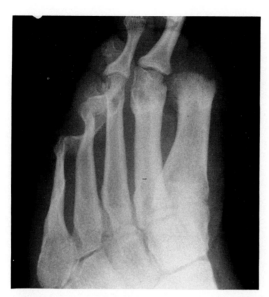

FIG 9–3.
Atrophic form of neuroarthropathy affecting the distal metatarsals. Notice the resorption of bone at this level.

been attained by Eloesser in 1917.[29] He sectioned the posterior nerve roots to the lower extremity in 38 cats. Of these specimens, 27 were later noted to have developed neuropathic joint changes. Other animals had joint injuries created either before or after the transection of the posterior nerve root. Eloesser noted that the animals that had the nerve roots sectioned first demonstrated greater degenerative changes within the joint. He concluded from this data that trauma was required in the insensitive limb for the initiation of a Charcot joint. This work was believed to confirm the neurotraumatic theory. With few exceptions, this was accepted as the means by which a Charcot joint developed.

In 1981 Brower and Allman reviewed the concepts regarding the cause of the Charcot joint.[30] This was prompted by several key observations following review of a number of cases. Brower and Allman noted that trauma could not account for the tremendous resorption of bone seen in a number of their patients, particularly patients whose upper extremity joints

were affected or in bedridden patients. Furthermore, in 32% of those patients studied the patients possessed joint pain and demonstrated no evidence of neurologic disease. Twenty-three percent of the patients had sustained spontaneous fractures without antecedent trauma or unusual activity. Eloesser's work was thought to be erroneous and poorly reasoned because all possible factors were not considered. Brower and Allman concluded that insensitivity alone could not account for the Charcot process; rather there had to be some underlying osseous abnormality as well. It was proposed that the weakened skeletal structure was related to autonomic neuropathy.

Reinhardt described four radiographic findings within the foot that preceded the onset of diabetes in a number of patients: pathologic fracture of the lesser metatarsal head resembling a Freiberg's infraction, ankylosis of the interphalangeal joints, collapse of the proximal phalanx of the hallux, and arthritic changes within the midfoot (Figs 9–4 and 9–5).[31] Most of these patients failed to demonstrate any evidence of sensory neuropathy and initially tested negative for diabetes, only to become diabetic later. A prediabetic phase with episodes of hyperglycemia may be the source of these injuries. It is reasonable to assume that the small unmyelinated autonomic fibers are most likely to be affected early in the disease process, thereby weakening bone and allowing these types of injuries to develop.[8, 23, 24] The presence of these findings should prompt one to refer the patient for appropriate evaluation to rule out diabetes and to take a proactive role in affecting the foot.

Later studies involving laboratory animals confirmed that trauma was a contributing factor in the development of neuroarthropathy, but not a primary factor.[32] Therefore, a relative weakness exists in the osseous tissues. The limb is then subjected to greater stresses due to mechan-

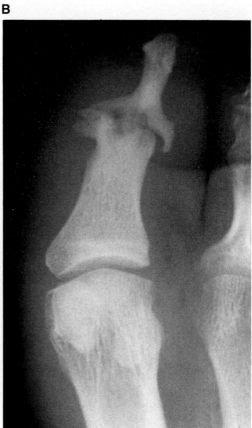

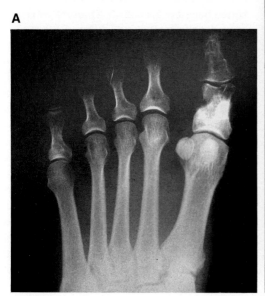

FIG 9–4.
A, previously undiagnosed diabetic female with changes in the hallux resembling fracture. **B,** ankylosis of the interphalangeal joint in the diabetic male.

ical imbalances that may be attributed to or aggravated by motor neuropathy. Sensory neuropathy will ensure that these destructive forces go unnoticed and places the osseous structures in greater jeopardy (Fig 9–6).

Limited Joint Mobility

Limited joint mobility may contribute to Charcot collapse. Diabetes results in a premature aging of collagen, which is mediated through a nonenzymatic binding of glucose to collagen. This increases the cross-links between the molecules and reduces elasticity. The hand was first noted to be affected by this process. Contractures develop at the interphalangeal joints, followed by reduced motion in active extension, then passive motion.[33] Limited joint mobility may be demonstrated clinically by the inability of the patient to completely flatten the palm and fingers on a tabletop. Another finding is the inability to completely approximate the fingers in a praying position (Fig 9–7).

Limited joint mobility has also been noted in the lower extremity. Patients with foot ulceration have been reported to possess a significant reduction in subtalar joint motion compared to control patients or other diabetics.[34, 35] These patients also demonstrate a significant association of limited joint mobility in the hand. Furthermore, limited joint mobility has also

B

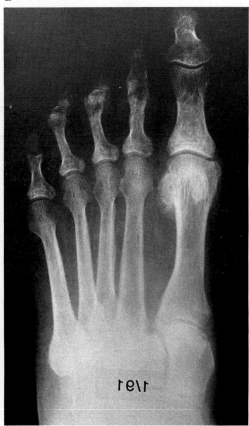

A

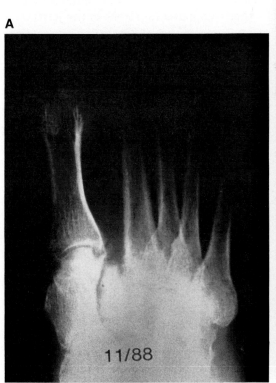

11/88

re\r

FIG 9–5.
A, patient seen with pain and swelling involving the midfoot demonstrating a partial LisFranc dislocation without antecedent trauma. Although there was no history of diabetes, the patient was sent for evaluation that proved to be negative. **B,** radiographic appearance more than 2 years later following conservative management. Several months prior the patient developed overt diabetes.

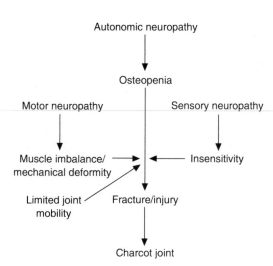

FIG 9–6.
Evolution of Charcot joints. (Modified from Heatherington VJ: The neuropathic foot. In McGlamry ED, Banks AS, Downey MS, editors: *Comprehensive textbook of foot surgery,* ed 2, Baltimore, 1992.)

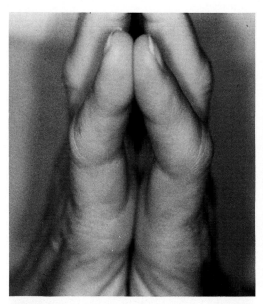

FIG 9–7.
The inability to approximate the fingers in a praying position is a simple clinical test for limited joint mobility. (From Banks AS, McGlamry ED: Charcot foot, *J Am Podiat Med Assoc* 79:213–235, 1989. Used by permission.)

been found in association with abnormally high plantar foot pressures.[35]

Just as these increased pressures render the neuropathic foot more susceptible to ulceration, the patient is similarly placed at a greater risk for fracture or

joint dislocation. Contractures that may have originally developed secondary to faulty biomechanics or motor neuropathy tend to become fixed and inflexible, further compounding stress to the joints.

MANAGEMENT OF THE ACUTE CHARCOT FOOT

The initial step in management of the acute Charcot foot is making an accurate diagnosis. The classic example is a foot that is grossly edematous, erythematous, and warm with good pedal pulses. Some patients who have this condition are mistakenly hospitalized with a presumptive cellulitis or thrombophlebitis. The severe edema and erythema that may accompany this acute phase may alarm individuals unfamiliar with Charcot joint disease, particularly physicians who believe that all diabetics have poor circulation (Fig 9–8). These patients may possess some level of pain that may be vague and poorly localized due to sensory neuropathy. This reinforces the unsuspecting physician's belief that this is not so much a localized process, but more general in nature. Accordingly, radiographs may not be performed.

A

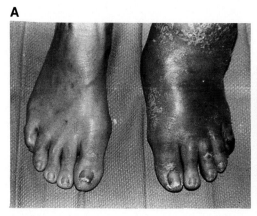

B

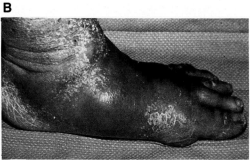

FIG 9–8.
A, B, clinical appearance of this patient with an acute Charcot episode. To the untrained clinician this may be mistaken for an acute phlebitis or cellulitis. (From Banks AS, McGlamry ED: Charcot foot, *J Am Podiat Med Assoc* 79:213–235, 1989. Used by permission.)

Even with more experienced practitioners a high index of suspicion is necessary to diagnose the more subtle initial findings that may be present. Not every patient will present with the classic symptoms mentioned here. Any diabetic who has either a painful or swollen extremity must be considered to potentially possess a Charcot foot, even if radiographs are negative. In some instances the initial phase of the process may be joint effusion. In others it may be a stress fracture or dislocation that has spontaneously reduced, and therefore, is not readily evident on radiographs. A very important clinical finding in those with an acute or impending Charcot process is an increase in the temperature to the extremity. Any increase in temperature to the foot should alert the clinician to institute protective measures.

Patients with either a confirmed or suspected acute Charcot episode should have the part immediately immobilized and weight-bearing eliminated. The goal is to heal any fractures and resolve any inflammation. This is best served with complete non-weight-bearing. Otherwise, healing and resolving the inflammation will be more difficult and prolonged. This stress may also allow the acute process to progress and involve other anatomic areas or render a foot with less ultimate stability. Crutches or a walker may be adequate to allow the patient continued ambulation while awaiting recovery. However, this may place additional stress on the contralateral extremity and increase the risk for potential complications at that level, including fracture and dislocation. Therefore, the temporary use of a wheelchair may prove most suitable to reduce the patient's overall risk.

Immobilization may take one of several forms. Initially the swelling may be extensive and several cast changes may be required prior to the permanent cast being applied. Serial Jones compression-type casts work well during this early acute period and once the edema has stabilized a more permanent device can be used. If the foot is flexible then one may manipulate the part to try and achieve a more favorable alignment during consolidation. The cast should be examined periodically to ensure a good fit and to identify any potential irritation.

Some individuals advocate the use of a total contact cast for this purpose. This well-fitted plaster device is a suitable means of assuring good immobilization with excellent molding capacity. The contact cast has been designed as a weight-bearing device. A complete description of this casting technique is included in Chapter 13. However, non-weight-bearing is still preferred by this author during the recovery period for the reasons previously outlined.

For physicians who are fearful of placing a neuropathic patient into a closed cast a bivalved cast may work well and allow periodic examination of the foot for any potential problems. This may be particularly helpful when there is a coexisting ulcer that will require attention. However, the bivalved cast will not provide the same degree of circumferential compression, and the tissue may become pinched when the cast is reapplied. Although this does not typically lead to cutaneous compromise, the localized congestion may impede healing of any adjacent ulcers.

Immobilization and non-weight-bearing should be continued until adequate consolidation of the osseous structures is demonstrated radiographically and until all clinical signs of inflammation have resolved. Clinically one will first notice the dissipation of erythema followed by a loss of edema. This is reflected by the return of normal color and skin lines to the foot. The warmth of the affected area will be the last component to resolve. Although otherwise the foot may appear truly recovered, one should wait until the temperature of the two extremities is symmetrical. Prior to this time, the structures

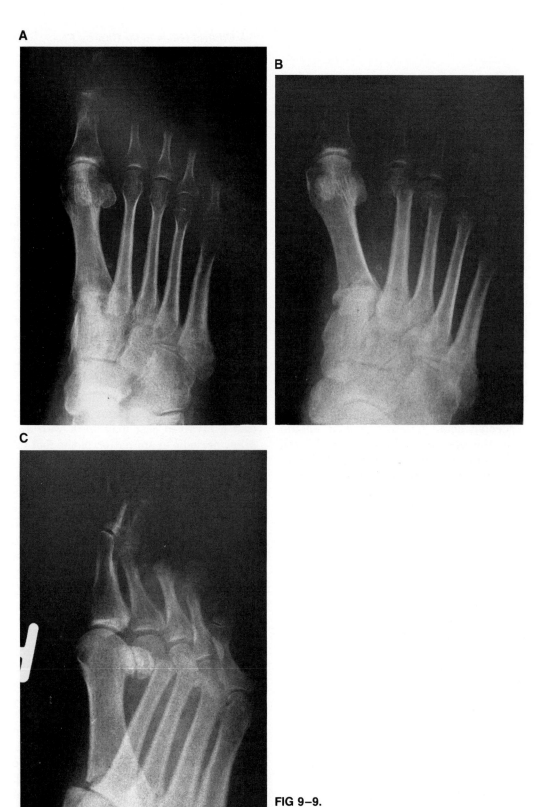

FIG 9–9.
A, radiographic appearance of this 42-year-old diabetic following removal of a below-knee cast and reinstitution of weight-bearing for a fracture of the fifth metatarsal base. The patient was sent to physical therapy where overly aggressive measures were instituted. **B, C,** several weeks later, appearance demonstrating fractures of the first metatarsal base and lesser metatarsal necks.

are still undergoing healing and any weight-bearing stress may risk further damage. Just as an increase in the temperature of the foot may be the harbinger of impending collapse, the complete dissipation of this thermal gradient represents complete resolution of the inflammation.

Once consolidation has been achieved and the inflammation has resolved, the patient may begin the progressive return to weight-bearing. This is a crucial period. Although there may be good radiographic evidence of healing, it may be difficult to accurately determine the ability of the osseous tissues to withstand full weight-bearing stress. In addition, the bone has been further weakened by disuse so that it may be difficult for the foot to abruptly adapt from a non-weight-bearing mode to unsupported weight-bearing without compromise. Therefore, some form of assisted support is used during a transition period. This may either be a weight-bearing cast or a removable brace. The patient is allowed restricted ambulation, aided by crutch or walker, for several weeks and then re-evaluated clinically and radiographically. The period of weight-bearing is then gradually increased and finally the patient is allowed to walk without the brace. In some instances a double upright brace may be used as a further protective measure for several months (Fig 9–9).

The rehabilitation process should be immediately discontinued if there is any evidence of an increased temperature to the part. Immobilization and non-weight-bearing are then reinstituted until the inflammation has subsided.

MANAGEMENT OF THE CHRONIC CHARCOT FOOT

Once the rehabilitation process is nearing completion the clinician must assess what measures will be required to reduce the likelihood of further complications within the foot. Several factors must be considered. For example, the osseous tissues may fuse during the process of healing and create a stable condition. If the position and alignment are sufficient, this is a favorable circumstance (Fig 9–10).

The overall configuration of the foot should be viewed and an assessment made of any prominences that will need to be accommodated. The natural inclination is to circumferentially build up around plantar protuberances to create a pocket within the orthotic device or innersole of the shoe. However, in the midfoot area this should be done in a judicious manner for if there is available motion within the joints distal to the prominence then aberrant stress may be applied across the dorsal joint interface. This will encourage greater plantar buckling and exacerbation of the deformity. Generally, when a large deep pocket is required it is safer to provide the bulk of the accommodation proximal to the prominence to avoid this wedging effect (Fig 9–11).

The patient should be closely examined for any evidence of equinus. If present, this powerful deforming influence must be accommodated or else the foot is left at infinitely greater risk. Even in static stance, the tight heel cord applies a constant bending force to the foot that will aggravate plantar weight-bearing pressures. Therefore, if this deformity is neglected one may find a greater risk of ulceration or else an acute Charcot episode. The majority of the effects of equinus may be alleviated by elevating the heel of the shoe so that when the patient is standing the achilles is not placed under undue tension. Commonly this will require a 1- to 1½-inch heel raise above the level of the sole.

External bracing is another modality often overlooked by many clinicians that affords an extra measure of protection for the foot at risk. The two types of braces generally used are the double upright and patellar tendon braces. Generally

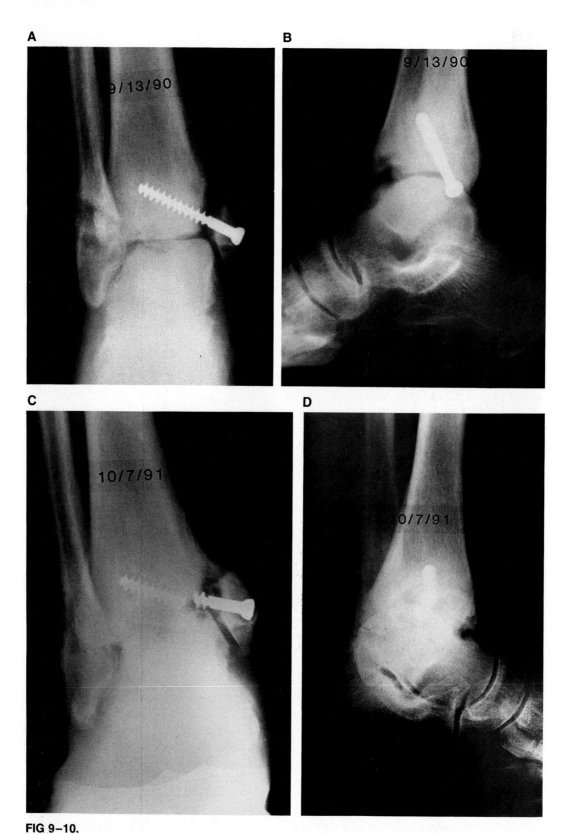

FIG 9–10.
A, B, diabetic male treated at another institution with this bimalleolar ankle fracture almost 7 months prior. **C, D,** acute Charcot episode 1 month later with im-paction of the talus. **E, F,** 5 months after cast immo-bilization and electrical bone stimulation. At this point the ankle has arthrodesed in good clinical alignment.

(Continued.)

E
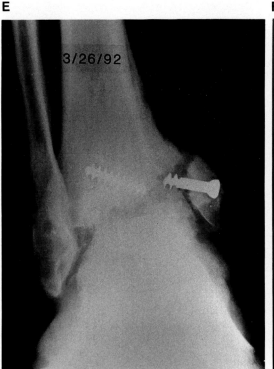

F
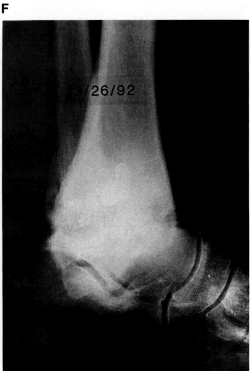

FIG 9–10 (cont.).
For legend see opposite page.

the double upright brace is fashioned with either limited or no ankle motion and may be combined with a rocker sole to further reduce bending stress. The patellar tendon brace acts similarly while also reducing some of the vertical loading force to the foot. However, these devices alone will not compensate for a tight heel cord. As discussed previously, additional measures regarding the shoe may be required (Fig 9–12).

The actual shoe selection will be based largely on the overall deformity and the required accommodation. Patients with primary sagittal plane collapse may do fine with a full-depth oxford if there is adequate space for an appropriate orthotic device or innersole. The foot demonstrating transverse plane abduction may be difficult to fit and may therefore require molded shoes.

The patient should be trained to ex-

amine the foot daily for any suspicious findings that might indicate an impending problem, particularly a localized increase in temperature.

SURGICAL TREATMENT OF CHARCOT FOOT DEFORMITIES

The gross deformity and instability that may accompany Charcot foot condition renders the patient more susceptible to ulcerations and infection. Even in the best of circumstances there will be some patients who fare poorly with appropriate conservative measures. These individuals may eventually undergo amputation as an expeditious means of alleviating an acute process or after futile attempts to prevent multiple complications in an otherwise hopelessly deformed foot.

Classic surgical intervention to sal-

A

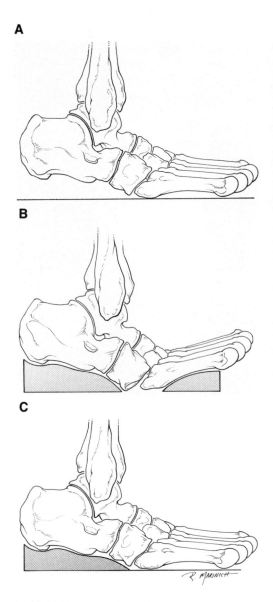

B

C

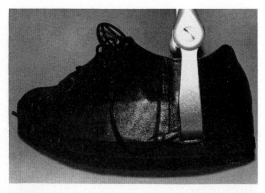

FIG 9–12.
Typical accommodative shoe for a patient with a chronic Charcot foot. This is a molded shoe with a slight rocker sole. Notice the heel raise incorporated into shoe for management of equinus. Double upright brace with no ankle motion is attached.

FIG 9–11.
A, lateral view of Charcot foot with equinus and hypermobility of the midfoot. **B,** the natural inclination when attempting to pad plantar prominence is to pad circumferentially around the area. However, if mobility is present, then deformity may only be accentuated. **C,** in these instances it is usually better to provide the bulk or all of the padding proximal to the prominence.

vage the limb has been avoided in the diabetic except for patients with infection, and then surgery has usually been ablative, but on a more limited extent. Many patients have succumbed to amputation of some form with little thought as to what could be done to prevent others from reaching the same outcome. Other diabetic patients possess significant foot deformities, yet receive only conservative care. Generally, this results from a fear on the part of the surgeon that this patient population will not recover from elective procedures successfully. However, the same patients may continue to recover well from multiple aggressive debridements for infection. Certainly in this modern day there must be a better way of assessing these patients, many of whom are placed at a great risk for complications due to the degree of foot deformity and the concomitant loss of sensation.

Perhaps the greatest concern for many physicians is the vascular supply to the lower extremity. Despite many years of misinformation, there is no objective evidence that diabetics are at a greater risk for the development of occlusive peripheral microvascular disease,[26] although this patient population is certainly at risk for large vessel compromise. There are a number of reliable noninvasive tests that can be performed to determine the vascular supply to the extremity. Unfortunately, contradicting many years of medical dogma is difficult. This has led most physicians to immediately dismiss any definitive treatment of diabetic foot deformities based on the errant belief that these patients do not possess the vascular capacity to heal. Most of these individuals misinform their patients without even discussing with them the option of undergoing an appropriate vascular evaluation. Furthermore, all authorities agree that good circulation is a prerequisite for the development of a Charcot foot. The data discussed earlier should confirm the circulatory capacity of the limb with neuroarthropathy. Once the physician understands the vascular capacity of the Charcot foot, further attention can be directed toward finding measures to reduce the risk for this patient population.

There are many surgical measures that may benefit the Charcot foot. Defining specific criteria for each procedure is difficult. However, basic guidelines may be established for consideration. Before determining which approach may be most advantageous, several need to be assessed.

The level of serum albumin and the total lymphocyte count appear to have a correlation with the potential for healing in diabetic feet, but the specifics have yet to be understood. Studies indicate that patients undergoing distal amputations (transmetatarsal or Symes) have distinct success when the total lymphocyte count is greater than 1,500/cu mm, and the serum albumin is either at least 3.0 mg/dl or 3.5 mg/dl preoperatively.[37, 38] In another study of diabetic patients undergoing transmetatarsal amputation, those who healed had an average albumin level of 3.6 compared to 3.08 for those with failed procedures. The total serum protein level appeared to demonstrate no specific correlation with the success of the procedure.[39]

The total lymphocyte count is thought to be somewhat representative of the patient's capacity to resist infection. The albumin level reflects the nutritional status of the patient. However, in patients with advanced nephropathy, albuminuria may decrease the level significantly despite an appropriate diet. What correlation these findings have with regard to elective surgical procedures has yet to be determined. Although the early evidence appears to demonstrate that these two values have some merit, other factors are also likely to be involved.

Serum glucose levels greater than 200 mg/dl have also been implicated with impaired wound healing.[40] Certainly from an elective surgical standpoint there should be good perioperative management of the serum glucose.

PROCEDURES

Biopsy

Chronic ulcerations may be present without overt radiographic or clinical evidence of infection. Surgery may be considered in patients who possess chronic ulcers that have not responded to aggressive local wound care and a period of *non-weight-bearing*. Despite the various modalities available to the physician for treating and protecting the ulcerated foot, the best possible scenario for healing is the complete alleviation of pressure from the extremity.

In those patients who fail to respond to a period of non-weight-bearing one should rule out the presence of a chronic osteomyelitis. The definitive diagnosis of osteomyelitis is made with a bone biopsy. Therefore, obtaining a specimen of bone from the area should be considered. When an open wound is present, one may consider obtaining the biopsy at a site removed from the ulcerative area to minimize the risk that the bacteria colonizing the wound will contaminate the bone cultures. The ulcer may be covered with an occlusive dressing such as Opsite to further reduce contamination.

However, there will be instances where the bone is not readily accessible from a distant site. In particular, accessing plantar midfoot ulcers from dorsal incisions may not allow for an accurate biopsy. In these instances the procedure may be performed through the plantar aspect of the foot with concomitant excision of the ulcer. In either event the most important goal is to ensure that the specimen is obtained from the appropriate area.

There may be some cases where a definitive diagnosis of either osteomyelitis or Charcot joint cannot be made solely on the radiographic appearance. Some patients may possess both conditions. Therefore, when a bone specimen is obtained, synovial tissue may also be taken for a biopsy. The characteristic microscopic appearance of the synovial tissue in patients with a Charcot joint will consist of multiple shards of bone and soft tissue embedded in the deep layers of the synovium.[41]

The author feels that a bone biopsy offers several advantages over other modalities that may be considered to rule out infection. A biopsy is a *definitive* means of diagnosing osteomyelitis. Although a variety of radionuclide scans are available for use, the specificity of each in the face of a Charcot foot can be seriously questioned. Technetium scans frequently provide false positive results in patients with Charcot deformity. The level of bone activity is usually quite high regardless of the presence or absence of infection. The author is familiar with several patients who have undergone bone scans at the request of other consultants, who subsequently recommended amputation solely based upon the high degree of uptake in the osseous tissue. Subsequent bone biopsy revealed no evidence of osteomyelitis, thus sparing the extremity.

Magnetic resonance imaging may offer a better noninvasive means of assessing the osseous tissues. However, the res-olution of the scans in the smaller bones of the foot may be somewhat lacking.

Exostosectomy

Reduction of an osseous prominence responsible for a current or potential ulceration is one of the indications for elective surgery in the Charcot foot. The sites most commonly affected are the midfoot or rearfoot areas. The most common pattern seen is the plantar dislocation of the cuneiforms or cuboid. As the triceps exert their deforming influence, the midfoot is wedged so that the proximal structures are forced plantarly with the distal segments or metatarsals assuming a more dorsal position. Intrinsic muscle atrophy eventually develops and reduces the soft tissue protection around these prominent areas. Persistent equinus continues to create extreme pressure across plantar aspect of the foot, particularly at the proximal side of the dislocation. As a consequence, significant compromise of the tissue may result.

A second type of plantar prominence occurs at the head of the talus. The site of primary dislocation in this instance is the subtalar and midtarsal joints. The talar head effectively adducts and significantly plantarflexes, which creates a medial bulge. At times the talus may completely dislocate from the calcaneus. A large degree of transverse plane deviation of the forefoot is usually evident. Because the talus usually maintains its alignment in the ankle mortise the full weight-bearing force is directed medially through the talar head and into the supporting surface.

A plantar medial prominence may be encountered when there is a lateral dislocation of the metatarsals upon the midfoot. Weight-bearing stress continues to be directed in a linear direction through the medial cuneiform, with the forefoot bearing an insufficient amount of weight.

An apparently simple way to alleviate

an osseous prominence is to perform an exostosectomy. However, one needs to assess the patient carefully prior to selecting this approach. The foremost consideration is to determine the overall stability of the foot. The foot must be consolidated and fairly rigid, otherwise further dislocation is likely and may negate the effects of the exostosectomy. If equinus is present then a tendoachillis lengthening should be performed. This will eliminate a powerful and destructive force from the foot. Equinus is usually intimately involved with the initial collapse, progression of further deformity, and an exacerbation of plantar pressure. Even in a stable foot an aggressive plantar exostosectomy could disrupt the osseous integrity enough to allow an uncompensated equinus to create further collapse.

The planal dominance of the collapse will also vary between patients. Some individuals will primarily demonstrate a sagittal plane deformity with little abduction or adduction. Others will have significant transverse plane involvement of a primary or secondary nature. Patients who have pure sagittal plane deformity will fare better with an exostosectomy than those with medial prominence due to significant abduction. In the foot with sagittal plane collapse one may adequately alleviate a problematic prominence of bone without an overly aggressive resection. However, to achieve a more favorable contour in a transverse plane deformity a greater excision of bone is usually required. Forefoot abduction may persist and weight-bearing will still be directed medial to the metatarsals. Although the prominence may be reduced, this medially directed vector of force may remain problematic unless the forefoot abduction is corrected.

Less often a significant degree of frontal plane rotation may also be noted. This usually manifests as a forefoot varus or an ankle varus deformity. Managing this component of deformity is more difficult with conservative or simple surgical measures.

Osseous prominences may create ulcers in these neuropathic feet despite appropriate conservative measures. Although it is usually preferable to have the ulcer healed prior to surgery, this is not always possible. With any nonhealing ulcer one must consider that there may be an underlying osteomyelitis. Usually it is almost impossible to achieve wound closure over infected bone.

However, factors other than infection may also preclude healing of a chronic ulcer. The chronic wound may have developed a mass of fibrotic tissue around the ulcer. This atrophic tissue may be present under an apparently granular ulcer bed, which misleads the clinician into believing that there is a good potential for healing. On the contrary, this fibrotic mass is avascular and impedes healing.

In some instances either the tendon sheath or joint capsule will have been compromised so that they are contiguous with the ulcer. Synovial fluid may now flow into the wound, macerating the tissue and increasing the local bacterial count. Wound healing will be difficult in this circumstance.

Osseous prominences may be treated surgically by exostosectomy. There are three basic ways to perform the surgery in the presence of an open wound. In some situations one may excise the offending portion of bone from an incision site removed from the ulceration as discussed previously. However, since the ulcer may be contiguous with the deep tissue or bone it may not provide any practical advantage. The bone removed should be submitted for biopsy and cultures. The ulcer may be debrided or excised and either allowed to granulate or closed primarily. The surgical incision is usually closed primarily.

Another technique involves the complete elliptical excision of the ulcer with resection of the offending bone through the same incision.[42] The wound is then closed primarily. Closed suction drainage can be used to reduce hematoma formation and allow the surgeon to culture the wound for any viable organisms. This technique offers two advantages: it may simplify the surgery and it directly eliminates any compromised tissue that might impede further healing. Furthermore, the initial primary closure will tend to reduce the overall time of disability.

The third means of exostosectomy consists of excising all soft tissue that is compromised or of questionable quality throughout the full extent of the wound. This may necessitate the removal of adjacent or contiguous tendon structures. Once the offending area of bone is reached the necessary amount of bone is resected and then submitted for microscopic evaluation. A specimen is also sent for bone culture. The wound is packed open pending pathologic evaluation of the bone.

Daily dressing changes are initiated on the second day following surgery. If the bone biopsies show there is no osteomyelitis then the wound may be closed primarily at a later time. However, at the time of surgery should the osseous tissues appear unviolated and good soft tissue integrity is present one may consider immediate primary closure. Should the bone later prove to contain osteomyelitis then the sutures may be removed to allow for any further care necessary.

Following surgery for an exostosectomy good supportive measures must be maintained to reduce the remaining stress to the foot. This is because other deformities will generally persist, albeit to a lesser degree.

Surgical Reconstruction

Surgical reconstruction of a Charcot foot is not new. However, few have seriously pursued this type of treatment, particularly in caring for diabetics. To a large extent this has been due to the miscon-

ceptions regarding the circulatory capacity of this patient population. Fear has prevailed over the indisputable evidence that patients with Charcot foot deformity possess good circulation. Although the process is not without risk, the alternative is usually even more unsettling. Even in this modern age many of these patients still undergo below-knee amputation for a Charcot foot. Those who do maintain the extremity usually are resigned to extremely limited activity.

Fusion of unstable joints or severely deformed feet provides a stable part that is in a much better position to accept weight-bearing stress. In many individuals this will eliminate recurrent ulcers, infection, further Charcot collapse, and in some instances loss of limb.

Lennox, in describing patients affected by leprosy, stated that surgery should not be delayed in a foot with bone and joint destruction where neuropathy is established.[43] The procedure of choice was noted to be arthrodesis, which was purported to stabilize the foot and "arrest an otherwise progressive condition." Early surgical intervention was advocated because success was more certain when there was a semblance of normal anatomy and prior to the development of gross deformity or destruction of osseous tissue. Lennox also cited Hodges as having successfully performed 15 triple arthrodeses in deformed lepromatous feet.

Harris and Brand[36] stated that they would consider fusion in a neuropathic foot where conservative measures had failed. Arthrodesis was generally successful when performed early in the disease process or at later intervals provided all of the diseased bone was resected. Immobilization generally took somewhat longer than comparable procedures in sensate feet. No follow-up or statistical information was provided.

Johnson[44] proposed more specific considerations for fusions in neuropathic joints. He emphasized the importance of awaiting the quiescent phase, adequate resection and good apposition of bone, supplementation with grafts when necessary, and effective prolonged immobilization until full healing was achieved. He felt that reconstruction of Charcot joints ". . . should be undertaken with great respect for the magnitude of the problem, but not with dread."

Johnson generally preferred tibial osteotomies as opposed to ankle arthrodeses. Triple arthrodeses and exostosectomies were deemed valuable in the foot. He proposed that, even if the joints did not fuse, the foot was aligned in a better position to withstand weight-bearing stress.

In their study of diabetic Charcot feet, Sinha et al,[1] noted that one of their patients underwent arthrodesis with equivocal results. However, these authors concluded that ". . . there is a need for evaluation of this form of treatment in a substantial number of patients with stable disease . . . ."

Warren indicated that it was advisable to surgically correct gross deformity when the foot could not be molded into a functional shape.[45] She later reported that she had performed over 4,000 surgical procedures in neuropathic patients due to a variety of diseases. Satisfactory results were noted in 39 of 48 patients who had undergone arthrodesis at the foot or ankle level at least 2 years prior to follow-up evaluation. She noted that arthrodesis failed only if external fixation was employed or if the patient was not immobilized an adequate period of time postoperatively.[46]

Charcot reconstruction as it related to diabetics was discussed by Banks and McGlamry.[47] Reconstruction was considered in patients where there was sufficient deformity or instability, when conservative care was unsuccessful, or where future complications could reasonably be anticipated. The prevention of below-knee amputation was considered a primary objective, especially in light of the dim future for most diabetic patients following the loss of limb.

Shibata et al. reported a fusion rate of 73% in Charcot ankle joints affected by leprosy.[48] The average follow-up period was 9 years. The authors noted that additional midtarsal destruction had been arrested and that none of the patients possessed ulcerations. Seven feet did develop ulcers postoperatively, but were managed with shoe modifications. Interestingly, even in the limbs where arthrodesis did not develop, the clinical symptoms were noted to resolve because it was possible to achieve the necessary stability with a brace.

Criteria for Reconstruction

There are no absolute criteria regarding patient selection for Charcot reconstruction, but rather a combination of factors are weighed in light of the patient's condition and prognosis. Foremost, one must consider factors that extend beyond the lower extremity; specifically the overall health of the patients, their diabetic control, metabolic and nutritional status, renal function, and cardiac status. Some of these patients will possess occult cardiac pathology, and a thorough evaluation by an internist or cardiologist is often revealing. In this same regard, the patient must be able to tolerate what is often an extended surgical procedure. The patient should also possess the functional capacity to truly benefit from the reconstruction.

Compliance with postoperative instructions, in particular the appropriate period of non-weight-bearing, is essential. Often, the convalescent period while the patient is awaiting surgery is a good way to determine the patient's reliability. Those who can follow instructions at this juncture are generally responsible enough to do so postoperatively.

In examining the lower extremity, one would prefer that any ulceration be healed prior to reconstruction. However, surgery in the presence of a clean, uninfected superficial lesion is not a contraindication. Deeper lesions are better treated by excision and removal of any offending osseous prominence. Once the wound is adequately healed then reconstruction can be performed.

The overall stability of the foot is important. If the foot is stable with mild to moderate sagittal plane deformity or mild transverse plane deformity, then the patient may be successfully managed with orthotic support, bracing, and *appropriate management of any coexistent equinus.* However, it may be preferable to perform a tendoachillis lengthening in patients who are surgical candidates.

From a conservative standpoint, greater amounts of sagittal plane deformity can be accommodated as opposed to transverse plane aberration. In either instance a key factor is the overall stability of the foot. This includes the joints affected by the Charcot process and adjacent areas. In some instances the pathologic joints will be fused, but significant hypermobility may exist at more proximal areas. If hypermobility exists at any level and cannot be suitably controlled then procedures to address this area may be indicated. Specifically, those joints that have sustained pathologic dislocation are at risk for further injury because the ligamentous structures can no longer provide stability. Any major tendon that inserts into the affected bone may actually serve as a deforming influence. This is particularly true with the tibialis anterior. Once subluxation occurs at the first metatarsocuneiform joint both weight-bearing and the active contraction of the tibialis anterior encourage further disruption. A similar occurrence may also be seen as the tibialis posterior contracts against a dislocated navicular.

More aggressive measures may also be required for stable deformed feet that have sustained ulcerations despite conservative measures. In many instances there is an ankle equinus that has not or cannot be adequately controlled conservatively. In other cases there is considerable osseous deformity.

The author continues to be favorably impressed with arthrodesing techniques for deformed Charcot feet that are not successfully treated by conservative measures. Although arthrodesing techniques are not always successful, most of these patients are able to resume meaningful weightbearing function without ulcerative problems. Furthermore, a number of patients who were to undergo amputation at other institutions have maintained their limbs (Figs 9–13 and 9–14).

The most common complication to date has been a variable loss of arch integrity once weight-bearing is resumed. This has been most notable in those individuals requiring greater amounts of bone grafting. Following a period of nonweight-bearing this process is generally arrested. Nonunions have been experienced on a limited basis and once again are directly correlated to the use of grafts. However, if the foot is positioned correctly, satisfactory function may still be attained with appropriate bracing. Complete failure of the surgery has also been noted in one case.

Tendoachillis Lengthening

An ankle equinus deformity will serve as a primary force that will create or aggravate a variety of foot problems in many patients. Therefore, tendoachillis lengthening may be advocated in several circumstances. Alleviation of the equinus deformity may assist in resolving chronic ulceration involving the plantar metatarsal area and reducing the frequency of cutaneous compromise. Tenotomy of the achilles alone has been noted to provide good long-term results in lepromatous feet where there is fixed deformity of the foot in conjunction with ulceration.[49] However,

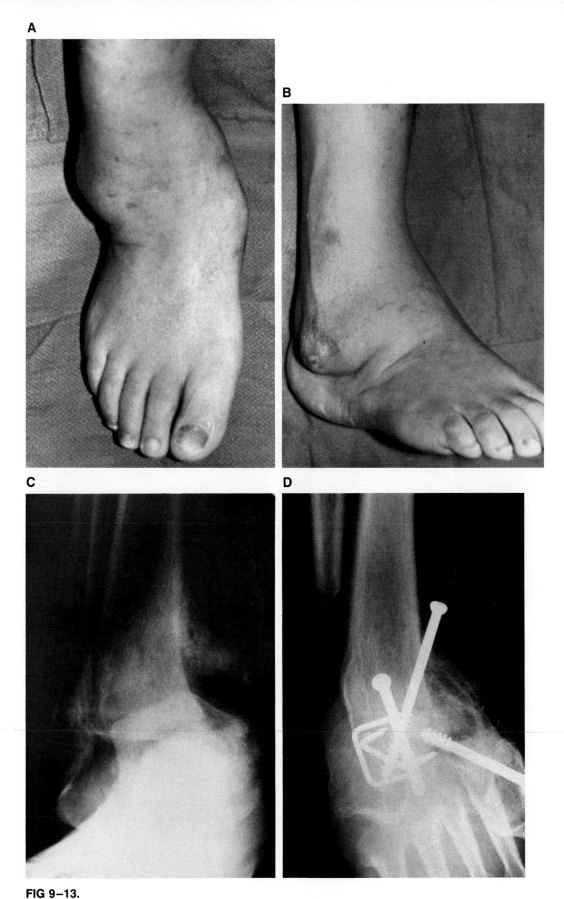

FIG 9–13.
A, B, clinical appearance of diabetic with frontal plane deformity and instability at ankle and subtalar levels. Despite bracing, repeated ulcerations develop when this man attempts to work or ambulate to any significant degree. **C,** preoperative radiograph further dem-onstrating degree of deformity. **D, E,** postoperative radiographs 7 months following pantalar arthrodesis. **F, G,** clinical appearance 7 months postoperatively. Patient at this time has returned to full-time work without limitations as a factory foreman.

(Continued.)

F

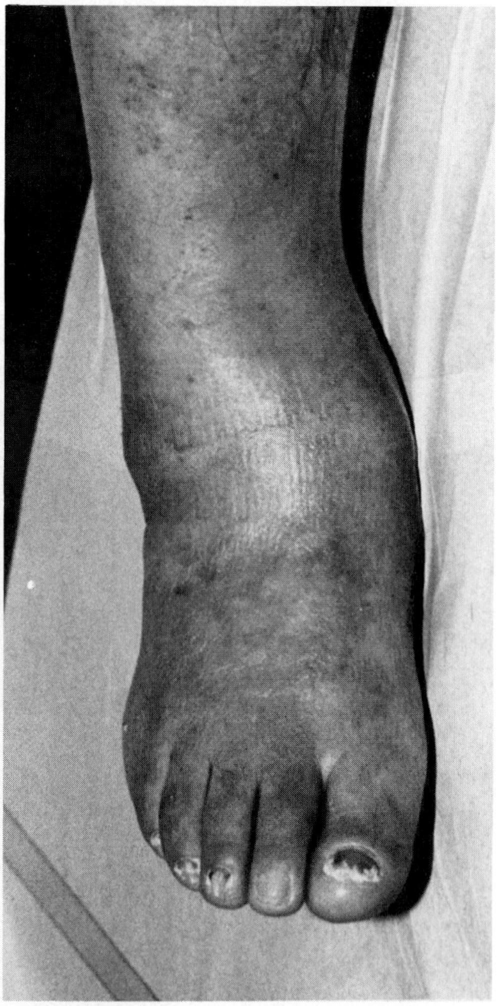

E

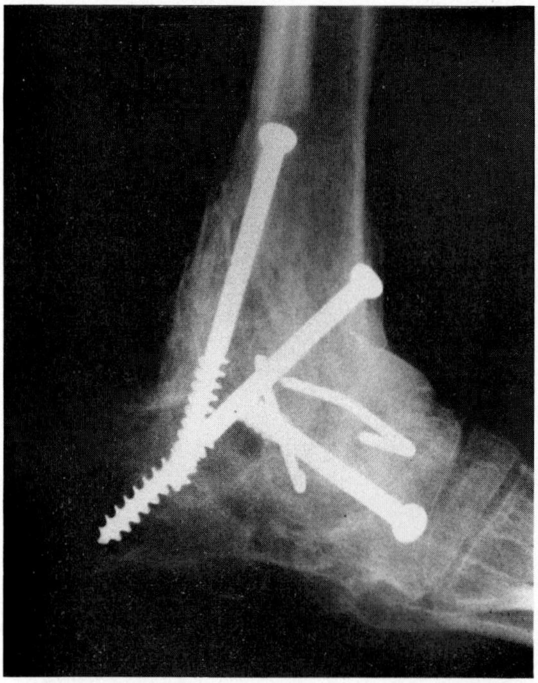

G

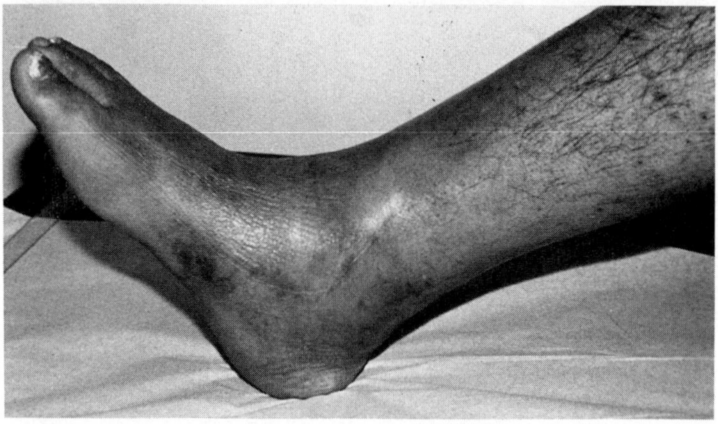

FIG 9–13 (cont.).
For legend see previous page.

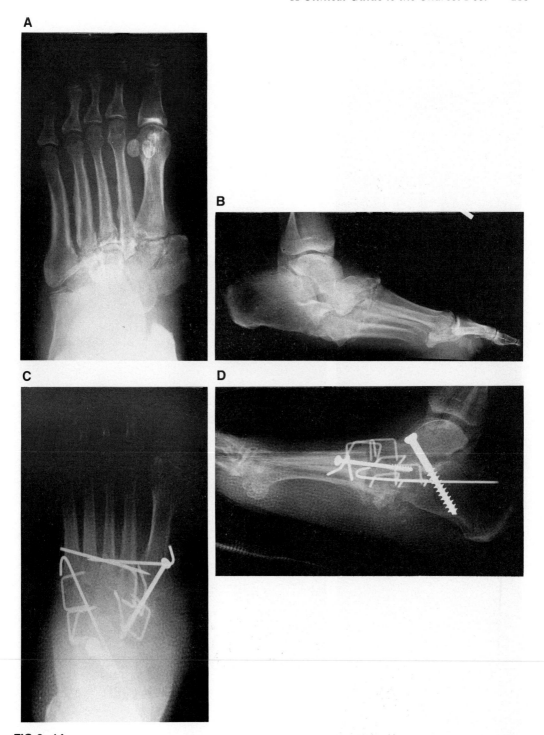

FIG 9–14.
This is the same patient shown in Fig 9–8. **A, B,** radiographic appearance following resolution of the acute process with severe deformity and instability. **C, D,** following reconstructive surgery. **E, F,** 20 months postoperative. The patient has been ambulating without complication since 6 months postoperatively. **G, H,** clinical appearance 22 months following surgery.

(Continued.)

E

F

G

H

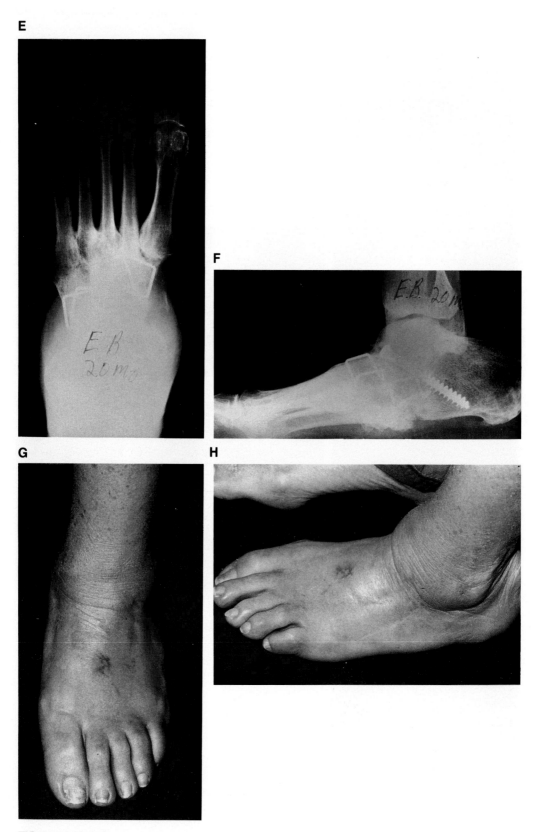

FIG 9–14 (cont.).
For legend see previous page.

in most patients there is still a suitable degree of extensor muscle strength, just simply a loss of normal muscle antagonism. Open lengthening of the achilles would tend to provide the same benefit of reducing excessive forefoot loading stress[43] without the excessive weakening and full loss of function expected with a complete tenotomy.

More frequently tendoachillis lengthening is used in conjunction with other surgical procedures. When performing an exostosectomy in a Charcot foot the equinus surgery is considered an integral part of the procedure.[43, 47] Although the exostosectomy alone may eliminate direct irritation, failure to alleviate the equinus will allow one of the primary causes of the Charcot condition to persist. One may choose to manage the equinus conservatively, but in most situations the presence of this condition is simply unrecognized. The tendoachillis lengthening is also considered an integral part of any arthrodesing procedures for Charcot deformity.[43, 47]

The author's preference for lengthening the heel cord is the open frontal plane technique. A more precise degree of correction may be attained with less chance of overcorrection when compared to either sliding or closed surgical approaches. The procedure may be performed with the patient in the supine position by externally rotating the leg and flexing the knee. This may be performed with local anesthesia with epinephrine in a 1:200,000 concentration for hemostasis, rather than using a tourniquet.

Many patients may never achieve complete restoration of muscle strength following this procedure. However, most patients do not feel this is a limiting factor with their activity. Any loss of propulsion is more than compensated by the salvage of the limb and the return to meaningful weight-bearing function.

CONCLUSION

Numerous advances have been made in understanding the factors that lead to a Charcot foot. The change in philosophy regarding the vascular capacity of these patients will impact favorably on a significant number of diabetics, including those with problems unrelated to the Charcot process. It is important for any physician to detect this condition at the earliest possible stage because that is when relatively minor forms of treatment may have maximum results. Treatment must also be based on an understanding of all three facets of the peripheral polyneuropathy. A review of previous material in light of today's objective findings has led to more advanced and definitive treatment protocols that should improve function and enhance the quality of life for many people.

Acknowledgment

Funding for the photographs and drawings within the text of this chapter was graciously provided by The Podiatry Institute.

REFERENCES

1. Sinha S, Munichoodappa CS, Kozak GP: Neuro-arthropathy (Charcot joints) in diabetes mellitus, *Medicine* 51:191–210, 1972.
2. Lippman HI, Perotto A, Farrar R: The neuropathic foot of the diabetic, *Bull NY Acad Med* 52:1159–1178, 1976.
3. Brown MJ, Asbury AK: Diabetic neuropathy, *Ann Neurol* 15:2–12, 1987.
4. Scarpello JHB, Martin TRP, Ward JD: Ultrasound measurements of pulse-wave velocity in the peripheral arteries of diabetic subjects, *Clin Sci* 58:53–57, 1980.
5. Boulton AJM, Scarpello JHB, Ward JD: Venous oxygenation in the diabetic neuropathic foot: evidence of arteriovenous shunting? *Diabetologia* 22:6–8, 1982.

6. Ward JD et al: Venous distension in the diabetic neuropathic foot (a physical sign of arteriovenous shunting), *R Soc Med* 76:1011–1014, 1983.
7. Edmonds ME, Archer AG, Watkins PJ: Ephedrine: a new treatment for diabetic neuropathic oedema, *Lancet* I:548–551, 1983.
8. Archer AG, Roberts VC, Watkins PJ: Blood flow patterns in painful diabetic neuropathy, *Diabetologia* 27:563–567, 1984.
9. Edmonds ME et al: Increased uptake of bone radiopharmaceutical in diabetic neuropathy, *Q J Med* 57:843–855, 1985.
10. Gilbey SG et al: Vascular calcification, autonomic neuropathy, and peripheral blood flow in patients with diabetic nephropathy, *Diabetic Med* 6:37–42, 1989.
11. Chantelau E et al: Effect of medial arterial calcification on O_2 supply to exercising diabetic feet, *Diabetes* 39:938–941, 1990.
12. Edmonds ME et al: Medial arterial calcification and diabetic neuropathy, *Br Med J* 284:928–930, 1982.
13. Clouse ME, Gramm HF, Flood T: Diabetic osteoarthropathy. Clinical and roentgenographic observations in 90 cases, *Am J Roentgenol* 121:22–34, 1974.
14. Goebel FD, Fuessel HS: Monckeberg's sclerosis after sympathetic denervation in diabetic and nondiabetic subjects, *Diabetologia* 24:347–350, 1983.
15. Kerper AH, Collier WD: Pathological changes in arteries following partial denervation, *Proc Soc Exp Biol Med* 24:493–494, 1926.
16. Duncan CP, Shim SS: The autonomic nerve supply of bone, *J Bone Joint Surg* 59B:323–329, 1977.
17. Trotman NM, Kelly WD: The effect of sympathectomy on blood flow to bone, *JAMA* 183:121–122, 1963.
18. Yu W, Shim SS, Hawk HE: Bone circulation in hemorrhagic shock, *J Bone Joint Surg* 54A:1157–1166, 1972.
19. Shim SS, Copp DH, Patterson FP: Bone blood flow in the limb following complete sciatic nerve section, *Surg Gynecol Obstet* 123:333–335, 1966.
20. Cundy TF, Edmonds ME, Watkins PJ: Osteopenia and metatarsal fractures in diabetic neuropathy, *Diabetic Med* 2:461–464, 1985.
21. Rundles RW: Diabetic neuropathy, general review with report of 125 cases, *Medicine* 24:111–160, 1945.
22. Martin MM: Charcot joints in diabetes mellitus, *Proc R Soc Med* 45:503–506, 1952.
23. Watkins PJ, Edmonds ME: Sympathetic nerve failure in diabetes, *Diabetologia* 25:73–77, 1983.
24. Fagius J: Microneurographic findings in diabetic polyneuropathy with special reference to sympathetic nerve activity, *Diabetologia* 23:415–420, 1982.
25. Guy RJC et al: Evaluation of thermal and vibration sensation in diabetic neuropathy, *Diabetologia* 28:131–137, 1985.
26. LoGerfo FW, Coffman JD: Vascular and microvascular disease of the foot in diabetes, *N Engl J Med* 311:1615–1619, 1984.
27. Flynn MD et al: Direct measurement of capillary blood flow in the diabetic neuropathic foot, *Diabetologia* 31:652–656, 1988.
28. Root ML, Orien WP, Weed JH: *Normal and abnormal function of the foot*, vol 2, Los Angeles, 1977, Clinical Biomechanics.
29. Eloesser L: On the nature of neuropathic affectations of the joints, *Ann Surg* 66:201–207, 1917.
30. Brower AC, Allman RM: Pathogenesis of the neurotrophic joint: neurotraumatic vs. neurovascular, *Radiology* 139:349–354, 1981.
31. Reinhardt K: The radiological residua of healed diabetic arthropathies. *Skeletal Radiol* 7:167–172, 1981.
32. Finsterbush A, Friedman B: The effect of sensory denervation on rabbits' knee joints. *J Bone Joint Surg* 57A:949–956, 1975.
33. Jelinek JE: Collagen disorders in which diabetes and cutaneous features coexist. In Jelinek JE, editor: *The skin in diabetes*, Philadelphia, 1986, Lea & Febiger.
34. Delbridge L et al: Limited joint mobility in the diabetic foot: relationship to neu-

ropathic ulceration, *Diabetic Med* 5:333–337, 1988.

35. Fernando DJS et al: Relationship of limited joint mobility to abnormal foot pressures and diabetic foot ulceration, *Diabetes Care* 14:8–11, 1991.

36. Harris JR, Brand PW: Patterns of disintegration of the tarsus in the anaesthetic foot, *J Bone Joint Surg* 48B:4–16, 1966.

37. Dickhaut SC, DeLee JC, Page CP: Nutritional status: importance in predicting wound healing after amputation, *J Bone Joint Surg* 66A:71–75, 1984.

38. Pinzur M, Kaminsky M, Sage R et al: Amputations at the middle level of the foot, *J Bone Joint Surg* 68A:1061-1064, 1986.

39. Sanders LJ, Dunlap G: Transmetatarsal amputation. A successful approach to limb salvage, *J Am Podiatr Med Assoc* 82:129–135, 1992.

40. McMurry JF: Wound healing with diabetes mellitus: better glucose control for better healing in diabetes, *Surg Clin North Am* 64:769–778, 1984.

41. Horwitz T: Bone and cartilage debris in the synovial membrane. Its significance in the early diagnosis of neuroarthropathy, *J Bone Joint Surg* 30A:579–588, 1948.

42. Leventen EO: Charcot foot—a technique for treatment of chronic plantar ulcer by saucerization and primary closure, *Foot Ankle* 6:295–299, 1986.

43. Lennox WM: The surgical management of foot deformities in leprosy, *Lepr Rev* 36:27–34, 1965.

44. Johnson JTH: Neuropathic fractures and joint injuries, *J Bone Joint Surg* 49A:1–30, 1967.

45. Warren G: Tarsal bone disintegration in leprosy, *J Bone Joint Surg* 53B:688–695, 1971.

46. Warren AG: The surgical conservation of the neuropathic foot, *Ann R Coll Surg Engl* 71:236–242, 1989.

47. Banks AS, McGlamry ED: Charcot foot, *J Am Podiatr Med Assoc* 79:213–235, 1989.

48. Shibata T et al: The results of arthrodesis of the ankle for leprotic neuroarthropathy, *J Bone Joint Surg* 72A:749–756, 1990.

49. Yosipovitch Z, Sheskin J: Subcutaneous achilles tenotomy in the treatment of perforating ulcer of the foot in leprosy, *Int J Lepr* 39:631–632, 1971.

James Jelinek, M.D.

Elliott Levy, M.D.

10   Radiologic Considerations for the Diabetic Extremity

RADIOLOGY OF THE DIABETIC FOOT

The last decade has witnessed the widespread application of new imaging modalities and techniques in the diagnosis and management of the diabetic foot. Early detection and monitoring of osseous changes that occur as a result of the neuropathy, devascularization, and infections commonly found in diabetic patients is the goal of radiologic imaging. Noninvasive and arteriographic vascular imaging have provided vascular, orthopedic, and podiatric surgeons with important preoperative predictors of wound healing and limb viability and guidance for planning reconstructive interventions. To appreciate the contribution and limitations of the radiologic modalities in the management of the problems of the foot in the diabetic patient, cne must understand the known pathophysiologic mechanisms of diabetes associated neuropathy, angiopathy, and bone destruction.

NEUROPATHIC BONE AND JOINT DISEASE

Neuropathic arthropathy is a slowly progressive form of joint and periarticular bone destruction seen in patients with peripheral neurosensory deficits of multiple etiologies. Previously common causes included syphilis, leprosy, and syringomyelia. Currently diabetes mellitus is the most common cause of neuroarthropathy. In the foot, the most commonly afflicted sites include the tarsometatarsal joints, metatarsophalangeal joints, and tibiotalar joints. The osseous destructive changes can occur without any specific antecedent trauma recognized by the patient, or, alternatively, the patient may recall a single relatively minor trauma after which the involved foot developed edema and erythema. Weight-bearing joints show bony eburnation and destructive changes concomitantly, including erosion and fragmentation of bone and marginal osteophytosis. Accelerated joint degeneration can result in joint dislocation (Fig 10–1) and development of intraarticular loose bodies. Clinically the neuropathic arthropathy must be distinguished from septic arthritis, osteomyelitis, cellulitis, or reflex sympathetic osteodystrophy.[1]

Neuropathic arthropathy may occur in an atrophic or hypertrophic form. The atrophic form rarely occurs in the lower extremities. The hypertrophic form exhibits more insidious progression, requiring months to years to develop. A particularly malignant version of hypertrophic neuropathic arthropathy has been reported in diabetic patients to occur 3 to 6 weeks after minor trauma.[2] This subject is discussed in greater detail elsewhere in this text.

A

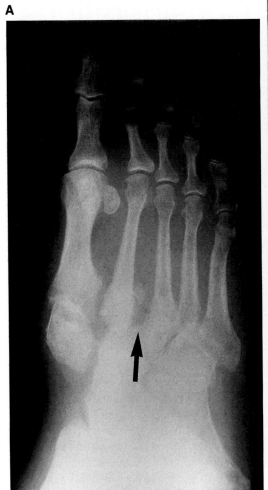

B

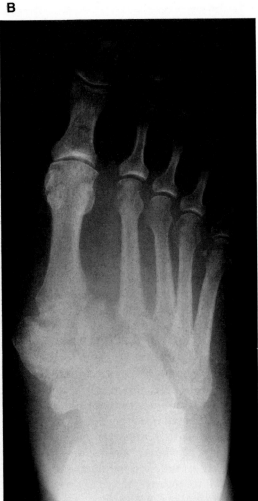

FIG 10–1.
Neuroarthropathy of the foot simulating a Lis-Franc dislocation of the metatarsal bases. **A,** Charcot's joint changes at the tarsometatarsal joints. Note abnormal distance between second and third metatarsals and significant abnormal appearance of the cuneiform bones. **B,** same patient now showing marked lateral dislocation of the second to fifth digits.

BONE INFECTION

Osteomyelitis is probably the most frequent subject of radiology consultation regarding the diabetic foot. Multiple imaging modalities are employed in the diagnosis and subsequent evaluation of acute osteomyelitis. The number and sequence of examinations must be specifically tailored to each individual patient. First, bone infection must be diagnosed as quickly as possible to begin intensive and prolonged antibiotic therapy or surgical intervention. Second, the extent of osseous destruction and soft tissue changes must be recognized to substantiate appropriate therapy. Finally, recurrence must be recognized in the setting of altered bony architecture.

Osteomyelitis in the diabetic adult most commonly arises from contiguous spread of soft tissue infection into the periosteum, with resulting extension through the medullary space. Osseous destruction is ordinarily limited by the cellular immune system elements and reparative process of the bone itself.[1] In the diabetic patient with compromised circulation, the effectiveness of these host defenses is significantly reduced and limb viability threatened.

A

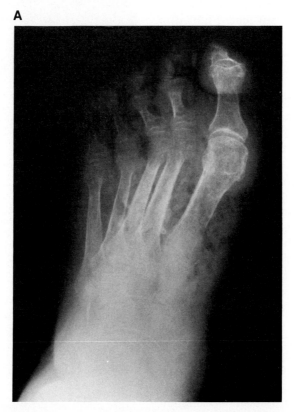

B

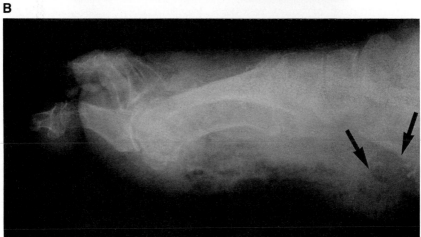

FIG 10–2.
Gas gangrene of the foot in a 73-year-old woman. **A,** extensive soft tissue gas is seen on the anteropos- terior view. **B,** a large plantar ulcer accompanies the subcutaneous gas *(arrows).*

RADIOLOGIC EVALUATION OF OSTEOMYELITIS

The radiologic evaluation of the foot of the diabetic patient with suspected osteomyelitis should begin with the plain film radiograph of the affected foot. Plain film radiography is accomplished using bone or magnification technique. Destruction of approximately 50% of the osseous mineral density must occur before bone destruction is detected radiographically. This degree of demineralization may require 10 to 14 days to develop.

A fundamental understanding of the pathophysiology of osteomyelitis is required to understand the plain film, radionuclide, and magnetic resonance imaging (MRI) appearances of osteomyelitis. Infection of bone typically involves one of three pathways. The first is hematogenous spread of infection, and this is most commonly seen in the pediatric population. The second is contiguous spread from local infection, such as spread from an infected ulcer to the bony structures. Finally, direct impregnation of bacteria into bone can occur with penetrating injury, such as a ballistic injury or as a result of stepping on a sharp object, such as a nail or thorn. In the foot, the most common route of contamination of bones results from contiguous spread of infection, especially in the diabetic foot. A soft tissue infection involves the skin, subcutaneous tissues, and deeper musculocutaneous and intracompartmental fascial structures (Fig 10–2). The first roentgen evidence of disease is swelling of the soft tissues with displacement or obliteration of normal fat planes adjacent to and between muscle compartments. When an organized collection of pus forms, this is considered an abscess. The presence of air may be diagnostic of a severe infectious process (see Fig 10–2). Direct extension to the bone initially affects the periosteum. The periosteum has a firm, fibrous attachment to the cortex and offers some degree of re-

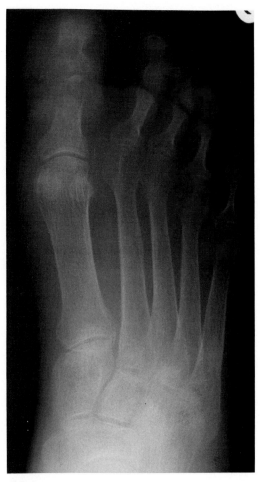

FIG 10–3.
Septic arthritis with accompanying osteomyelitis of the interphalangeal joint of the great toe showing destructive changes of the adjacent bony structures and marked soft tissue swelling. Note the indistinct poorly defined borders of the bones and loss of normal bone cortex.

sistance to the spread of infection. However, once there is extension of infection to the periosteum (infectious periostitis), there is progressive disruption of the periosteum and, hence, disruption of osseous blood flow that extends from the periosteum.[1] After this there is much less resistance to penetration of the deeper osseous structures.

Radiographic evidence of osteomyelitis is usually lacking until approximately 50% of bone has been resorbed (Fig 10–

3). Frequently this requires days to weeks. The earliest radiographic signs of infection are found within the soft tissues, and this is where attention should be first directed.

The initial bony changes of contiguous spread of infection from the soft tissues into the bone are seen as loss of definition and sharpness of the outer bony cortex. This is followed by progressive patchy and poorly defined lucency of the bone cortex. In response, the bone may develop fine periosteal bone formation (Fig 10–4), and this may be the initial radiographic finding of osteomyelitis.[1] When deeper penetration into the marrow space has occurred, one begins to see rarefaction of the bony structures (see Fig 10–3). If an acute focus of osteomyelitis progresses, a more rapid appearance of bone destruction becomes apparent, typically resulting in a ragged, poorly defined, moth-eaten appearance. Within the area of osteomyelitis, however, are intermingled areas of more normal appearing bone. The plain film radiographic demonstration of osteomyelitis underestimates the actual extent of infection within the bone. Subsequent appearance of the osteomyelitis may take several forms. If an infectious process becomes subacute or chronic, it may develop a relatively well-defined margin, a so-called Brodie's abscess. Typically the lucent defect of the osteomyelitis is lined by a rim of sclerosis with a fading margin of sclerosis into the normal bone. If there is evidence of bony destruction, a focus of dead bone can be seen among the osteo-

A

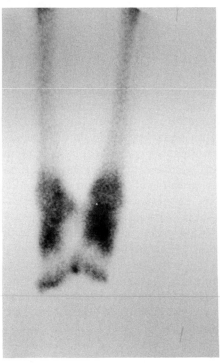

B

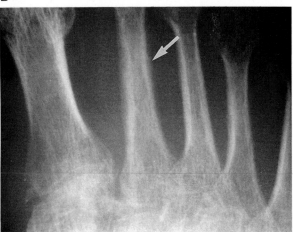

FIG 10–4.
Osteomyelitis of the metatarsals. **A,** Technetium–methylene diphosphonate bone scan demonstrating increased activity in the region of the midmetatarsals. **B,** close-up plain film radiograph demonstrates early osteomyelitis showing loss of normal sharp cortical line along the lateral aspect of the second metatarsal. The cortex and periosteum of the lateral aspect of the second metatarsal shows a fuzzy border and a subtle periosteal reaction. Compare with the lateral aspect of the first metatarsal.

myelitis and surrounded by a rim of granulation tissue. This devitalized sclerotic bone within the infectious process is referred to as a sequestrum.

Plain radiographs will also identify the presence of fractures, bony fragmentation and joint subluxation associated with neuropathy, vascular calcifications, and gas in severe soft tissue infections. Bone resorption and periosteal reaction require intact vascular supply to bone, and absence of reactive demineralization is a poor radiographic prognostic sign. However, other more sensitive imaging modalities are frequently needed to detect acute osteomyelitis before plain radiographic changes become evident.

Imaging of the bones of the lower extremities using radiopharmaceuticals has evolved as a primary radiologic technique for the diagnosis of osteomyelitis. Radioisotope examinations are minimally invasive, requiring only the intravenous injection of small quantities of radiopharmaceuticals. The studies are limited only by the availability of the pharmaceuticals, relatively poor spatial resolution, and length of time required to complete the examination. The most commonly employed radioisotope, technetium-99m, is readily obtained from a benchtop molybdenum generator universally found in licensed hospital and outpatient facilities. Minimal patient preparation is required for most types of examinations.

Radioisotope bone scanning is most frequently performed to diagnose acute osteomyelitis. The presence of cellulitis, recent fracture, degenerative joint disease, or skeletal metastases affects the distribution of the agent and therefore the specificity of the study, depending on the radiopharmaceutical administered. Frequently correlation with other imaging modalities is required to determine the extent of involvement, particularly in the setting of chronic osteomyelitis, neuroarthropathy, or fracture.

The localization of the various pharmaceuticals is dependent on several physiologic factors, but all such agents are imaged by their radioactive decay, in which gamma photons are emitted and detected by a gamma camera calibrated for the desired photon energy level. The images generated by the gamma camera detection crystals have limited anatomic resolution compared with computed tomography (CT) or MRI. The most commonly employed radioisotopes in clinical practice include ^{99m}Tc, gallium-67 citrate, and leukocytes labeled with indium-111.

The various imaging modalities are frequently compared by their sensitivity and specificity in detecting pathology. The sensitivity is defined as the ratio of the true positive examination results to the number of confirmed true positive and false negative study results (or the ability to correctly identify those who have the disease). The specificity is defined as the ratio of the true negative examination results and the confirmed true negative and false positive examination results (or the ability to identify correctly those who do not have the disease).

Three phase bone scanning is more than 90% sensitive for osteomyelitis. Specificity is high (95%) in the absence of coexisting bone pathology, but the average specificity is considerably less when other causes of osseous destruction and repair are present (33%).[3] Studies using alternative agents or summation examinations employing multiple imaging agents have been used to increase the specificity of nuclear bone imaging. Readers desiring more extensive discussions of the role of nuclear medicine in the diagnosis of osteomyelitis are referred to the excellent reviews by Schauwecker[3] and Handmaker and Leonard.[4]

TECHNETIUM-99M

Technetium-99m is most commonly administered in the form of ^{99m}Tc methylene diphosphonate (Tc-MDP) and hydroxymethylene diphosphonate (Tc-

HMDP). Both agents are produced in kits requiring only the addition of the ^{99m}Tc isotope obtained from the generator. The radiopharmaceutical is intravenously injected and is rapidly distributed throughout the intravascular space then into the extracellular fluid. Concentration in foci of active new bone formation occurs over several hours related to osteoblastic activity in response to bone injury. Images of the normal skeleton show diffuse uptake in the axial and appendicular skeleton, with slightly increased activity in the joints of the elderly.

The ^{99m}Tc bone scan is performed in stages or phases, organized to maximize the distinction between pathologic bone uptake and less specific uptake from other causes discussed later on. The first phase images, or flow phase, are obtained of the suspected area immediately after injection at several second intervals. The second phase images, or blood pool images, are obtained 5 minutes after injection. Delayed images are obtained 3 to 4 hours after injection when renal excretion has reduced the extraosseous radiopharmaceutical levels. The flow and blood pool phase images reveal initially increased delivery of the agent as a result of increased hyperemia caused by inflammation, infection (osteomyelitis, cellulitis), trauma, or tumor. The delayed images reveal increased uptake in pathologic bone independent of early hyperemic factors, allowing distinction of cellulitis from osteomyelitis (see Fig 10–4). Uptake has been observed to continue after 4 hours following injection in infected bone and improved resolution using a four-phase study, including imaging 24 hours after injection has been observed in the feet of patients with peripheral vascular disease.[5,6]

LEUKOCYTES LABELED WITH GALLIUM-67 AND INDIUM-111

Gallium-67 citrate differs from ^{99m}Tc in several important respects: (1) the imaged photons are emitted with multiple higher energies, (2) the isotope is employed directly without binding to molecular complexes for the desired imaging properties, (3) the isotope is produced in the cyclotron and is more expensive to obtain, and (4) routine imaging requires longer delays between injection and imaging. The localizing mechanisms for ^{67}Ga citrate are not known, although ^{67}Ga uptake at sites of infection is currently thought to be caused by specific leukocyte uptake and chemotaxis and bacterial iron metabolism because ^{67}Ga is an iron analog with regard to extracellular proteins. Gallium-67 imaging for bone infection is hampered, however, by significant diffuse uptake in bone marrow and by nonspecific low levels of uptake in all sites of bone remodeling in response to fractures, neuropathic changes, or prostheses.[7,8]

Indium-111-labeled leukocyte scans are increasingly being performed in preference to ^{67}Ga scans as a second examination to increase the specificity of the ^{99m}Tc bone scan. The ^{111}In isotope is obtained from a cyclotron and is used to label autologous white blood cells (WBCs) from the patient to be studied. Leukocyte counts of greater than 5,000 cells/mm^3 are required for adequate labeling, and complete cell preparation requires 2 hours. The In isotope binds to cytoplasmic components. The WBCs are then injected intravenously and are distributed throughout the intravascular space. Cumulative circulation time is estimated to be 7 hours. Imaging routinely begins 24 hours after injection, allowing for diminution of the generalized systemic blood pool activity. Images may be obtained as early as 4 to 6 hours in instances of severe infection. Localization of the labeled leukocytes to foci of bone infection is relatively specific despite the presence of coexisting conditions stimulating bone remodeling such as fracture.[9–11] Localizing infection in the bones of patients with diabetic arthropathy and cellulitis using ^{111}In-labeled leukocytes is less specific and may require a combined ^{99m}Tc bone scan and ^{111}In-labeled WBC study approach. In this manner, Schauwecker et al.[12] were able to localize infection to the bone or adjacent tissues in 89% of the patients with neuropathic osteopathy in the feet. Uptake resulting from rapidly progressive new onset neuroarthropathy may obscure acute bone infection uptake using combined ^{99m}Tc-^{111}In scanning.[13]

False positive^{111} In-labeled WBC scans have been reported in instances of rheumatoid arthritis and healing fractures. Usually these pathologic conditions result in relatively diminished affinity of labeled leukocytes and appear as foci of relatively diminished uptake compared with osteomyelitis.[14] Sensitivity of 93% and specificity of 95% for the detection of osteomyelitis in the setting of diabetes mellitus, fracture nonunion, recent surgery, and overlying soft tissue infection has been reported for ^{111}In-WBC scans.[15] These authors report overlying soft tissue infection as the most common reason for misdiagnosis of osteomyelitis. Potential for false positive results exists if ^{111}In-WBC scanning is performed immediately after a ^{99m}Tc bone scan showing focally increased uptake. For this reason, ^{111}In imaging should be performed before or 48 hours after ^{99m}Tc scanning. The major disadvantages of ^{111}In imaging are that it is usually done in conjunction with a ^{99m}Tc bone scan (requiring several days of imaging time) and the fact that cyclotrons are not widely available, even less available than MRI.

The radiopharmaceutical agents vary in their affinity for foci of chronic osteomyelitis. Technetium-99m bone scans may show focally increased uptake up to 2 years after successful treatment. In contrast, ^{67}Ga uptake returns to normal levels after treatment. The relative intensity of uptake in foci of chronic infection of ^{67}Ga and ^{111}In-WBCs appears to be approximately equal. Indium-67–WBC scanning has been recommended over combined ^{99m}Tc-^{67}Ga imaging, with a reported overall accuracy of 83% vs. 57%.[16]

Agents currently under investigation include ^{99m}Tc-labeled hexamethylpropyleneamine oxime (HMPAO) and ^{99m}Tc- or ^{67}In-labeled antigranulocyte antibodies. The former enjoys the advantage of easy kit preparation and the possibility of single photon emission computed tomography (SPECT) scanning, whereas the latter does not accumulate in the marrow space to the same extent as ^{111}In-labeled WBCs. The advantage of radiolabeled antigranulocyte antibodies may be more important in the axial rather than appendicular skeleton, however.

MAGNETIC RESONANCE IMAGING OF MUSCULOSKELETAL INFECTION

Magnetic resonance imaging, by virtue of unique physical imaging properties, has assumed an important role in the diagnosis of osteomyelitis in the axial and appendicular skeleton. Body tissue placed in a strong external magnetic field and subjected to specific radiofrequency signals generates proportional, unique, radiofrequencies that are received and used to reconstruct an image of the tissue. The signal pattern is dependent on the water (proton) content of the tissue and the nature of the incipient radiofrequency applied. Images generated are labeled according to the "pulse sequence" (i.e., the pattern of applied radiofrequencies directed toward the tissue studied). The most commonly used pulse sequences are T_1- and T_2-weighted images. T_1-weighted images relate to net magnetization of the tissue, whereas T_2-weighted images rely on interaction between adjacent molecules. Qualitative signal intensity determines image contrast. Multiplanar MRI images provide excellent tissue contrast and spatial resolution, and this modality has assumed particular importance in the diagnosis and extent of osteomyelitis.

MRI imaging of osteomyelitis and neuroarthropathy is based on the change in bone marrow signal intensity that results from the increased water (proton) content secondary to edema, inflammation, or infection. Normal bone marrow shows increased signal intensity relative to the bone cortex and therefore appears bright or white on T_1-weighted images and as a more intermediate (gray) signal intensity on T_2-weighted images. The low-proton content of bone cortex results in low signal intensity or black on imaging sequences. Fibrous and muscular tissues have intermediate to low signal intensities with the various imaging sequences.

A

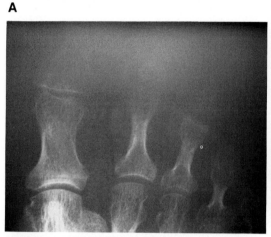

B

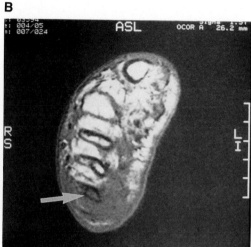

C

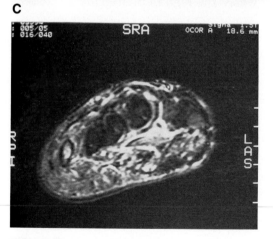

FIG 10–5.

Osteomyelitis of the fifth phalanx. **A,** coned-down plain film radiograph demonstrates severe osteopenia of the phalanges. No discrete foci of osteomyelitis is seen, though the fifth digit is osteopenic and not visible. **B,** coronal T_1-weighted image through the proximal phalanges demonstrates a discrete area of cellulitis laterally, which extends around the fifth digit, and there is replacement of the normal fat by low signal intensity.

C, coronal T_2-weighted image with fat suppression. Note that normal fat signal intensity has been entirely suppressed. There is diffuse edema within the foot that correlates with the clinical examination. The fifth phalanx demonstrates markedly increased signal intensity within the central marrow consistent with the patient's osteomyelitis. Radionuclide bone scan has had demonstrated diffuse cellulitis but not osteomyelitis.

A

B

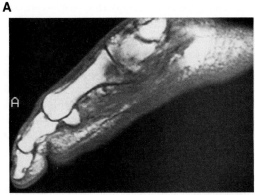
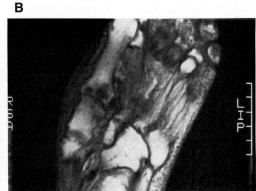

FIG 10–6.

A, sagittal T₁-weighted image demonstrated marked skin thickening and cellulitis along the plantar surface of the foot deep to the first tarsometatarsal joint. Note the area of bone involvement along the inferior aspect of the joint in continuity with the area of cellulitis. There is evidence of a discrete focus of osteomyelitis present within the cuneiform and first metatarsal bone. **B,** axial T₁-weighted image through this same region demon-

strates the septic joint between the cuneiform and the first metatarsal bone. It also demonstrates that there are two foci of osteomyelitis within the base of the first metatarsal bone and minimal involvement of the distal cuneiform. Note the relationship to the extensive cellulitis also present along the far medial aspect of the foot.

Infected bone marrow shows poorly marginated areas of lower signal intensity on T₁-weighted images that show corresponding increased signal intensity relative to normal marrow on T₂-weighted images (Figs 10–5 to 10–7).[17–22] This difference in marrow signal intensity is accentuated on short tau inversion recovery (STIR) or in fat-suppressed T₂-weighted images where the high to intermediate intensity

A

B

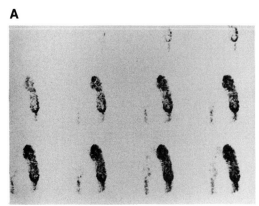
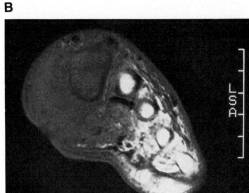

FIG 10–7.

Cellulitis and osteomyelitis demonstrating the value of MRI in evaluating extent of infection. **A,** radionuclide bone scan demonstrating marked increased uptake in the medial forefoot. **B,** coronal T₁-weighted images demonstrating the exact extent of severe infection of the medial aspect of the foot. The small ulcer crater is seen along the plantar surface medially with a large diffuse abscess and cellulitis that encases and in-

volves the distal phalanx of the great toe. Note also evidence of early involvement of the anterior compartment and diffuse skin thickening seen throughout the foot. The second through fifth digits are spared of osteomyelitis. The most lateral extent of the osteomyelitis along the plantar surface of the foot is sharply delineated, being confined to the medial compartment.

of marrow fat is suppressed to a darker shade (see Fig 10–5). As infection spreads, subperiosteal accumulation of pus and violation of muscle and fascial planes occurs. Subsequently, adjacent intraosseous infection may be documented by decreased signal intensity on T_1-weighted images and increased signal on T_2-weighted images. The excellent spatial resolution of MRI allowed the highest sensitivity and specificity for the diagnosis of osteomyelitis compared with radionuclide bone scintigraphy and plain radiographic imaging in the series by Yuh et al.[18]

Accurate diagnosis of the extent of osteomyelitis within a bone and involvement of soft tissues, fascial compartments, and joints with infection is important for careful surgical planning. Mason et al.[19] found good correlation between the extent of the intramedullary disease seen on their MRI images with serial sections of amputated specimens. Fibrotic marrow was found to show low signal intensity on T_1-weighted images without corresponding increased signal intensity on T_2-weighted images, whereas osteomyelitis showed lower signal intensity on T_1-weighted images and increased signal on T_2-weighted images.

Modic et al.[20] point out that the observed marrow changes with osteomyelitis are not specific for infection and that altered signal intensity may be also seen in bone tumors, dysplasia, bone infarction, trauma, or neoplasm. Complete clinical correlation, including specific history of antecedent surgery, trauma, prior infection, and often plain radiographic correlation, is essential for relevant MRI interpretation. Careful evaluation of margins, shape, size, and extent of the disease process may allow a more confident diagnosis of infection over these other etiologies.[23]

In addition to the improved sensitivity and specificity of MRI compared with radionuclide scanning in the evaluation of patients with osteomyelitis, MRI more precisely defines extent of infection within the soft tissues and the bone (see Fig 10–7). Furthermore, the focus of infection can be directly imaged and anatomically localized with respect to muscle compartments, neurovascular structures, joint spaces, and degree of involvement of each individual bone (see Fig 10–6). This precise anatomic resolution cannot be matched by current radionuclide studies.

An important consideration in ordering any test is cost. Current MRI examinations are very expensive. However, when one considers the cost of the serial ^{99m}Tc bone scans or a combination of a ^{99m}Tc bone scan and ^{111}In (or ^{67}Ga) bone scans, the difference between radionuclide imaging and MRI becomes minimal. If surgical intervention is required, improved anatomic visualization of infectious involvement and its relationship with vital structures may favor the use of MRI over the use of radionuclide bone scanning. MRI may help in the preoperative planning of the extent of disease present and the degree of surgical resection required. Increasing numbers of orthopedic and podiatric surgeons are using MRI in the preoperative planning of complex infectious and neoplastic processes.

ANGIOGRAPHY

The frequent concomitant presence of severe peripheral vascular disease in patients with diabetes complicates the course and management of the soft tissue and bone disease discussed. Mild to moderate peripheral vascular disease causes primary symptoms and signs, including intermittent claudication, whereas chronic severe ischemia may be associated with poor wound healing, ulceration, and, most severely, gangrene. Poor arterial inflow limits the effectiveness of the cellular and humoral immune system and the delivery of antibiotics. Pulsatile blood flow has been believed to be required to assure complete wound granulation and healing.

Evidence for vascular disease is initially derived from physical examination of the peripheral pulses, plain radiographic demonstration of vascular calcification, and noninvasive vascular diagnostic examination. Noninvasive or angiographic examinations are recommended in the following clinical settings: (1) patients presenting with relatively minor surgical indication (i.e., bunionectomy with diminished pedal pulses); (2) patients with chronic, poorly healing cellulitis or osteomyelitis; and (3) patients with "foot" or "calf" pain with exertion (intermittent claudication), together with evidence of trophic skin changes or nonpalpable pedal pulses. Patients requiring surgical intervention who have significant peripheral vascular disease are preoperatively evaluated to determine likelihood for successful postoperative healing. Chronic cellulitis or osteomyelitis in the diabetic lower extremity may be considered a limb-threatening situation requiring a revascularization procedure for limb viability.

Noninvasive Doppler and color flow sonographic imaging are routinely performed as a screening examination before angiography. Doppler sonography provides the absolute ankle or digital brachial systolic pressure index and the presence of pressure gradients and abnormal flow patterns (Doppler waveforms) localizing arterial obstruction or occlusion to specific anatomic levels. Color flow and Doppler sonography has been employed in attempts to preangiographically distinguish patients who may benefit from percutaneous transluminal angiography as opposed to surgical bypass grafts.

Measurement of systolic blood pressure at the ankle is a simple, reproducible noninvasive method of assessing the arterial inflow to the foot. Doppler interrogation of the dorsalis pedis and posterior tibial artery is performed after inflation of a pneumatic cuff placed around the ankle. The systolic occlusion pressures at these two sites should not differ by more than 10 mm Hg. The ankle systolic occlusion pressure is compared with the brachial pressures in the ankle-brachial index. The index is therefore normalized by division by the current central aortic pressure and can be used to monitor improvement after vascular intervention. The ankle-brachial index is generally a reliable measurement, compromised only by medial arteriosclerotic calcification, which prevents arterial luminal collapse and yields spuriously high systolic "occlusion" pressures.

Abnormal ankle-brachial systolic indices generally correlate with severity of vessel wall calcification, and segmental pressure gradients obtained in the leg correlate well with the level of obstruction.

Toe systolic occlusion pressure has been measured as an index for predicting healing of diabetic foot ulcers and successful postsurgical wound healing. Several studies have been performed comparing absolute ankle and toe systolic pressures and toe plethysmography to predict successful amputation wound or ischemic ulcer healing in the diabetic foot. Significant variability in the absolute pressures required at the ankle and toe for successful healing has been observed because, in part, of medial calcification of the pedal arteries and differences in measurement techniques.

Ankle pressures less than 80 mm Hg in diabetic patients often suggest that ischemic foot ulcers or postoperative wounds will not primarily heal, and arteriography should be performed to determine the optimal revascularization procedure. Arteriograms should be obtained in cases with abnormal ankle-brachial index even if ankle pressures are in excess of 80 mm Hg; improvement in inflow despite persistent pedal vascular disease may allow successful wound or ulcer healing. Apelqvist et al.[24] reported in their series of 314 diabetic patients that ankle pressures of less than 40 mm Hg were inconsistent with primary healing, and a toe pressure of greater than 45 mm Hg correlated with a primary healing rate of 85%. These authors could not define an upper systolic toe or ankle pressure limit above which an amputation was not required.

An understanding of the invasive nature of arteriography and the risks associated with the intra-arterial or intravenous administration of iodinated contrast material must guide the clinician in optimal patient selection and preparation. Administration of iodinated vascular contrast material can be associated with mild or more severe adverse reactions. Newer

contrast agents with lower osmolarity have been developed with a significant (threefold to fivefold) reduction in both mild and severe reactions. The frequency of adverse or allergic reactions has been recently reviewed in a large series of patients by Katayama et al.[25] and Schwab et al.[26]

Peripheral angiography is performed most commonly via percutaneous puncture of the common femoral artery, followed by introduction of a polyethylene catheter over a guidewire into the arterial lumen. The guidewire is removed, and iodinated contrast material is injected. Conventional radiographic or digital subtraction images of the abdomen, pelvis, and lower extremities are obtained. Digital

A

B

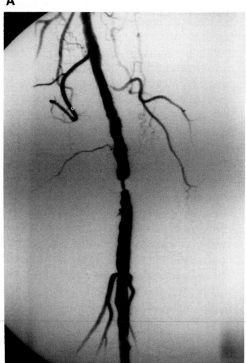
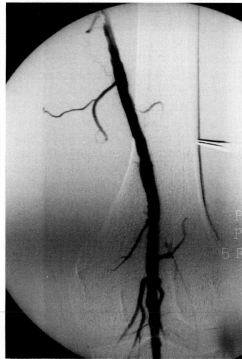

FIG 10–8.
Angioplasty study showing marked improvement of blood flow to the foot in a patient with poorly healing ulcer. **A,** severe stenosis is present within the superficial femoral artery at the level of the adductor canal. The patient had infected, nonhealing ulcers of the medial aspect of the foot. Healing had been delayed sec-

ondary to ischemia. **B,** angiogram after angioplasty of the superficial femoral artery shows excellent postangioplasty result. The patient had palpable pulses after the procedure, and the patient's infected ulcers healed without complications.

subtraction angiography offers the potential for angiographic images using smaller quantities of iodinated contrast material. Images captured by the fluoroscopic image intensifier are stored in computer memory after the "mask" or preinjection image data are "subtracted," improving the resolution of the opacified vessels. Digital subtraction images are degraded by patient motion.

Normal arteries show smooth, gradually tapering luminal caliber. Atherosclerotic vessels show severe luminal irregularity, focal stenoses, or complete occlusion (Fig 10–8). Collateral vessels will be opacified and may reconstitute proximally occluded primary vessels.

The aorta and iliac arteries are considered to be the inflow vessels to the lower extremities, whereas the infrainguinal arteries are considered the "runoff" vessels. Usually both legs are studied simultaneously; in addition to establishing a baseline examination of the asymptomatic extremity, the frequent bilaterally symmetric nature of the atherosclerosis may demonstrate an underlying focal stenosis as the cause for a longer segmental occlusion in the ipsilateral extremity. Stenoses and occlusions have a greater tendency to occur at sites of luminal angulation, bifurcation, or increased flow turbulence. The superficial femoral artery is often occluded at the adductor canal level, with reconstitution of the popliteal artery distally (see Fig 10–8). Proximal or inflow occlusive disease is more commonly examined first in preparation for either distal surgical bypass or an individual angioplasty procedure. The pedal circulation is often specifically examined with conventional or digital subtraction images for patency of the dorsal and plantar arches and for possible distal bypass anastomosis sites, including the dorsalis pedis, posterior tibial, or common plantar arteries.

Atherosclerosis of the lower extremities in the diabetic patients most commonly occurs in the femoral-popliteal segment as in the nondiabetic patient. The diabetic patients frequently have severe disease or occlusion of the popliteal trifurcation vessels as well.

DIRECT TREATMENT OF THE ISCHEMIC DIABETIC FOOT

The variety of contemporary multidisciplinary approaches to chronic leg ischemia have recently been presented as a complete summary and list of recommendations in the Consensus Document II.[27] This publication represents the combined understanding and philosophical approach endorsed by numerous international professional societies, including the World Health Organization. Critical leg ischemia in diabetic and nondiabetic patients is defined by either of two criteria, "persistently recurring ischemic rest pain requiring regular adequate analgesia for more than 2 weeks, with an ankle systolic pressure less than or equal to 50 mm Hg and/or a toe systolic pressure of less than or equal to 30 mm Hg, or ulceration or gangrene of the foot or toes, with an ankle systolic pressure of less than or equal to 50 mm Hg or a toe systolic pressure of less than or equal to 30 mm Hg."[27] Direct treatment, including revascularization, requires a team approach by the podiatrist, vascular surgeon, internist, interventional radiologist, and diabetologist, regardless of the initial referral pattern. The role of the interventional radiologist will be discussed in this section with particular reference to angioplasty.

Percutaneous transluminal angioplasty (PTA) consists of the direct recanalization of a stenosed or occluded artery using direct balloon inflation within the diseased segment under fluoroscopic guidance (see Fig 10–8). Access to the vascular segment under treatment is achieved using the percutaneous arteriographic technique. Angioplasty procedures have very low complication rates, do not require general anesthesia, have significantly shorter patient recovery time, and rarely preclude future surgical procedures. For these reasons, PTA should be considered the first revascularization option for amenable lesions.

Angioplasty and surgical bypass procedures have been compared by examining long-term patency rates for lesions according to their site and length. Angioplasty compares most favorably with bypass surgery for focal stenoses in the iliac and femoral arteries. The patency rate after treatment of occlusions longer than 3 cm by angioplasty alone is less favorable than comparable bypass surgery. The advent of newer hydrophilic guidewires and low-profile balloons, together with adjunctive thrombolytic therapy, has increased the initial technical success rate for angioplasty treatment of long segment occlusions of the iliac and femoral arteries.

Absolute contraindications for PTA include aortic occlusion, thrombosed popliteal aneurysms, and severe hemorrhagic disorders.[27] Acute complications that may require surgery occur in 3% or fewer catheter procedures. Long-term patency rates are diminished in longer occluded segments or vessels demonstrating diffuse atherosclerotic changes.

Treatment goals and technical success for revascularization procedures must be considered on an individual patient basis. Patients who are poor operative candidates or who are nonambulatory may benefit from PTA for less optimal lesions or extensive atherosclerotic disease if a shorter patency rate will allow wound healing.

REFERENCES

1. Resnick D, Niwayoma G: Osteomyelitis, septic arthritis, and soft tissue infections: mechanisms and situations. In *Bone and joint imaging,* Philadelphia, 1979, WB Saunders, pp 728–755.

2. Soman-Kovacs DS, Braunstein EM, Brandt KD: Rapidly progressive Charcot arthropathy following minor joint trauma in patients with diabetic neuropathy, *Arthritis Rheum* 33:412–416, 1990.

3. Schauwecker DS: The scintigraphic diagnosis of osteomyelitis, *AJR* 158:9–19, 1992.

4. Handmaker H, Leonard R: The bone scan in inflammatory osseous disease, *Semin Nucl Med* 6:95–105, 1976.

5. Israel O, Gips S, Jerushalmi J, et al: Osteomyelitis and soft tissue infection: Differential diagnosis with 24 hour/4 hour ratio of Tc-99m-MDP uptake, *Radiology* 163:725–726, 1987.

6. Alazraki N, Dries D, Datz F et al: Value of a 24-hour image (four phase bone scan) in assessing osteomyelitis in patients with peripheral vascular disease, *J Nucl Med* 26:711–717, 1985.

7. Glynn TP: Marked gallium accumulation in neurogenic arthropathy, *J Nucl Med* 22:1016–1017, 1981.

8. Hetherington VJ: Technetium and combined gallium and technetium scans in the neurotrophic foot, *J Am Podiatr Med Assoc* 72:458–463, 1982.

9. Maurer AH, Millmond SH, Knight LC et al: Infection in diabetic osteoarthropathy: use of indium labeled leukocytes for diagnosis, *Radiology* 161:221–225, 1986.

10. Schauwecker DS, Park HM, Mock BH et al: Evaluation of complicating osteomyelitis with Tc-99m-MDP, In-111 granulocytes, and Ga-67 citrate, *J Nucl Med* 25:849–853, 1984.

11. Wukich DK, Abreu SH, Callaghan JJ et al: Diagnosis of infection by preoperative scintigraphy with indium-labeled white blood cells, *J Bone Joint Surg* 69A:1353–1360, 1987.

12. Schauwecker DS, Park HM, Burt RW et al: Combined bone scintigraphy and indium-111 leukocyte scans in neuropathic foot disease, *J Nucl Med* 29:1651–1655, 1988.

13. Seabold JE, Flickinger FW, Kao SCS et al: Indium-111–leukocytes/technetium-99m-MDP bone and magnetic resonance imaging: difficulty of diagnosing osteomyelitis in patients with neuropathic osteoarthropathy, *J Nucl Med* 31:549–556, 1990.

14. Abren SH: Skeletal uptake in indium-111 labeled white blood cells, *Semin Nucl Med* 19:152–155, 1989.

15. McCarthy K, Velchik MG, Alavi A et al: Indium-111–labeled white blood cells in the detection of osteomyelitis complicated by a pre-existing condition, *J Nucl Med* 29:1015–1021, 1988.

16. Merkel KD, Brown ML, Dewanjee MK et al: Comparison of indium labeled leukocyte imaging with sequential technetium-gallium scanning in the diagnosis of low grade musculoskeletal sepsis, *J Bone Joint Surg* 67A:465–476, 1985.

17. Unger E, Moldofsky P, Gatenby R et al: Diagnosis of osteomyelitis by MR imaging, *AJR* 150:605–610, 1988.

18. Yuh WTC, Corson JD, Baraniewski HM et al: Osteomyelitis of the foot in diabetic patients: evaluation with plain film, 99m-Tc-MDP bone scintigraphy, and MR imaging, *AJR* 152:795–800, 1989.

19. Mason MD, Zlatkin MB, Esterhai JL et al: Chronic complicated osteomyelitis of the lower extremity: evaluation with MR imaging, *Radiology* 173:355–359, 1989.

20. Modic MT, Pflanze W, Feiglin DHI et al: Magnetic resonance imaging of musculoskeletal infections, *Radiol Clin North Am* 24:247–258, 1986.

21. Beltran J, Noto AM, McGhee RB et al: Infections of the musculoskeletal system: High field-strength MR imaging, *Radiology* 164:449–454, 1987.

22. Wong A, Weinstein D, Greenfield L et al: MRI and diabetic foot infections, *Magn Reson Imaging* 8:805–809, 1990.

23. Berquist TH: Magnetic resonance imaging of the foot and ankle, *Semin Ultrasound CT MR* 11:327–342, 1990.

24. Apelqvist J, Castenfors J, Larsson J et al: Prognostic value of systolic ankle and toe blood pressure levels in outcome of diabetic foot ulcer, *Diabetes Care* 12:373–378, 1989.

25. Katayama H, Yamaguchi K, Kozuka T et al: Adverse reactions to ionic and nonionic contrast media: a report from the Japanese committee on the safety of contrast media, *Radiology* 175:621–628, 1990.

26. Schwab SJ, Hlatky MA, Pieper KS et al: Contrast nephrotoxicity: a randomized controlled trial of a nonionic and an ionic radiographic contrast agent, *N Engl J Med* 320:149–153, 1989.

27. Chronic critical leg ischemia—consensus document, *Circulation* 8(4):1–26, 1991.

11 _____ Magnetic Resonance Imaging of the Diabetic Lower Extremity

David P. Mayer, M.D.

Youssef M. Kabbani, D.P.M.

The diagnosis of diabetes and the myriad of associated conditions are a constant challenge to clinicians and radiologists. This is especially true in the diagnosis of diabetic foot infections.

Diabetes is the third leading cause of morbidity in the United States.[1] The actual number of patients who carry the diagnosis of diabetes in the United States is estimated at 12 million,[1] and there is said to be a significant segment of the population that remains undiagnosed.[2] Gestational diabetes alone accounts for 86,000 new cases annually.[3] Most of the patients diagnosed with diabetes are more than age 40 years, and approximately 2.5 million of them are more than age 65 years.[4]

Research and data compiled from the past 20 years indicate that foot infections are the most common cause of sepsis and hospitalization of patients with diabetes mellitus[5, 6] because of a host of complications associated with diabetes affecting the extremities. Some of these complications of diabetes include atherosclerosis, neuropathy (autonomic and otherwise), and immunopathy. Although several processes may be contributory, none is more important than vascular disease. It is estimated that anywhere from 16% to 58% of all patients with diabetes have peripheral vascular disease.[7] Approximately 40,000 amputations each year are performed on diabetic patients.[7] About 15% of diabetics have ischemic ulcers on their

ankles and feet, and gangrene occurs each year in 5 of 1,000 diabetic individuals.[7]

Neuropathy, immunopathy, and angiopathy often complicate the evaluation and early diagnosis of diabetic foot infections. In these patients, the infection is often more extensive than it initially appears and can rapidly progress and may even become fatal if not promptly diagnosed and treated. Morbidity in these patients may result from a trivial soft tissue infection, which itself has an incidence of about 30% in this population group.[8]

PATHOGENESIS OF DIABETIC FOOT INFECTIONS

Neuropathy

Studies have shown that approximately 50% of patients with insulin-dependent diabetes mellitus manifest symptoms of diabetic neuropathy.[9]

Neuropathy in diabetes may manifest as a distal symmetric polyneuropathy, a proximal motor neuropathy, a focal neuropathy, or a combination of all three types.[10] The cause of these neuropathies has recently been linked to diabetic metabolic disturbances.[11] Insulin therapy and better glycemic control restores nerve conduction in velocity, but the relation between long-term control of hyperglycemia and the clinical severity of neuropathy has yet to be proved. Neuropathy most frequently occurs in middle-aged diabetics

161

and is not necessarily related to the severity of insulin deficiency.[12]

Neuropathy contributes to the increased risk of infections in patients with diabetes mellitus. Sensory impairment results in ulcerations that are potential routes of entry for bacteria and subsequent infection. The association of infections with an ulceration in the foot and ankle in patients with diabetes mellitus may be as high as 68%.[9]

Immunopathy

The diminution of the immune response in patients with diabetes mellitus may correlate with the degree of hyperglycemia and probably the duration of the disease. On a cellular level, hyperglycemia has been shown to reduce granulocyte function.[13] Chemotaxis, as well as phagocytosis of the granulocytes, has been shown to be reduced in diabetics.[14] In addition, decreased fibroblastic activity and collagen synthesis have been shown to occur in diabetics, thus leading to impaired wound healing.[15] However, humoral immunity in patients with diabetes appears to be normal.

Angiopathy

Peripheral vascular disease (PVD) is 20 times more common in diabetics than in nondiabetics.[1] It is estimated that there is a sixfold increase in the incidence of PVD 20 years after the onset of diabetes.[7] Furthermore, the incidence of gangrene is 20 times more prevalent in diabetics than in nondiabetics.[7]

Macrovascular, as well as microvascular, disease accounts for the major of morbidity and mortality in the diabetic population. PVD develops at a younger age in the diabetic population and tends to be equal between men and women. The disease affects primarily the vessels below the knee, which, in turn, produces arch and digital claudication.

Microvascular involvement in patients with diabetes has been shown to occur at the capillary basement membrane level.[16, 17] Clinically, changes in the integument are most expressive of the pathology of the microvasculature occurring in the diabetic foot. The skin becomes shiny and atrophic, the nails become thickened, and there is loss of digital hair.

Given all these pathophysiologic processes occurring simultaneously, it is therefore essential to use the most effective diagnostic modalities to make the correct diagnosis. Plain radiographs, scintigraphy, and computed tomography (CT) all have been used in the diagnosis of diabetic foot infections. The sensitivity and specificity of each of these modalities vary widely.

RADIOGRAPHIC EVALUATION OF THE DIABETIC FOOT

Because osteomyelitis in the diabetic is most frequently caused by contiguous soft tissue infection, plain radiographs coupled with the clinical findings offer helpful clues in excluding osteomyelitis.[18] Ulcerations are frequently visible on plain films, and bony involvement may be demonstrated. Radiolucencies associated with bony destruction, along with soft tissue infection, are frequent findings. Other findings may include osteosclerosis, cortical thickening, and periosteal new bone formation.[19] Finally, gas is sometimes demonstrated by plain film radiography, and when present, it offers significant additional diagnostic information.

The limitations of plain film radiography in diagnosing infections, especially in the diabetic, are many. X-ray changes lag behind the infectious process by as much as 10 to 21 days.[20] Initially bone marrow alterations in response to infection are also radiographically undetectable (Fig 11–1). Later, the destructive changes of osteomyletis may become

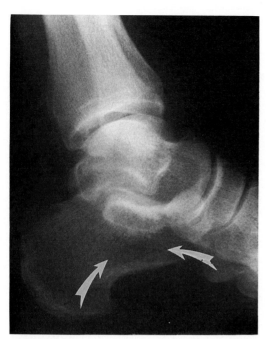

FIG 11–1.
Lateral radiograph of a patient with symptoms localizable to the calcaneus. The *two curved arrows* delineate an area of relative lucency in the middle to anterior calcaneus. This area later proved to have a focus of osteomyelitis.

invisible. Furthermore, differentiation of osteomyelitis from bony neurotrophic changes in the diabetic offers the greatest challenge.[18] Specifically, neurotrophic destructive bony changes, cortical thickening, and sclerosis manifesting with or without an associated ulceration can be impossible to differentiate from osteomyelitis. In a comparative study on the detection of osteomyelitis in the diabetic foot, radiography was found to be 75% specific and sensitive.[21] Thus, radiology serves as the first step in the diagnosis of foot and ankle complications of diabetes.

SCINTIGRAPHY OF THE DIABETIC FOOT

Scintigraphy has been effectively used in the detection of osteomyelitis in the general and the diabetic population. The techniques include scans of leukocytes labeled with technetium-99m, with gallium-67, and indium-111. The sensitivity and specificity of these techniques vary,[21–27] especially when used in the diagnosis of diabetic foot infections.[28–31]

Technetium-99m pyrophosphate scans have been used to differentiate cellulitis from osteomyelitis.[29] Blood pool images aid in this effort, because cellulitis is said to appear as diffuse uptake on blood pool images and osteomyelitis appears as a focal uptake on both early and delayed images (Fig 11–2, A and B). Omara[69] showed ^{99m}Tc studies to be 76% sensitive, 99% specific, and 93% accurate on diagnosing osteomyelitis vs. 76% accuracy for routine radiographs.[66]

Both ^{67}Ga and ^{111}In scans have been reported to have increased sensitivity in the detection of osteomyelitis.[22, 26, 28, 30, 31] Leukocytes labeled with ^{111}In seek the site of infection and may allow for differentiation of cellulitis and osteomyelitis from other processes (Fig 11–2, C).

Some recent comparative studies on the effectiveness of scintigraphy as a diagnostic modality in the evaluation of diabetic foot infections are not as favorable. In their study of various techniques for the evaluation of diabetic foot infections, Unger et al.[32] found scintigraphy to have 100% false positive specificity in diabetics who have coexistent cellulitis, chronic skin ulcers, other soft tissue infections, periostitis, and neurotrophic changes. The limited spatial resolution and lack of direct visualization of the bone marrow as well as difficulty in distinguishing between a soft tissue infection vs. diabetic osteoarthropathy and osteomyelitis were some of the problems cited.

Although ^{111}In scans has improved the sensitivity of scintigraphy for infection, poor spatial resolution and inability to delineate the soft tissues from bony involvement has lead to high false positive results.[28, 33] Furthermore, the technique has been cited as being ineffective in demon-

A

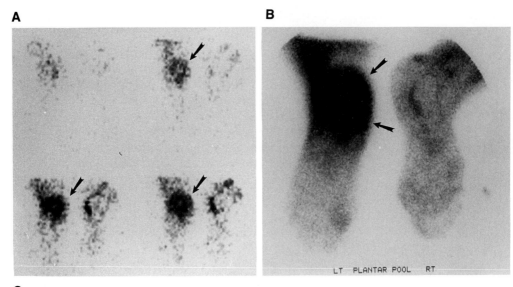

B

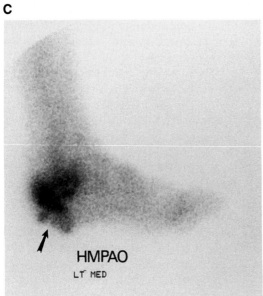

C

FIG 11–2.

A, four images from the angiographic (flow) phase of the ^{99m}-Tc pyrophosphate scan of a patient with a osteomyelitis of the left calcaneus. The *straight arrows* show the area of increased uptake in the calcaneus. **B,** a single blood pool radionuclide scan shows an area of marked increase in uptake in the region of the hind foot consistent with what proved to be calcaneal osteomyelitis. **C,** lateral view of the ankle showing uptake in the calcaneus consistent with osteomyelitis using ^{111}In-labeled leukocytes.

A

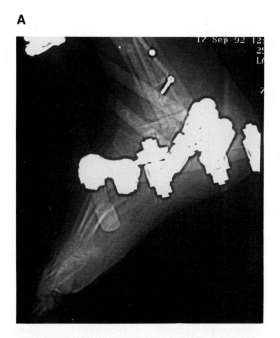

B

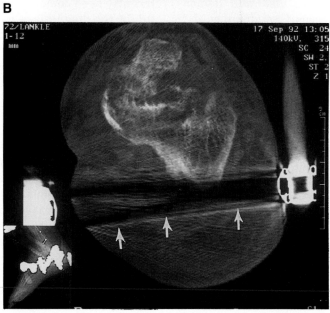

FIG 11–3.
A CT localizer image in **A** and a direct coronal image of the same patient. It should be noted that on the localizer there is an extensive amount of metal that precluded satisfactory plain film radiography. However, in **B** with the judicious choice of scan planes (direct coronal plane), and despite the loss of satisfactory imaging along the dorsal aspect of the midfoot *(straight arrows)*, much information can still be obtained concerning changes in the osseous structures.

strating chronic osteomyelitis.[34] There are other limitations include a prolonged labeling process and questionable potential long-term radiation harm to the lymphocytes.[35] Thus, other imaging modalities may be required to yield additional diagnostic information in these patients.

COMPUTED TOMOGRAPHY OF THE DIABETIC FOOT

The literature is limited concerning utilization of CT scanning in the evaluation of the diabetic foot.[36–38] Nevertheless, CT has been shown to be of some value in the detection of musculoskeletal infections.[39–41] Cortical destruction and periosteal involvement are well demonstrated by CT. Medullary and soft tissue extension can also be identified. Soft tissue pathology and gas are also well demonstrated in many cases. Chaudnaui et al.,[42] in their study on the experimental detection of osteomyelitis and abscesses, found CT to be 52% sensitive and 100% specific in the detection of abscesses. Furthermore, CT was 66% sensitive and 97% specific in the detection of osteomyelitis, and it had an acceptable accuracy of about 78% overall. Disadvantages of CT include its limited utility in patients with metallic implants, which may yield inadequate imaging (Fig 11–3). In addition, there is the potential toxicity of the iodinated intravenous contrast agent[43] required for enhanced CT scanning.

Computed tomography of the foot and ankle in patients with potential osteomyelitis requires the finest possible techniques. Acquiring images in small fields of view and imaging only a single limb at a time should be carried out with scanning in at least two orthogonal planes. In our series (unpublished data) at least 70% of patients can be positioned to allow direct sagittal imaging. In addition, it is essential that the planes of section be optimized to lie orthogonal to the structure under

study. Images that are acquired in an oblique fashion are more difficult to interpret, and partial volume averaging artifacts may become more pronounced under those circumstances.

Furthermore, for optimal imaging it is essential to acquire the images using a high-resolution bone algorithm (edge enhancement), as well as to reconstruct the images using a soft tissue algorithm. When these techniques are used, subtle areas of proliferative bony change, erosion, and fragmentation can be detected more easily.

MAGNETIC RESONANCE IMAGING TECHNIQUES FOR THE DIABETIC FOOT

Magnetic resonance imaging (MRI) has recently been demonstrated to be successful for the diagnosis of marrow space disease and the demonstration of diabetic foot infections.[21, 43–45] The superb soft tissue contrast of MRI has become an invaluable diagnostic tool. Several other attractive features of MRI are its ability to image in any (desired) plane without the use of ionizing radiation, excellent resolution, safer contrast agent, and the capability to perform magnetic resonance angiography.

Like CT scanning, imaging of the foot and ankle in patients with a potential infection also requires optimization of technique. Imaging with a single limb allows much increased resolution. With current technology, a send/receive extremity coil will produce satisfactory images. In the future, technologic advances, including phased array and quadrature extremity surface coils, will allow augmented image quality and increased throughput.

Images must be obtained in at least two planes of sections that are orthogonal to the structures under examination.[46] This is a general rule of thumb in MRI, which is particularly important in the foot and ankle where the anatomy is especially complex. In our facility, we use fields of view (FOV) that are never more than 16 cm (160 mm). The typical imaging FOV is 14 cm for the ankle and midfoot, whereas the forefoot studies require FOV between 8 and 10 cm. As higher matrices become available and the signal/noise ratio is enhanced with additional surface coils using technologies such as phased array or quadrature imaging, as well as fast imaging techniques, it may be possible to acquire the images with a larger field of view with a correspondingly higher matrix to allow better coverage of the foot and ankle without significant loss of resolution.

In general, MRI has among the highest contrast of any diagnostic imaging modality. There are now additional techniques to augment the already inherently high contrast seen in conventional T_1- and T_2-weighted spin-echo images, as well as with gradient-echo studies. These techniques include fat saturation, which can be used before contrast with T_2-weighted images or after contrast with T_1-weighted images. In addition, Short T_1 Inversion Recovery (STIR) can be used to augment contrast by effectively adding together the differences between the T_1-weighted image and the T_2-weighted image of pathological vs. normal tissues. This technique is especially high in sensitivity but relatively low in specificity, as well as frequently low in resolution and signal/noise ratio when compared with conventional spin-echo or other techniques.

Routine imaging of the forefoot is typically done at our facility with dual 3-in. coils that can be phased array or conventional.[47] Alternatively, if a phased array extremity surface coil is available, this produces a particularly high signal/noise ratio and can be used with the forefoot as well. In general, with the smaller fields of view there are smaller voxels (volume element), and thus there are greater demands on the system to produce enough signal so as to maintain satisfactory im-

age quality; hence, improved surface coils or other techniques may be required.

Routine techniques employed for midfoot and ankle MRI in our facility include sagittal T_1-weighted images using a 256 by 512 matrix with a 16-cm FOV. After this, using a 14-cm FOV, axial T_1 and T_2-weighted images are acquired. A sagittal T_2-weighted fat saturated or STIR series are also acquired using fast spin-echo techniques. This technique requires approximately 2 minutes to acquire and is extraordinarily sensitive for small amounts of fluid signal intensity material that typically accompany inflammatory processes or bone injuries. After this, 14-cm FOV images in the coronal plane using fast spin-echo, proton density and T_2-weighted images are acquired. Fast spin echo is a technique recently introduced that dramatically decreases the acquisition time for T_2-weighted spin-echo type of images. This technique allows higher resolution in less time than previously required for conventional spin-echo imaging.

In cases in which there is suspected abscess or osteomyelitis, contrast is typically administered after initial T_1, T_2, and fat saturation T_2-weighted images. On precontrast T_1-weighted images, the typical focus of osteomyelitis is lower in signal intensity than the secondary normal fatty marrow (Fig 11–4, A and B). On a T_2-weighted image, this area becomes increased in signal intensity (Fig 11–4, C). On T_2-weighted fat saturation images in which the signal intensity from the background fatty marrow is suppressed, the area of inflammatory change (which has an increased amount of free water) is significantly increased in relative signal intensity and hence rendered more obvious (Fig 11–4, D).

When contrast is administered, it should be administered using bolus techniques. After this, T_1-weighted images are acquired. On postcontrast T_1-weighted images without fat saturation, there is rel-

A

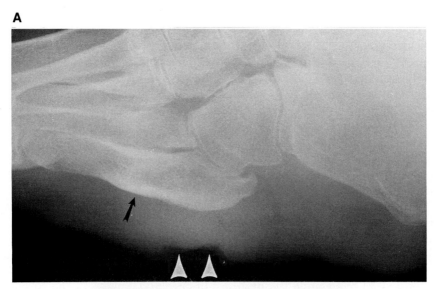

B

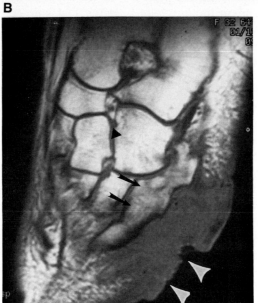

FIG 11–4.

A, the arrowheads show a focal defect in the skin with some overlying increase in density of the subcutaneous fat adjacent to the base of the fifth metatarsal. The base of the fifth metatarsal shows some inhomogeneity of density and some sclerosis of the cortices *(straight arrow)*. **B,** parasagittal T_1-weighted MR image. The ulceration in the skin is also well demonstrated (see *arrowheads*). In addition, the subcutaneous fat is diffusely lower in signal intensity consistent with induration, edema, or cellulitis. The normal marrow space signal of the cuboid *(black arrowhead)* is contrasted with a lower signal intensity of the marrow space of the fifth metatarsal *(black arrows)*. In the proper clinical setting, this lowered marrow signal intensity on the T_1-weighted image should always be considered suspicious for osteomyelitis. **C,** T_2-weighted coronal image. The high signal from the marrow space of the base of the fifth metatarsals *(straight arrow)* is contrasted with that of the normally low signal intensity of the marrow space of the cuneiforms *(little arrows)*. **D,** T_2-weighted fat saturation image. Notice the diminished signal/noise ratio (increased graininess) on the image that occurs when there is less signal coming from the marrow spaces secondary to a cancellation of the signal from the fat protons. However, the diffusely increased signal intensity from the area of inflammatory change within the proximal half of the fifth metatarsal is well demonstrated consistent with osteomyelitis.

C

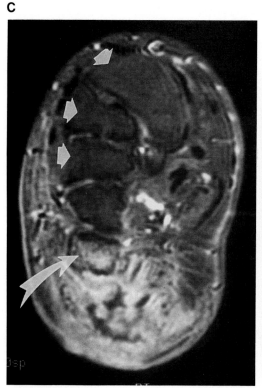

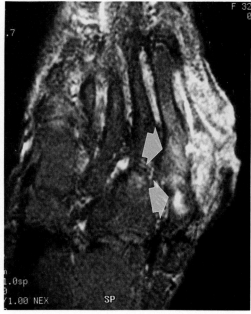

FIG 11–4 (cont.).
For legend see opposite page.

ative enhancement at the area of osteomyelitis. However, the fatty marrow tissue will itself enhance briskly after gadopentate dimeglumine (Gd-DTPA) administration. Thus, the relative difference between the inflammatory tissue and the enhancing fat may be limited. To increase the relative conspicuity of the area of inflammatory change from that of the background normal marrow, one can use fat saturation techniques. With fat saturation T_1-weighted post-^{67}Ga enhancement images, the relative conspicuity of the inflammatory area is significantly increased as the background fatty marrow signal is suppressed (Fig 11–5).

Patients who have pacemakers, ferromagnetic aneurysm clips, cochlear-stimulating devices, and other implanted electrical devices, as well as patients who have shrapnel fragments within their bodies should be excluded from the MRI scanner.[48] In addition, patients who have had extensive internal metallic fixation may not be candidates for MRI because the image quality will be sufficiently degraded by the presence of metal to preclude a diagnostic study. However, whereas in CT scanning the metal will cause a marked artifact that frequently produces near total obscuration of the image, in MRI the presence of internal metallic fixation may obscure only a portion of the image and leave a substantial amount of useful information in the remainder of the study.[49]

It should also be noted that as a routine consequence of podiatric and orthopedic surgery throughout the body, microscopic metallic fragments are frequently deposited into the surgical bed. This causes characteristic artifacts in which

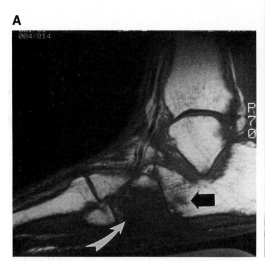

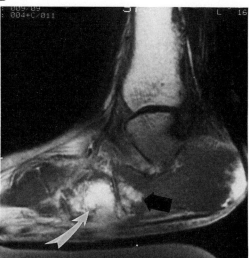

FIG 11–5.

A, T₁-weighted sagittal image through the calcaneus, cuboid, and base of the fourth metatarsal. The *curved arrow* shows very low signal intensity from the cuboid. **B,** T₁-weighted postcontrast fat saturation technique image. The *white curved arrows* in **A** and **B** show an area of extensive osteomyelitis affecting the cuboid.

The area of involvement is of a diminished signal on conventional T₁-weighted image and is briskly enhanced on the postcontrast T₁-weighted fat saturation images. *The black arrow* in **A** and **B** shows an area of osteomyelitis affecting the anterior aspect of the calcaneus as well.

there is an area of low signal surrounded by a halo of higher signal. This does not typically produce sufficient deterioration of the image to preclude a satisfactory diagnostic study.[49] The artifact will be most pronounced on gradient echo examinations because of the so-called susceptibility artifact. The images least affected by these metal-induced artifacts are those produced by fast spin-echo techniques, which are relatively less sensitive to susceptibility artifacts.

Findings

Edema

In several studies on MRI of the diabetic foot, nonspecific edema was noted to be a frequent finding.[21, 45, 50] The edema is usually found localized within both the dorsal and the plantar compartments of the foot (Fig 11–6). The exact etiology of this phenomenon is not known. Some theorize that associated diabetic neurop-

athy results in uneven weight bearing, resulting in stasis and fluid accumulation as a possible cause.[21]

Edema, which is obviously made up of excess water, appears as diffusely increased signal intensity on T₂-weighted images within the superficial or deep compartments. If the edema is limited in extent, it frequently manifests with a branching pattern. In one study this finding was particularly prevalent deep to the plantar aponeurosis, between the flexor digitorum brevis and the plantar fascia.[45] Because this finding is nonspecific, edema may be difficult to differentiate from the findings of cellulitis on MRI. However, the distortion of the subcutaneous tissues seen in infectious processes can aid in the differentiation between noninfectious edema and cellulitis.[51]

Cellulitis

Cellulitis is a deep infection of the skin, resulting in a localized area of ery-

A

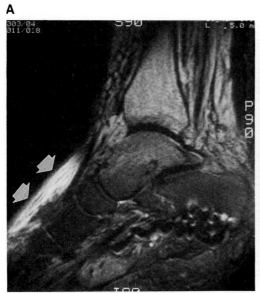

B

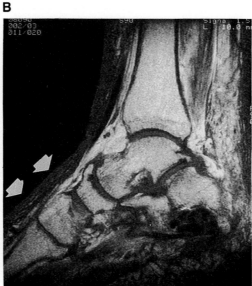

FIG 11–6.

The *small white arrows* denote an area of diffusely diminished signal intensity on the T_1-weighted image **(B)** affecting the dorsal aspect of the midfoot with associated increased in signal intensity on the T_2- weighted image **(A)** within the same region. This represents an area of noninfectious edema along the dorsal aspect of the foot in a diabetic patient.

thema. In adults, cellulitis most frequently affects the lower legs and is a frequent finding among diabetic patients. Although cellulitis is considered a clinical diagnosis, cellulitis can easily mask an abscess or osteomyelitis in patients with diabetes mellitus. In addition, because cellulitis is managed with antibiotics and local therapies, differentiating it from a deep abscess or osteomyelitis is crucial, especially when the patient's condition is complicated by vascular and neurological compromise.

On T_1-weighted MRI images, the normal high signal intensity of the subcutaneous fat and intermuscular fatty septa is replaced by intermediate signal intensity of the inflammatory process (Fig 11–7).[52] On proton density–weighted spin-echo MRI pulse sequences (short TE, long TR), cellulitis appears as a diffuse area of intermediate signal within the subcutaneous tissues. The area appears indistinct and is poorly marginated. The soft tissues may appear thickened as well. On T_2-

weighted MRI pulse sequences, cellulitis takes on a markedly increased signal intensity that is typical of inflammatory processes in which there is increased free water in the tissue. Morphologically, cellulitis has poor margination, which is quite helpful in differentiating it from an abscess. Gd-DTPA enhancement may further aid in the diagnosis, as cellulitis, abscess, and sinuses tracts have been shown to enhance, whereas frank pus and necrotic areas will not enhance.[45]

Abscesses and Deep Soft Tissue Infections

Soft tissue infections are the most common infections in the diabetic.[53] Deeper soft tissue infections may result from puncture wounds or pressure ulcerations. Web space and nail bed infections may result in a potentially life-threatening deep plantar space infection if not treated effectively. The complex anatomy of the plantar spaces may allow for the infection to spread beyond the confines of

A

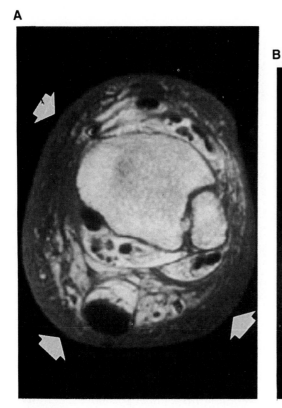

B

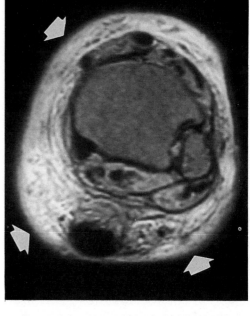

FIG 11–7.
Axial T₁- **(A)** and T₂-weighted **(B)** images through the ankle just proximal to the plane of the ankle joint. There is diffuse diminution in signal on the T₁-weighted im-ages of the subcutaneous tissues. The changes in the subcutaneous fat are confluent. This is consistent with the patient's extensive cellulitis.

the plantar space to involve the lower leg.[54]

On T₁-weighted MRI images abscesses appear as localized low signal intensity (slightly less in signal intensity than muscle) collections surrounded by a low intensity rim. The presence of a well-defined collection may yield a "mass effect" on adjacent structures and thus aid in the differentiation from cellulitis alone (Fig 11–8, A and B).[50] On T₂ and STIR pulse sequences, the abscess collection appears as a high signal intensity mass, well marginated, and predominantly homogeneous (Fig 11–8, C and D). The collection may even appear higher in signal than the surrounding edema on these images.[50] The ability to precisely locate these high signal intensity lesions in multiple planes

with excellent resolution, and the ability to evaluate for other associated tissue involvement makes MRI the modality of choice when these lesions are imaged. After Gd-DTPA contrast enhancement, the rim of the lesion will enhance and thus yield a zone of higher signal intensity, but the pus itself does not enhance. T₁-weighted, contrast-enhanced fat saturation images, which lower the signal intensity of the subcutaneous and deep fat, as well as the signal from fatty marrow, will show water-based lesions such as cellulitis and abscess to even better advantage when compared with conventional contrast-enhanced, T₁-weighted images (Fig 11–8, E and F).

Gas within an abscess appears as low signal intensity focus on all pulse se-

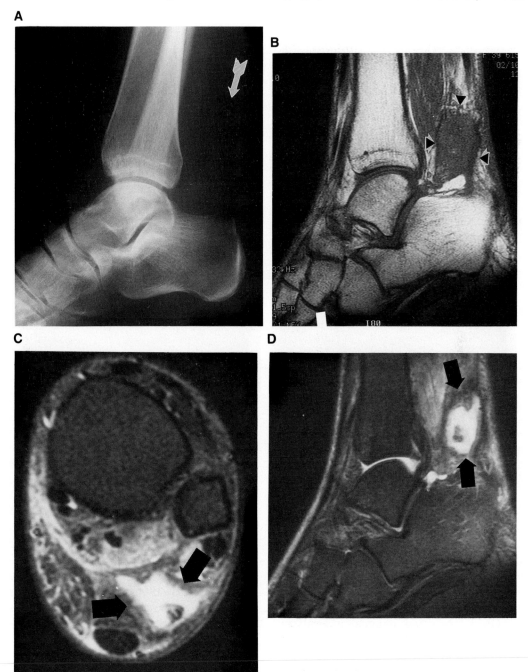

FIG 11–8.
Lateral radiograph **(A)** and sagittal T_1-weighted image **(B)**. On the lateral radiograph *(small arrow)* there is a subtle area of increased density projected in Kager's triangle. On the T_1-weighted image **(B)** the arrowheads denote an area of diminished signal intensity within Kager's triangle surrounded by relatively normal high signal intensity fat. FSE axial T_2-weighted images **(C)** and sagittal fat saturation FSE T_2-weighted images **(D)**. The arrows denote the abscess, which is a region of high signal intensity centrally with a relatively low signal intensity periphery. Axial T_1-weighted conven- tional spin-echo image **(E)** and T_1-weighted axial fat saturation post-⁶⁷G enhancement images **(F)**. In **E** the abscess is diffusely diminished in signal intensity *(small white arrows)*. This can be contrasted with the high signal of the subcutaneous fat along the posterior and medial aspect of the ankle *(curved white arrow)*. In **F,** the pus within the center of the abscess is rela- tively lower in signal intensity *(double-headed arrow)*. The abscess wall briskly enhances denoted by the *small black arrows*.

(Continued.)

E

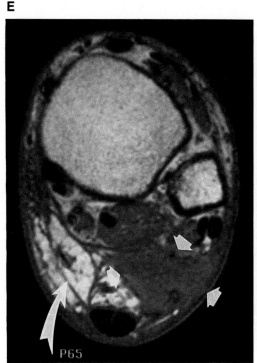

F

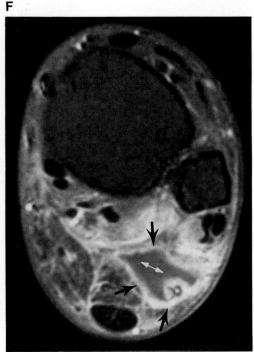

FIG 11–8.
For legend see previous page.

quences. Foreign bodies such as metal will appear as low signal intensity foci frequently surrounded by an incomplete high signal intensity halo. Some pulse sequences (especially gradient echo scans) may have partially prominent susceptibility artifacts, which are usually very low in signal intensity from the gas and metal (Fig 11–9).

Ulcerations

On T_1-weighted images, ulcerations appear as defects of low signal intensity in the skin and in the subcutaneous tissues. The soft tissues appear thickened. Sinus tracts extending from the ulcer bordering on bone are well demonstrated as linear low signal intensity bands on T_1-weighted images. On T_2-weighted images, there is frequently higher signal from the tissues surrounding the ulceration (Fig 11–10).

Acute Osteomyelitis

Direct extension or contiguous spread of infection are the most common sources of bone infection in diabetics (Fig 11–11). In one study, 68% of diabetic patients with foot infections were associated with an ulceration.[8] Osteomyelitis as a complication of diabetic foot problems occurs in about 13% of patients admitted to hospitals for diabetic foot problems in the Kozak et al.[55] series and as many as one third of all diabetic foot infections in the Waldvogal-Vasey[56] series.[57] About one fourth of diabetic osteomyelitis is said to be secondary to vascular insufficiency.[58]

Osteitis

Osteitis is an infection of bone tissue that does not penetrate the medullary cavity. Osteitis may result from direct puncture wounds or from underlying ulcerations, both of which are encountered

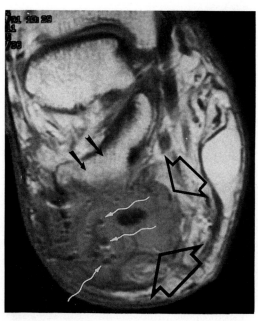

FIG 11–9.
Coronal proton density image through the midfoot. The small black arrows indicated the calcaneus. An abscess is present in the plantar aspect (delineated by *open black arrows*). Within the abscess are punctate areas of low signal intensity with an incomplete high signal intensity halo *(curved white arrows)*. The *curved white arrows* denote tiny gas bubbles within the abscess. The low signal with surrounding halos are a manifestation of susceptibility artifact.

more frequently in diabetic patients than in the general population. When soft tissue infection extends to bone, it may induce a periosteal reaction or periostitis. At this stage the osteitis may be on an infectious or noninfectious basis. Cortical extension from the inflammatory process may extend into the medullary cavity, thus causing osteomyelitis.

Periosteal elevation and irritation are commonly seen in acute cases of osteomyelitis. On MRI, periosteal elevation ap-

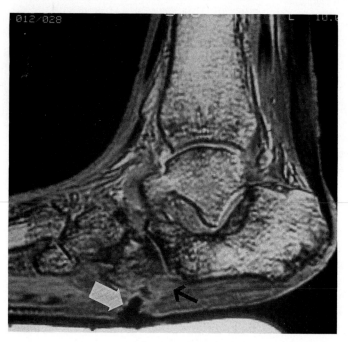

FIG 11–10.
Gradient-echo image performed in a volumetric acquisition with contiguous 2-mm slices (TE = 10 ms; TR = 25 ms; flip angle = 30 degrees). The *white arrow* denotes an ulceration in the skin underlying the cuboid. The *small black arrow* denotes a subtle area of increased signal intensity in the adjacent subcutaneous tissue on this image, which is very slightly T_2 weighted.

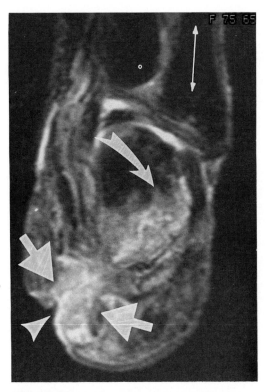

FIG 11-11.
Image from a STIR coronal study through a patient with a focal ulceration *(white arrowhead)* with adjacent reactive changes in the soft tissues of the plantar aspect of the hind foot. The *double-headed arrow* in the distal fibula shows the markedly diminished signal emanating from the normal marrow fat in the STIR technique. The *curved arrow* shows an area of osteomyelitis within the calcaneus.

pears as a single linear low signal intensity band paralleling the cortex. High signal intensity alterations between the periosteal and the cortex represent pus or inflammatory edema suggestive of infective osteitis.

On T_1-weighted images, periosteal irritation is noted as a very low signal intensity abnormality bordering the surface of the involved bone. Areas of cancellous bone involvement also appear as low signal intensity focus against the high intensity background of normal marrow fat.

On T_2-weighted and STIR images, periosteal involvement manifests as areas of increased signal intensity set against a background of the normally low signal intensity of the adjacent normal cortex (Fig 11-12, A).[50] Extension beyond the cortical margin involving the subchondral bone plate and marrow space is highlighted as an increased signal intensity region, suggesting extension of the infectious process.

Once the infection extends into the medullary cavity, significant inflammation results, and progression of this process is followed by marrow replacement. This produces a characteristic decreased signal intensity on T_1-weighted images and increased signal intensity on T_2-weighted and STIR pulse sequences (Fig 11-12, B and C). These changes are thought to result from a decrease in the fat content and an increase of the water content of the infected bone (Fig 11-13).[50] Cortical disruption as a result of the infectious process is often associated with soft tissue involvement, which aids in the diagnosis.

Most of the literature reviewed on MRI of osteomyelitis indicates that this signal intensity pattern is not 100% specific for this process. This is consistent with our experience. Other acute processes involving the medullary cavity also cause nonspecific inflammation of the bone marrow, thus yielding similar MRI signal intensity patterns as seen in osteomyelitis. Specifically, occult fractures, metastasis, and ischemic necrosis[59] result in edema and signal intensity patterns as may be similar to osteomyelitis. In these situations, MRI results should be correlated with the clinical findings, as well as radiographs, other diagnostic imaging modalities, and laboratory tests, such as sedimentation rate and complete blood cell differential count. Unger et al.[32] found MRI to be 92% sensitive and 96% specific and showed an overall accuracy of 94% in the diagnosis of osteomyelitis. The use of contrast enhancement may yet prove to help differentiate between pathological processes that produce increases in free

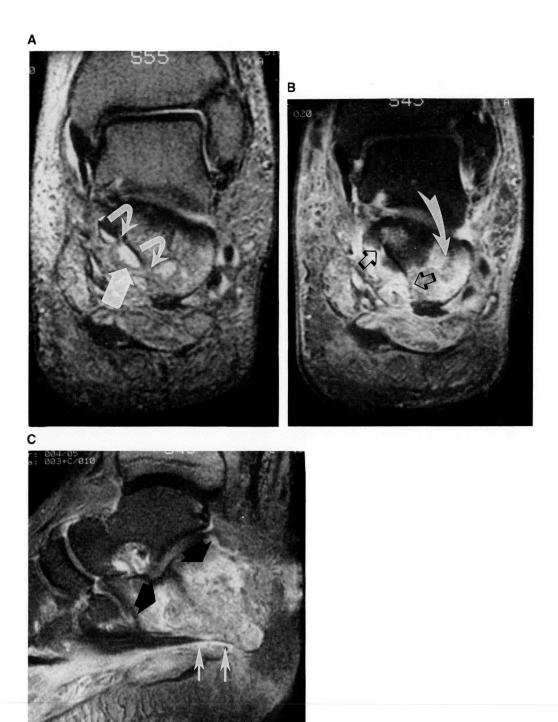

FIG 11–12.
Coronal conventional T_2-weighted image **(A)** and coronal T_2-weighted fat saturation image **(B)**. The *curved arrows* in **A** denote two areas of abnormally increased signal intensity of the dorsal medial cortex of the calcaneus. The *straight arrows* shows a pocket a fluid signal intensity material, representing abscess associated with these areas of osteitis. On the T_2-weighted fat saturation image **(B)**, the *two open black arrows* show the areas of abnormally increased signal intensity of the cortex to even greater advantage. The adjacent increase in signal within the marrow space *(curved white marrow)* shows a region of osteomyelitis associated with an area of cortical osteitis. **C,** sagittal image also using T_1-weighted fat saturation techniques. The *small straight arrows* show an area of inflammatory change adjacent to the plantar cortex of the calcaneus. The cortex itself shows patchy increase in signal intensity. The diffuse increase in signal of the marrow space *(small black arrows)* shows an extensive area of osteomyelitis.

A   **B**

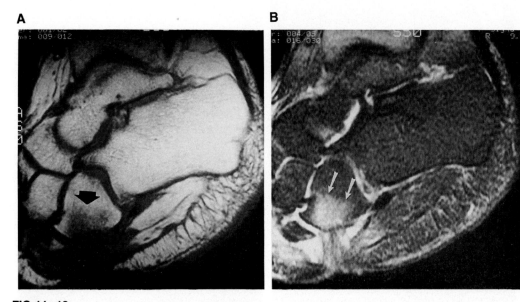

FIG 11–13.
Sagittal T_1- **(A)** and T_2-weighted **(B)** fat saturation images. The cuboid shows a focal area of diminished signal intensity *(black arrows)* in **A,** which is a T_1weighted noncontrast-enhanced image. This represents an area of replacement of the normal marrow

fat with hematopoietic and inflammatory elements. On the T_2-weighted fat saturation image **(B)**, the area of osteomyelitis is well demonstrated as well *(white arrows).*

water within the marrow space on a noninfectious basis vs. osteomyelitis.

Chronic Osteomyelitis

Chronic osteomyelitis is often a sequelae of long-standing ischemic or neurotrophic ulcerations. Indeed, approximately 25% of diabetic osteomyelitis is secondary to vascular insufficiency.[58] Chronic osteomyelitis may also result from hematogenous spread, after surgery, or as a result of open or closed fractures and puncture wounds. A frequent diagnostic challenge is the ruling out of osteomyelitis in a diabetic foot with associated Charcot's changes.

Chronic osteomyelitis can be diagnosed solely by standard radiographs. The classic secondary changes of this process as seen on radiographs include sequestra, involucra, sinus tracts, and cloacae. Unfortunately, these same changes may be also noted in noninfectious chronic Charcot's joint changes, causing a diagnostic dilemma when radiography, scintigraphy, and CT are used.[60]

On T_2-weighted pulse sequences intramedullary foci of active infection are demonstrated as regions of increased signal intensity. These areas may be separated from healthy bone by a low intensity rim. The increased signal intensity within the medullary bone may be secondary to an intramedullary abscess or granulation tissue. Resolution of the infection results in normalization of the intramedullary signal on T_1-weighted images, possibly because of the replacement of the abnormal hematopoietic marrow by normal fatty marrow on resolution of the infection (Fig 11–14).[32]

Sequestra are devitalized pieces of bone and usually cortical in origin. They appear as low signal intensity bodies similar to cortical bone on T_1- and T_2-weighted images. If they are of cancellous origin, they appear slightly higher in signal intensity. Usually they are irregularly shaped and may be surrounded by an outer low intensity rim secondary to pus on T_1-weighted images.[52] On T_2-weighted images, the pus will be of a higher signal intensity.

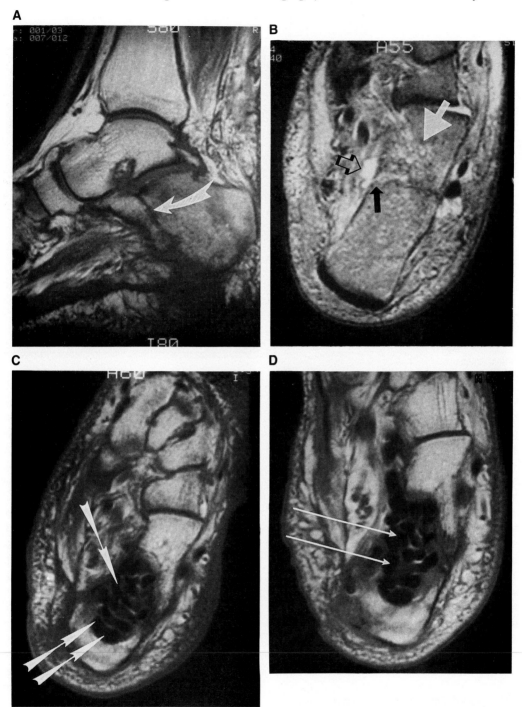

FIG 11–14.
A, sagittal T$_1$-weighted image. The changes of chronic osteomyelitis are identified by manifest of inhomogeneity of signal intensity throughout the calcaneus. In addition, a fracture line is identified *(curved white arrow)*. **B,** which is an axial T$_2$-weighted image, is an adjacent area of pus *(open black arrow)* seen in the area of focal disruption in the cortex of the calcaneus *(small black arrow)*. The signal within the calcaneus is abnormally increased on this T$_2$-weighted image *(white arrow)* consistent with the patient's known osteomyelitis. Surgical therapy was required to correct this chronic osteomyelitis. In **C** and **D** axial T$_1$-weighted and axial T$_1$-weighted images respectively, the focus areas of low signal within the surgical defect *(straight arrows)* represent the low signal from antibiotic impregnated methyl methacrylate beads. On the post-contrast scans there is only scant enhancement identified consistent with successful therapy.

(Continued).

E

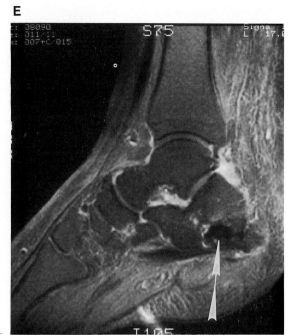

FIG 11–14 (cont.).
For legend see previous page.

Sinus tracts appear as high-signal intensity, linear-shaped foci extending from the bone to the skin. Within these tracts, pus and necrotic debris may be demonstrated.

Finally, the cortices along with the soft tissues surrounding the osteomyelitis bone also demonstrate characteristic changes associated with chronic osteomyelitis. On T_1-weighted images the cortices are thickened and of low signal intensity. The soft tissues such as the subcutaneous tissues and septae appear intermediate in signal intensity and may be obliterated. Surrounding muscles may be edematous and thus reveal an increased signal intensity on T_2-weighted images.

EVALUATION OF THE DIABETIC CHARCOT FOOT: CHARCOT VS. OSTEOMYELITIS

Although there are various etiologies for neuropathic arthropathy, diabetes mellitus is by far the most common cause. It has been estimated that about 50% of di-

abetics manifest with some clinical evidence of neuropathy.[9] Neuroarthropathy in diabetics involves primarily the foot and ankle and may have an incidence between 5% and 10% in these patients.[9]

In their large series at the Joslin Clinic, Frykberg et al.[61] reported on the frequency of foot and ankle involvement by the neuropathic process. The tarsometatarsal joints were most frequently involved, followed by the first metatarsal phalangeal joint and then the ankle joint. They noted 20% bilateral involvement regardless of sex.[61] Similarly, bilateral involvement has been reported by Cofield et al.[62] in 1983, but in their cases the metatarsal-phalangeal joint was more commonly involved. Ulcerations adjacent to areas of bony involvement also had a significant incidence of 87% in the Cofield et al.[62] study.

Frequently it is the complications associated with diabetic neuropathic arthropathy that contribute a significant degree to the morbidity and mortality in patients with diabetes mellitus. Loss of joint sensory innervation and proprioception may result in spontaneous fractures, progressive articular, and periarticular destructive changes leading to deformity and soft tissue injuries resulting in skin ulcerations, tendon and ligament tears, as well as soft tissue and bony infections, all potentially leading to loss of a limb (Fig 11–15).

The radiologic findings of neuropathic arthropathy of the feet can be categorized based on the area of involvement of the disease process.[62] Diaphyseal involvement manifests with specific radiographic findings. These include periosteal reaction, osteoporosis or osteosclerosis, and thickening or thinning of the bone. Metaphyseal periarticular or articular areas radiographically may manifest with subluxation or dislocation, cartilage loss, bony fragmentation, sclerosis or resorption,

prominent effusion, loose bodies, and debris.

Charcot joints associated with ulceration often manifest with soft tissue swelling and osteoporosis of the adjacent bone. Although this manifestation may aid in the diagnosis of an infected Charcot joint, it is by no means a reliable method.[60] Further diagnostic imaging studies are often required to evaluate for the presence of osteomyelitis in these individuals.

ROLE OF SCINTIGRAPHY FOR CHARCOT'S FOOT

Scintigraphy has been used to aid in diagnosing possible osteomyelitis in diabetic Charcot's feet.[63–65] The results have varied with the different techniques.

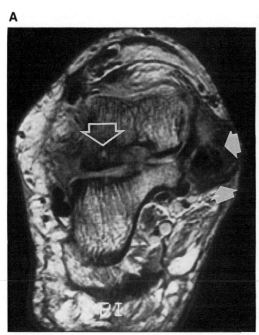

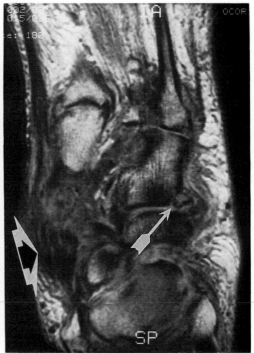

FIG 11–15.
A, proton density coronal through the plane of the sustentacular tali. The *small white arrows* denote swelling of the sheath and enlargement and disruption of the posterior tibial tendon. The *white open arrow* shows an area of diminished area of signal intensity in the talus opposite the calcaneus consistent with sclerotic changes in the bone. These findings are in a 53-year-

old obese woman who is diabetic and has a Charcot foot. **B,** the *broad arrow* shows marked disruption of the posterior tibial tendon with chronic and presumed superimposed acute changes. The *long white arrow* shows an area of fragmentation in the proximal, lateral, and dorsal aspect of the cuboid.

Some investigators have showed that ^{99m}Tc phosphate scans can be used to separate osteomyelitis from diabetic neuroarthropathy.[66] Osteomyelitis in the diabetic patients showed increased activity in the arterial phase of the flow study, whereas neurotrophic joints with soft tissue pathology showed increased venous flow. The sensitivity and specificity of the scans for osteomyelitis was 94% and 79%, respectively, in one series.[67] However, Maurer et al.[28] found that the ^{99m}Tc phosphate scan was only 56% sensitive for osteomyelitis in the diabetic neuropathic joints.

Leukocyte labeling with ^{111}In has improved the specificity of nuclear studies in diagnosing osteomyelitis in neuroarthropathic feet.[64–66, 68] The technique has been shown to be 89% specific in these instances.[28] Indium scintigraphy was even more sensitive in diagnosing soft tissue abscesses.[28] In general, it is believed that a negative ^{111}In white blood cell–labeled scan in the presence of positive ^{99m}Tc and ^{67}Ga scan in Charcot joints reliably excludes infectious complications.

Despite these favorable results obtained using ^{111}In scanning, many authors admit that it is difficult to reliably separate bony from soft tissue infections using this technique. Poor spatial resolution is also a major limitation of the method. The close proximity of infected soft tissues to bone in the foot is yet an additional problem.[43] Another is the low count rates available with leukocyte imaging. Finally, other limitations include false negative images secondary to altered leukocyte migration seen in diabetes, antibody interference, and parasitic infections.[28]

CT FOR THE DIABETIC NEUROARTHROPATHY

CT evaluation of Charcot joint reveals bone and articular fractures and displacement. Significant sclerosis and fragmentation are usually demonstrated as well. Multiple minute fragments of bone and cartilage are seen suspended within the soft tissues. Joint effusions are demonstrated as areas of relatively low attenuation on CT studies. Subchondral bone fragmentation and fracture orientation are also well depicted by CT (Fig 11–16).

CT should be performed with high-resolution techniques and multiplanar acquisition. This can guide therapy in two ways. Were surgery to be attempted, the surgeon will have a better knowledge of the orientation of the osseous structures, as well as the degree of fragmentation that can profoundly change the surgical approach (Fig 11–17). Moreover, when other studies suggest the presence of osteomyelitis such as radionuclide examination or MRI using conventional CT guidance techniques, a needle can be placed into the area of concern either within the medullary space of the bone or in the adjacent soft tissue spaces. Thus, the tissue of osteomyelitis or soft tissue infection can be clarified without need for open surgical biopsy.

MRI FINDINGS IN DIABETIC NEUROARTHROPATHY

Old fracture lines may have low signal on both T_1- and T_2-weighted images, with adjacent marrow signal being normal. However, acute spontaneous neuropathic fractures may show abnormally diminished signal of the marrow signal on the more T_1-weighted images, with increased marrow signal on the T_2-weighted scans. These findings are similarly seen with osteomyelitis (Fig 11–18). Thus, there may be overlap. The use of contrast enhancement may be helpful in separating out areas of active inflammatory changes from those that are posttraumatic in nature (posttraumatic lesions have an increased amount of free water), which will produce a higher signal on T_2-weighted

A

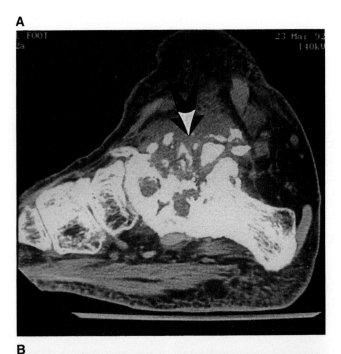

B

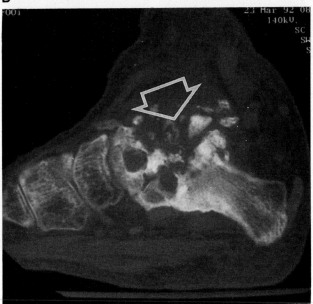

FIG 11–16.
Direct sagittal CTs with soft tissue **(A)** and bone windows **(B)**. Direct coronal soft tissue **(C)** and bone **(D)** images through the ankle on a diabetic patient with advanced changes as a result of Charcot's joints. The combined *black and white arrow* in **A** and the *open white arrow* in **B** show the marked fragmentation of the talus with the destruction of the articular surfaces on both sides of the subtalar joint. **C,** direct coronal image through the tibia *(small black open arrow)* and fibula *(small black arrow)* showing marked destruction of the ankle joint. The *curved arrow* denotes the fragmented talus; the *black arrows* denote the subtalar joint. In **D,** which is a direct coronal image more anteriorly positioned than **C,** the distal tibial *(open white arrow)* lies in close proximity to the subtalar joint as a result of a near total destruction of the talus. The posterior facet of the subtalar joint is indicated by the *open white arrows* located medially and laterally. The small remaining articular surface of the talus is indicated by the *small black arrows*.

(Continued.)

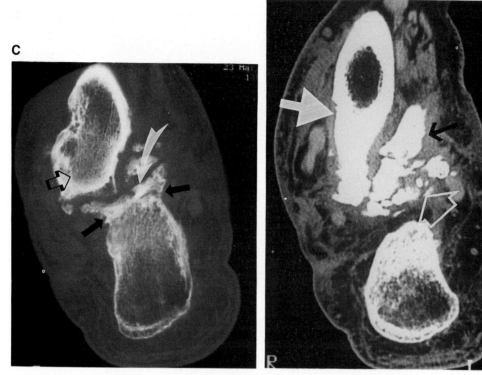

FIG 11–16 (cont.).
For legend see previous page.

FIG 11–17.
Direct sagittal CT scan after attempted surgical repair for Charcot's foot (same patient as in Fig 11–16). The metallic fixation rods are indicated by the *small black arrows*. These internal fixation rods run in a mediolateral orientation. The *long black arrows* indicate allograft bone that has been placed in an attempt to stabilize the ankle joint.

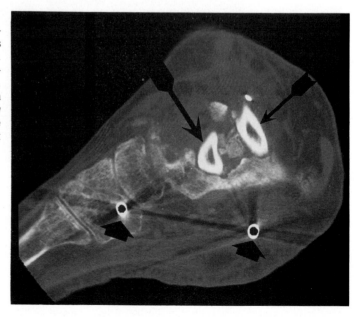

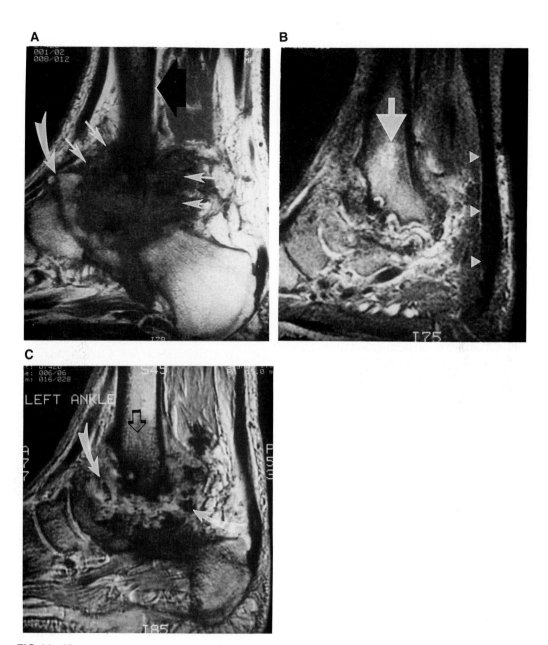

FIG 11–18.

A, sagittal T$_1$-weighted image. The *black arrow* denotes the distal tibia. The *small white arrows* both anteriorly and posteriorly denote the region of the fragmented and destroyed talus. Anteriorly, a tiny piece of the talus remains. It is subluxed with respect to the navicular bone *(curved arrow)*. Sagittal T$_2$-weighted **(B)** and gradient-echo **(C)** images in the same area. The fragmentation of the talus is best demonstrated on the gradient echo image (see areas of low signal intensity) denoted by *curved arrow*. Low signal in the distal tibia *(open black arrow)* could represent sclerosis or replacement of the normal red marrow with hematopoietic or inflammatory tissue. In **B,** a T$_2$-weighted image, this area is of an increased signal intensity, which is consistent with an accumulation of fluid signal intensity material. Without contrast enhancement or other correlative studies, osteomyelitis cannot be ruled out *(white arrow)*. The *white arrowheads* denote thickening of the Achilles tendon, which has accompanied the destructive changes in the ankle joint.

images but should not yield brisk enhancement on the postcontrast scans.[45] The clinical setting, including the laboratory findings (elevated sedimentation rate, white cell count, etc.), as well as patient symptoms, may help separate out osteomyelitis from a case where there is only acute trauma associated with a Charcot foot. In addition, a subtle differential point between noninfectious diabetic neuroarthropathy vs. osteomyelitis may be the relatively extensive area of increased signal intensity on T_2-weighted scans in the noninfected scans without a corresponding area of diminution signal on the noncontrast T_1-weighted scans.[50]

Another differential point between osteomyelitis and changes to diabetic neuroarthropathy may be the relative absence of adjacent soft tissue changes, as well as absence of associated periosteal and cortical bone changes. Because most cases of osteomyelitis and septic arthritis develop within the bones and joints of diabetic patients and are thereby secondary to direct as opposed to hematogenous spread, there is very commonly an adjacent abnormality extending from the skin to the deep spaces of the foot and ankle. This is contrasted with noninfectious diabetic neuroarthropathy in which changes are predominantly medullary.[50] The reverse situation in which there is concern on T_1-weighted images (lower signal in the marrow spaces, as well as abnormal radiographs) in the absence of abnormal signal on the T_2-weighted images, should effectively rule out the presence of osteomyelitis.[48]

RECOMMENDATIONS

In routine cases of possible infection involving the foot and ankle, conventional radiographs should be initially obtained. For patients in whom there is relatively little likelihood of coexistent soft tissue infection and where osteomyelitis is a con-

cern, radionuclide imaging is a satisfactory next diagnostic tool. In complicated cases in which there are likely soft tissue changes only or soft tissue plus possible bony inflammatory disease, or in those patients in whom other diagnostic modalities are equivocal, MRI with conventional and contrast-enhanced techniques may well be of value. CT should be used in those patients who are contraindicated for MRI, when biopsy is required, or when specific information concerning bony structures or loose calcific bodies is required.

REFERENCES

1. Gibbons GW, Freeman D: Vascular evaluation and treatment of the diabetic. In *Clinics in podiatric medicine and surgery: The diabetic foot,* Philadelphia, 1987, WB Saunders, p 377.
2. The Carter Center of Emory University: Closing the gap: The problem of diabetes mellitus in the United States, *Diabetes Care* 8:391, 1985.
3. American Diabetes Association: Gestational diabetes mellitus, *Ann Intern Med* 105:461, 1986.
4. Levin ME: Understanding your diabetic patient. In *Clinics in podiatric medicine and surgery: The diabetic foot,* Philadelphia, 1987, WB Saunders, p 315.
5. Whitehouse FW: Infections that hospitalize the diabetic, *Geriatrics* 28:97–99, 1973.
6. Pratt TC: Gangrene and infection in the diabetic, *Med Clin North Am* 49:987–1004, 1965.
7. Kilo C, Dudley J: Diabetes and peripheral arterial disease, *Geriatr Med Today,* 7(1):63–70, 1988.
8. Corn DB, O'Keefe RG, McCarty DJ: Soft tissue infections of the foot and ankle, *J Am Podiatr Assoc* 67:508–514, 1977.
9. Jahss MH, Lusskin R: Miscellaneous peripheral neuropathies and neuropathy like syndromes. In Jahss MH, editor: *Disorders of the foot and ankle: Medical and surgical management,* Philadelphia, 1991, WB Saunders, p 2129.

10. Joseph WS, LeFrock JL: The pathogenesis of diabetic foot infection: Immunopathy angiopathy and neuropathy, *J Foot Surg* 26(suppl 1):7–11, 1987.
11. Greene DA, Lattimer S, Ulbrecht et al: Glucose induced alterations in nerve metabolism: Current perspective on the pathogenesis of diabetic neuropathy and future directions for research and therapy, *Diabetic Care* 8:290, 1985.
12. Cahill GF, Arky RA, Perlman AJ: Diabetes melitus. In Cahill GF, Arky RA, Perlman AJ, editors: *Scientific medicine,* New York, 1987, Scientific American, Inc, pp 1–19.
13. McMurry JF: Wound healing with diabetes mellitus: Better glucose control for wound healing, *Surg Clin Med North Am* 64(4):769–777, 1984.
14. Molenaar DM, Palumbo PJ, Wilson WR et al: Leukocyte chemotaxis in diabetic patients and their nondiabetic first degree relations, *Diabetes* 25:880–887, 1976.
15. Goodson WH III, Hunt TK: Wound healing and the diabetic patient, *Surg Gynecol Obstet* 149:600–608, 1979.
16. Williamson JR, Kilo C: Current status of capillary basement membrane disease in diabetes mellitus, *Diabetes* 26:197, 1977.
17. Kilo C et al: Muscle capillary basement membrane changes related to aging and to diabetes mellitus, *Diabetes* 21:881, 1972.
18. Mendelson EB, Fisher MR, Deschler TW et al: Osteomyelitis in the diabetic foot: A difficult diagnostic challenge, *Radiographics* 3:248–261, 1983.
19. Greenfield CB: *Radiology of bone diseases,* Philadelphia, 1975, JB Lippincott Co, p 343.
20. Bowadkapour A, Gaine VD: Radiology of osteomyelitis, *Orthop Clin North Am* 14:21–37, 1983.
21. Yuh WT, Corson JD, Baraniewski HM, et al: Osteomyelitis of the foot in diabetic patients: Evaluation with plain film Tc-99 MDP bone scintigraphy and MR Imaging, *AJR* 152:795–800, 1989.
22. Merkel KD, Brown ML, Dewanjee MK et al: Comparison of indium-labeled leukocyte imaging with sequential technitium-gallium scanning in diagnosis of low-grade musculoskeletal sepsis, *J Bone Joint Surg* 67A:465–476, 1985.
23. Skankiamakis GN, Al-Sheikh W, Heal A et al: Comparison of scintigraphy with In-111 leukocyte and Ga 67. In diagnosis of occult sepsis, *J Nucl Med* 23:618–626, 1982.
24. Park NW, Wheat LJ, Siddiqui AR et al: Scintigraphic evaluation of diabetic osteomyelitis: Concise communication, *J Nucl Med* 23:569–573, 1982.
25. Handmaker H: Acute hematogenous osteomyelitis: Has the bone scan betrayed us? *Radiology* 135:787–789, 1980.
26. Duszynsici D, Kuhn J, Asfani E et al: Early radionuclide diagnosis of acute osteomyelitis, *Radiology* 117:337–340, 1975.
27. Al-Shieklh M, Skakianakis GM, Mnaymineh W et al: Subacute and chronic infections: Diagnosis using In-111 Ga67 and Tc99m MDP bone scintigraphy and radiography, *Radiology* 155:501–506, 1985.
28. Maurer AH, Millmond SH, Knight LC et al: Infection in diabetic osteoarthropathy: use of indium labeled leukocytes for diagnosis, *Radiology* 161:221–225, 1986.
29. Seldin DW, Heiken JP, Feldman F, et al: Effects of soft tissue pathology in detection of pedal osteomyelitis, *J Nucl Med* 26:988–993, 1985.
30. Lartos G, Brown ML, Sutton RT: Diagnosis of osteomyelitis of the foot in diabetic patients: Value of 111 in leukocyte scintigraphy, *AJR* 157:527–531, 1991.
31. Keenan AM, Tindel NL, Alavi A: Diagnosis of pedal osteomyelitis in diabetic patients using current scintigraphy techniques, *Arch Intern Med* 149:2262–2266, 1989.
32. Unger E, Moldofsky P, Gatenby R et al: Diagnosis of osteomyelitis by MR imaging, *AJR* 150:605–610, 1988.
33. McAfee JG, Samin A: In-111 labeled leukocytes: A review of problems in imaging interpretation, *Radiology* 155:221–229, 1985.
34. Datz FL, Thorne DA: Effect of chronicity of infection on the sensitivity of the In-111 labeled leukocyte scan, *AJR* 148:809–812, 1986.

35. Thakur ML, McAfee JG: The significance of chromosomal abbreviations in indium 111 labeled leukocyte, *J Nucl Med* 25:922–927, 1984.

36. Sartoris DJ, Devine S, Resnick D et al: Plantar compartmental infection in the diabetic foot: The role of computed tomography, *Invest Radiol* 20:772–784, 1985.

37. Sartoris DJ, Resnick D: Computed tomography of podiatric disorders: A review, *J Foot Surg* 25(5):394–403, 1986.

38. Williamson B, Teates C, Philips C et al: Computed tomography as a diagnostic aid in diabetic and other problem feet, *Clin Imaging* 13(2):159–163, 1989.

39. Hermann G, Rose JS: Computed tomography in bone and soft tissue: Pathology of the extremities, *J Comput Assist Tomogr* 3:58–66, 1979.

40. Kahn JP, Berger PE: Computed tomographic diagnosis of osteomyelitis, *Radiology* 130:503–506, 1979.

41. Wing VW, Jeffrey RB, Federle MP et al: Chronic osteomyelitis examined by CT, *Radiology* 154:171–174, 1985.

42. Chaudnaui VP, Beltran J, Morris CS et al: Acute experimental osteomyelitis and abscesses: Detection with MR Imaging versus CT, *Radiology* 174:233–236, 1990.

43. Beltran J, Campanini DS, Knight C et al: The diabetic foot: Magnetic resonance imaging evaluation, *Skeletal Radiol* 19:37–41, 1990.

44. Wang A, Weinstein D, Greenfield L et al: MRI and diabetic foot infections. *Magn Reson Imaging* 8:805–809, 1990.

45. Moore TE, Yuh WTC, Kathol MH et al: Abnormalities of the foot in patients with diabetes mellitus: Findings on MRI imaging, *AJR* 157:813–816, 1991.

46. Pykett IL, Newhouse JH, Gerdinardo BS et al: Principles of nuclear magnetic resonance imaging, *Radiology* 143:157–168, 1982.

47. Beltran J, Watu AM, Musure JC et al: Ankle: Surface coil MR imaging at 1.5T, *Radiology* 101:203–209, 1986.

48. Pavileck W, Geisinger M, Castle L et al: The effects of nuclear magnetic resonance on patients with cardiac pacemakers, *Radiology* 147:149–153, 1983.

49. Lackman RW, Kaufman B, Han JS et al: MR Imaging in patients with metallic implants, *Radiology* 157:711–714, 1985.

50. Deutsch AL: Bone and soft tissue infection. In Deutsch A, Mink J, Kerr R editors: *MRI of the foot and ankle,* New York, 1992, Raven Press, pp 199–222.

51. Mason MD, Zlatin MD, Esterhai JL et al: Chronic complicated osteomyelitis of the lower extremities: Evaluation with MR imaging, *Radiology* 173:335–359, 1989.

52. Tang JSH, Gold RH, Bassett LW et al: Musculoskeletal infection of the extremities: Evaluation with MR imaging, *Radiology* 166:205–209, 1988.

53. Axler DA: Microbiology of diabetic foot infections, *J Foot Surg* 26(suppl 1):3–6, 1987.

54. Tan JS, Flanagan PJ, Donovan DL et al: Team approach in management of diabetic foot infections, *J Foot Surg* 26(suppl 1):12–16, 1987.

55. Kozak GP, Rowbotham JL: Diabetic foot disease: A major problem. In Kozak GP, Hoar CS, Rowbotham JL, et al, editors: *Management of diabetic foot problems,* Philadelphia, 1984, WB Saunders, pp 1–8.

56. Waldvogal FA, Vasey H: Osteomyelitis: The past decade, *N Engl J Med* 303:360–370, 1980.

57. Maggiore P, Echols RM: Infections in the diabetic foot. In Jhass MH, editor: *Disorders of the foot and ankle: Medical and surgical management,* Philadelphia, 1991, WB Saunders, pp 1937–1957.

58. Bamberger DM, Daus GP, Gerding DN: Osteomyelitis in the feet of diabetic patients. Long term results prognostic factors and the role of antimicrobial and surgical therapy, *Am J Med* 83:653–660, 1987.

59. Vogler JB, Murph WA: Bone marrow imaging, *Radiology* 168:679–693, 1988.

60. Quinn SF, Murray W, Clark RA et al: MR imaging of chronic osteomyelitis, *J Comput Assist Tomogr* 12:113–117, 1988.

61. Frykberg RG: Osteoarthropathy. In *Clinics in podiatric medicine and surgery: The diabetic foot,* Philadelphia, 1987, WB Saunders, pp 351–359.

62. Cofield RH, Morrison MJ, Beabout JW: Diabetic neuroarthropathy in the foot: Patient characteristics and patterns of radiographic change, *Foot Ankle* 4:15–21, 1983.
63. Splittgerder GF, Stiegehoff DR, Buggy BP: Combined leukocyte and bone imaging used to evaluate diabetic osteoarthropathy and osteomyelitis, *Clin Nucl Med* 14:156–160, 1989.
64. Schauwecker DS, Park HM, Burt RW et al: Combined bone scintigraphy and indium 111 leukocyte scans in neurotrophic foot disease, *J Nucl Med* 29(10):1651–1655, 1988.
65. McCarthy K, Velchik MG, Alavi A et al: Indium 111 labeled white blood cells. In the detection of osteomyelitis complicated by a preexisting condition, *J Nucl Med* 29:1015–1021, 1988.
66. Seldin DW, Heiken JP, Feldman F et al: Effect of soft tissue pathology on detection of pedal osteomyelitis, *J Nucl Med* 26:988–993, 1985.
67. Berquist TH, Brown ML: Infection. In Berquist TH, Brown ML, editors: *Radiology of the foot and ankle,* New York, 1989, Raven Press, pp 277–313.
68. Seabold JE, Slickinger FW, Kao SCS et al: Indium-111 leukocyte/technetium 99m-MDP bone and magnetic resonance imaging, difficulty in diagnosing osteomyelitis in patients with neuropathic osteoarthropathy, *J Nucl Med* 31:549–556, 1990.
69. Omara RE, Wilson GA, Burke AM: Skeletal imaging in osteomyelitis, *J Nucl Med* 24:71, 1983.

12 — Cutaneous Manifestations of the Lower Extremities in Diabetes Mellitus

Daniel J. McCarthy, D.P.M., Ph.D.

Diabetes mellitus (DM) affects 11 million Americans.[1] This multifactorial disease frequently complicates podiatric presentations, which in turn may exacerbate the systemic conditions.

The skin is the largest organ of the human body having many complex functions.[2] It is sensitive to enzymatic and hormonal influences, and an understanding of the anatomy and physiology is necessary to appreciate the effects of DM relative to the integument.

In general, the skin is not always structurally altered in terms of thickness in adult-onset diabetes mellitus (AODM). However, skin thickness is demonstrably thickened in many patients.[3, 4] The skin of juvenile-onset diabetics frequently differs from that of adult onset diabetes in that the integument assumes a more pale and translucent quality.[5]

ANATOMICAL CONSIDERATIONS

The skin is composed of an epidermis and a dermis that covers the subcutaneous strata. The epidermis is characterized by four layers: the strata basale, spinosum, granulosum, and corneum (Fig 12–1). The strata lucidum, sometimes referred to in the literature appears to be an artifact of fixation.

The stratum basale lies upon a basement membrane that delineates the dermis below from the epidermis above. The basement membrane is a trilamilar structure derived from both epidermal and dermal components. Keratinocytes of the stratum basale have a dominant ovoid nucleus and a relatively sparse cytoplasm.[6] Basal cells are characterized morphologically as low columnar and have relatively few subcellular organelles. Such cells are polarized at right angles to the free surface of the skin (Fig 12–2). Whenever vesicles or bullae form in diabetic states, they are characterized as being suprabasilar or subbasilar or intraepidermal or intradermal.

The stratum spinosum is so named because of the desmosomes that surround the cells. The term intercellular bridges used in older literature is a misnomer.[6] Actually, two adjacent hemidesmosomes come together at the intercellular space to form a tight junction. In disease states, there is frequently disruption of the tonofilament-desmosome-complex (TDC), and widening of the intercellular spaces occurs. In thick skin conditions of AODM, the stratum spinosum is said to be acanthotic or thickened relative to what is considered to be normal. The so-called prickle cells become progressively oriented more parallel to the free surface of the skin and the nucleus becomes more attenuated. The cytoplasm contains a complexity of subcellular organelles including mitochondria, rough endoplasmic reticulum,

191

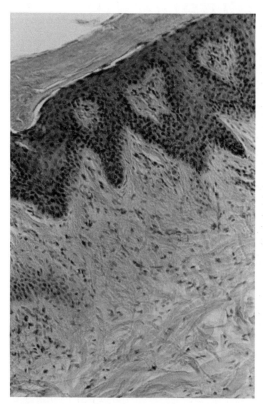

FIG 12–1.
Epidermis and dermis of the skin demonstrating all strata. Hematoxyia and eosin preparation at light microscopy level *(LM).*

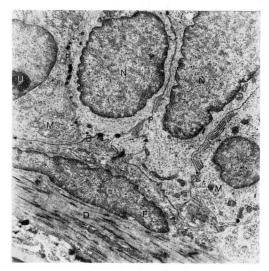

FIG 12–2.
Polarized orientation of stratum basal. Transmission electron micrograph. *N* = nucleus; *M* = mitochondria; *P* = plasma membrane; *F* = fibroblast; *D* = dermis; *B* = basement membrane.

free ribosomes, Golgi apparatus, vesicles and, Odland bodies (lamellar granules). These many structures are involved in the normal processes of keratinization[7] and may become deficient in the skin of diabetic patients.

The stratum granulosum lies above the stratum spinosum and beneath the stratum corneum. It is deeply basophilic on hematoxylin- and eosin-stained microscopic slides because of clumps of keratohyaline. These irregular electron-dense clumps mesh with tonofilaments as enzymatic processes relating to keratinization are completed.

The stratum corneum demonstrates a more or less homogeneous matrix. Nuclei are not present and subcellular organelles are absent within the cytoplasm. Cells have a brick-like orientation as the free surface of skin is approached. The intercellular spaces are relatively widened and filled with a proteinaceous substance so as to provide for an essentially water-tight layer. In disease states, this layer can be greatly thickened (lichenification) or atrophic.

The dermis in DM is altered in much the same way as in aging. Dermal collagen is thickened most probably as a result of increased cross linkages from nonenzymatic glycosylation.[8] The stabilization of proteins is said to produce a browning process, which can affect keratin of the epidermis and collagen of the dermis.[9] Elastic fibers of the dermis are numerically reduced and tend to clump in DM.[10]

The skin is generally thickened in diabetes, but increased collagen synthesis is not a feature of this condition.[11] The relatively inflexible thickened dermis underlies an epidermis which has fewer anchoring fibrils at the basement membrane level. Such weaknesses may predispose diabetics to cutaneous injury and sloughing.[10]

Dermal microvasculature is faulty in DM in that blood vessel walls are thickened and demonstrate increased deposition of periodic-acid-Schiff (PAS) positive substances in or about the basement membranes of vessels.

The increased predisposition of diabetic skin to injuries from traumatic events together with impaired microvasculature in the dermis and subcutaneous tissue make the lower extremities vulnerable to various degenerative problems.

BIOCHEMICAL CONSIDERATIONS

Glucose as well as galactose, ribose, mannose, fructose, and fucose may glycosylate proteins. The process of nonenzymatic glycosylation is one of attachment of carbohydrate to protein.[12] Glycosylation consists of the covalent linkage of the double bonded oxygen on glucose with a nitrogen atom, either on the α-amino group of the N-terminal amino acid or on the ε-amino group of lysine. This condensation step, resulting in Schiff base, is a reversible reaction.[1]

A series of reactions reconfigures the molecules to form glucose derived intermolecular crosslinks. The glycosylation of dermal collagen results in the nonglycosylation of dermal collagen which in turn results in the nonenzymatic browning effect seen in diabetics.[1] This cutaneous event correlates directly with Hba_1 levels and therefore relates to the level of control of the diabetic blood glucose levels. Increased cross-linking, packing and stiffening of collagen occur during the browning effect so as to produce connective tissue abnormalities that can be measured by fluorescent techniques.

The morphology of the human skin in health and disease is determined by a biochemically driven equipotential system. Cohen[13] in 1969 postulated a derivative of fibroblast homogenates as stimulator of epidermal mitosis. He designated the un-defined substance as the dermal influencing factor. The author had just completed a study using the Human Fibroblastic Growth Factor (HFGF) in the treatment of diabetic foot ulcerations. This dermal fibroblast product has been shown experimentally to stimulate epithelialization, collagenation and revascularization. Mitosis of the stratum basale and stratum spinosum, therefore, occur as a result of fibroblast-derived dermal influences which direct epidermal proliferation on a biochemical basis.

The epidermis, however, has present within its cells a substance known as the epidermal chalone. Vorhees and Duell[14] believed that psoriasis, a highly proliferative epidermal disease characterized by scaling and short cell transit time might be a defect of the adenyl-cyclase-cyclic AMP cascade. The epidermal chalone, $3' \times 5'$ adenosine monophosphate, exists essentially as an *inhibitor* of epidermal cell mitosis and proliferation.

Whenever epidermal cells are stripped away or otherwise injured, the epidermal chalone is relatively reduced and the dermal influencing factor is free to stimulate epidermal mitosis. Conversely, when the epidermis is thickened, the chalone exists in abundance and essentially "advises" the epidermal cells not to undergo further mitosis.

The balance between epidermal chalone and the dermal influencing factor determines the overall thickness of the skin and the relative thicknesses of the suprapapillary stratum Malpighi and stratum corneum.[15] When the two biochemical factors of cell proliferation are in balance, the epidermal-dermal interface of the skin tends to be more or less featureless. If, however, fibroblastic signals are appreciably increased, cells of the suprapapillary Malpighi stratum increase and the epidermal-dermal interface is expanded by extensions of the rete ridges (pegs) into the dermis.[16] The pars papillaris is heavily populated by fibroblasts that orient at right angles to the free surface of the skin in the inflammatory situations characteristic of the pedal lesions heloma durum and tyloma.[17]

Heloma durum and tyloma (corns and calluses) are not necessarilly statistically related to DM. However, these common foot complaints constitute a serious threat to life and limb of poorly controlled diabetics. In heloma durum, a circumscribed area of significantly thickened stratum corneum is found in association with a hypertrophied and eburnated phalangeal head. Acanthosis of the stratum spinosum and gross hypertrophy of the rete ridges also characterize the lesion (Fig 12–3).[17]

DM is, in part, a disease of enzymatic malfunction. Glycosylation and the browning effect are known to be active in DM, and it is likely that there are other biochemical systems deleterious to the skin.

Heloma durum causes significant pain and patients often, in desperation, attempt to obtain relief, by paring the cornified tissue. Inadvertant cuts into the dermis and subcutaneous interphalangeal skin can lead to serious infection.

The use of commercial corn cures can be equally dangerous. Such medications erode and undermine the involved epidermal tissues and again infection is a likely

possibility.[18] In the presence of diabetic microangiopathy, ischemia and gangrene are imminent.

The formation of an adventitious bursa beneath helomata and the hypertrophic phalangeal head is a not-infrequent complication of helomas. In such circumstances, the involved digit may become edematous and inflamed. Fistula formation is a real possibility and infection can be extended into the joint proper.

Osteomyelitis of small digital bones in association with heloma durum in diabetics can become an irreversible condition requiring amputation. The serious sequelae that accompany heloma durum in DM give importance to the palliative care provided by the skillful podiatrist.

Tylomata (calluses) are histologically similar to helomata. These morphologically variable skin lesions are usually associated with the plantar surface of the foot that is normally much thicker than the integument of the toes. Distinctive hypertrophic epidermal ridging of the epidermal dermal interface normally characterizes the submetatarsal and heel regions.[15] Such areas are prone to excess callus formation and hyperkeratosis, parakeratoses, hypergranulosus, and acanthosis can be seen affecting the epidermis when such tissues are examined microscopically.

Tyloma beneath the metatarsophalangeal joints usually have a biomechanical cause. Hyperdeclination of a metatarsal or hypertrophic osseous changes of a particular metatarsal head can cause the formation of nucleated tyloma or the so called intractible plantar keratosis (IPK). The plantar conical shaped skin lesions are heloma-like and are found within a more generalized callus. In diabetes mellitus, trophic changes involving the skin and subcutaneous tissues result in poor vascularization and innervation. Tylomata of the skin of the plantar aspect of the foot, therefore, can be placed at considerable risk (Fig 12–4).

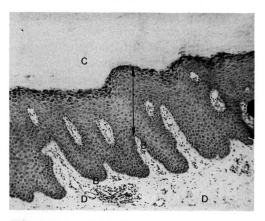

FIG 12–3.
Hypertrophic skin of heloma durum. *C* = stratum corneum; *D* = dermis, *B* = basement membrane.

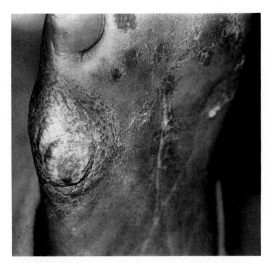

FIG 12–4.
Submetatarsal head five with tyloma formation in diabetic. Skin is cracked and at risk for invasion of pathogenic bacteria.

Heloma and tyloma reflect intermittant but continuing pressure to the foot's integument. When the pressures involved become unremitting, the skin may break down and ulcerate. Heloma and tyloma, so involved, become the primary focus for cellulitis, deep space infections, osteomyelitis and septicemia.

Surgical interventions to correct the primary bony involvements leading to heloma and tyloma are entirely justifiable for well controlled diabetic patients. Interphalangeal joint arthroplasties for heloma and distal or proximal elevating metatarsal osteotomies for tylomas should be offered to selected diabetic patients to prevent morbid sequelae. Such intervention assumes a level of good health and the relative absence of serious microangiopathy or neuropathy.

Tylomata develop in response to point pressures and shearing forces related to weight-bearing and walking. Diabetic dermatological conditions including tyloma and heloma often require more conservative nonsurgical types of intervention. Biomechanical devices (foot orthotics) then become important to the treatment plan. Modern technology has produced a number of materials designed to alleviate shock, shear, torque, and similar forces and the podiatric physician can help diabetic patients greatly through their use. The Mobility Shoe manufactured by Markell Co. (504 Saw Mill River Road, Yonkers, NY 10702), for example, employs Velcro and plastazote together with special soft leather to make a light, roomy, flexible shoe that minimizes insults to the diabetic skin brought about by walking.

Tyloma can occur at alternate locations to the plantar metatarsaphalangeal regions of the foot. Diabetics often have deep calluses circumscribing the plantar aspect of the heels. These deep seated lesions often form cracks and fissures that may break the skin. Once again, an avenue of infection is provided that can become painful and threaten the well-being of diabetic patients.

Pinch calluses, poro keratosis, heloma molle, heloma milliare, heloma vasculaire, and heloma neurofibrosum are other hyperkeratotic types of foot lesions that affect diabetic patients and the general population. As with tyloma and heloma durum, these complaints lend themselves to self treatment which involve cutting or chemical cautery. Consequently, they also become potential sites for cutaneous ulcerations or portals for the introduction of infecting microorganisms so dangerous to diabetic patients.

The skin as described earlier demonstrates several specialized modifications known as the adnexa: Nails, hair, sudiferous, and sebaceous glands are among such structures. All of them are subject to inflammatory and infectious processes that can adversely compromise patients with DM. Of the adnexa of skin, the nails have greatest potential for diabetic complications. However, these complications are not restricted to the diabetic population.

Nails occupy the dorsal distal aspects of the fingers and toes. They constitute the largest sheet of keratin existing within the body and are of importance to the practice of clinical medicine because nails can reflect the general status of an individual over the past several months.[19] Nails develop a nail plate from a matrix situated dorsal to the ungual or distal phalange itself. This germinal tissue lies posterior to the lunula (half moon) and is inferior to the cuticle and eponychium covering the most proximal portions of the nail structures.

The nail hyponychium is the area under the free edge of the nail: The lateral nail folds constitute the ungualabia. The nail bed demonstrates a limited strata of epidermis (there is no stratum corneum in the presence of a keratinized nail plate), and the dermis is characterized by longitudinal grooves and ridges.

As the nail tissue proper is formed, epidermal cells demonstrate intracellular edema, nucleolysis and finally shrinkage.[21] The vascular and nerve supply at the distal parts of fingers and toes is formed by an elaborate anastimosis from dorsal and central aspects of the respective digits.

Onychocryptosis is that condition in which the free edge or lateral margins of the nail plate penetrates the contiguous epidermis anterior or laterally (Fig 12–5). These complaints are not peculiar to diabetic patients, but they do have potentially serious implications in the disease. Faulty footgear, improper nail care, and injury are causes of onychocryptosis and these factors should be avoided. Inverted nails and hypertrophied ungualabia are frequently inherited traits, so that periodic nail care by the podiatric physician is required.

When the nail plate penetrates the contiguous soft tissues, inflammation and pain develop. Eventually, pathogenic microorganisms can produce pus, and granulation tissue (in the form of "proud flesh") which can envelop the involved ungual-

abia. Such complications need to be quickly treated in diabetics because infection can elevate blood glucose levels and diabetic control is lost. Digital infections can lead to deep space infection and gangrene can develop in the presence of microangiopathy.

Simple total avulsion of the nail plate or more conservative excision of the offending nail plate border can quickly achieve adequate incision and drainage of infected onychocryptosis. Proud flesh can be debrided and cauterized with silver nitrate. Soaks and/or continuous wet dressings of Burow's solution are useful in reducing inflammation and broad-spectrum systemic antibiotics can be used if infection is a problem.

When onychocryptosis is a recurring problem and the patient is in reasonably good health and control, diabetics need not be denied surgical intervention for permanent correction of this vexing nail problem. The Winograd or Frost type of procedure is well suited for situations when hypertrophy of the ungualabia and incurvation of the nail plate exist together. I tend to avoid nail matrix phenolization in diabetic patients because of the degree of chemical destruction of soft tissues that results.

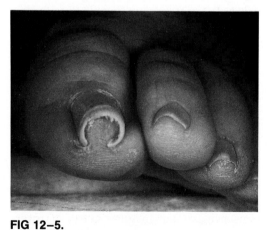

FIG 12–5.
Onychemycosis with hypertrophy of unqualabia of great toe in diabetic patient.

PARONYCHIA

Paronychia (whitlow) is that condition of the nail matrix and contiguous deeper structures that is associated with progressive inflammation and suppuration. Such conditions evolve from the more benign onychia (onychitis). In DM, such inflammatory foci can lead to serious more proximal involvements such as deep space infections and gangrene in the extremity.

Onychia and paronychia usually develop from traumas to the forefoot that range from foreign-body penetration (e.g., thorns or splinters) to stubbing of the toes. The role of constricting footwear should not be overlooked. This factor can be a significant problem when parathesia or anesthesia of the foot is a complication of diabetes. Parasitic infestation of the nail groove has been reported on occasion.

Candida species are often involved in the initial stage of diabetic paronychia, but staphylococcal, streptococcal, pseudomonas species as well as coliform bacilli are frequently cultured from lesions.

In the presence of polymicrobial infection within the narrow confines of the lateral and posterior toe nail folds of diabetics, it is important that adequate incision and drainage be established in diabetic paronychia. Expert clinical evaluation determines if total nail avulsion is indicated. In well-controlled DM with adequate circulation, atraumatic avulsion provides the most expeditious drainage. In compromised diabetics more conservative approaches should be considered. Careful excision of offending nail spicules and debridement of necrotic or abscessed ungualabia may be the most judicious approach.

Astringent wet dressings of aqueous aluminum subacetate or povidine iodine are indicated and broad-spectrum antibiotics may be required. Bed rest, elevation, and even hospitalization are viable options. Onychia and paronychia in dia-

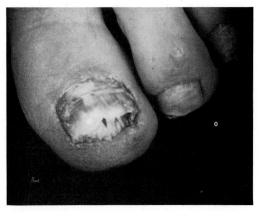

FIG 12–6.
Onychogryphosis of hallucal nail *(A)*.

betic patients shoud be regarded as potentially dangerous lesions and treated as such.

Onychomycosis (tinea unguium) is that involvement of the nail plate or nail bed caused by certain pathogenic fungi (Fig 12–6).[20] The condition was once considered rare but now seems to be much more common.[21] Patients with DM often demonstrate this complaint, but it is probably not true that elevated levels of glucose or other carbohydrate nutrients support fungal growth more than is true of the normal population. Hypertrophied and pithey nail plates in diabetics can be removed without trauma by using 20% to 40% urea under occlusive dressing.[23] Podiatrists are experienced in the conservative reduction of thickened onychomycosis by atraumatic mechanical means when the diagnosis is confirmed by laboratory means.

Caution must be used when diabetics are given oral systemic antifungal medications because of immunodeficiency factors as well as nephro and hepatic toxicity, which occurs occasionally.

Local antifungal medications can be considered for topical use in onychomycosis. Sulfonazole, chlotrimazole, miconazole, and econazole can be locally effective antifungal medications for some fungal nail infections. Other local medications efficacious in onychomycosis will be discussed in the context of diabetic tinea pedis.[22]

Because of the chronic nature of fungal infections and the immune compromised nature of diabetic patients as well as the adverse conditions inherent in wearing foot gear (darkness, moisture, warmth) the prognosis for recovery from onychomycosis is generally poor. Minimal repeated trauma to the toes, peripheral neuropathy, vascular embarrassment of the distal parts of the foot are additional factors which hinder recovery from fungal nail infections.

Onychogryphosis and onychauxis (ram's horn nail and club nail respectively) represent those conditions of toe nails in which there is gross hypertrophy of the nail plate (Fig 12–7). The nail assumes an exaggerated curvature in long-standing cases in onychogryphosis.[24] These two morphologically related nail conditions are in no way pathognomonic to DM, but they do have special significance and relevence in DM.

The etiology of onychauxis can be hereditary when it is known as pachyonychia. However, onychauxis is more often traumatic in origin. Such trauma includes infection which can involve the nail matrix. Such events stimulate hyper-

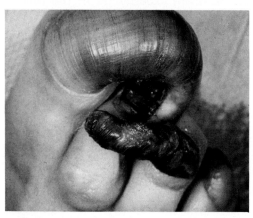

FIG 12–7.
Onychogryphosis of the hallucal nail in diabetic.

trophy of the involved dermal papillae which in turn induce proliferation of epidermal cells which contribute to the nail plate substance (epidermal chalone imbalance).

In DM, nail matrix infections are fairly common as are various external insults to the nail plate. Hypertrophic alterations of the nail plate are further accelerated by the bulk of the nail itself and a vicous cycle ensues which creates more and more nail mass over time.

The danger in onychauxis and onychogryphosis in diabetes mellitus is that bulky deformed nails will injure adjacent toes so as to penetrate the skin and allow for pathogens to become established. Moreover, the continuous pressure on the hypertrophied nail plate can produce ulceration of the toes with all of the morbidity that that entails to diabetics.

Periodic podiatric intervention can abort these potentially serious diabetic sequelae. Krausz advises soaking affected nail plates with 1% aqueous cresol (U.S.P.) for several minutes after which a nail nipper is used to reduce as much of the nail's bulk as possible. Finally, the nail plate is further smoothed and shaped with a podiatric burr and electric drill. Such treatment can be dangerous to the therapist if aerosols are inhaled.[25] Total nail avulsion with matrixectomy can be considered in well controlled diabetics.

The subject of onychopathy is involved and much of it beyond the scope of the present study. Five of 31 conditions listed by Krausz[24] have special significance in diabetes mellitus. Two more nail presentations need to be discussed in concluding this subject.

Onychyphemia is that condition in which bleeding occurs under the nail plate. Trauma is usually etiologic and for this reason, diabetics who are often insensate need to observe their feet regularly. Contusion and hematoma formation together with attendant pain require that blood be allowed to escape. This can be accomplished with a 1/16-in. dental burr and electric drill. A heated straightened out paper clip pressed against the free surface of the nail can also be employed. Of course, special attention to asepsis and postoperative dressings needs to be observed. Petechia are small dark spots of organized blood elements; vibex are transverse streaks beneath the nail plate.[24]

Beau's lines are transverse furrows associated with the nail plate. They give evidence of earlier pathological disturbances involving the nail matrix. Their initial appearances are seen within the lunula and Beau's line progress distally with the forward growth of the nail plate. Diabetics demonstrating Beau's lines should be questioned concerning trauma, onychia, nervous shocks or inflammatory diseases which may have induced a sudden arrest of proliferation of normal nail cells. Since nail plates regrow from the matrix in about 180 days, one can mathematically estimate the approximate time of the earlier pathologic event.[24] Beau's line have diagnostic significance, but no treatment is indicated.

ATHLETES FOOT IN DIABETES MELLITUS

Athletes foot is the term commonly used to describe a variety of superficial skin conditions related for the most part to fungal infections. Tinea pedis is a more precise term which I associate with the more limited group of organisms known as dermatophytes. *Epidermorpyton flococosum, Microsporum ferrungineum, Microsporum audouni, Trichophyton concentricum, Trichophyton mentagrophytes, Trichophyton interdigitale, Trichophyton soudanese,* and *Trichophyton rubrum* constitute the currently known anthropophilic dermatophytic organisms affecting diabetic patients.[22] In this sense diabetics do not differ from the general population complaining of tinea pedis.

Immunodeficiencies associated with diabetes make tinea pedis potentially more troublesome among diabetic patients and may delay resolution of foot infections almost indefinitely. Moreover, the problem of misdiagnosis of conditions that mimic tinea pedis leads to mistreatment which further complicates matters. Candida species can present as a vesicular foot infection which can mimic dermatophytic involvements. This is also true of so-called gram negative athletes foot caused by the bacteria *Proteus* species and *Pseudomonas* species.

PSEUDOMONAS

Because diabetics are much more unresponsive to conventional "shot gun" treatment approaches for skin infections, it is imperative that therapy begin with a precise diagnosis.[22] Classic KOH preparations of skin scrapings for microscopic examination constitutes the first step in diagnosis. Appropriate cultures using Sabouraud's dextrose agar without antibiotics is the first-line culture media for fungi. If bacteria are etiologic, blood agar or phenyl ethyl alcohol blood agar are best used. Dermatophyte test medius (DTM) can be used, although the medium is prepared to demonstrate only the presence of dermatophytes and false positive results are not uncommon.[22]

Diabetics often have foot problems which predispose to dermatophytic involvement. In addition to the immunocompromised state, hyperhidrosis and dry, scaly or cracked skin can devitalize diabetic skin and favor the establishment of fungus infections. These factors can be so significant in DM that opportunistic organisms can become etiologic. *Aspergillus niger* became established in one brittle diabetic patient with multiple systems disease as a black fungating patch on the plantar aspect of the foot (Fig 12–8). Subsequent ulceration and cellulitis ulti-

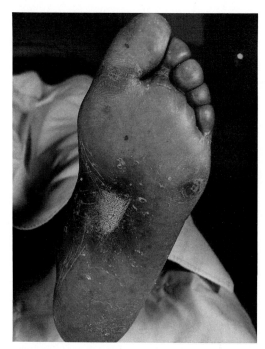

FIG 12–8.
Longitudial arch presentation of non-dermatophyte. *Aspergillus niger* in immune compromised diabetic patient.

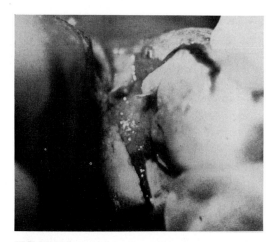

FIG 12–9.
Interdigital fissure in tinea-like lesion caused by Pseudomonas species.

mately led to below-the-knee amputation in this very complicated case.

The most frequent presentation of tinea pedis amongst diabetics, as it is in the general population, is that which occurs interdigitally[22] with soggy, white macerations which are often malodorous occur. Such intertrigenous macerations may fissure to allow for the entry of secondary pathogens. Pseudomonas species mimics interdigital lesions in diabetics (Fig 12–9). Lesions appear initially as more or less benign skin defects, but they may progress to act as the portal of entry for serious pyogenic foot pathogens. The area between the fourth and fifth toes is an especially vulnerable site for deep space infections in diabetics.

Vesicles and pustules are usually not present within the moccasin-type distribution of hyperkeratotic pattern lesions of the plantar surface of the foot (Fig 12–10). *Trichophytron rubrum* is most

frequently present in such lesions in which the interdigital lesions most often are absent. Physicians should be alert to the fact that *Candida* species may also simulate moccassin type distributions of clinical tinea pedis. Hyperkeratotic forms of tinea pedis also exist in combinations with vesicular forms or alone (Fig 12–11).

A subacute vesicular type of tinea pedis exists that involves the dermatophytes in general, but most often is caused by *Trichophytron mentagrophytes*. Lesions characteristically are observed on non-weight-bearing areas of the soles of the feet but they may derive from intertrigenous areas as well.[22]

Diabetics are frequently involved in acute or subacute vesicular conditions that may spread to the entire plantar surface of the foot. Such extensive involvements can easily be secondarily infected by bacterial pathogens with subsequent ulceration, cellulitis, deep space infection, and lymphangitis. Dermatophyte infections of a prolonged nature may also lead to ID reactions indicating sensitivity to the fungi on a systemic basis.

Treatment of the diabetic patient with dermatophytosis relates to the severity of the infection. Hospitalization is often indicated when poor diabetic control, poor general health, and immunocompromized state coexist along with advanced secondarily infected tinea pedis.

The secondary bacterial pathogens are of initial concern. Broad-spectrum intravenous antibiotics, bed rest and elevation, supportive therapy, and judicious debridement to establish adequate drainage are required. Continuous wet dressing or wet-to-dry antiseptic and/or astringent wet dressings are helpful. Again, careful culturing and sensitivity testing are required and changes in microflora are evaluated to adjust antibiotic coverage as needed over time. As soon as the dominant pathogens are known, the narrowest spectrum effective antibiotic should be selected for use.[22]

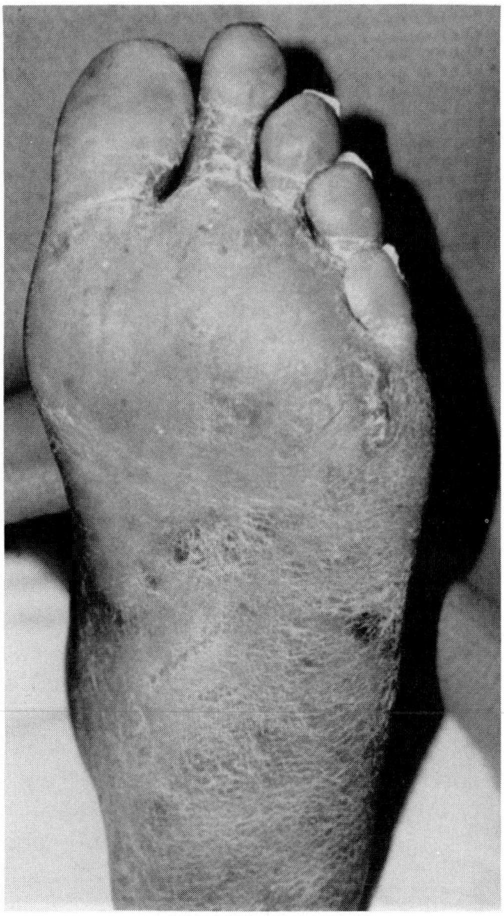

The aggressive treatment plan just described would not be necessary if acute secondarily infected states were totally avoided by using simple common sense measures early on. Diabetics need constant reinforcement to ensure proper foot hygiene. Maceration and hyperhidrosis of the foot are always problems when adverse conditions, such as hot humid weather, occur. Exposure to fungi and their spores under minimal trauma to the foot as can occur in athletic activity should alert diabetics to the need for special attention to the feet. Diabetics should avoid exposure to dyes and man-made materials in hosiery and shoes. Many times, contact dermatitis can appear as an acute eruption that closely mimicks tinea pedis

FIG 12–10.
Vesicular eruption of tinea pedis with moccasin-like distribution.

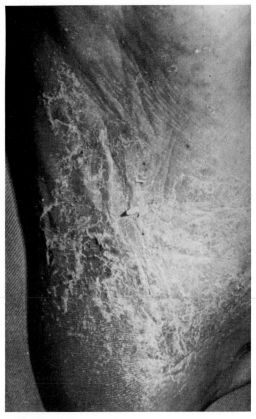

FIG 12–11.
Dry scaling type of hyperkeratotic tinea pedis.

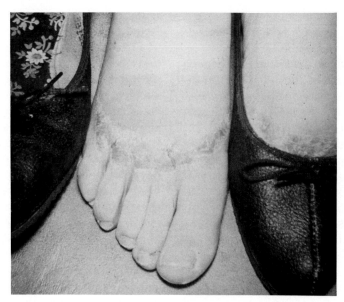

FIG 12–12.
Contact dermatitis due to shoes may mimic tinea pedis. (Courtesy of Dr. L. Levy.)

(Fig 12–12). Treating dermatitis as tinea pedis can exacerbate the reaction.[6] This is especially true for diabetics with immunodeficiencies. Correct diagnosis and an appropriate treatment plan for diabetics with tinea pedis are necessary. Herein lies the danger in self treatment using over the counter (OTC) preparations. This statement does not deny the efficacy of OTC drugs when their use is indicated and appropriate. Iodochlorohydroxyguinol is antifungal and to a limited extent, antibacterial.[22] The 3% cream or ointment is commercially available with hydrocortisone (Vioform HC) or without hydrocortisone (Vioform). Povidine iodine is active against fungi, bacteria, and yeasts. It is somewhat toxic in open wounds and is best known as Betadine.

Castellani's paint is a deeply staining fuchsin dye in a vehicle containing alcohol, acetone, phenol, and resorcinol. It is fungicidal, dehydrating, and most beneficial in interdigital complaints.[22]

Tolnaftate is the most popular of OTC products that are used to hinder the development of fungal hyphae. The powder form is useful in treatment and in prophylaxis in foot infections caused by dermatophytes. Tolnaftate is marketed as Tinactin and Dr. Scholl products. Recurrence rates are comparatively high with topical tolnaftate.

Undecylenic acid is comparable to tolnaftate in activity and is available as liquid and ointment. The product has astringent properties and is marketed under the name Desenex.

Miconazole nitrate has broad efficacy against fungi, some gram-positive bacteria, some saprophytic fungi, and *Candida Albicans.*[22] This imidazole is available without prescription as Micatin cream (spray liquid, powder, or powder alone).

There are many products that are fungicidal or fungistatic, which cannot be discussed in this limited format. Keratolytic products are useful in physically removing the infected stratum corneum in athlete's foot. Whitfield's ointment contains 3% salicylic acid and benzoic acid in an emollient base. It has been used widely for many years in dry, scaly tinea pedis.[22]

Solutions of acetic acid, aluminum chloride, ammoniated mercury, benzethonim chloride, aluminum acetate, zinc salts, and the potassium permanganate solutions popular in World War II are all commonly used formulations used in treating tinea pedis. Diabetics need to be cautioned in their use to prevent complications from improper treatment.[23]

Amphotericin B is a polyene that is used in deep mycotic infections. It is used intravenously and topically as a 3% cream. Many prescription preparations with special efficacy are available for use. Imidazole and triazole derivatives make up most of the available market currently available for topical use.[26, 27]

Ciclopitrox is efficaceous for dermatophyte infections and for *Candida Albicans*. It is available by prescription as Loprox.

Clotrimazole is an imidazole (triazol) derivative that is antifungal and selectively antibacterial that can be combined with betamethasone as Latrisone for increased antiinflammatory effects.[22] Clotrimazole alone is available in cream form as Lotrimin and Mycelex.

Econazole nitrate is marketed as Spectazole, which is an imidazole active against dermatophytic and some other fungi as well as some bacteria. The product also has antiinflammatory properties.

Haloprogen has comparable activity as tolnaftate but has additional coverage for *Candida Albicans*. It is available on prescription as Halotex. Allylamine-class drugs include naftinidne (Naftine), which is a synthetic antifungal medication available as a 1% cream. It has no antibacterial activity but is active in vitro against *Candida* species.[22]

Nystatin is a polyene antifungal that inhibits membrane steroid biosynthesis that is selective for the yeast-like fungi *Candida albicans*.[22] It is used therapeutically or prophylactically in cream, ointment, and powder as Mycostatin and Nystat.

Other prescription drugs active for use as broad spectrum antifungals include sulconazole (Exeldern) and oxiconazole (Oxistat) and terkonazole. Diabetics need to deal with dermatophytic and other fungal foot infections swiftly and effectively. Once resolved, appropriate prophylactic measures should be taken.[28]

Treating dermatophytic infections in diabetics may require the use of oral antifungal antibiotics such as griseofulvin and ketoconazole when the usual local therapies have been ineffective. Griseofulvin is an oral agent that interferes with mitotic division within pathogenic dermatophytic fungi.[22]

Ketoconazole is also an oral antibiotic that acts as an inhibitor of membrane biosynthesis in fungal development. Griseofulvin is not effective against yeasts, while ketoconazole is active against *Candida* species and the dermatophytes.[29]

Diabetic patients are often at risk from renal and hepatic complications. Therefore patients taking oral antifungal antibiotics need to be carefully monitored for kidney and liver function. Patients should be told about the side effects of these drugs.

Griseofulvin and ketoconazole have been marketed for some time in the United States. Several oral antibiotics have been efficaciously used in Europe that have yet to be approved for treatment of fungus infections by the Food and Drug Administration (FDA).

Fluconazole is one such drug. It is active in vitro against the dermatophytes and *Candida* species.[22] It is inactive against *Aspergillus* species and many fungal pathogens in vitro. However, its efficacy in animal models can be impressive.[30]

Itraconazole has a wide spectrum of antifungal antibiotic activity in vitro. It is a drug of the azole class acting to block sterol biosynthesis. It is currently in use for deep mycotic infections, against *Candida* species, the dermatophytes and other fungi such as *Aspergillus* and yeasts. Oral dosages up to 200 mg bid are documented.[31] Side effects are reported in 5% to 8% of cases; the side effects include gastrointestinal complaints, headache, edema, rash, and impotence. Diabetics need to be concerned with polyuria and elevation of liver enzymes.[31]

The newer allylamine class of antifungal drugs include naftifine and terbinafine. They specifically inhibit squalene epoxidase, thereby interfering with ergosterol biosynthesis.[32] Terbinafine (Lamasil) was shown to be effective against dermatophytes, as well as many molds and yeasts including some *Candida* species. Side effects attributable to the drug itself were not reported as yet in double-blind studies. New systemic antifungal drugs are necessary in diabetic patients because of the development of griseofulvin resistance among some dermatophytes.

Heloma, tyloma, dermatophytosis, and the onychopathies are admittedly mundane podiatric problems. However, they deserve the most meticulous attention from patients with DM and from physicians who treat these problems. If not properly treated, these problems could become serious. Thus, one could conclude that podiatrists are responsible for both life and limb of these patients.

Most studies concerning diabetic dermatology do not deal with the pedal lesions just discussed. Rather, a number of lesions that seem to be related to diabetes make up the bulk of the literature and these topics need to be reviewed at this point.

ACANTHOSIS NIGRANS

Acanthosis nigrans are warty pigmentations of the skin that occur in the flexure folds of the lower extremity and elsewhere in the body.[33] These hyperpigmented elevated lesions are markers for a heterogenous group of endocrine disorders that have insulin resistance as markers and therefore have special significance in DM. Additionally, they may give indication of a possible association with malignant neoplasia[34] most often referable to the gastrointestinal tract. When diabetes is not present, as is often the case, the lesions of acanthosis nigrans are associated with other endocrine diseases or obesity.

Greater insulin resistance and raised insulin levels characterize diabetics demonstrating acanthosis nigrans (AN).[35] Two syndromes are recognized. Type A syndrome is linked with genetic defects in the receptor function or in postreceptor pathways and may show hyperandrogenism.[36] Type B syndrome is characterized by circulating antibodies to the insulin receptor.[36]

Structurally similar receptors for insulin and insulin-like growth factors (IGF) have been demonstrated in human keratinocyte monolayer cell cultures. Therefore it is possible that increased binding of insulin to these IGF receptors may induce mitogenic signals within the epidermis to promote keratinocyte cell proliferation as is observed in AN.[37] Alternatively, it is possible that insulin-like growth factors or androgens given as replacement therapy can produce acanthosis nigrans.[33]

Soft fibroma and skin tags are frequently observed in obese diabetics along with the lesions of AN. While these lesions have only cosmetic implications, it is interesting to speculate that they all may relate to excess of growth factors of one type or another.[33]

Histologically, AN resembles verruca and some hard and soft nevi that make up the differential diagnosis. There is hyperkeratosis and acanthosis together with a mild degⁱee of hyperpigmentation. Dermal papillae are evenly elongated, hyperplastic, and may arborize. However, AN does not produce a centripetal configuration of the rete pegs as does verrucae. The epidermis assumes a serrated and papillomatoses configuration in AN.

CHEIROARTHROPATHY

Diabetic thick skin and stiff joints have been called cheiroarthropathy, although not without some controversy. This condition mimicks scleroderma in some respects. Thickening of the skin with consequent limitation of flexion and extension of the toes and fingers can be demonstrated early on by placing the palms of the hands together using the so-called prayer maneuver.

Cheiroarthropathy may be a reversible condition. It is not correlated to diabetic browning or to nonenzymatic glycosylation.[33,38] It is possible that cheiroarthropathy is an outcome of prolonged poorly controlled hyperglycemia and is considered by some to be a marker for ophthalmic lesions and renal impairment.[33]

The pseudoscleroderma of cheiroathropathy is sometimes referred to as diabetic scleredema. The thickened skin is most often accompanied by nonpitting induration (Figs 12–13 and 12–14). If the limbs are extensively involved, joint contractures can result. Most patients so involved are obese. Microscopically, the dermis demonstrates thickened collagenic fibers with hyaluronic acid interspersed (Fig 12–15).

The author studied in some detail the scleredema of Buschke in 1986.[39] This rare condition most often follows an infectious episode. In the case studied there was a threefold thickening of the dermis in which collagenic fibers replaced most of the matrix. The brittle diabetic patient went on to develop many ulcerations of the extremities that led ultimately to cellulitis, septicemia, and ultimately to below-the-knee amputation in spite of all of the medical interventions used.

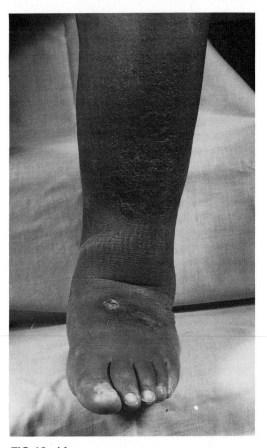

FIG 12–14.
Frontal view of scleredema of Buschke demonstrating coexisting dorsal cutaneous ulcer.

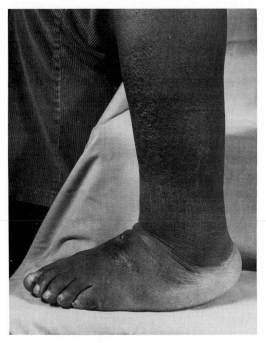

FIG 12–13.
Scleredema of Buschke in brittle diabetic.

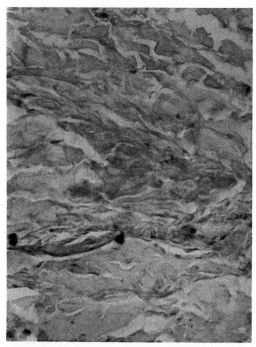

FIG 12–15.
Collagenic fibers of threefold-thickened dermis in scleredema of Buschke, hematoxylin, and eosin preparation light, microscopy.

The syndrome of limited joint mobility (LJM) in cheiroarthropathy may relate as much to the microvascular complications of diabetes as to the thickening of the skin. Increased nonenzymatic glycosylation of keratinocytes of the stratum corneum of the foot's plantar surface may account for the thickened skin and other foot abnormalties including neuropathic ulcerations and callus formation.[40]

DIABETIC BLISTERS

Diabetic blisters (bullosis diabeticorum, diabetic bullae) are a fairly uncommon and curious phenomenon observed in patients with DM (Fig 12–16). Reported cases are published singly from time to time, but as many as 30 cases have been reported in a single investigation.[41] The blisters occur spontaneously on the extremities in a more or less symmetrical fashion. They measure from several millimeters to several centimeters in diameter. The cause of such lesions has not been established, but trauma has been excluded as a cause.[1, 42]

Bullae may occur on the dorsum of the feet where shoe pressure is a problem. Lesions resolve spontaneously over a period of 2 to 5 weeks.[43] In areas of the body that do not receive pressure and where bullae do not create pain, it is prudent to permit resolution over time. However, when spontaneous rupturing of bullae becomes a distinct possibility as can result from the shoe's compression on the mass, it seems prudent to aspirate the sterile fluid from the tense bullae without deroofing the lesion. Once performed, a sterile covering should be provided.

Two types of bullae can be observed among diabetics. The first class involves intraepidermal cleavage with healing occurring spontaneously and without scarring or acantholysis. Bullae of the second class may be hemorrhagic and the healing process can be complicated by mild atrophy of the involved skin and scarring. Skin cleavage in such instances occurs subepidermally.

A third class of blisters have been observed in a very limited number of patients: lesions that appear on sun-exposed, deeply tanned skin of diabetics. Lesions are tender, but nonscarring and cleavage is suprabasilar.[44]

The lesions of diabetic blisters and bullae may demonstrate different levels of epidermal cleavage, but they all seem to relate to poorly controlled diabetes. Calcium and magnesium imbalances, immunological factors, renal disease, vascular and neurological insufficiency in the presence of dermal rigidity have all been implicated in diabetic blistering. Alterations in collagen with loss of anchoring fibrils within the skin also appear to be involved in the development of diabetic blisters and bullae.

GRANULOMA ANNULARE

Granuloma annulare occurs in localized and generalized forms. If the condition occurs locally, no established relationship with DM has been established.[35] However, in older diabetic populations some association between DM and granuloma annulare is likely, although the precise cause is unknown.[45]

Lesions occur as ring-like (annular) individual papules that tend to coalesce. Central portions of the ring consist of hyperpigmented spots that in the feet usually have a purplish coloration.[33] Alternatively, the center of the annular configuration may have normal skin or may be a uniform plaque that has formed from coalesced papules.[46]

Nonannular eruptions can occur in which coalescing papules occur in scattered fashion, but this is not usually seen on the lower extremities. In one study of 100 patients with granuloma annulare, 47 women and 24 men demonstrated foot lesions. Of these cases, 5 affected the soles of the feet, 12 cases were on the toes, 22 cases involved the ankle, and 30 were seen on other areas of the foot.[46]

Histologically, an annular arrangement of skin structures is characteristic just as it is true of the gross appearance. Individual papules of the peripheral ring are composed of palisading (elongated parallel rows) granulomas within the pars reticularis. However, the level of the lesion is variable and may extend to the subcutaneous level. The central portion of the lesion is characterized as necrobiotic, and a low power[47] examination is useful in appreciating the overall morphology of the individual, usually small, papule.

The central area of necrosis may lack nuclei altogether. It may contain connective tissue elements in bundles or necrosis may be more complete, leaving a stringy hematoxylinophilic material. The granulomatous wall is variable in terms of composition and quantity. Cells are stellate or fusiform and tend to orient centripetally

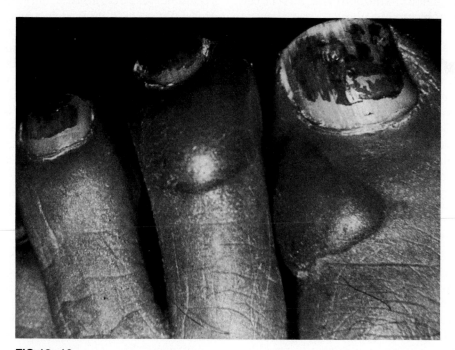

FIG 12–16.
Bullosis diabeticorum involving great and second toes of diabetic patient.

about the variable necrotic center. A lymphocytic infiltrate may or may not be present.[47]

Granuloma annulare in its generalized form is often associated with DM. It also may have some inexplicable connection with malignancies. It seldom regresses spontaneously, so some form of treatment should be attempted. Potassium iodide, systemic antifungals and antibiotics, systemic vitamins (A and E) antituberculosis agents, tars, colchicine, radiation therapy, and nonsteroidal antiinflammatory agents were all shown to be ineffective in one study.[46] Antihistamines and azathioprine are occasionally useful.

Intralesional glucocorticosteroids and to a lesser extent, topical and systemic glucocortical costeroids, are effective. Chlorambucil was effective in each of six cases studied. Freezing, dapsone, and antimalarials were also shown to be partically effective in the treatment of granuloma annulare.[46] As is always the case, the overall medical status in DM directs the choice of treatment plan.

INFECTIONS

Uncontrolled DM provides a fertile field for the establishment of skin infections. Some of these concerns have already been addressed e.g., dermataphytosis, candidiasis, and paronychia. Diabetes produces faulty neutrophilic chemotaxis, phagocytosis, and microbial killing.[33] Additionally, cell mediated immunity is deficient, related in part, to hyperglycemia.[48] There is, however, no evidence of impairment of specific cutaneous defenses such as changes in the normal skin flora or defects in Langerhan's cell function.[33]

Microorganisms, many of which are pathogenic, can always be recovered from normal skin. The outermost strata of skin, the stratum corneum, normally provides an effective barrier that separates the body's hostile environment from its complex and sensitive internal milieu.[49] Unfortunately, the integrity of skin is often disturbed or disrupted in diabetics. Hyperhidrosis, dry cracked skin, neurovascular deficiencies, peripheral neuropathy, ischemia, and adnexal malfunction are but a few factors leading to decreased skin resistance and increased morbidity from skin infections among diabetics.

The normal resident microflora of the skin of diabetics is that of the normal population. Aerobic and anaerobic species are so represented.[50] *Staphylococcus, Micrococcus, Corynebacteruim, Brevibacterium, Propionibacterium* and *Pitysosporum* species can usually be cultured from intact skin, hair follicles, and the pilosebaceous glands of the lower extremities.

Transient bacteria that tend to change with the external environment as well as opportunistic microbes can join the normal skin microflora to complicate skin infections affecting the lower extremities of diabetics. Gram-negative rods such as *Pseudomonas aeruginosa,* proteus and klebsiella species, escherichia and enterobacter species and others can be transient or opportunistic on wet and dry skin.[50] Gram-positive cocci including enterococcal, streptococcal species as well as gram-positive rods such as *Bacillus, Clostridium* and *Propionibacterium* species can colonize the skin and infect the skin of diabetic feet and legs.[50]

Scratching can inoculate the skin of diabetics with potential pathogens. Abrasions, lacerations, insect bites, etc., which might have been innocuous to the normal patient, become dangerous to the immunocompromised diabetic.

Bacterial infections of the skin are classified as primary and secondary pyodermas. *Staphylococcus aureus* or group A *Streptococcus* are almost always etiologic in primary pyodermas. Interaction between the host skin and bacteria that colonize the skin, which is essentially intact or at most traumatized by mild excoriation or laceration, produce most of the clinical disease observed.[50] In such instances immediate appropriate antibiotic therapy will arrest most primary pyodermas in diabetics.

Streptococcal primary pyodermas must be initiated by a break in the skin. It is characterized by spreading erythema and local skin necrosis, which may lead to lymphangitis and cellulitis. It is important to remember that kidney disease can follow streptococcal skin infections and diabetics are at increased risk in this respect.[51]

β-Hemolytic streptococci may produce nonbullous impetigo that progresses from a macular lesion to a vesicle. Other species of staphylococci and streptococci may be secondarily implicated. Vesicles ooze and become crusted; lesions can then coalesce to form large patches.

Hyperpigmentation can remain for a time on resolution of impetigo, but scarring does not usually occur.[51] Impetigo is a childhood affliction, but it can be seen in some immunocompromised diabetic patients.

Depressed atrophic scars do develop following ecthyma. Pustules surrounded by erythema and induration follow the appearance of the primary lesion that is a vesicle. This primary pyoderma occurs in the upper dermis and lower epidermis as opposed to the subcorneal lesions of impetigo. Erysipelas and cellulitis represent deeper forms of skin infections which represent a progression on to secondary pyodermas (Fig 12–17).

Erysipelas is heralded by a tender, warm, erythematous, edematous, enlarging hard plaque of the skin.[51] Regional adenopathy, fever, chills, and malaise accompany the local signs and symptoms.

The plaques of erysipelas are sharply defined and may contain petechiae. Vesicles and bullae may also appear. Streptococcal organisms usually cause erysipelas. Consequently, it must be assumed that a break in the skin is necessary to

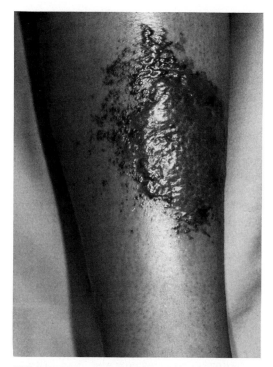

FIG 12–17.
Streptococcal erysipelas in patient with diabetes mellitus. (Courtesy of Dr. Marc Brenner.)

permit the entry of the pathogen. Treatment is symptomatic and by specific antibiotic as defined by culture and sensitivity testing. Long-term therapy is often required.

Cellulitis is a secondary pyoderma involving the deep dermis and subcutaneous tissues. Skin ulcers, exogenous or endogenous eczema, and interdigital fissures, allow for the entry of any one of a number of microorganisms; *Clostridium Perfingens* and many *Staphylococcal* and *Streptococcal* species are etiologic. Diabetic cellulitis is often of polymicrobial nature and aggressive intervention may be required. Hospitalization for several days is usually required for diabetics with cellulitis. Elevation and compresses on the involved limb are indicated.[6] Selection of a proper antibiotic may require consultation with an infectious disease specialist. Third-generation cephalosporins and an aminoglycoside given intravenously along with appropriate monitoring of hepatic and renal functions may be indicated. Appropriate home therapy over an extended period of time is sometimes required after clinical resolution of cellulitis of the lower extremities in diabetics.

LYMPHANGITIS

Lymphangitis is an acute pyogenic inflammation of lymphatic vessels most often caused by group A streptococci. Lymphatics normally collect a complex intercellular fluid known as lymph. Involved vessels are thin walled lacking a distinct muscularis. Lymph from the extremities are returned to the heart via the cysterua chylae.

The initial appearance mimics a cellulitis from which the condition frequently develops. Wounds, abrasions, and interdigital fissures can also lead to lymphangitis, which is characterized by red streaks that outline the course of involved lymphatic channels. As the subcutaneous infection progresses proximally, lymph nodes can be enlarged and palpably tender. Chills, fever, and malaise can occur with remarkable rapidity in diabetics as bacteremia becomes established. It is important to select the proper antibiotic when sensitive Streptococcal species are etiologic.

Staphylococcal skin infections, unlike streptococcal involvements, need not break the skin to cause pathogenicity. Staphylococcal infections tend to become more widespread quickly in diabetics. Penicillinase-producing cocci are frequently a nosocomial infection, making hospital acquired infections difficult to treat.

Bullous impetigo is usually a penicillin resistant skin infection produced by group N coagulase positive styphylococci, phage type 71.[51] Primary lesions are first vesicular then become bullous. Bullae spread outwardly while collapsing in the center of the lesion. Bullae may rupture leaving a burn like area. Thin brown crusts develop as exudates dry in this fairly contagious condition.[51]

Scalded-skin syndrome (SSS) is a painful erythema of skin characterized by large bullae that precede the peeling away of large portions of epidermis.[51] The disease usually is restricted to the newborn, but immunocompromised diabetic patients can be involved. The clinical appearance is similar to that of toxic epidermal necrolysis (TEN), which is characterized by deeper subepidermal blistering and is most often caused by reactions to medication. Microscopic examination, history, and physical examination establish the differential diagnosis.

Folliculitis is a skin condition fairly common among diabetics that occurs in superficial and deep forms. Superficial folliculitis demonstrates dome-shaped pustules pierced by hair, which is surrounded by a small rim of erythema.[51]

Erythematous indurated nodules that may obliterate the follicles and are tender to palpation characterizes deep folliculitis. Established furuncles become suppurative and often rupture in a week or two.[51] Folliculitis is treated by warm compresses, incision and drainage and topical or systemic antibiotics, as directed by culture and sensitivity testing.

Chronic furunculosis may be an initial sign of DM and diseases such as lymphoma, agammaglobinemia, as well as in leukocytic defects.[51] Physicians who treat DM should be aware of this characteristic of chronic furunculosis.

Substance abuse can be a source of pyoderma. Toxic substances injected by drug addicts have been shown to lead to skin infection, dermopathy, ulcerating nodules, and atrophic scars.[52] Substance abusers have been known to use the foot as a site of injection. Nutritional habits and poor hygiene, as seen among alcohol abusers, can contribute to pyodermas. Abusers of alcohol are subject to trauma and a degree of immunodepression that can also lead to additional skin infections in this population.[53]

The subject of skin infections cannot be closed without mention of phycomycetes species that do well in high glucose media provided by DM.[1] Opportunistic organisms can become established in neuropathic and immunocompromised diabetics particularly when trauma, ulcerations on nonhealing surgical wounds precede the infection.[1] Culture and histologic examination are diagnostic in such instances. Deep mycotic infections by a variety of organisms as well as common fungi and yeasts including *Candida* species can be primary as well as secondary pathogenic invaders in pyodermas of the lower extremities.[1]

Another skin infection is that of erythrasma caused by rod-shaped bacillus

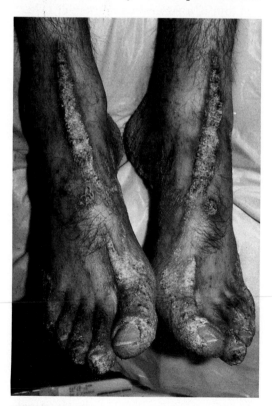

FIG 12–18.
Hypertrophic lichen planus. (Courtesy of Dr. Lee Sander.)

Corynebacterium Minutissemum. In the foot, such infections mimic scaling macerating tinea infections that occur interdigitally. Wood's light examination is most helpful diagnostically and the oral administration of erythromycin can be curative.[53]

LICHEN PLANUS AND OTHER PSORIAFORM DISORDERS

Lichen planus (LP) has been associated with DM on a statistical basis.[54] It is a relatively common papulosquamous skin disease that occasionally affects the skin of diabetics, although the precise biochemical linkage remains obscure.[55] Polygonal flat lesions of a purplish hue are characteristic of the primary lesions of LP.[56] Grayish-white cross hatching (Wickham's striae) is characteristic of scales. This pruritic inflammatory dermatitis affects men and women in a bilaterally symmetrical fashion (Fig 12–18). Nail changes can be seen in approximately 10% of LP patients.[57] Such changes include thinning, grooving, onycholysis, subungual keratosis, and pterygium.

Viral, psychogenic, drug sensitivity, immunodeficiencies, and exogenous toxicity are among the suspected causes of lichen planus in diabetics.[56]

Evidence for an immune deficiency role in lichen planus stems from observations that the T-cell lymphocytic infiltration observed in the dermis of lesions as well as levels of IgA and IgM and immunoglobulin deposits in the involved skin are increased.[58] Moreover, a LP specific antigen has been isolated in the suprapapillary stratum Malpighi.[59]

Histologic analysis of LP demonstrates hyperkeratosis, hypergranulosis, acanthosis, saw-toothed alterations of rete pegs, degenerative liquifaction of the stratum basale, colloid bodies of lower epidermis, and lymphocytic and histiocytic infiltrate of the dermis.[56]

Treatment for LP is largely symptomatic because most lesions clear spontaneously. Systemic corticosteroids are used for severe LP reactions but overly aggressive use of this class of medications in diabetics should be carefully monitored. Pruritis can be relieved by antihistamines and topical fluorinated steroids.

Lichen sclerosus et atrophicus is an antiimmune condition said to be somehow related to latent DM.[60] This skin disease is characterized by ivory white papulous elements that may affect any cutaneous body surface, but is mainly associated with the genitalia. It is mentioned here for the sake of completeness.

LIPODYSTROPHY

The lipodystrophies comprise a group of uncommon skin disorders in which there is partial or total absence of subcutaneous fat. Such lesions have been associated with dermatological abnormalities associated with DM.

LIPOHYPERTROPHY

Hypertrophic reactions of adipose tissue have been associated with repeated injections of older insulins, particularly of highly purified pork products.[61] The condition can be seen as a large sheet of fatty tissue. Alternatively, lipohypertrophy may appear in the form of mobile anaesthetic nodules.[33] Because this condition relates to large accumulations of poorly disseminated quantities of insulin, it is unlikely to occur in the foot.

LIPATROPHY

Loss of adipose tissue in the form of atrophic plaques may occur at the sites of insulin injection.[33] The mechanism of this phenomenon is that lipolytic compo-

nents of some insulin preparations or immunocomplex-mediated inflammatory processes cause the release of lysosomal enzymes that break down fat cells.[62] Lipatrophy relates to insulin injection; therefore, this diabetes-related skin condition is not likely to occur in the foot.

NECROBIOSIS LIPOIDICA

Necrobiosis lipoidica diabeticorum juvenalis is a term often used for this diabetes-related condition. However, it is not necessarily related to DM nor is it confined to juveniles. Therefore, it will simply be called necrobiosis lipoidica (NL) for purpose of this discussion. Fifty percent of all patients with NL have coexisting diabetes.[63] In this sense, necrobiosis lipoidica can be said to be unequivocally related to DM and is a cutaneous marker of D.M.[34] On the other hand, only 0.3% of all patients with diabetes will ever develop necrobiosis lipoidica.[64]

Lesions of necrobiosis lipoidica may be solitary or multiple and is three times more likely to occur in females than among male patients. Initially, NL appears as a circumscribed, erythematous papule. Radially evolving lesions demonstrate atrophic telangiectatic centers and have hard, depressed, waxy yellow-brown surfaces.[1] Active lesions demonstrate erythematous raised peripheral borders. Minor trauma induces ulceration in about one third of cases.

Most lesions appear along the thin-skinned tibial crest of the midleg (Fig 12–19), although other areas of the body are not necessarily spared. The histopathology of necrobiosis lipoidica is that of necrotizing neutrophilic vasculitis. Adnexal structures and dermal collagen undergo degenerative changes.[65] Later alterations are granulomatous in nature with sclerosis of the lower reticular dermis. A yellow coloration is due to fatty deposits in the papillary dermis. Small-vessel throm-

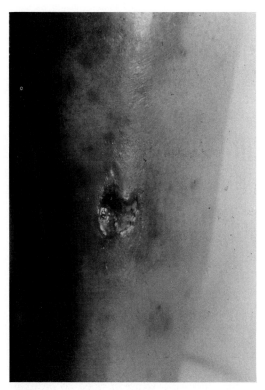

FIG 12–19.
Necrobiosis lipoidica diabeticorum. (Courtesy of Dr. Thomas Delauro.)

bosis and abnormal platelet function results in dermal collagen degradation.[33] The pathophysiology of necrobiosis lipoidica is not well understood. However, intralesional injections of corticosteroids or topical applications of steroids have proven to be beneficial.[1]

Diabetics with necrobiosis lipoidica need to be cautioned about the dangers of trauma and consequent ulceration. Skin grafting may be necessary in poorly healing necrotizing lesions.

PEMPHIGOID

Bullous pemphigoid generally involves the elderly and occurs more frequently in diabetics.[66] Peripherally disposed urticated erythematous plaques evolve into subepidermal blisters where IgG immune antibodies can be demonstrated on paralesional skin biopsy.[67] The lamina lucida of the epidermal basement membrane, and patient serum are the locations for antibodies that may initially be derived from degenerative collagen changes within the dermis.

Patients with DM who have extensive itching or blistering need careful evaluation to differentiate staphylococcal bullous impetigo and the bullae of drug sensitivities of bullous pemphigoid. Skin biopsy for histology, immunofluorescence, circulating autoantibodies, as well as blister fluid culture and immunology and porphorin studies are all essential for accurate diagnosis of the blistered diabetic patient. Bullosis diabeticorum is localized and transient with a high recurrence rate while pemiphigoid is extensive and persistent.[33]

Bullous pemphigoid can be a severe and acute skin disease requiring hospitalization. Systemic corticosteroids are useful and dosages of prednisone ranging from 100 to 500 mg daily may be required.[68] However, because gastrointestinal bleeding, hyperglycemia, opportunistic infection, and psychosis are potential side effects when steroids are used, great care and caution needs to be taken with diabetic patients. Azathioprine or cyclophosphamide may be used along with prednisone to reduce the effective concentration of steroid required.[68]

PSORIASIS

Psoriasis is a papulosquamous disease of the skin that may have an association with DM.[33] Genetic factors predispose to psoriasis, which are known to be closely linked to the major histocompatibility (HLA) antigen.[69] HLA-B 27, HLA-Bw17, HLA-Bw16, HLA-Bw37, HLA-B8, HLA-B27, HLA-Cw6 are HLA antigens which have been shown to be associated with psoriasis.[69] HLA-B8 is associated with persistant palmar-plantar pustulosis.[70] Alterations affecting the immune system are common to DM, psoriasis and a number of diabetic related conditions already discussed.

Pathogenesis of psoriasis involves a sharp increase in epidermal replication and maturation and keratinocyte mitosis. Hyperkeratosis, parakeratosis, and acanthosis are histologic features of psoriasis with cell transit time reduced from 28 days to 3 to 4 days in the disease. Manipulations within cyclic AMP pathways are involved in regulation of epidermal cell proliferation as well as in vascular response.[71]

The extensor skin surfaces of the lower extremities show a special affinity for psoriatic lesions along with other body locations. Well-defined, rounded, erythematous, dry, scaling plaques of varying size are characteristic of psoriasis. Silvery-white or grayish white scales cover the plaques that emerge from solitary pinkish or red macules.[70] Auspitz's signs are small bleeding points that make themselves evident upon removal of the scales. Psoriatric erruptions may occur at the site of skin trauma, a response known as isomorphic or Koebner's phenomenon.

Erythematous papules and pustules as well as thick fissured plaques occur extensively on the soles of the feet in psoriasis. Such lesions allow for the portal of entry of pathogenic bacteria in diabetics and the combination of pyoderma within a devitalized skin can lead to serious complications.

The histopathology of psoriasis as revealed by biopsy confirms the diagnosis. Rete pegs are elongated and thickened at the epidermo-dermal interface. The acanthotic supra papillary Malpighi stratum underlies the hyperkeratotic and parakeratotic stratum corneum. There is agranulosis and the dermal papillae are narrow and atrophied. Munro's microabscesses are small collections of neutrophils localized within the stratum corneum that are typical to psoriasis. Pustular forms of psoriasis are characterized by large, rounded intraepidermal unilocular pustules containing polymorphonuclear leukocytes that may erode into the dermis.[69]

Psoriasis also affects the nails as well as joints of the feet as an inflammatory peripheral arthritis, or spondylitis, or both. Psoriasis is a complex disease and an indepth discussion of it is beyond the scope of this study as is a discussion of all of the many therapuetic plans available.

Photochemotherapy (PUVA) has been successful in treating psoriasis as has been the use of oral steroids. Glucocorticosteroids, keratolytics, anthralin, and coal tar ointments have all been used to advantage. Cytotoxic agents such as 5-fluorouracil (5 FU) and systemic methotrexate have also been used. However, in dealing with diabetic patients with psoriasis, care and caution need to be exercised so as not to exacerbate either condition.

SHIN SPOTS

Shin spots occur on the thin-skinned areas covering the crest of the tibia of the leg and occur in nondiabetic as well as diabetic patients. Such lesions are pigmented and atrophic in appearance.[33] It has been suggested that they may be the sequelae of diabetic blisters.[72]

Paralesional vacuolization has been noted around nonspecific papular and excoriated lesions of the extremities of older diabetics, which may be part of a spectrum of aging and such phenomenon may be involved in diabetic shin spots.[33]

SKIN TAGS

Skin tags are soft fibromata that are common skin lesions associated with obesity and DM.[34] One study associated skin tags with three fourths of the diabetic population.[73] Aside from the statistical interest, skin tags have only cosmetic significance. Acrochordon or skin tags are outward evaginations of skin having an inner core of papillary dermis covered by all of the epithelial strata. Most consist of one hyperplastic papillae although others seem to be papilloma-like or appear as sessile flat seborrheic warts.[46] If such lesions appear on the foot in places traumatized by footwear, they may be excised in diabetics when the underlying disease is well controlled.

FLUSHING

Ten to thirty percent of patients using the oral hypoglycemic drug chlorpropamide experience flushing 15 minutes after the ingestion of alcohol. Headache, tachycardia, and shortness of breath accompany this reaction, which usually subsides within 1 hour.[74]

Autonomic neuropathy with defective reinnervation may cause decreased sweating in one area with compensatory hyperhidrosis elsewhere is a condition that can occur in diabetics.[75] Inappropriate localized facial sweating can occur during the ingestion of food.[76] Obviously, physicians treating the lower extremities are not involved with these symptoms, but the basic mechanisms of hyperhidrosis are of interest in DM and the phenomenon itself needs to be understood.

SYSTEMIC ALLERGIC REACTIONS

Maculopapular rashes may occur when oral hypoglycemic agents such as sulfonylureas, tolbutamide, and chlorpropanide are prescribed.[77] Generalized erythema, morbilliform eruptions, urticarial lesions and occasional photosensitive reactions can also occur. Sulfonylurea drug

reactions may resolve spontaneously but switching to another oral hypoglycemic agent is recommended.[35]

Systemic allergic reactions as severe as anaphylaxis have been reported from the use of older pork and beef insulins. Impurities in these preparations are probably the allergens that can produce varying degrees of immunological response.[33]

Practitioners treating diabetic complaints involving the lower extremities need to be aware of these allergic reactions, although it is unlikely that symptoms of these reactions will involve the foot or leg. Other treatment-related skin conditions in DM such as lipoatrophy and lipohypertrophy have been dealt with previously in this book.

VITILIGO

Vitiligo is a skin condition characterized by symmetrical patches of depigmentation.[33] Its occurrence is higher among insulin-dependent diabetics than in noninsulin-dependent diabetics, but it does not appear to have any significant relationship to any HLA-type autoimmune disease. Wood's light is reflected from patches of vitiligo because of the reduction of skin pigmentation.[78]

PRURITIS

Pruritis is said to be the most common of all dermatologic complaints.[79] It is not a disease in and of itself but is rather a symptom that can be a marker for internal diseases including DM. Hypothyroidism and hyperthyroidism are other endocrine disorders characterized by generalized itching. Chronic renal failure, obstructive biliary disease, lymphoma, leukemia, polychythemia rubra vera, multiple myeloma, iron deficiency, and psychiatric, and idiopathic causes must also be considered.[79]

Diabetic patients complaining of generalized itching should be carefully evaluated to rule out the possibility of coexisting systemic illness (Fig 12–20). Diabetics, as is true of the general population, deal with itching by scratching or rubbing the offending skin. This activity may result in excoriations which can become secondarily infected. Lichenification is that thickened, leatherlike appearance of the integument which also demonstrates exaggerated skin markings as a result of chronic repetitive scratching. Picking at the skin in a repetitive fashion results in prurigo nodularis.[79]

Xerosis, or dry skin, is common in diabetics and pruritis is one of its symptoms. Rehydration through the use of topical emollients can be partially successful in dealing with xerosis.

Idiopathic pruritis is a common condition, which, as the name suggests, has no known etiology. Functional changes of sensory end organs of the skin of diabetics may be implicated.[80] Scratching the arch of one foot using the great toe of the contralateral foot can cause excoriations that become inoculated with the nail's microflora and a diabetic pyoderma can ensue.

Psychological problems have been cited for itching of unknown cause. However, this possibility should be considered only after all other possibilities for the itching have been ruled out.[79] The subject of diabetic dermatology is that of dermatology in general. Podiatric dermatology has several unique subjects that have been discussed previously.

Other general dermatologic entities discussed are those that are classically associated with DM. Other conditions such as yellow skin and yellow nails might have been cited since they are associated with DM.[1] Sebaceous gland disorders have been loosely associated with diabetes because some patients exhibit excess sebum production with resultant acne-like eruptions.[80]

Odd diabetic complications, such as perforating collagenosis, where altered

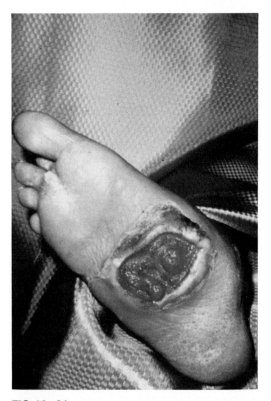

FIG 12–21.
Severe plantar foot ulceration in the insensitive diabetic with charcot joint. (Courtesy of Dr. Brenner.)

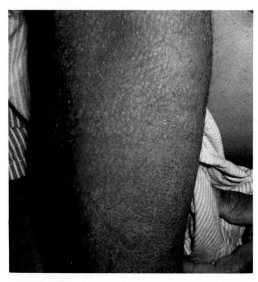

FIG 12–20.
Dry, pruritic skin in diabetic.

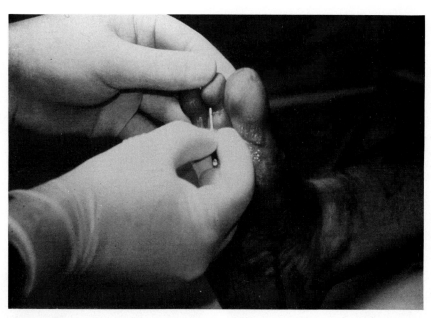

FIG 12–22.
Biopsy is frequently required in diabetic foot conditions.

collagen is eliminated through the epidermis[81, 82] could have been discussed.

A discussion of the dermatology of DM would not be complete without mention of mal perforans of the lower extremities. This subject is discussed in detail, elsewhere in this volume in a different context.

The skin is a large and complex organ. When it is violated, as in the case of cutaneous ulceration in diabetics, life and limb may be threatened. Ulcers may occur in association with hematologic disorders, granulomatous disease, vasculitis, and arterial and venous vascular diseases, as well as in a number of miscellaneous causes. Those ulcerations that occur in association with DM can be especially vexing since macro and microvascular disease as well as peripheral neuropathy are usually involved.[83]

The anesthetic foot of diabetes does not appreciate the degree of trauma to which it is exposed and injured. Weight-bearing foci of the skin may break down, form bullae, and ulcerate (Fig 12–21). These regions often are preceded by the formation of heloma and tyloma. Local fibrosis, necrosis and purulent exudation are features of diabetic foot ulcerations. Deep space infection and osteomyelitis may ensue with consequent loss of life or limb.

Healing of diabetic mal perforans, when and if it comes, occurs with considerable difficulty. Those factors that predispose to ulceration tend also to obstruct normal healing processes. Proper healing also depends on accurate diagnosis. Diabetics can be host to cutaneous malignancies which can ulcerate and they may have deep mycosis that lead to ulceration. Therefore, biopsy and culture may be necessary in assessing diabetic ulcerations (Figs 12–22 and 12–23).

Diabetic ulcers are often infected by polymicrobial flora and require broad spectrum antibiotics (Fig 12–24). Often, opportunistic microbes are involved as are gram-negative organisms and anaerobic bacteria that require expert deep culture techniques and appropriate media. In fulminating conditions, diabetics may need hospitalization, which should

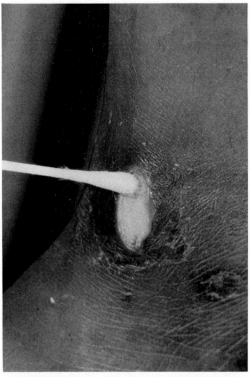

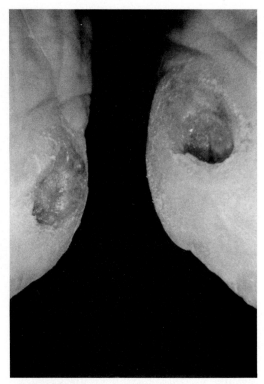

FIG 12–23.
Culture and sensitivity testing is essential in treating diabetic ulcerations, as well as all other foot infections.

FIG 12–24.
Bilateral mal perforans of the heels of diabetic with polymicrobial involvement.

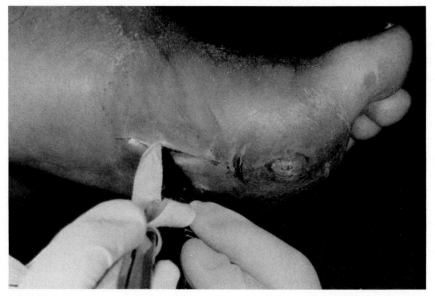

FIG 12–25.
Incision and drainage is a common requirement for deep space infections in diabetic patients.

not be delayed.[84] Incision and drainage of deep space infection extending from a diabetic ulcer is not an uncommon requirement of infected diabetic patients (Fig 12–25).

Supportive systemic therapy is frequently required for diabetic mal perforans. Attempts at vasodilitation or to otherwise improve local tissue repair can be instituted. Trental (Hoechst-Roussel, Sommerville, NJ) has been used to enhance erythrocyte flexibility in Europe. FDA approval for this use has yet to be achieved in the United States.

Evaporating wet dressings and tepid soaks with astringents and antiseptics are of use therapeutically as well as for analgesic purposes. Wet-to-dry dressings may mechanically debride ulcer surfaces as the dry dressing is removed from the lesion during dressing changes. Proteolytic enzymes may assist in the chemical debridement of ulcerations.[84]

Immobilization of the anesthetic limb in the form of total contact casting has been used in treating diabetic ulcers.[85] Soft crusts, unna boots and ace bandaging may also be useful. Hyperbaric oxygen has been suggested as therapeutic for ulcers. (See chapter on HBO therapy in this text.)

Hydrophilic beads of Dextranomer (Debrisan, Johnson and Johnson Co., New Brunswick, NJ) can be used as a powerful desiccant to remove debris, bacteria and, exudates from ulcer surfaces.

Surgical osteotomies to remove bone pressure can be useful in healing ulcerations.[86] Saucerization of bone and other surgical approaches to remove osteomyelitic bone may be required.

Several specialized dressing materials are presently marketed for ulcer care. Occlusive dressings are available that remain in situ for a week or more. When infection is not a problem, such dressings allow tissue fluids and the body's own proteolytic enzymes and nutrients to promote healing in ulcerations. Dressings are available that are impermeable as well as permeable to atmospheric oxygen.[87]

Biological dressings which are compatible to host tissues are available for use as xenografts. The xenografts provide dressing to ulcer surfaces and protect naked nerve endings to provide comfort for healing ulcers. Porcine (pig) and fetal calf skins have been used in this manner.[88, 89] All of the above mentioned techniques for ulcer management have their place when used appropriately. It is of the utmost importance that each wound be thoroughly evaluated prior to initiating any treatment protocol.

SUMMARY

Dermatological considerations in patients with DM are many and varied. Practitioners need to know the many ramifications involved. A high index of suspicion needs to be exercised in the differential diagnosis of diabetics who have problems other than DM. Once the assessment is correctly made, an effective therapeutic plan can be implemented.

REFERENCES

1. Huntley AC: Cutaneous manifestations of diabetes mellitus, *Dermatol Clin* 7:531–545, 1989.
2. McCarthy DJ: The skin. In McGlamry ED, editor: *Fundamentals of foot surgery,* Baltimore, 1987, Williams & Wilkins.
3. Hanna W et al: Pathologic features of diabetic thick skin, *J Am Acad Dermatol* 16:546–553, 1987.
4. Rosenbloom AL: Diabetic thick skin and stiff joints, *Diabetologia* 32:74–76, 1989.
5. Braverman IM: *Skin signs of systemic disease,* Philadelphia, 1981, WB Saunders.
6. McCarthy DJ, Montgomery R: *Podiatric dermatology,* Baltimore, 1986, Williams & Wilkins.

7. Zelickson AS : *Ultrastructure of normal and abnormal skin,* Philadelphia, 1967, Lea & Febiger.

8. Buckingham BA et al: Scleroderma like syndrome with non-enzymatic glycosylation of collagen in children with poorly controlled insulin dependent diabetes, *Paediatr Res* 15:626, 1981 (abstract).

9. Kennedy L, Baynes JW: Non-enzymatic glycosylation and chronic complications of diabetes. An overview, *Diabetologia* 26:93–98, 1984.

10. Goodfield MJD, Millard LG: The skin in diabetes mellitus, *Diabetologia* 31:567–575, 1988.

11. Seibold JR et al: Collagen synthesis and collagenase activity in dermal fibroblasts from patients with diabetes and digital sclerosis, *J Lab Clin Med* 105:664–667, 1985.

12. Kirschenbaum DM: Glycosylation of proteins. Its implications in diabetic control and complications, *Pediatr Clin North Am* 31:611–621, 1984.

13. Cohen J: Interactions of the skin, *Br J Dermatol* 81(supp.3):46–59, 1969.

14. Vorhees JJ, Duell EA: Psoriasis as a possible defect of the adenyl cyclase-cyclic AMP cascade, *Arch Dermatol* 104:352–358, 1971.

15. McCarthy DJ, Habowsky JEJ: The epidermo-dermal interface of the human foot as compared with the composite body. In Clark TE, editor: *Yearbook of podiatry 1978–1979,* Mt Kisko, New York, 1979, Futura Publishing.

16. McCarthy DJ, Habowsky JEJ: Alterations in skin morphology in heloma durum utilizing maceration technique for examination of epidermal-dermal interface, *J Am Pod Assoc* 65(8):303–307, 1972.

17. McCarthy DJ, Habowsky JEJ: Histochemistry and anthropometric analysis of heloma durum, *J Am Pod Assoc* 65(1):4–18, 1975.

18. Bartolomei FJ, McCarthy DJ: Digital ulceration secondary to a "medicated corn pad" containing 40% salicylic acid, *Curr Podiatr* 8:25–26, 1984.

19. Beaven DW, Brooks SE: *Color atlas of the nail in clinical diagnosis,* St Louis, 1984, Mosby–Year Book.

20. Bates JE: Onychomycosis, *J Natl Assoc Chirop* 37(10):47, 1947.

21. Saborand R: *Topographical dermatology,* New York, 1906, Rebman.

22. Page JC: *Athletes' foot: evolving concepts in the diagnosis and treatment of pedal infections,* New York, 1991, Ortho Phamaceutical (monograph).

23. Port MS, Sanicola KF: Nonsurgical removal of dystrophic nails utilizing urea ointment occlusion, *J Am Pod Med Assoc* 70(10):521–523, 1980.

24. Krausz C: Onychopathy. In McCarthy DJ, Montgomery R, editors: *Podiatric dermatology,* Baltimore, 1986, Williams & Wilkins.

25. Abramson et al: Serologic profiles following prolonged inhalation of onychomycotic aerosols, *Bacteriol Proc* 399, 1983.

26. Cleary JD, Taylor JW, Chapman SW: Imidazoles and triazoles in antifungal therapy, DICP, *Ann Pharmacol* 24:149–152, 1990.

27. Jones HE: Consensus of the role and positioning of the imidazoles in the treatment of dermatophytosis, *Acta Derm Venereol* 121:139–146, 1986.

28. Abramson C, McCarthy DJ: Athletes' foot infections. In Abramson C, McCarthy D, Rupp M, editors: *Infectious diseases of the lower extremities,* Baltimore, 1991, Williams & Wilkins.

29. Van der Bossche H, Willemsens G, Cools W: Inhibition of ergosterol synthesis in *Candida albicans* by ketoconazol, *Arch Int Physiol Biochim* 87:849–851, 1979.

30. Graybill JR: Azole therapy of systemic infections. In Holmberg K, Meyer RD, editors: *Diagnosis and therapy of systemic fungal infections,* New York, 1989, Raven Press.

31. Denning DW et al: Itraconazole therapy of fungal infections: endemic and opportunistic mycoses In Holmberg K, Meyer RD, editors: *Diagnosis and therapy of systemic fungal Infections,* New York, 1989, Raven Press.

32. Smith EB, Nopadon N, Newton RD: A clinical trial of topical terbinafine (a new allymine antifungal) in the treatment of tinea pedis, *J Am Acad Dermatol* 23:790–794, 1990.

33. Goodfield MJD, Millard LG: The skin in diabetes mellitus, *Diabetalogia* 31:567–575, 1988.

34. Meuer M, Roef–Markus S: Diabetes mellitus and skin diseases, *Curr Probl Dermatol* 20:11–23, 1991.

35. Kahn CR, Flier JS, Bar RS: The syndromes of insulin resistance and acanthosis nigrans: insulin receptor disorders in man, *N Engl J Med* 294:739–745, 1976.

36. Flier JS: Insulin receptors and insulin resistance, *Ann Rev Med* 34:145–150, 1983.

37. Misra P et al: Characterization of insulin-like growth factor -I-/somatomedin-C receptors on human keratinocyte monolayers, *J Invest Dermatol* 87:264–267, 1986.

38. Lyons TJ, Kennedy L: Non-enzymatic glycosylation of skin collagen in patients with type 1 (insulin dependent) diabetes mellitus and limited joint mobility, *Diabetologia* 28:2–5, 1985.

39. Saunders M, Herzberg A, McCarthy DJ: Sclerederma of Buschke of the lower extremities, *J Am Pod Med Assoc* 76(9):496–501, 1987.

40. Delbridge L et al: Non-enzymatic glycosylation of keratin from the stratum corneum of the diabetic foot, *Br J Dermatol* 112:547–554, 1985.

41. Cantwell AR, Martz W: Idiopathic bullae in diabetics. Bullosis diabeticoium, *Arch Dermatol* 96:42, 1967.

42. Edwards JR, Tillman DB, Miller ME: Infection and diabetes mellitus, *West J Med* 130:515–521, 1979.

43. Rocca F, Pererya E: Phylctenar lesions in the feet of diabetic patients, *Diabetes* 12:220–222, 1963.

44. Bernstein JE, Medenica M, Soltani K: Bullous eruption of diabetes mellitus, *Arch Dermatol* 115:324–325, 1979.

45. Cunliffe WJ: Necrobiotic disorders. In Rook A et al, editors: *Textbook of dermatology,* vol 11, Oxford, 1986, Blackwell Publishers.

46. Dabski K, Winkelmann RK: Generalized granuloma annulare: clinical and laboratory findings in 100 patients, *J Am Acad Dermatol* 20(1):39–47, 1989.

47. Pinkus H, Mehregan AH: *A guide to dermatohisto-pathology,* New York, 1969, Appleton-Century Crofts.

48. MacCuish AC et al: Cell mediated immunity to human pancreas in diabetes mellitus, *Diabetes* 23:693–697, 1974.

49. Witkowski JA: Pathogenesis of skin infections. In Abramson C, McCarthy DJ, Rupp M, editors: *Infectious diseases of the lower extremities,* Baltimore, 1991, Williams & Wilkins.

50. Terleckyj B, Abramson C: Microbial ecology of the foot and ankle. In Abramson C, McCarthy DJ, Rupp M, editors: *Infectious diseases of the lower extremities,* Baltimore, 1991, Williams & Wilkins.

51. Witkowski JA: Bacterial skin and soft tissue infections. In Abramson C, McCarthy DJ, Rupp M, editors: *Infectious diseases of the lower extremities,* Baltimore, 1991, Williams & Wilkins.

52. Kallick C: *Diagnosis of infected lesions associated with abscesses and ulcerations,* (series 11), Indianapolis, 1978, Eli Lilly.

53. Brenner MA: Pyodermas in *Podiatric dermatology,* Baltimore, 1986, Williams & Wilkins.

54. Jolly M: Lichen planus and its association with diabetes mellitus, *Med J Aust* 59:990–992, 1972.

55. Shuttleworth D, Graham-Brown RAC, Campbell AC: The autoimmune background of lichen planus, *Br J Dermatol* 115:199–203, 1986.

56. Sanders, LJ: *Psoriasform disorders.* In *Podiatric dermatology,* Baltimore, 1986, Williams & Wilkins.

57. Samman PD: The nails in lichen planus, *Br J Dermatol* 73:288–292, 1961.

58. Flamenbaum HS, Safai B, Siegel FP: Lichen planus in two involved hosts, *J Am Acad Dermatol* 6:918–920, 1982.

59. Olsen RO, Duplessis D, Barrong C: Lichen planus dermopathy: demonstration of a lichen planus specific epidermal antigen in affected patients, *J Clin Path Immunol* 10:103–106, 1982.

60. Garcia-Bravo et al: Lichen sclerosis et atrophicus. *J Am Acad Dermatol* 19(3):482–485, 1988.

61. Alberti KGM, Hockaday TDR: Diabetes mellitus. In Weatheral DJ, Ledingham

JGG, Warrell DA, editors: *Oxford textbook of medicine,* Oxford, England, 1986, University Press.

62. Edidin DV: Cutaneous manifestations of diabetes mellitus in children, *Pediatr Dermatol* 2:161–179, 1985.

63. Smith JG Jr: Necrobiosis lipoidica: a disease of changing concepts, *Arch Dermatol* 74:280–285, 1956.

64. Huntley AC: The cutaneous manifestations of diabetes mellitus, *J Am Acad Dermatol* 7:427–455, 1982.

65. Ackerman AB: *Histologic diagnosis of inflammatory skin diseases: a method of pattern analysis,* Philadelphia, 1978, Lea & Febiger.

66. Chuang et al: Increased frequency of diabetes in patients with bullous pemphigoid: a case control study, *J Am Acad Dermatol* 11:1099–1102, 1984.

67. Jordan RE et al: Basement membrane zone antibodies in bullous pemphigoid, *JAMA* 200:751–756, 1967.

68. Moschella SL, Hurley HJ: *Dermatology,* ed 2, vol 1, Philadelphia, 1985, WB Saunders.

69. Sanders LJ: Psoriasiform disorders (106–112). In McCarthy DJ, Montogomery R, editors: *Podiatric dermatology,* Baltimore, 1986, Williams & Wilkins.

70. Ward JM, Barnes RMR: HLA antigens in persistent palmoplantar pustulosis and its relationship to psoriasis, *Br J Dermatol* 99:477–483, 1983.

71. Voorhees JJ, Chambers DA, Duell EA: Molecular mechanisms in proliferative skin disease. *J Invest Dermatol* 67:442–450, 1976.

72. Kuruia A, Roberts P, Whitehead R: Concurrence of bullous and atrophic skin lesions in diabetes mellitus, *Arch Dermatol* 103:670–675, 1971.

73. Margolis J, Margolis LS: Skin tags—frequent sign in diabetes mellitus, *N Engl J Med* 294:1184, 1976.

74. Wilkin JK: Flushing reactions: consequences and mechanisms, *Ann Intern Med* 95:468–476, 1981.

75. Martin MM: Involvement of antonomic nerve fibers in diabetic neuropathy, *Lancet* 264:560–565, 1953.

76. Watkins PJ: Facial sweating after food: a new sign of diabetic neuropathy, *Br Med J* 1:583–587, 1973.

77. Almeyda J, Baker H: Drug reactions: adverse cutaneous reactions to hypoglycemic reagents, *Br J Dermatol* 82:634–637, 1970.

78. McCarthy DJ: Dermatologic diagnostic techniques. In McCarthy DJ, Montgomery R, editors: *Podiatric dermatology,* Baltimore, 1986, Williams & Wilkins.

79. Duncan WC, Fenske NA: Cutaneous signs of internal disease in the elderly, *Geriatrics* 45(8):24–30, 1990.

80. Fenske NA, Lober CW: Structural and functional changes of normal aging skin, *J Acad Dermatol* 15:571–585, 1986.

81. Cohen MD, Auerbach R: Acquired reactive perforating collagenosis, *J Am Acad Dermatol* 20(2):287–289, 1989.

82. Rapine RP, Herbert AA, Duecker CR: Acquired perforating dermatosis, *Arch Dermatol* 125:1074–1078, 1989.

83. O'Keefe RG, Pikscher I: Ulcers of the lower extremities. In McCarthy, DJ, Montgomery R, editors: *Podiatric dermatology,* Baltimore, 1986, Williams & Wilkins.

84. McCarthy DJ: Therapeutic considerations in the podiatric care of ulcerations. In Dockery G, editor: *Dermatology of the lower extremities,* vol 3, *Clinics in podiatric medicine and surgery,* Philadelphia, 1986, WB Saunders.

85. Singelton EE, Cotton RS, Shelman HS: Another approach to the long term management of the diabetic neurotrophic foot ulcer, *J Am Pod Assoc* 65:242–247, 1978.

86. Martin WJ, Weil LS, Smith SD: Surgical management of neurotrophic ulcers in the diabetic foot, *J Am Pod Med Assoc* 65:365–373, 1975.

87. McCarthy DJ, Montgomery R: Polyurethane in the management of ulcerating lesions of the lower extremities, *J Am Pod Med Assoc* 73:1–9, 1983.

88. McCarthy DJ, Axler DA: The efficacy of porcine skin grafts for non-healing ulcers. *J Am Pod Med Assoc* 68:86–95, 1978.

89. McCarthy DJ: *Practical podiatric medicine. Management of dermal ulcerations and wound complications,* Evanston, Illinois, 1981, Arthur Retlaw and Associates.

13 Outpatient Management of Pedal Complications

Stephen J. Kominsky, D.P.M.

A myriad of problems are associated with the lower extremities of people with diabetes. These complications can be categorized into two major groups: those of the vascular type and those of the neuropathic type. There is also a large population of patients that exhibit complications from both groups.

There have been volumes of material published over the years regarding the physiology, etiology, philosophy, and treatment of every one of the potential complications that could exist in the lower extremities of diabetics. Some of this material has been based on statistical data, some on anecdotal experiences, and some on conjecture. There are many different philosophies regarding problems in the lower extremity of the diabetic patient, and until the management of these problems is fully understood, the complications will continue to exist.

This chapter is critical to the understanding of the overall management of the diabetic foot because most problems that develop can be managed on an outpatient basis.

COMPLICATIONS

As mentioned repeatedly throughout this textbook, there are a great many categories of complications that develop in the lower extremity of people with diabetes. The major classifications can be broken down into neuropathic, vascular, dermatologic, traumatic, infectious (including iatrogenic infections), and biomechanical. Within each of these major headings are subclasses of complications, i.e., neuropathic ulcers, Charcot joint, etc.

This chapter will approach these conditions in a logical sequence beginning with the underlying thread that links all of these complications together: neuropathy. In the presence of neuropathy, any one of the other problems may develop.

Biomechanical deformities will be mentioned at the end of this chapter as complications of diabetes, but the specific discussions relative to pressures will be mentioned in Chapter 3.

NEUROPATHY

It is important when considering outpatient management issues to include neuropathy. When evaluating a diabetic patient for neuropathy, it is helpful to think of neuropathy as occurring along a spectrum. At one end of the spectrum there is a very painful condition, known as hyperesthesia, or painful neuropathy, and at the other end of the spectrum is hypoesthesia, or painless neuropathy. Fortunately, sensory deficit occurs far more frequently than does the hyperesthesia. At least with hypoesthesia the patient is not suffering in pain. Unfortunately in our society, we are taught subconsciously to ignore medical problems if they do not hurt. As a result, many patients do not react to a problem on the foot, even when it is clearly a problem, simply because it does not hurt.

This is where the role of patient education from both the physician and nurse, plays a major factor in the prevention of limb morbidity.

Hyperesthesia

Patients presenting with hyperesthesia are often distraught and depressed. Pain from this neuropathic condition is most frequently described as "electric shocks," or "fire," or as "a tingling sensation." In addition, patients complain that their symptoms occur most often during the night when they are asleep. It is not uncommon for them to be awakened with this terrible, burning pain.

Acute painful neuropathy may be associated with profound weight loss, depression, impotence, and anorexia.[8] Typically the onset is gradual, developing over the course of a year. Although the pain is usually most severe in the soles of the feet, pain often times radiates proximally up the legs. Another common feature is the increased sensitivity to light touch (clothing or linens). This is probably the reason for an increase in the frequency of symptoms at night.

Treatment for this complex syndrome is often doomed to fail and very frustrating for the patient and practitioner. Painful neuropathy usually resolves between 6 to 18 months after the initial onset of the symptoms.

Treatment of Painful Neuropathy

None of the currently available treatments are 100% effective in resolving the symptoms. In fact, most are only able to provide symptomatic relief. Many different pharmacologic agents have been used over the years to treat the symptoms for this condition. See Table 13–1 for a listing of these agents by category. Table 13–2 is a suggested treatment approach to painful neuropathy, as recommended by Belgrade

TABLE 13–1.

Pharmacologic Agents Used to Treat Neuropathy

Experimental status
  Aldose reductase inhibitors
  Myoinositol
  Ganglioside
  Nerve-sprouting enhancers
  Vitamin B12
Tricyclic antidepressants
  Amitriptylene (Elavil, Endep)
  Imipramine (Janimine, Tofranil)
  Desipramine (Norpramin)
  Doxepin (Adapin, Sinequan)
  Nortriptyline (Aventyl Hcl, Pamelor)
Anticonvulsants
Topical agents
  Capsaicin .025%, .075%
Nonsteroidal anti-inflammatory drugs
Opioid analgesics
Local anesthetics
Behavior modification techniques
  Hypnosis
  Biofeedback
  Relaxation
Physical therapy/orthosis
Surgery
  Tarsal tunnel release

et al. This table provides a step-by-step approach with specific recommendations about medications and dosages.

Experimental treatments with aldose reductase inhibitors (sorbinil), myoinositol, ganglioside, nerve-sprouting enhancers, and vitamin B12 are intended to correct dearrangement in neural tissues. Thus far, early animal models are showing positive results, but no definitive long-term studies have been done on human models.[8]

There is one new area that is showing some promise on a small percentage of patients. Capsaicin .075%, (tradename Axsain), is a topical cream, which when applied three times daily, provides symptomatic relief to some patients. Initially, the cream causes a burning sensation at the site of application, but on the patients where it provides relief, this increased sensitivity is reported to last for only 2 to

3 days. Although this has yet to be documented, there has been some clinical observation on the part of this author as to its effectiveness.

In 1991, Dellon published a paper whereby he was able to demonstrate that in 67% of his patient population with painful neuropathy, he was able to relieve their symptoms by performing a tarsal tunnel release surgery. The theory was that as a result of the biochemical changes associated with diabetes, the posterior tibial nerve enlarged (swelled) within its tunnel and, as a result, became impinged. By releasing the tunnel, the nerve was decompressed and the pain resolved.

I have performed this procedure 20 times thus far for this precise diagnosis, and I have had a 97% resolution of patient discomfort. The 3% was at least a diminution of pain, as compared to a complete resolution of pain.

TABLE 13–2.

Suggested Treatment Strategy*

Patients with mild pain:
1. Relaxation techniques.
2. Physical measures; orthosis, blanket cradles on the bed, TENS units.
3. Mild medications at bedtime, i.e., anti-inflammatory or acetaminophen with codiene.

Patients with moderate to severe pain (assuming that there are no medical contraindications):
1. Amitriptyline 10 to 25 mg 1 to 2 hours before bedtime. Dosing depends on age, weight, and condition of the patient. Dose should be increased in 10 to 25 mg increments once or twice a week as side effects allow until the patient can tolerate 150 mg night-time dose. It may be necessary to change to Desipramine or Nortriptyline if the anticholinergic or sedative effects of amitriptyline are limiting.

If pain persists:
Begin carbamazepine at 100 mg bid and titrate up to 600 to 800 mg/day or until side effects occur.
At this point, if pain still exists, consider use of other drugs that are listed in Table 13–1.

*From Belgrave MJ, Lev BI: Diabetic Neuropathy; helping patients cope with their pain, *Postgrad Med* 90(5):263–270, 1991. Used by permission.

THE INSENSITIVE FOOT

At the other end of the neuropathic spectrum is the hypoesthetic foot, or the insensate foot. This form of peripheral neuropathy occurs far more frequently than the painful neuropathic foot. This condition is of greater concern because it leads to the ultimate breakdown and destruction of the diabetic foot.[2, 4, 7, 9, 10] Peripheral neuropathy with insensitivity is the silent destroyer, because in most cases the patient is unaware that neuropathy exists. On many occasions, this author has seen patients with grossly infected wounds that are red, draining, and swollen. When questioned as to why they let it get to that stage, the typical response is, "I didn't think that it was this serious, because it doesn't hurt."

Brand originally described the four mechanisms under which the diabetic foot is destroyed in the presence of neuropathy.[30] (This is discussed in great detail in Chapter 8.) These four mechanisms are as follows: (1) the direct mechanical disruption of tissue, leading to infection; (2) a small amount of pressure over a long period of time, which leads to tissue ischemia; (3) a moderate amount of force, over a short time, which leads to inflammation, and destruction of tissue via enzymatic necrosis; and (4) by infection via any one of the first three routes. For any of these pathologic sequences to occur, the foot must be insensitive, otherwise the condition would be very painful, and the patient would respond appropriately to the painful stimulus.

Although to date there is no specific treatment for insensitivity, (see neuropathy chapter), it is of the utmost importance from the limb salvage perspective that these patients be seen and evaluated on a regular basis. In addition, proper education as to the methods of self examination by the physician and diabetes educator serves as a prophylactic means in the prevention or treatment of complications.

OUTPATIENT MANAGEMENT OF COMMON CONDITIONS

The Plantar Ulcer

The most common complication of the diabetic foot that may potentially lead to the foot's demise is the plantar ulcer. Ulcers on the foot have been described for many centuries, and only really understood in the last 30 years. Commonly referred to as the mal perforans, it occurs on the bottom of the foot under a weight-bearing surface. Many papers have been written to describe the cause of the plantar ulcer, and why it occurs under bony prominences (see Chapter 8). Boulton et al.,[11] Duckworth et al.,[12] and Betts, et al.[13] discuss the changes in the dynamic foot pressures once peripheral neuropathy has developed. Boulton concludes that most abnormal loadings occur under the metatarsal heads.

The diabetic foot ulcer is the leading cause of diabetic hospitalization in the United States and Great Britain.[14, 15, 16] The treatment of this problem is estimated to cost several billion dollars per year in the United States.[17]

Numerous studies have been performed using gait plates or other dynamic computerized gait analysis systems to evaluate the position of the plantar ulcer relative to forces on the foot. Vertical and horizontal forces have been studied in detail. I.A.F. Stokes et al. found that ulcers on the bottom of the foot are found most commonly under the second, third, or fourth metatarsal head.[18] G.C. Cterctko et al. stated that diabetic patients with or without neuropathy, and with or without a history of ulceration, transmitted proportionally less force through the toes than normal individuals, and therefore transmitted a greater force through the metatarsal heads.[19] Duckworth and Boul-

ton conclude that abnormally high pressures are more common in patients with neuropathy.[20] All of the authors cited here agree that plantar ulcers occur at the point(s) of maximum loading.

The reason for this, it is postulated, has to do with the presence of motor neuropathy. If there is a loss of intrinsic muscle power, that is, the lumbricals and interossei, the digits will be less stable against the supporting surface. Secondary to this, the toes contract dorsally, which places a retrograde force against the metatarsal head in a plantar direction. As a result of this increased load, the vertical force through that metatarsal head increases significantly. Once the pathomechanics of the plantar ulcer are understood, steps can be taken to correct the stress and heal the ulcer.

Evaluation of the Plantar Ulcer

Wagner in 1981 established the most widely used system for evaluating the plantar ulceration.[21] He took into account the depth of the lesion relative to the extent of tissue involvement and the presence of necrotic, or infected tissue (Table 13–3). This is an excellent system for categorizing ulcers on the foot and guides the treatment regime in accordance with the severity of the problem. There are many occasions when surgery is not needed and the ulcers can be treated conservatively (Table 13–4).[22] There are other classification systems that rely on temperature and others that classify based on whether the limb is ischemic, or neuropathic, and well perfused.[23, 24]

The ulcer itself must be carefully examined. The dimensions of the ulcer should be recorded in the patients' records to monitor any change in size. The diameter and the depth should be determined. There are several ways to do this. A measuring device with millimeter increments can be used to obtain an actual measurement of the diameter or the

TABLE 13–3.

Wagner Grading System for Diabetic Foot Lesions*

Grade 0	No open lesions; may have deformity or cellulitis
Grade 1	Superficial ulcer
Grade 2	Deep ulcer to tendon, capsule, or bone
Grade 3	Deep ulcer with abscess, osteomyelitis, or joint sepsis
Grade 4	Localized gangrene—forefoot or heel
Grade 5	Gangrene of entire foot

*From Wagner FW: The dysvascular foot: A system for diagnosis and treatment, *Foot Ankle* 2:64, 1981. Used by permission.

TABLE 13–4.

Wagner Classification Treatment Protocol*

Grade 0
  Proper shoes/orthotics
  Education
  Palliative podiatric care
  Prophylactic surgery
  Prevention
Grade 1
  Antibiotic therapy
  Wound care
  Radiographs
  Stress corrective techniques (see text)
  Surgery
Grade 2
  Antibiotic therapy
  Evaluate wound dimensions
  Radiographic evaluation
  Surgery as needed
Grade 3
  Hospitalize for IV antibiotic therapy
  Deep aggressive debridement with diagnosis for osteomyelitis
  Metabolic control
  Plastic surgical closure as needed
Grade 4
  Local amputation as determined by amount of necrosis and vascularity
Grade 5
  Major amputation required

*Wagner FW: Treatment of the diabetic foot, *Comp Ther* 10:29, 1984.

length and width of an oblong ulcer. A tracing of the ulcer can be made and placed into the chart to provide a visual aid to the patient. A sterilized piece of x-ray film is a simple and inexpensive way to make a tracing for the chart. Many patients may not be able to appreciate measurements in millimeters, but they would easily be able to appreciate the dimensions of the ulcer if they saw a tracing. If the tracings are repeated on each visit, the chart will provide a visual record of the patient's progress. This technique provides a psychological benefit as well because it is an excellent way to give positive feedback to the patient. This may encourage the patient to continue with the treatment.

There are computer software programs available that can scan the ulcer to provide the dimensions, but they are not readily available and are very expensive. Some practitioners use gel impression casting to make a three-dimensional model of the ulceration. This is an excellent way to appreciate the size of the lesion, but in a busy practice or clinic this is not a practical method.

Once the size of the ulcer is recorded, the depth should be evaluated. This should be done with a sterile measuring device to record this aspect of the lesion. In addition to recording the depth of the base of the ulcer, the ulcer should be probed to determine if there are any sinus

tracts present. A sterile, blunt nasal probe is an excellent tool for this purpose. The probe should be gently pressed against the base of the ulcer all around its perimeter and across the center of the lesion. Another way to visualize the depth of the ulcer, or to visualize the presence of sinus tracts is to take an x-ray with the probe in place. If a sinus is present, the x-ray will confirm whether the probe makes contact with bone or penetrates into a joint space (Fig 13–1). This information is helpful when determining a treatment plan. If a nasal probe is not available, the stick of a sterile cotton swab is very useful.

The presence of a sinus tract may require a change in the treatment plan. If the sinus probes to bone, the bone should automatically be considered con-

A

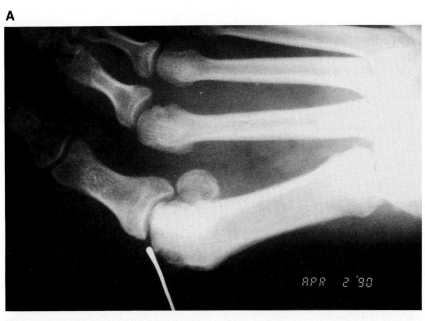

B

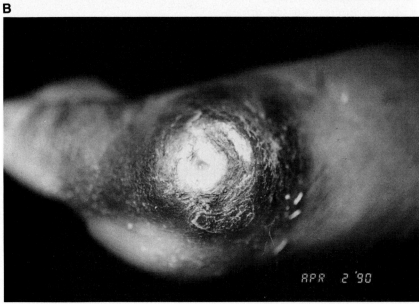

FIG 13–1.

A, probe inserted into the joint capsule to determine the depth of the sinus tract. This is helpful when determining whether bone has been exposed to the outside environment. **B,** closeup of the sinus tract on the bunion of the patient in **A.** Notice the hyperpigmentation of the soft tissue around the tract. This is usually indicative of a chronic inflammatory situation. Also notice the very discreet hole in the center of the picture. This is where the probe was inserted. No anesthesia is necessary when doing this since these patients are completely neuropathic.

taminated, due to its exposure to the environment (Fig 13–2). Often, with a chronic ulcer, the bone is infected, not just contaminated, which partially or fully explains the reason for the ulcer not healing. With a bone infection, treatment centers on antibiotics and perhaps surgical debridement. The decision to operate on the infected bone should be based on several factors, including the degree of bony destruction (i.e., if the bone is infected in several pieces (sequestrum) (Fig 13–3), it is too late for that section of the bone to heal); the vascular status of the foot and the location of the bone in the foot; (i.e., phalanx vs. tarsal bone). For a more com-

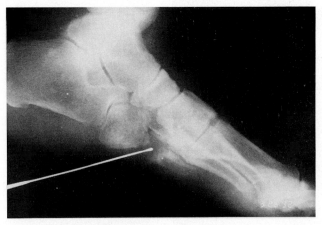

FIG 13–2.
A probe is inserted through a plantar ulceration to determine the depth and extent of the lesion.

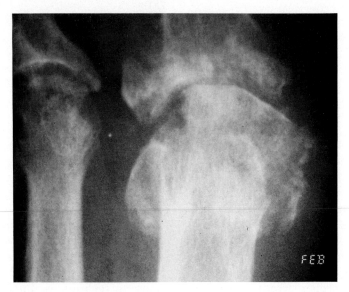

FIG 13–3.
This is an x-ray demonstrating osteomyelitis whereby the bony destruction has caused pathologic fractures of the base of the phalanx, and the metatarsal head. Sequestrum is present in this photo.

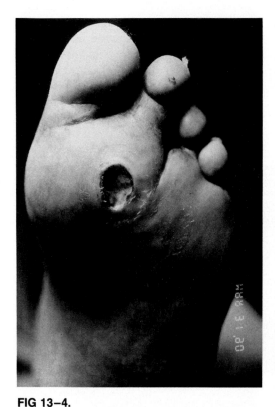

FIG 13–4.
This ulcer beneath the second metatarsal looks innocent enough, but the base of the lesion as well as the surrounding signs point to the presence of an infection. The tissue in the base is gray as opposed to red; the surrounding tissue is inflamed, and a probe inserted into this lesion penetrates to the second metatarsal head.

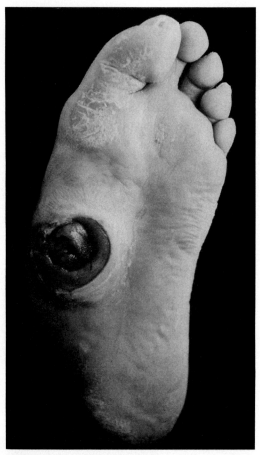

FIG 13–5.
This is an example of a noninfected ulceration. Even though it is quite large and has been present for quite awhile, there are no "cardinal signs" of infection, including no bony involvement.

plete discussion on the decision to operate on the osteomyelitic bone, see Chapters 15 and 16.

There are other important characteristics to be considered when evaluating an ulcer. The quality of the tissue in the base of the ulcer is a window to the healing potential of that wound. If the base of the wound appears clean (free from purulence), and exhibits healthy red granulation tissue, the chances are very good that the ulcer is not infected and will go on to heal with the proper stress correction. However, if grayish fibrous tissue is present, it is likely that either the foot is not well perfused (that is, has poor circulation), or that the wound is infected (see

Fig 13–4). The infection in this case may be either soft tissue, or bone, or both. If the base of the ulcer has that appearance, further investigation should be carried out.

If there is a suspicion of an infection, then the proper steps should be taken to fully evaluate that condition. These would include obtaining a culture of the wound and performing one of the radiographic imaging techniques. Initially, plain film x-rays would be the simplest and most cost effective. If questions persist after x-ray evaluation regarding the extent of the bony involvement, other imaging techniques should be considered including nuclear scans or magnetic resonance imaging (MRI). Once the determination is made as to whether the wound is infected, proper treatment may be initiated. For proper culturing techniques, and the actual management of infections, see the section in this text on infections.

For an infected wound the decision must be made as to whether surgical debridement and hospitalization for intravenous antibiotics are necessary, or whether the condition can be treated on an outpatient basis. A superficial infection localized to the ulcer site generally responds well to local wound care and oral antibiotics (Fig 13–5). (See chapter in this text regarding proper antibiotic therapy). It is imperative that proper culture techniques be used to obtain reliable information as to the offending organism(s). This procedure is critical in determining the appropriate antibiotic.

If hospitalization is necessary, (see chapter on medical management of infections), surgical debridement of the ulcer or abscess may be necessary (Fig 13–6). Once this wound has been converted to a noninfected condition, then outpatient management may begin.

Treatment of the Plantar Ulcer

In 1978 Brand[25] discussed four mechanisms whereby the diabetic foot may be destroyed. The mechanism that leads to the development of the plantar ulcer is described as a moderate amount of force to the plantar surface of the foot over an extended period of time leading to soft tissue inflammation. This inflammation in turn may lead to enzymatic necrosis of soft tissue, which leads to the development of the plantar ulcer. Earlier in this chapter, the concept of vertical force, and prominent metatarsal heads was discussed rel-

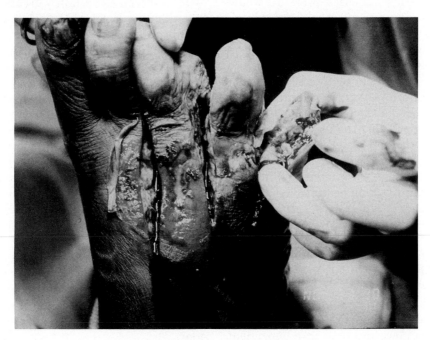

FIG 13–6.
The patient in this photo came to the emergency room with what she thought was an infected fifth toe. What was discovered was that she had an infection which occupied several compartments in the foot. Aggressive surgical management was initiated, and salvage of the foot was accomplished.

ative to ulcer development. To manage the plantar ulcer once it has developed, one must recognize the underlying pathomechanics. As just described, this has to do with repetitive force to a bony prominence over an extended period. If the proper stress corrective techniques are used, the ulcer should heal as long as the wound is not infected and the blood supply is adequate (Table 13–5).

BED REST

Because eliminating weight-bearing stress from the bottom of the foot is essential for healing the noninfected plantar ulcer, bed rest is a logical therapy. Walking, any amount, could potentially undo all of the benefit that bed rest has provided to that point. Dependency of the limb, after bed rest, would increase the fluid volume in the foot, which would immediately increase the tissue hydrostatic pressure. This increased pressure would have an adverse affect on the ulcer's healing.

Historically, patients with plantar ulcers were admitted to the hospital for bed rest and therapy. In today's economic climate, hospitalization for plantar ulcers that are not infected is unnecessary, and is often rejected by the utilization review person in the hospital. Fortunately, there are other alternatives for stress relief to the sole of the foot. Patient compliance is a significant issue in bed rest therapy because patients who don't "feel sick" resume activity too quickly.

CRUTCHES

Crutches require the same high level of patient compliance that bed rest does. They also place the limb in a dependent position without accounting for the increase in edema. Patients who use crutches selectively or discard them

TABLE 13–5.

Methods of Stress Relief to the Plantar Surface of the Foot

Bedrest
Crutches
Wheelchair
Ambulatory total contact cast
Accommodative padding/orthotics
Accommodative shoeing

prematurely, risk significant setbacks. Crutches are also very difficult for geriatric patients to handle. Therefore the use of crutches to relieve pressure on the bottom of the foot is favorable for a very small select group of patients.

SHOES, ORTHOTICS, ACCOMMODATIVE PADDING

All of these devices are reviewed for purposes of this discussion. However, they will be discussed in much greater detail, individually, in their respective chapters within this text.

An important function of the shoe in this patient population is to house the accommodative, protective device within the shoe itself. The shoe can be used to rebalance the foot and compensate for a biomechanical problem. In the presence of motor neuropathy, several biomechanical deformities can develop. These include a drop-foot, a varus foot, a cavus foot, and several other possibilities. (These biomechanical deformities are discussed in the chapter on biomechanics.) One should not take a shoe that fits properly, i.e., the correct size, and place an accommodative device within it. There are many different modifications that can be made to the shoe to reduce weight-bearing stress on the sole of the foot and on the dorsum of the toes.

The basic shoe to start a patient on is the extra depth shoe (Fig 13–7). This type of shoe is made by several different manufacturers and is available in several different styles. The purpose of the extra depth is to provide a deeper toe box in the front end of the shoe to prevent the shoe from rubbing on the tops of the toes (Fig 13–8). Greater pressure on the dorsum of a contracted toe could also potentially increase a retrograde force on the metatarsal head, which creates a plantar ulceration or prevents it from healing.

The extra depth also allows more room within the body of the shoe. This provides a greater space to place a molded orthosis. (The materials, and theory behind orthotics for the diabetic foot are discussed in greater detail in their respective chapters within this text.) In concept, the purpose of the molded orthotic for the diabetic insensitive foot is to provide softness within the shoe against the foot, and to increase the surface area against the sole of the foot. For example, a 150-lb person standing on a one inch square block of wood, is exerting 150 pounds per square inch (psi) of force against the tissue under that wooden block. But, if the 1-inch square was expanded to a 5-inch square, the force would be reduced to 30 psi. Therefore, the concept of placing a molded orthotic into a shoe is to increase the surface area against the foot, thereby reducing the psi of force by a significant number. Once this is accomplished, the repetitive stress that would cause a plantar ulcer to develop is nullified. If an ulcer is already present, the stress reduction may be sufficient to allow for healing.

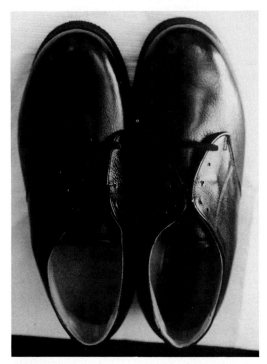

FIG 13–7.
Standard "extra-depth" shoes, worn to accommodate custom molded insoles, as well as a foot with digital deformity.

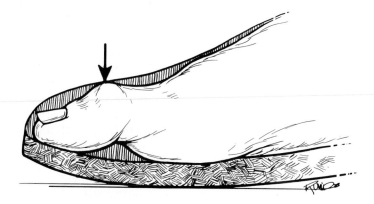

FIG 13–8.
Cross sectional view of a toe within the toebox of a shoe. The arrow indicates the area of irritation of the shoe onto the top of the toe. If this continues for a long enough time, a digital ulcer will develop.

Rocker soles affixed to the outsole of a shoe are another means to reduce stress to the bottom of the foot. Schaff, and Cavanagh in 1990, published a paper discussing the effect of the rocker bottom shoe on plantar pressure distribution in the diabetic insensitive foot.[26] Their findings were favorable with respect to the use of rocker bottom soles for treating ulcers in most locations on the foot. They found that there was an increase in pressure in the heel and no reduction of pressure under the fifth metatarsal head. These findings were consistent with those of Sims and Birke.[27] The decisions involved in using the rocker bottom sole are complex and require some expertise and understanding of lower-extremity biomechanics. Consultation with an experienced pedorthist may be helpful for someone with little knowledge of shoes and biomechanics. This concept is discussed fully in the respective chapter within this text.

AMBULATORY TOTAL CONTACT CAST

This is a very effective device for reducing the vertical forces on the sole of the foot. This cast was originally described in Sri Lanka in the 1930s by an orthopedist named Milroy Paul. He used it initially for the treatment of ulcers associated with Hansen's disease. In India, in the 1950s, Paul Brand began using this casting technique for similar patients. After several modifications and some experience, Brand brought this technique to the United States in the early 1960s.[28, 29]

As mentioned previously, plantar ulcerations are directly related to stress on the sole of the foot and occur most often under a bony prominence. The total contact cast is a form of an occlusive dressing that allows the patient to ambulate but at the same time reduces the forces on the bottom of the foot.

This is accomplished in several different ways. The cast forces the person wearing it to shorten his or her stride length during gait. This reduces the gait's velocity, thereby reducing the vertical forces on the foot. The cast also eliminates ankle joint motion in the sagital plane, which eliminates the propulsive phase of the gait cycle.[10, 29] By accomplishing this, the vertical forces on the forefoot are greatly reduced. Most forefoot ulcerations occur under the metatarsal heads and are dynamic in nature. If the propulsive phase of gait can effectively be eliminated, the lesions will heal and recurrence may be prevented.

The greatest effect of the total contact cast is its ability to increase surface area against the plantar surface of the foot. By molding the cast material to the contour of the foot and leg, all of the skin surface area is in contact, which in turn increases the surface area and results in a greatly reduced vertical force at the site of the bony prominence.

This benefit, in combination with the others previously mentioned, makes the total contact cast an excellent tool for treating the diabetic foot. In addition, where the other techniques for stress relief mentioned earlier (bedrest, crutches, shoes, orthotics and padding) all require a great degree of patient compliance, the total contact cast reduces (but does not eliminate) the need for strict compliance.

There are several other benefits for using this casting technique as therapy for the plantar ulcer. Because of the construction of this cast, the toes are encased within fiberglass, thus protecting the foot from injury by foreign objects. Additionally, due to its intimate contact with the foot and leg, the cast has the ability to reduce pedal and leg edema significantly. As a result, the first cast usually needs to be removed after 48 hours. If it is not, and the original fit of the cast on the leg has changed (due to a reduction of edema), the

TABLE 13–6.

Indications for the Use of the Ambulatory Total
Contact Cast

1. To immobilize the foot, to diminish the forces of
   weightbearing.
2. To reduce the vertical forces of gait, to allow the
   plantar ulcer, or the pre-ulcerous lesion to heal.
3. To immobilize the post-operative surgical foot.
4. To allow for consolidation of the Charcot foot
   (neuroarthropathy).
5. To reduce pedal and lower leg edema.

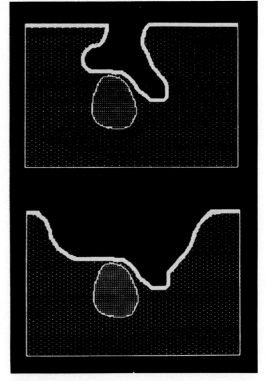

FIG 13–9.

In this representation, the diagram at the *top* shows
an ulcer that is more deep than it is wide. The concern
is that the surface may epithelialize, before the deepest
recess of the wound fills in. The *lower* diagram represents the proper condition, whereby the ulcer is
wider than it is deep. This is the way the ulcer should
be at the time of total contact casting.

cast may "piston" (slide) on the leg, causing friction and irritation, which might
cause a wound. Edema should be reduced
when treating these patients because the
edema causes an increase in tissue hydrostatic pressure. If this is not recognized,
the resultant high pressure may go on to
cause a breakdown in the soft tissue, leading to further damage.

Due to a reduction in the vertical
forces of gait, and the elimination of the
propulsive phase of the gait cycle, the total
contact cast may also have a place in postoperative immobilization of the foot. Ambulation after foot surgery in a total contact cast would place minimal force on the
surgical site.

Other indications for the total contact
cast include immobilization during the
consolidation phase of treatment for the
acute charcot joint (Table 13–6).

Contraindications to the Use of the Total Contact Cast

There is a very specific set of contraindications to follow when one is considering
the use of this casting technique. If the
cast is not applied correctly, or if the cast
is used in the wrong circumstance, the results could be devastating. Careful attention must be used when applying this
technique.

The number one contraindication to
this technique is in the case of an infected
wound. This cast should not be applied to
an infected ulcer or bone. The environment inside of the cast is dark, warm, and
moist, which are the perfect conditions for
bacteria to thrive. Also, if an infection is
present, the condition could not be monitored properly because the entire cast is
closed around the foot. Therefore, if an infection is even suspected one should wait
until the condition is resolved before initiating this therapy.

Another condition that must be met
when using the total contact cast is that
the ulcer must be wider at the surface
than it is deep (Fig 13–9). If this is not
the case, the surface could epithelialize

before the deepest recess has a chance to granulate. This premature closing of the ulcer would leave a cavity beneath the skin, thus increasing the potential for abscess formation. In the case where the surface opening of the ulcer, or sinus tract, is very narrow, it must be opened surgically. This in many instances can be done in an office setting.

Other contraindications to the contact cast include claustrophobia. Also skin sensitivities to any of the components of the cast, especially the adhesive on the felt or on the tape may cause dermatologic reactions. Diabetic dermopathy, which may already exist, is a contraindication to the use of this cast.

See Table 13–7 for the complete list of contraindications to the use of this casting technique.

Lastly is the issue of patient cooperation. Even though these patients are insensate, there is still an ability to perceive a problem with the cast (Fig 13–10). The patient has to be trusted to call the office if that perception exists. In addition, this technique is time intensive, and requires a commitment from the patient in terms of the number of visits and length of time spent in the office.

THE HEALING SANDAL

For the occasions when a patient may not be the ideal candidate for use of the total contact cast, an alternative is the healing sandal. First developed at the USPHS hospital in Carville, Louisiana, by Brand and his colleagues, the healing sandal applies the principles of total contact with the plantar surface of the foot, while at the same time using a rocker sole on the outsole of the shoe. There are many different versions of the healing sandal, but they all have in common the basic principles of unloading the area of greatest pressure.

The innersole of the sandal is lined with layers of molded plastizote of varying

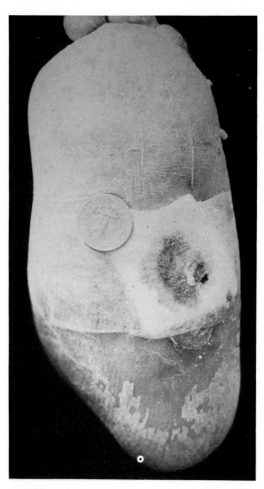

FIG 13–10.
In this example, a patient who was completely insensate perceived a problem within the total contact cast. The cast was removed, and on the bottom of the foot was a quarter. Had the doctor not removed the cast to examine the foot, the pressure from the quarter would have led to the development of another ulceration.

TABLE 13–7.
Contraindications for the Use of the Total Contact Cast

1. Patient noncompliance.
2. Presence of active infection.
3. Presence of an active dermatologic condition, or sensitivity to a component of the cast.
4. Claustrophobia.
5. Presence of an ulcer that is more deep than wide.

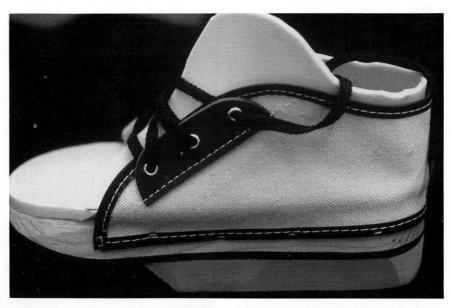

FIG 13–11.
A healing sandal may be made from a basic surgical shoe, and then modified with a plastizote inlay and a rocker sole when necessary. This is a good alternative to the cast situations where a patient cannot be casted.

densities to achieve the total contact. By molding the material, each part of the foot is in contact, which in turn increases the surface area, thereby decreasing the force under the area of high stress. The purpose of the rocker sole is to displace the forces of gait away from the forefoot, and the metatarsal parabola. (Fig 13–11). If one is successful in accomplishing both of these, the patient may ambulate with very little force on the bony prominence, thus allowing the area to heal.

This sandal may be used as a transition device, when going from the total contact cast to the definitive shoes, or may be used in place of the total contact cast if any of the contraindications to the cast exist. For the actual fabrication of the sandal, see the chapter on shoes and orthotics in this text.

Application of the Total Contact Cast

Prior to the actual application of the cast, several steps are carried out. All of the toenails must be debrided to protect the toes from irritation. If the nails are elongated or onychauxic, irritation to the adjacent toe may occur. In the insensate lower extremity especially inside of a cast, this could be a catastrophic problem; therefore, proper nail care is important. The next step is to hydrate the skin with an emollient cream or lotion. There are many different products that work well for this. Examples would include vitamin E lotion, cocoa butter lotion, and aloe vera lotion. This is especially important in the patients exhibiting autonomic neuropathy with anhidrosis, where the skin may be dry and susceptible to fissuring.

Once these preliminary steps are completed, the ulcer must be addressed. Measurement, probing, and debridement must be completed prior to this stage. At this point, a thin dressing is applied simply to cover the wound. There should be no circular bandaging around the foot, like a gauze roll, because the physician cannot see the foot inside of the cast. This type of dressing could potentially cut into the skin or reduce the blood flow to the foot if it is too tight. A 2 × 2, or 4 × 4 taped to the foot with paper tape is sufficient in most cases. Any of the antibiotic ointments are acceptable to apply to the wound just prior to casting. It is far more important to be concerned with what is taken off of the ulcer, i.e., pressure, than what is being put on.

At this point, the patient should be in the prone position to begin applying the cast. The prone position provides two advantages over the supine position. The first is that the posterior calf muscle mass shifts more proximally on the leg, which allows a better fit of the cast to the foot and the leg. Second, with the patient prone, it is easier to place the foot at a 90° position, relative to the leg. This position will allow the patient to ambulate more comfortably (Fig 13–12).

For the actual step-by-step application of the cast, see Table 13–8. When this casting technique was first developed, the entire cast was made of plaster. Now, it is easier and faster to use synthetic materials for the outer layers of the cast. This material provides a more durable and stronger cast. It also allows the patient to bear weight sooner than if it were all plaster.

Complications Associated With the Total Contact Cast

If the cast is applied according to the very specific guidelines that have been established, the potential for complication is reduced significantly. When considering complications using this technique, two areas stand out.

The first category is complication associated with the items on the list of contraindications. If any of those contraindications is disregarded, the likelihood of complication is increased.

The other category of complication associated with the total contact cast has to do with extrinsic factors. For example, overly aggressive removal of the cast with the cast saw could cause abrasion or lac-

eration to the skin. Wrinkles of the stockinette inside of the cast (Fig 13–13) may cause irritation to the skin, thus leading to further problems. If the patient walks on the cast prior to the material hardening, the plantar surface of the cast could collapse, creating an indentation against the bottom of the foot. Since the patient is neuropathic, this complication would go unperceived unless it is detected prior to the patient leaving the office. This particular problem is more prevalent with plas-

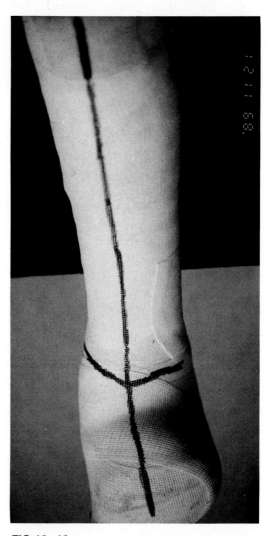

FIG 13–12.
This photo is that of a contact cast after it has been completed. The lines represent where the cast saw should cut in order to facilitate its removal. Note: the toes are completely enclosed within the cast.

TABLE 13–8.

Application of the Total Contact Cast

I. Preparation of the foot.
   A. Debride toenails.
   B. Hydrate the skin with emollient.
   C. Place cotton between toes to absorb moisture.
   D. Ulcer: debride as necessary. Ulcer must be wider at the surface than it is deep. Apply ointment of choice, with a light dressing. *No circlage bandaging.*
II. Apply cotton stockinette to the leg.
   A. Should be snug, with no wrinkles.
   B. Fold stockinette dorsally over the toes, and tape it in place.
   C. Make a cut in the stockinette at the ankle joint level; tape it closed.
III. Apply a 3-inch wide strip of adhesive felt to the anterior aspect of the leg, along the crest of the tibia. The edges of the felt should be well skived. The felt should be ⅛-inch-thick. It should extend from the dorsum of the toes, to the tuberosity of the tibia.
IV. A circular piece of felt should be cut large enough to cover both malleoli, then taped in place. Once again, the edges should be skived.
V. A 4-inch-square × 1-inch-thick piece of foam is taped in a dorsal to plantar fashion across the tips of the toes.
VI. A 4-inch × 5-yard roll of gypsona plaster is applied at this stage to the foot and leg. It should extend from the base of the toes to the proximal extent of the felt. Care needs to be taken so as to eliminate all bulges and folds of the plaster, especially on the bottom of the foot. *It is important that the assistant be instructed to only use the flat surfaces of the hands, and avoid using fingertips.* Indentations in the material may go unperceived in the neuropathic foot.
VII. Apply a 3-inch-roll of fiberglass to cover the gypsona layer.
VIII. A ¼-inch-piece of plywood, fashioned into the shape of the foot, is placed on the bottom of the foot so as to be perpendicular with the long axis of the leg. If it needs to be adjusted to make it perpendicular, pieces of fiberglass can be used to "shim" the board.
IX. A rubber walking heel is placed on the plywood platform, just proximal to the metatarsal heads. It should be affixed to the board as it would in a regular cast.
X. Complete the rest of the cast with 3-inch- and 4-inch-roles of fiberglass, covering the foam over the toes. One to two more rolls of material are usually used at this point.
XI. The patient needs to remain in the office for approximately 30 minutes to allow for drying, and to be sure that the fit is acceptable.

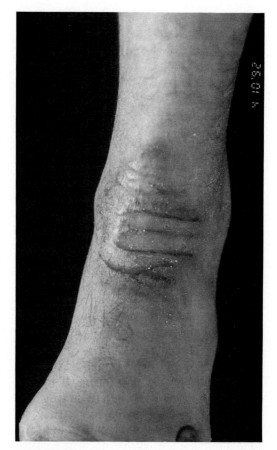

FIG 13–13.
This photograph demonstrates a complication of casting a patient with the total contact cast. The wrinkles of the skin come from stockinette in the cast "rolling up," and not being pulled smooth during the application phase. If this problem is allowed to remain, the pressure against the skin would certainly cause a breakdown of the soft tissue.

ter casts. Therefore, to prevent this problem, the patient should wait in the office for approximately 30 minutes prior to ambulating. If only plaster materials are available, the patient should remain non-weight-bearing on the casted limb for 24 hours.

Removal of the Total Contact Cast

Because there is no padding in this cast, removal must be slow and meticulous. The purpose of the adhesive felt strip along the front of the leg is to provide a safe place for the cast saw to be introduced. This should be the only place that the saw blade penetrates through the material. If there is overzealous use of the cast saw, the chances of laceration to the foot or leg are high. The cut with the saw should extend from the top edge of the cast along the tibial crest, to the tip of the toes. Once the material has been cut, the cast spreader may be inserted and the edges gently separated.

As with the application of this cast, it takes some practice and skill to master this technique. It is advisable to practice removal of this cast before trying it on a patient.

Total contact cast therapy is not for every patient or for every clinician. This is a high-risk procedure and requires expertise in working with casting materials. In addition, careful patient selection is critical. The application of the cast, preparation of the foot, and removal of the cast are extremely time consuming. If the office and staff are not set up to do this procedure, the results can be very frustrating. Inexperienced physicians should attend a hands-on workshop for this casting technique. If a workshop is not available, contact a colleague who has some experience. This is a highly successful approach to treating a frustrating condition.

OUTPATIENT MANAGEMENT OF THE CHARCOT JOINT

Lower-extremity inflammation is exacerbated by continued ambulation. Therefore, successful treatment must focus on eliminating the stress of weight-bearing. This can be accomplished in the same ways that were discussed in the section on the plantar ulcer.

Due to the contact cast eliminating the propulsive phase of the gait cycle and increasing the surface area (thereby decreasing the pounds per square inch), the contact cast is an effective means to treat the Charcot foot while it is healing. The goal of this technique is to allow the involved joints to consolidate. Once this is accomplished, bracing, shoeing, and surgical intervention may be considered. The total contact cast can convert the acute Charcot condition to the chronic condition.

It is not uncommon for the patient with a Charcot joint to be in a total contact cast for 6 to 8 months (Fig 13–14). The process of consolidation is a slow one and often takes a long period of time. These casts should be changed every several weeks to monitor the condition of the soft tissue, as well as repeat serial radiographs. At each cast change visit, skin temperatures should be recorded in the chart, so that the change from the acute Charcot condition to the chronic one can be monitored.

The other techniques to reduce stress on the foot may also be applied in the Charcot condition. Some are more effective than others, and each should be considered for its merits and shortcomings. Treatment of the Charcot joint is covered in detail in this text.

THE DIGITAL ULCERATION

Digital ulcers are very common in the insensitive foot. Ulcers on the dorsum of the toe are caused by shoe pressure. Hammertoes (cock-up toe) develop as a result of a biomechanical muscle imbalance. The intrinsic muscles in the forefoot responsible for stabilizing the toes against the ground cease to function in a normal fashion. Occasionally this is due to a biomechanical fault, but most commonly in the diabetic population this is due to motor neuropathy. Once the digital deformity develops, it becomes the site of shoe irritation within the toebox of the shoe.

The steps of progression to develop a digital ulceration are very similar to the plantar ulcer. First, a bony prominence has to exist. In this case, the prominence is the dorsally protruding toe. Secondly, the source of irritation in this case is not the pressure of walking but instead the pressure and friction of a shoe against the dorsum of the toe. In the sensate foot, this condition is very painful, and the patient has the ability to respond to the painful stimulus. Usually, a shoe change or a visit to the podiatrist's office to have the corn debrided is the next step in these situations. In the cases of the insensate foot, where the protective feedback mechanism has been interrupted, there is no perception of pain, so the process continues. As a result of the chronic inflammation due to friction, the tissue breaks down via the process of enzymatic autolysis, and an ulcer develops (Fig 13–15). If the process is not interrupted at this stage or if the patient does not recognize that a problem exists, a localized infection of the toe may occur. Because a digital ulcer begins as a corn on the toe, it is imperative that the physician examines the feet of these patients each time they come into the office.

It is even more important that the physician counsels patients on shoes and shoe fit, especially in the presence of hammertoe deformities because most of these complications can be prevented.

There are two other locations where digital ulcerations may develop. The first is on the tip of the toe, due to a mallet toe, whereby the position of the toe is such that all of the pressure of walking is placed onto the tip of toe. The cycle of the development of this lesion is the same as in the case of the dorsal digital ulcer. The difference is the location and the nature of the forces acting on the toe. If an adjacent toe has been removed, the forces affecting the remaining toes may be shifted sufficiently to cause a lesion to develop on the tip (Fig 13–16).

Another type of digital ulceration occurs on the side of the toe, and arises as a result of pressure and friction from an adjacent toe. Often, these begin as a soft corn, but due to constant friction in the presence of neuropathy the inflammatory response eventually contributes to the

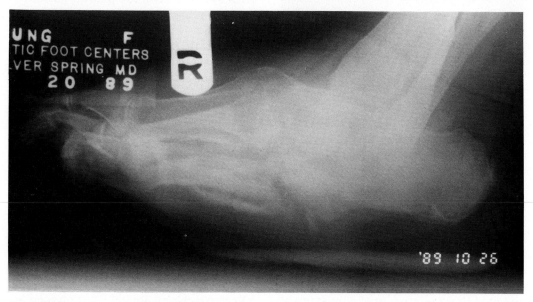

FIG 13–14.
This lateral radiograph represents a Charcot collapse of the mid-tarsal joint. This condition was treated with a total contact cast for 7 months. This process was monitored with serial radiographs and skin temperatures. Casts were changed approximately every 3 to 4 weeks.

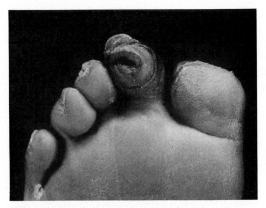

FIG 13–16.
Following a partial hallux amputation, the pressure of weight-bearing increased on the tip of the second toe, thereby causing this ulceration to develop. This occurs only in the presence of sensory neuropathy.

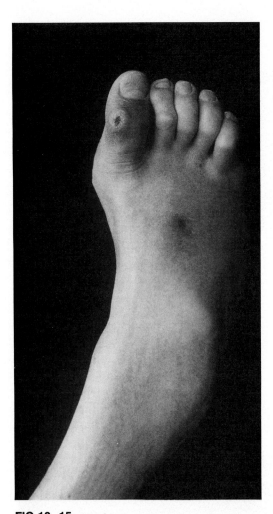

FIG 13–15.
Ulceration on the dorsum of the hallux as a result of digital deformity. This patient represents a severe case of motor neuropathy secondary to diabetes. As a result of this muscle imbalance, the "hallux hammertoe" has developed. In a conventional shoe, which does not provide ample toebox clearance, friction led to the development of this lesion.

breakdown of the skin, leading to the development of the ulcer. A common location for an ulcer to develop in the presence of a bunion is on the medial side of the second toe. This is directly related to the abduction of the hallux, with a juxtaposition against the second toe. In the presence of sensory neuropathy, this pressure goes undetected and eventually leads to tissue breakdown and ulceration (Fig 13–17).

When this scenario occurs, a prophylactic bunionectomy, or at the minimum, an accommodative pad should be applied to reduce the destructive forces. Too often, though, the problem goes unnoticed until the patient develops a bone infection and potential amputation ensues.

Another location where the digital ulcer may occur is on the plantar surface of the hallux. Increased pressure in this area is common in the case of hallux limitus. As a result of the inability of the first metatarsophalangeal joint to dorsiflex during toe off, there is a slight abductory twist that develops, which places an increased stress on the plantar surface of the hallux. Due to this increased pressure, insensate patients may develop an ulceration in this location.

The standard evaluation for an ulcer should be performed for this lesion as it would be for any ulcer. Treatment of this lesion should focus on the biomechanics of the joint. These forces may be compensated for with the use of orthotics, preferably an accommodative device (Fig 13–18), or may be addressed surgically. The procedure chosen should focus on increasing the motion of the first metatarsophalangeal joint to decrease the force on the plantar surface of the toe.

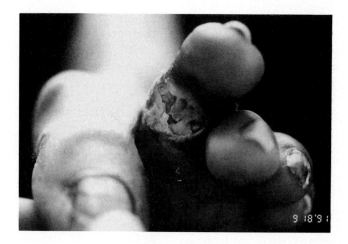

FIG 13–17.

This ulcer developed on the medial side of the second toe as a result of a bunion deformity. The juxtaposition of the hallux against the second toe caused pressure which was unperceivable by the patient due to sensory neuropathy. The first time that this patient was examined by her physician, pieces of bone were extruding through the wound.

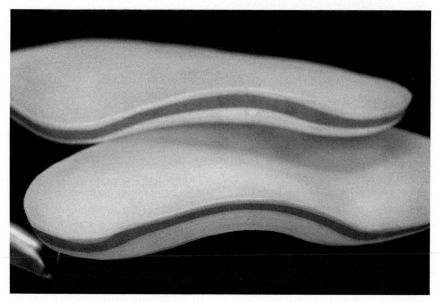

FIG 13–18.

This pair of tri-density molded orthotics are made from a plaster mold of the patient's feet. The purpose of these devices is to"accommodate" areas of high pressure on the plantar surface of the foot. This is provided by increasing surface area by achieving "total contact." These are also known as "total contact inlays."

Treatment of the Digital Ulcer

Evaluation of this ulcer should be identical to an ulcer on the plantar surface of the foot. The size, the depth, and the characteristics of the ulcer should be determined. The ulcer should then be examined to determine if it is infected. This should be done both by clinical evaluation (as mentioned in preceding sections), and by radiographic means.

If the ulcer is infected, the determination as to the proper course of action should be made based on criteria as established in the chapter on infections. A simple localized infection of the soft tissue can easily be managed on an out-patient basis with proper oral antibiotics. If the infection is widespread, or if the bone is infected, the patient may need to be admitted to the hospital for treatment.

Once the infection is resolved, the most important aspect in treatment is the recognition of the underlying problem. This involves the biomechanics of the deformity, the style and fit of the shoe, and the life-style (occupation and activity level) of the patient. After these components are evaluated, proper steps may be taken to avoid recurrence of the lesion or transfer of the ulcer to an adjacent toe.

This discussion brings about the notion of prophylactic surgery as an attempt to prevent these problems from developing in the first place, or prevent them from recurring after they have resolved. The concept of prophylactic surgery is philosophical, and is based on one's perspective on elective surgery in the diabetic population. There is a chapter in this text devoted to this important topic.

There are many other complications in the diabetic population that can be managed on an out-patient basis. Biomechanical deformities such as dropfoot, varus foot, or cavus foot may lead to the development of other problems and must be reckoned with. Dermatologic conditions plague the lower extremities of millions of diabetics. Many of these skin conditions can progress to become serious problems if left untreated.

All of the maladies discussed in this chapter will lead to the development of other problems if the maladies are neglected. Therefore these complications are discussed in great detail in this text.

REFERENCES

1. Boulton AJM et al: Impaired vibratory perception and diabetic foot ulceration, *Diabetic Med* 336–339, 1986.
2. Delbridge L, Appleberg M, Reeve TS: Factors associated with development of foot lesions in the diabetic, *Surgery* 93: 78–83, 1993.
3. Deanfield JE, Daggett PR, Harrison MJG: The role of autonomic neuropathy in diabetic foot ulceration, *J Neurol Sci* 47:203–210, 1980.
4. Harrison MJG, Faris IB: The neuropathic factor in the etiology of diabetic foot ulcers, *J Neurol Sci* 28:217–223, 1976.
5. Birke JA, Sims DS: Plantar sensory threshold in the ulcerative foot, *Lepr Rev* 57:261–267, 1986.
6. Wound healing: alternatives in management. In Hampton G, Birke J: *Treatment of wounds caused by pressure and insensitivity.*
7. Harati Y: Diabetic peripheral neuropathies, *Ann Intern Med* 107:546–559, 1987.
8. Belgrave MJ, Lev BI: Diabetic neuropathy; helping patients cope with their pain, *Postgrad Med* 90(5):263–270, 1991.
9. LoGerfo FW, Coffman JD: Vascular and microvascular disease of the foot in diabetes; implications for foot care, *N Engl J Med* 311:1615–1619, 1984.
10. Coleman W, Brand PW, Birke JA: The total contact cast; a therapy for plantar ulceration on insensitive feet, *J Am Podiatr Med Assoc* 74:548–552, 1984.
11. Boulton AJM et al: Abnormalities of foot pressure in early diabetic neuropathy, *Diabetic Med* 4:225–228, 1987.
12. Duckworth T et al: The measurement of pressures under the foot, *Foot Ankle* 3:130–141, 1982.

13. Betts RP, Franks CI, Duckworth T: Analysis of pressure and loads under the foot. Part II: quantitation of the dynamic distribution, *Clin Phys Physiol Meas* 1:113–124, 1980.
14. Gibbons GW, Eliopoulos GM: *Infections in the diabetic foot,* Philadelphia, 1984, WB Saunders.
15. Edmons ME: The diabetic foot: pathophysiology and treatment, *Clin Endocrinol Metab* 15:889, 1986.
16. Boulton AJM, Bowker JH: The diabetic foot. In Olefsky JM, Sherwin R: *Diabetes mellitus: management and complications,* New York, 1985, Churchill Livingstone.
17. Financing Diabetes into the 90s. Conference of the Health Care Financing Association, December 1989 Washington, D.C.
18. Stokes IAF, Faris IB, Hutton WC: The neuropathic ulcer and loads on the foot in diabetic patients, *Acta Orthop Scand* 46:839–847, 1975.
19. Cterctko GC et al: Vertical forces acting on the feet of diabetic patients with neuropathic ulceration, *Br J Surg* 68:608–614, 1981.
20. Duckworth T et al: Plantar pressure measurements and the prevention of ulceration in the diabetic foot, *J Bone Joint Surg* 67B:79–85, 1985.
21. Wagner FW: The dysvascular foot: a system for diagnosis and treatment, *Foot Ankle* 2:64, 1981.
22. Wagner FW: Treatment of the diabetic foot, *Compr Ther* 10:29, 1984.
23. Williams H, Hutchinson K, Brown G: Gangrene of the feet in diabetics, *Arch Surg* 108:609, 1974.
24. Edmons ME: The diabetic foot; pathophysiology and treatment, *Clin Endocrinol Metab* 15:889, 1986.
25. Bauman JH, Brand PW: Measurement of pressure between the foot and shoe, *Lancet* 23:629–632, 1963.
26. Schaff PS, Cavanagh PR: Shoes for the insensitive foot: the effect of a "rocker bottom" shoe modification on plantar pressure distribution, *Foot Ankle* 11:129–145, 1990.
27. Sims DS, Birke JA: Effect of rocker sole placement on plantar pressures. (Abstract) Proceedings of the Twentieth Annual Meeting of the United States Public Health Service Professional Association, 1985, Atlanta.
28. Kominsky SJ: The ambulatory total contact cast. In Frykberg R, editor: *The high risk foot in diabetes mellitus,* New York, 1991, Churchill Livingstone.
29. Brike J, Sims DS, Buford WL: Walking casts: effect on plantar foot pressures, *J Rehabil Res Dev* 22:18, 1985.
30. Bauman H, Girling JP, Brand PW: Plantar pressure and trophic ulceration, *J Bone Joint Surg* 45B:652, 1963.

SUGGESTED READINGS

Banks A, McGlammery ED: Charcot foot, *J Am Podiatr Med Assoc* 79:213–235, 1989.
Beach K et al: Progression of lower-extremity arterial occlusive disease in type II diabetes mellitus, *Diabetes Care* 11(6):247–253, 1988.
Beltran J et al: The diabetic foot: magnetic resonance imaging evaluation, *Skeletal Radiol* 19:37–41, 1990.
Berquist T et al: Magnetic resonance imaging: application in musculoskeletal infection, *Magnet Reson Imag* 3:219–230, 1985.
Bier R, Estersohn H: A new treatment for Charcot joint in the diabetic foot. *J Am Podiatr Med Assoc* 77:63–69, 1987.
Birke JA et al: Methods of treating plantar ulcers, *Phys Ther* 71:116–122, 1991.
Burden AC et al: Use of the "Scotchcast boot" in treating diabetic foot ulcers, *Br Med J* 286:1555–1557, 1983.
Cahill G: Current concepts of diabetes. In: *Joslin's diabetes mellitus,* ed 12, Philadelphia, 1985, Lea & Febiger.
Calhoun J, Mader J: Infection in the diabetic foot, *Hosp Pract* March 30:81–104, 1992.
Cohn B, Brahms M: Diabetic arthropathy of the first metatarsal cuneiform joint; introduction of a new surgical fusion technique, *Orthopaedic Review* 16, 1987.
Coleman WC: The relief of pressures using outer shoe sole modifications. Proceedings of the International Conference on Biomechanical and Clinical Kineseology of the Hand and Foot, Madras, India, 1985.
Consensus statement: report and recommendations of the San Antonio Conference on

Diabetic Neuropathy, *Diabetes,* 37:1000–1004, 1988.

Cunha B: The diabetic foot: case study in infectious disease, *Emergency Med* September 30:1004–1007, 1988.

Davis J: The use of adjuvant hyperbaric oxygen in the treatment of the diabetic foot, *Clin Podiatr Med Surg* 4, 1987.

Dickhaut S, DeLee J, Page C: Nutritional status: importance in predicting wound healing after amputation, *J Bone Joint Surg* 66A:71–75 1984.

Drury D, Blair V: Total contact casting for the treatment of plantar neuropathic foot ulcers, *Ostomy/Wound Management* 33, 1991.

Durham J et al: Impact of magnetic resonance imaging on the management of diabetic foot infections, *Am J Surg* 162:150–154, 1991.

Edmonds ME: The diabetic foot: pathophysiology and treatment, *Clin Endocrinol Metab* 15:889–916, 1986.

Edmonds ME et al: Improved survival of the diabetic foot: the role of a specialised foot clinic, *Q J Med* 60:763–771, 1986.

Erdman K et al: Osteomyelitis: characteristics and pitfalls of diagnosis with MR imaging, *Radiology* 180:533–539, 1991.

File T, Tan J: Treatment of bacterial skin and soft tissue infections, *Surgery* 172:

Florkowski GM et al: Clinical and neurophysiological studies of aldose reductase inhibitor ponalrestat in chronic symptomatic diabetic peripheral neuropathy, *Diabetes* 40:129–133, 1991.

Fortes Z et al: Direct vital microscopic study of defective leukocyte-endothelial interaction in diabetes mellitus, *Diabetes* 40:1267–1273, 1991.

Frykberg R: Neuropathic arthropathy: the diabetic Charcot joint, *Diabetes Educator* Winter:17–20, 1984.

Gandsman E et al: Differentiation of Charcot joint from osteomyelitis through dynamic bone imaging, *Nucl Med Communications* 11:45–53, 1990.

Gillespie W, Allardyce R: Mechanisms of bone degradation in infection: a review of current hypothesis, *Orthopedics* 13:407–410, 1990.

Gold R, Hawkins R, Katz R: Bacterial osteomyelitis: findings on plain radiography,

CT, MRI and scintigraphy, *Am J Radiol* 157:365–370, 1991.

Grim P et al: Hyperbaric oxygen therapy, *JAMA* 236:2216–2220, 1990.

Guy RJC et al: Evaluation of thermal and vibration sensation in diabetic neuropathy, *Diabetologia* 28:131–137, 1985.

Helm P, Walker SC, Pullium G: Recurrence of neuropathic ulceration following healing in a total contact cast, *Arch Phys Med Rehabil* Nov. 72:967–970, 1991.

Irwin S et al: Lesions due to "small vessel disease," *Br J Surg* 75:1201–1206, 1988.

Kathol M et al: Calcaneal insufficiency avulsion fractures in patients with diabetes mellitus, *Radiology* 180:725–729, 1991.

El-Khoury G, Kathol M: Neuropathic fractures in patients with diabetes mellitus, *Diagn Radiol* 134:313–316, 1980.

Knight D et al: Imaging for infection: caution required with the Charcot joint, *Eur J Nucl Med* 13:523–526, 1988.

Knighton D, Fylling C, Doucette M: Wound healing and amputation in a high risk diabetic population, *Wounds: Compend Clin Res Practice,* 107–114, 1989.

Knighton D et al: Classification and treatment of chronic nonhealing wounds, *Ann Surg* 204:322–330, 1986.

Knighton D et al: Amputation prevention in an independently reviewed at-risk diabetic population using a comprehensive wound care protocol, *Am J Surg* 160, 1990.

Kucan J, Robson C: Diabetic foot infections: fate of the contralateral foot, *Plast Reconstr Surg* 77:439–441, 1986.

Krentz A et al: Spontaneous fractures in patients with diabetic neuropathy, *J R Coll Physicians Lond* 23:111–113, 1989.

Laing PW, Cogley DI, Klenerman L: Neuropathic foot ulceration treated by total contact casts, *J Bone Joint Surg* 74:133–136, 1991.

Lipsky B et al: Outpatient management of uncomplicated lower extremity infections in diabetic patients, *Diabetes Spectrum* 4:790–797, 1991.

Martin J et al: Radical treatment of mal perforans in diabetic patients with arterial insufficiency, *J Vasc Surg* 12:264–268, 1990.

Mooney V, Wagner W: Neurocirculatory disorders of the foot, *Clin Orthop* 53–61, 1977.

Moore T et al: Abnormalities of the foot in patients with diabetes mellitus: findings on MR imaging, *Am J Radiol* 157:813–816, 1991.

Myerson M et al: The total-contact cast for management of neuropathic plantar ulceration of the foot, *J Bone Joint Surg* 74A:261–269, 1992.

Newman L et al: Unsuspected osteomyelitis in diabetic foot ulcers, *JAMA* 266:1246–1251, 1991.

Pecorara R et al: Chronology and determinants of tissue repair in diabetic lower-extremity ulcers, *Diabetes* 40:1305–1313, 1991.

Quinn S et al: MR imaging of chronic osteomyelitis, *J Comput Assist Tomogr* 12:113–117, 1988.

Rice J: Diabetic infection, ulceration and gangrene, *J Am Podiatr Med Assoc* 64:774–781, 1974.

Scartozzi G, Kanat I: Diabetic neuroarthropathy of the foot and ankle, *J Am Podiatr Med Assoc* 80:298–303, 1990.

Sindrup S et al: Concentration-response relationship in imipramine treatment of diabetic neuropathy symptoms, *Clin Pharmacol Ther* 509–515, 1990.

Splittgerber G, Spiegelhoff D, Buggy B: Combined leukocyte and bone imaging used to evaluate diabetic osteoarthropathy and osteomyelitis, *Clin Nucl Med* 14:156–160, 1989.

Stevens MJ et al: Selective neuropathy and preserved vascular responses in the diabetic Charcot foot, *Diabetologia* 35:148–154, 1992.

Subbarao J et al: Diabetic neuro-osteoarthropathy: rehabilitation of a patient with both ankle joints involved and associated skin problems, *Orthop Rev* 15:471–478, 1986.

Tang J et al: Musculoskeletal infection of the extremities: evaluation with MR imaging, *Radiology* 166:205–209, 1988.

Tur E, Yosipovitch G, Bar-On Y: Skin reactive hyperemia in diabetic patients: a study by laser Doppler flowmetry, *Diabetes Care* 14:958–962, 1991.

Wheat J et al: Diabetic foot infections: bacteriologic analysis, *Arch Intern Med* 146:1935–1940, 1986.

Wound Care Center. New frontiers in the care of diabetic foot ulcers. Paper presented at the Thirty-fifth Annual American Diabetes Association Post Graduate Meeting, Palm Springs, Calif, 1990.

Yuh W et al: Osteomyelitis of the foot in diabetic patients: evaluation with plain film, Tc-MDP scintigraphy, and MR imaging, *Am J Radiol* 152:795–800, 1989.

14 _____ Medical Management of the Diabetic Inpatient

Robert E. Ratner, M.D.

Michelle F. Magee, M.D.

When the individual with diabetes requires hospitalization for treating lower-extremity disease, it is necessary to consider two global perspectives. First, what is the effect of the underlying lower-extremity disorder and its treatment on overall glycemic control? Second, what is the impact of the acute diabetic state on the ability to resolve the underlying foot pathologic condition? Throughout this chapter, we will attempt to address both the effects of the diseased foot on diabetes and the effect of diabetes on the foot.

METABOLIC STRESS RESPONSES

When an individual develops lower-extremity disease, manifested by skin ulceration, infection, or gangrene, a generalized stress response is initiated. Elevations in counter regulatory hormones including epinephrine, glucagon, cortisol, and growth hormone are noted at the time of hospitalization and throughout the course of acute illness. The effect of these counter regulatory hormone elevations is to significantly accelerate catabolism, hepatic gluconeogenesis, and lipolysis. The end result of these metabolic processes is to raise circulating serum glucose, free fatty acids, and ketone body levels. The rise in circulating substrate levels further fuels the hyperglycemia and blunts the islet cell response via the mechanism of glucose toxicity.[1] As lower-extremity dis-

ease progresses to involve either sepsis or gangrene, circulating acidosis ensues, either from lactate or ketone body accumulation. Acidosis leads to impairment in peripheral insulin sensitivity, progressive insulin resistance, and further impairment in controlling circulating glucose and other substrate levels. This initiates a cycle of acute illness inducing hyperglycemia and hyperglycemia subsequently impairing the physiologic response to that illness (Fig 14–1). This is exemplified by the finding of infection as the most common precipitating cause of ketoacidosis.[2]

Difficulty in achieving glycemic control is further exacerbated by the total disruption in typical daily activities and diet and the use of pharmacologic interventions. Increases in insulin requirements are typically noted upon presentation of an acute illness in the diabetic population. Efforts to bring blood glucose levels under control are made more difficult by the artificial environment forced on a hospitalized diabetic. Dramatic changes in dietary intake result from decrease in appetite secondary to illness, the dietary prescription, and the palatability of hospital food. Meals are frequently interrupted by medical tests and often cancelled if a nothing by mouth (NPO) order is written to prepare for a specialized test or surgery. How much insulin will be given and how often it will be given to the patient are now taken out of the individual's control. Instead, administration of the insulin will

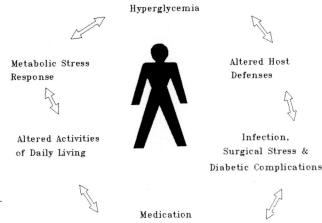

FIG 14–1.
The vicious cycle of hyperglycemia and diabetic complications.

be dependent on physician's orders and nursing availability. The ideal situation of administering subcutaneous insulin 30 to 60 minutes prior to a meal is seldom possible in a hospital. The effect of acute illness and hospitalization is the significant change in insulin requirements, dietary intake, and activity. This leads to dramatic fluctuations in glucose control and may lead to hyperglycemia.

GLUCOSE TOXICITY

The cycle (see Fig 14–1) is "closed" by the effect of hyperglycemia and overall uncontrolled diabetes on the progression of diabetic complications. As previously described in Chapter 1 of this text, hyperglycemia has been correlated with a higher incidence of lower-extremity gangrene,[3] peripheral vascular disease,[4] and peripheral neuropathy.[5] These underlying complications predispose to the development of ulcers, which serve as portals of entry for bacterial infection, leading to sepsis and gangrene.

Hyperglycemia affects the body's ability to fight infection.[6] Rayfield et al demonstrated a direct correlation in the overall prevalence of infection with mean plasma glucose levels in more than 240 diabetic patients. The mechanism by which hyperglycemia contributes to infec-

tion remains hotly debated. Evidence exists to support defects in neutrophil function at the level of chemotaxis,[7] adherence,[8] phagocytosis,[9] and intracellular microbiocidal activity.[10] There appears to be a reversible component to this dysfunction with return to baseline on control of circulating serum glucose levels.[8]

Once the skin integrity in the lower extremity has been interrupted, wound healing is dependent on numerous factors including:

1. Removal of the traumatic cause of skin breakdown (e.g., pressure due to biomechanical abnormalities);
2. Adequacy of blood flow;
3. Absence of infection;
4. Appropriate fibroblast and connective tissue proliferation; and
5. Maintenance of a noncatabolic, euglycemic state.

The process of wound healing takes place in two phases. The first, or inflammatory phase, is characterized by vascular events leading to hemostasis and vasodilatation and cellular events countering infection. The second phase is the proliferative or regenerative phase, in which growth of new capillaries, collagen, and epithelial cells takes place.[11] Weringer et al demonstrated decreased neovascularization and fibroblast proliferation with diminished collagen synthesis in the wounds of diabetic animals.[12] This resulted in a dramatic reduction in the tensile strength of the wound, which could be reversed or prevented by insulin administration and control of the circulating glucose levels. Insulin administration increases the number of leukocytes and fibroblasts and the amount of collagen in the wound margins. Diabetes interferes at multiple levels of wound repair, thus providing for a continuous portal of entry for subsequent wound infection.[13]

GLUCOSE CONTROL

Because of the deleterious effects of hyperglycemia on progression of lower-extremity disease, it is imperative that glycemic control be achieved in both the acute and chronic setting of diabetic foot disease. This must always be tempered by the potential risk of hypoglycemia in patients in whom nutritional intake may be impaired. Although no absolute cutoff for hyperglycemia can be established, available data would suggest that maintenance of serum glucose levels below 200 mg/dl will optimize granulocyte function and improve wound healing.[14] Maintaining serum glucose levels at 200 mg/dl or less will prevent diabetic ketoacidosis and hyperosmolar nonketotic states. These levels allow sufficient leeway to minimize the risk of hypoglycemia. In the otherwise healthy individual who can recognize early signs and symptoms of hypoglycemia and is able to ingest rapid-acting carbohydrates to correct hypoglycemia, attempts to maintain near normoglycemia in the hospital can be undertaken. In patients whose oral caloric intake is compromised or in patients in whom hypoglycemia may be devastating because of underlying autonomic neuropathy, cardiovascular or cerebrovascular disease, the

goals of therapy must be liberalized to the 150 to 200 mg/dl range.

GLYCEMIC MONITORING

Maintenance of glycemic control requires ongoing assessment of nutritional intake (both enteric and parenteral), activity (physical therapy or strict bed rest), concomitant medications (e.g., steroids), and blood glucose measurements. Bedside capillary blood glucose monitoring (CBGM) is now available in most hospitals and allows for rapid and accurate determination of blood glucose levels throughout the day. Such monitoring is imperative for both assessing the efficacy of insulin therapy and determining adjustments in insulin.[15] Urine glucose determinations have no role in the management of the hospitalized patient. Urine ketone testing is an important adjunct to metabolic monitoring during acute illness and stress. This testing should be done if serum glucose determinations exceed 240 mg/dl.[16] Although valuable for assessment of long-term control and for subsequent diabetes education and motivation,[17] the use of glycated hemoglobin or albumin is not necessary in the acute inpatient setting. Results of glycated hemoglobin cannot be used for short-term manipulation of insulin regimens.[18]

INSULIN ALGORITHMS

Using data from CBGM, multiple insulin algorithms can be implemented.[19] The greatest error committed in the inpatient setting is discontinuing regular doses of depot insulin in the patient whose caloric intake is unpredictable. Insulin requirements *rise* in the setting of acute illness due to the catabolic and stress-related phenomena associated with acute illness. Thus in the patient with insulin dependent diabetes it is imperative to maintain depot insulin therapy and closely monitor glucose results to assess the need for supplemental doses. In the type II patient, caloric restriction actually may lower the amount of insulin or eliminate the need for depot insulin or oral hypoglycemic agents.

Sliding scale insulin regimens have been used by generations of medical and surgical house officers for glycemic control, even though the underlying hypothesis they are based upon is nonphysiologic, relying upon retrospective treatment of blood glucose levels. It is more physiologic, and thus preferable, to give insulin in anticipation of upward glycemic excursions and prospectively keep glucose levels within an individual's target range. "The objective is not to let the patient become repeatedly sick and then try to treat the problem that we have allowed to occur."[20] From personal observation, sliding scale insulin seldom achieves adequate glycemic control and typically prolongs hospital stay for 48 hours or longer until an appropriate discharge dose of insulin can be determined. This does not mean that supplemental regular insulin should not be given if the blood glucose is dangerously high, as will be discussed in greater detail subsequently.

Appropriate insulin adjustments may be made according to a multitude of insulin algorithms. Daily determinations of insulin doses can be made based upon the glycemic response to the preceding day's insulin regimen. The patient's anticipated caloric intake and activity must also be taken into account (Table 14–1). Supplemental regular insulin may be given in addition the typical depot preparations to prevent ketosis, electrolyte imbalance, and hyperglycemic emergencies. Such sick-day doses should be incorporated into subsequent insulin administration to prevent recurrent hyperglycemic excursions (Table 14–2).

TABLE 14–1.

Insulin Adjustment for Basal Insulin Regimen

The goals for blood glucose control are:
 Fasting less than _____
 All others less than _____

Guidelines to increase insulin:
Be sure the blood sugar is higher than acceptable before making the appropriate adjustment.

If the blood sugar:	Increase:
Before breakfast is over _____	Evening NPH/Lente by _____ units
Before lunch is over _____	Morning regular by _____ units
Before dinner is over _____	Morning NPH/Lente by _____ units Evening regular by _____ units
Before bedtime is over _____	

Guidelines to decrease insulin:
Determine if the low blood glucose may be due to any of the following:
 a. a skipped meal
 b. eating less at a meal than usual
 c. an increase in exercise
 d. an inaccurate amount of insulin
If there is no explanation for an insulin reaction or a blood glucose less than _____, decrease the appropriate insulin dose the next day according to the following guidelines.

For a reaction or low blood glucose:	Decrease:
Between 2 a.m. and breakfast	Evening NPH/Lente by _____ units
Between breakfast and lunch	Morning regular by _____ units
Between lunch and supper	
Between supper and 2 a.m.	Morning NPH/Lente by _____ units Evening regular by _____ units

DIABETIC EMERGENCIES

Subcutaneous depot insulin is inadequate therapy in the setting of acute hyperglycemic emergencies such as diabetic ketoacidosis (DKA) or hyperosmolar nonketotic states (HONC). These metabolic derangements may stem directly from in-

TABLE 14–2.

Sick Day Guidelines With Insulin Adjustment

Monitoring
1. Test blood glucose every 4 hours or at least 4 times a day (before each meal and at bedtime).
2. Keep a record of results.
3. Test urine Ketones every 4 hours if blood sugar is greater than 240 mg/dl.
4. Record results.

Medication
Always give the usual dosage of insulin. Extra regular insulin may be needed because the stress of being sick can raise blood glucose levels.

Instructions for taking extra insulin during sick days
I. Blood glucose should be checked at least every 4 hours. If blood sugar is greater than 240 mg/dl give additional regular insulin *at that time.*
   A. *If there are no ketones* in the urine give 10% of the daily dose of insulin as a supplement dose. Follow these guidelines to calculate the dose of extra insulin:
      1. Add up the total daily insulin dose:
         Morning _____
         Prelunch _____
         Predinner _____
         Bedtime _____
         _____
         Total daily insulin dose
      2. Multiply the total daily insulin dose by 10%:
         _____ total daily insulin dose × .10 = _____ the dose of *extra* regular insulin
   B. *If there are ketones present in the urine,* give 20% of the daily dose of insulin as a supplemental dose. Follow these guidelines to calculate the dose of extra insulin:
      1. Add up the total daily insulin dose:
         Morning _____
         Prelunch _____
         Predinner _____
         Bedtime _____
         _____
         total daily insulin dose
      2. Multiply the total daily insulin dose by 20%:
         _____ total daily insulin dose × .20 = _____ the dose of *extra* regular insulin
II. Look at this example to see how a sick day may be handled based on 3 insulin doses:

Time	Blood Sugar	Urine Ketones	Usual Insulin Dose	Extra Insulin Dose	Total
8:00 A.M.	251	Negative	4uR + 25uN	4uR	8uR + 25uN
12:00 P.M.	306	Moderate	_____	9uR	9uR
4:00 P.M.	296	Small	6uR	9uR	15uR
10:00 P.M.	200	Negative	10uN		10uN

fection or gangrene in the lower extremity or may result from the withholding of depot insulin in the patient who is acutely ill, but kept NPO. DKA is a condition characterized by marked dehydration, electrolyte depletion, and an anion gap metabolic acidosis. Despite intervention, DKA accounts for approximately 10% of reported diabetic deaths, with the precipitating factor (e.g., sepsis) frequently being the cause of death.[21] Aggressive management of both the ketoacidosis and the underlying precipitating factor is imperative. Table 14–3 provides a protocol for the management of patients with DKA. It is imperative that the precipitating factor for DKA be identified and appropriately treated to minimize morbidity and mortality.

HONC states are conditions charac-

TABLE 14–3.

Protocol for Therapy of Diabetic Ketoacidosis

Nothing replaces close observation of the patient.
  I. Fluids (patients are usually 5 to 8 liters depleted on average).
    A. 2 to 3 liters of 0.9% NaCl should be given over first 2 hours to replace ECF volume.
    B. When BP is stable and urine flow adequate, 0.45% NaCl can be used to replace free water deficit.
    C. 5% glucose is added when plasma glucose falls to 250 to 300 mg/dl to prevent hypoglycemia. This is continued until ketosis clears and patient is able to take po fluids. Increase dextrose concentration to 10% if glucose falls below 150 mg/dl and patient is still ketotic.
  II. Potassium (in general, 100 to 200 mEq will be required over the first 24 to 36 hours).
    A. Ensure adequate urine output and exclude hyperkalemia prior to replacement.
    B. Replacement therapy ordinarily becomes necessary about 4 hours into treatment as plasma levels begin to fall. Should be given 20 to 40 mEq per hour as KCl.
    C. If the initial potassium concentration is normal or low, replacement should be started immediately.
  III. Phosphate (generally 60 to 80 mM depleted).
    A. Replacement is not normally required during the acute phase of treatment.
    B. Indications for its use include left ventricular dysfunction, evidence of rhabdomyolysis, or failure to clear mental confusion despite improvement in circulating volume, hyperosmolarity and acidosis.
    C. Dose to be administered in these circumstances is approximately 1 mM/kg body weight to be given over 8 to 12 hours. The phosphate content of commercially available preparations vary. Potassium phosphate solution contains 4.4 meq/ml of K+ and 3.0 mM/mL of phosphate. The sodium phosphate solution contains 4.4 meg K$^+$/mL and 3.0 mM PO$_4$/mL.
    D. Potential complications of phosphate therapy include symptomatic hypocalcemia, hypomagnesemia, and metastatic calcium phosphate deposition.
  IV. Bicarbonate.
    A. Not necessary unless severe acidosis (pH less than 6.9) or dangerously low serum bicarbonate (5 mEq/L or less).
    B. Sodium bicarbonate can be given as 1 to 2 ampules (total of 44 to 48 mEq) in 1 liter of 0.45% normal saline per hour. If used, the infusion of bicarbonate should be stopped when the pH reaches 7.0 in order to avoid late metabolic alkalosis.
  V. Insulin (use only regular insulin during acute phase).
    A. Low dose continuous IV infusion.
       A continuous infusion of regular insulin at a dosage of 0.1 to 0.15 units per kg body weight per hour is given through a constant infusion pump. There is no need for a bolus injection preceding the drip. (Allow 30 mL of insulin-containing fluid to run through the plastic tubing prior to connecting it to the patient. This avoids the necessity of adding plasma or albumin to prevent insulin binding to the plastic).
    B. Continue insulin regimen until ketosis has resolved (pH > 7.30 and/or serum bicarbonate greater than 18 mEq/L with closed anion gap). Patients can then be started on regular insulin 20 to 25% of their usual total daily dose subcutaneously every 4 hours. The IV insulin regimen should be maintained for 30 minutes after regular subcutaneous insulin is given. The following morning, the patient may be restarted on their usual daily dose of intermediate insulin supplemented by regular insulin as needed.

terized by severe hyperglycemia and hyperosmolarity in the absence of significant ketoacidosis. Although there is a significant crossover between DKA and HONC, plasma glucose levels tend to be higher in HONC and the acidosis, resulting from lactate accumulation rather than ketone bodies, is considerably milder. It is typically patients with type II diabetes who develop HONC, although they may rarely develop significant ketosis. Mortality remains extremely high for HONC, as high as 10% to 20%.[22] Aggressive management of HONC is imperative, as is the investigation of its underlying precipitating cause (Table 14–4).

PERIOPERATIVE MANAGEMENT

Inpatient management of diabetic lower-extremity disease frequently requires surgical intervention. In the perioperative period, it is desirable to maintain glucose

TABLE 14–4.

Protocol for Therapy of Hyperosmolar Non-ketotic State

Hyperosmolarity produces the symptoms, but volume depletion or too rapid a fall in glucose produces the morbidity and mortality.
I. Fluids (patients are usually 10 to 12 liters depleted).
    A. 2 to 3 liters of 0.9% NaCl should be given over the first 2 hours to replenish ECF volume.
    B. Normal saline should be maintained until blood pressure and perfusion pressure have been normalized. At this point, 0.45% NaCl can be used to replace the free water deficit and correct the hyperosmolarity.
    C. 5% glucose is added to the IV solutions when plasma glucose falls to 250 to 300 mg%.
    D. 50% of the fluid deficit should be replaced within the first 12 hours of therapy with the remainder replaced more slowly over the following 24 hours.
II. Insulin (these patients are usually exquisitely sensitive to exogenous insulin).
    A. Subcutaneous or intramuscular injections during the acute phase of therapy are of marginal value due to poor perfusion pressures and failure to absorb from the depot.
    B. Low dose continuous IV infusion.
    A continuous IV infusion of regular human insulin is given at a rate of 0.05 units per kg per hour via a constant infusion pump. There is no need for a bolus injection preceding the drip. All drips should be piggy-backed into IV hydration.
    C. Decrease insulin infusion rate by 50% when plasma glucose falls to 250 to 300 mg/dl.
    D. Cerebral edema is associated with hypoglycemia or a too rapid reduction in plasma glucose, so great care must be taken in controlling the insulin infusion rate and subsequent fall in plasma glucose.
    E. Some patients may require no insulin therapy at all to correct the hyperglycemia and may correct with rehydration alone.
III. Potassium.
    A. Ensure adequate urine output and exclude hyperkalemia prior to replacement.
    B. Replacement therapy should be given as KCl at approximately 20 to 40 meq/hour.
IV. Bicarbonate.
    A. There is no indication for its use unless lactic acidosis has resulted in a pH <7.00
V. Heparin.
    A. Large vessel arterial thrombosis and embolization are common complicating events in HONC.
    B. If clinical evidence of thrombosis exists, full dose heparin anticoagulation is indicated (30,000 to 45,000 units daily by continuous infusion).
    C. In the absence of clinical evidence of thrombosis, low-dose heparin (5,000 units three times per day) may be given as prophylaxis.

levels in the 140 to 200 mg/dl range to prevent acute metabolic complications of diabetes, maintain fluid and electrolyte balance, and optimize wound healing and white blood cell function.

Whenever possible, surgery should be scheduled after glucose, fluid and electrolyte status have been optimized. Preoperative assessment of cardiovascular disease and autonomic neuropathy are imperative to prevent perioperative problems. Of course, emergency situations may preclude the opportunity to perform such interventions and surgery should proceed with greater perioperative observation and aggressive intervention. When possible, surgery for a diabetic patient should be performed on an elective basis.

Perioperative management of plasma glucose can be achieved using a variety of algorithms. In the individual who is diet- or oral agent-controlled, it may be possible to obtain adequate glycemic control simply by omitting glucose from intravenous fluids administered perioperatively.[23] In the patient requiring insulin for glycemic control in the preoperative state, more aggressive perioperative management is likely to be required. The use of subcutaneous insulin regimens typically results in inadequate glycemic control due to variable absorption from the subcutaneous depot.[24]

A variety of intravenous regimens have also been used that prevents the problem associated with peripheral ab-

TABLE 14–5.

Intravenous Insulin Infusion Regimen for
Perioperative Diabetic Control

Patients qualifying for this protocol:

1. All insulin requiring diabetics undergoing surgical
   procedures under general anesthesia.
2. Diabetics on oral agents or those who are diet
   controlled, who are found to have a serum glucose in excess of 300 mg/dl in the recovery
   room.
3. All patients who are found to have serum glucose
   levels in excess of 300 mg/dl in the recovery
   room regardless of prior history of hyperglycemia
   or diabetes mellitus.

Therapeutic intervention:

1. If the patient was insulin requiring preoperatively,
   the patient will have a dextrose containing IV begun between 7 and 8 a.m. on the morning of surgery with insulin infused through a piggyback apparatus at a rate of 0.02 units of regular human
   insulin per kilogram per hour. This is most easily
   accomplished by placing 50 units of insulin in a
   500 cc bag of normal saline and running the infusion through a continuous infusion pump at the
   appropriate rate. If approximately 20 to 30 cc of
   this fluid are run through the tubing, all of the insulin binding sites on the plastic will be saturated
   and the insulin recovery rate will be essentially 95
   to 100%.
2. All patients found to have glucose values in excess of 300 mg/dl in the recovery room will be
   started on 0.02 units regular human insulin per kg
   per hour via continuous infusion in D5 containing
   IV solutions as described above.
3. Therapy will continue until the patient is taking
   PO feedings at which time appropriate oral or
   subcutaneous therapy of the patients diabetes
   will be instituted approximately 2 to 4 hours prior
   to the discontinuation of the insulin infusion.

Monitoring:

1. All patients should be monitored for serum glucose upon arrival in the recovery room and on an
   every 2 hour basis thereafter. This can be accomplished either with the use of automated lab
   techniques or more conveniently by the use of a
   reflectance meter.
2. No alteration or interruption of this protocol will be
   undertaken as long as the serum glucose remains greater than 150 mg/dl and less than 250
   mg/dl. If the glucose exceeds these limits, the infusion may be altered in the appropriate direction
   by 20% for an almost immediate effect.

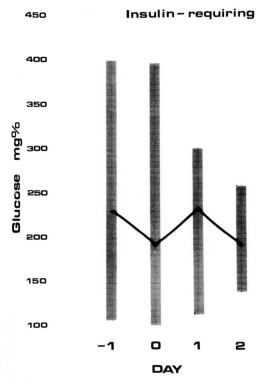

FIG 14–2.

Glucose response to intravenous infusion therapy in
the peri-operative period in type I diabetes. Twelve
patients were begun on therapy pre-operatively, while
seven were identified and begun on therapy in the
recovery room.

sorption and allows minute-by-minute
control of plasma glucose levels. No single
protocol has been shown to be superior due
to the difficulties associated with controlling for confounding variables.[25, 26] An intravenous (IV) insulin infusion regimen
for perioperative diabetic control used by
the authors is provided in Table 14–5. In
initial pilot studies, this protocol proved
easily achievable with no technical errors
in its implementation. Serum glucose control was quickly achieved with institution
of the IV regimen either preoperatively
or upon identification of hyperglycemia
in the immediate postoperative period.
Twelve type I patients were identified and
started on the protocol preoperatively, and
seven were identified and begun on the
protocol postoperatively in the recovery

room. Mean glucose for those started pre-operatively was 184 mg/dl for the day of surgery. Those begun postoperatively had a mean glucose of 361 mg/dl at initiation of therapy, but showed progressive declines to 202 and 168 mg/dl over the ensuing two postoperative days (Figs 14–2 and 14–3). Type II patients were begun on the protocol on six occasions when recovery room glucose determinations exceeded 300 mg/dl. As can be seen in Figure 14–4, glucose control progressively improved. No episodes of symptomatic hypoglycemia were encountered and the infusion protocol was able to be maintained for as long as the patient remained NPO (62 patient-days total and up to 7 days in a single patient in this study).

RISK FACTOR INTERVENTION

Inpatient management of the individual with diabetic lower-extremity disease is ideal for the assessment and management of underlying risk factors. Cigarette smoking has been associated with lower-extremity disease[27] and significantly more morbidity and hospitalization than in nonsmoking diabetic patients.

Control of hypertension and hyperlipidemia clearly reduces subsequent risks of cerebrovascular and cardiovascular disease, and it may also play a significant role in the treatment of peripheral vascular disease and exacerbation of diabetic lower-extremity disorders. Assessing the causes of lower-extremity disease includ-

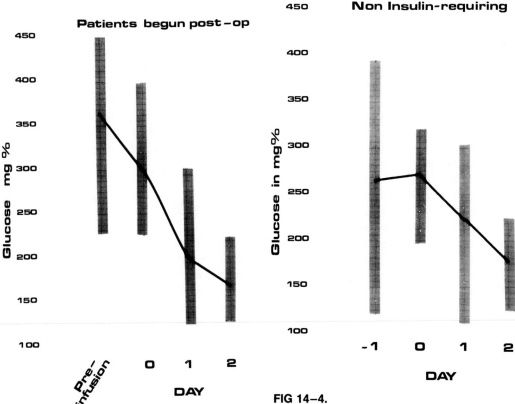

FIG 14–3.
Glucose response to intravenous insulin infusion therapy begun in the post-operative period on day 0 in patients with type I diabetes.

FIG 14–4.
Glucose response to intravenous insulin infusion therapy in the peri-operative period in non-insulin requiring type II diabetes. All patients were found to have glucose values > 300 mg/dl in the recovery room prior to initiation of IV insulin infusion therapy.

ing neuropathy, peripheral vascular disease, and infectious processes is covered in greater detail in other chapters. Appropriate evaluation and intervention are imperative to prevent subsequent tissue breakdown and recurrence of diabetic foot ulceration.

COEXISTING DIABETIC COMPLICATIONS

Other complications may also affect the care of diabetic foot disease. For example, the presence of diabetic nephropathy must be kept in mind when evaluating fluid and electrolyte status, as well as in anticipation of giving contrast media to evaluate peripheral vascular disease. The presence of a serum creatinine in excess of 2 mg/dl is a relative contraindication to the use of contrast media. As many as 75% of such patients will have significant deterioration in renal function following IV contrast injection and 30% will experience irreversible renal failure.[29] Even the use of modern, low osmolar contrast media has failed to significantly alter the incidence of progression to renal insufficiency in such a situation.[30] Newer imaging techniques are currently being introduced that may eliminate the need to use such dyes. Meanwhile, a consideration of underlying renal status is imperative prior to evaluative arteriography in the individual with diabetic lower-extremity disease. Provisions for treating both acute and chronic renal failure must be made prior to use of contrast dye in these patients.

The presence of autonomic neuropathy is both a poor prognostic indicator and a potentially complicating factor in the inpatient management of the individual with diabetes. Three-year mortality has been found to be 50% in this population.[31] Autonomic neuropathy may contribute to the pathogenesis of lower-extremity disease as a result of either anhydrosis or vasomotor disturbances in the feet. Acute complications in the inpatient setting due to autonomic neuropathy may include hypoglycemic unawareness, the acute development of a neurogenic bladder and urinary retention, and profound difficulty in glucose control resulting from gastroparesis diabetocorum. In addition, the presence of orthostatic hypotension will have its most profound manifestation in the individual who has been maintained at bed rest either postoperatively or in an effort to prevent weight-bearing on an injured lower extremity. Efforts for early mobilization postoperatively may be hampered by the absence of postural accommodations and subsequent hypotension in the individual with diabetic autonomic neuropathy.

The presence of coronary disease must be considered in anyone with long-standing diabetes mellitus. Even in the absence of typical angina, individuals with diabetes may have significant coronary artery disease complicating acute illness. Preoperative evaluation of underlying cardiac function is imperative with close follow-up care, and aggressive intervention is indicated in the presence of abnormalities.

EDUCATION

Hospitalization provides the opportunity for aggressive educational intervention for patients with diabetic lower-extremity disease. Lower-extremity disease occurs due to the interplay of trauma, neuropathy, altered biomechanics, vascular insufficiency, and infection. Treatment of any apparent infection, ulceration, or vascular insufficiency is primary in the acute care setting, but it fails to alter the underlying pathophysiology that resulted in the ulceration in the first place. This has been underscored by the high prevalence of lesions in the contralateral leg following amputation for diabetic lower-extremity disease and the ultimate contralateral amputation in 50% of cases.[32] Appropriate intervention to correct biomechanics, improve foot care, and perhaps revascularize the lower extremity is critically important to reduce recurrent disease.[33]

Diabetic foot disease results in hospitalization more often than any other diabetic complication,[34] with 16% of all hospital admissions and 23% of total hospital days attributable to foot disease.[35] Current medical practice patterns fall short of the standards of foot care adopted by the American Diabetes Association.[36] Meeting these standards of care and reducing risk factors for amputation have been projected to yield a 50% reduction in amputations within the diabetic population.[37] Meeting these standards and achieving the desired goal is best accomplished by use of a multidisciplinary team of health-care professionals who can provide both acute care for diabetes and its complications. Instruction in self-management techniques and preventive measures (such as the use of orthotic devices or specialized shoes) to prevent recurrence or progression of diabetic lower-extremity disease will also help reduce the number of amputations. Health-care professionals who provide specialized foot care can reduce the incidence of both major amputations and minor operations. Such strategies reduce both the need and the duration of inpatient management.[38]

REFERENCES

1. Leahy JL, Bonner-Weir S, Weir GC: B-cell dysfunction induced by chronic hyperglycemia, *Diabetes Care* 15:442–455, 1992.
2. Muller WA, Faloona GR, Unger RH: Hyperglucagonemia in diabetic ketoacidosis. Its prevalence and significance, *Am J Med* 54:52–57, 1973.
3. West KM: *Epidemiology of diabetes and its vascular lesions,* New York, 1978, Elsevier.
4. Keen H, Jarrett R, editors: *Complications of diabetes,* London, 1975, Edward Arnold.
5. Service FJ et al: Near normo-glycemia improves nerve conduction and vibration sensation in diabetic neuropathy, *Diabetologia* 28:722–727, 1985.
6. Rayfield EJ et al: Infection and diabetes: the case for glucose control, *Am J Med* 72:439–450, 1982.
7. Mowat AG, Baum J: Chemotaxis of polymorphonuclearleukocytes from patients with diabetes mellitus, *N Engl J Med* 284:621–627, 1971.
8. Bagdade JD, Stewart M, Walters E: Impaired granulocyte adherence: a reversible defect in host response in patients with poorly controlled diabetes, *Diabetes* 27:677–681, 1978.
9. Wierusz-Wysocka B et al: The influence of increasing glucose concentrations on selected functions of polymorphonuclear neutrophils, *Acta Diabetol Lat* 25:283–288, 1988.
10. Marhoffer et al: Impairment of polymorphonuclear leukocyte function in metabolic control of diabetes, *Diabetes Care* 15:256–260, 1992.
11. Rosenberg CS: Wound healing in the patient with diabetes mellitus, *Nurs Clin North Am* 25:247–261, 1990.
12. Weringer EJ et al: Effects of insulin on wound healing in diabetic mice, *Acta Endocrinol* 99:101, 1982.
13. Dunn JM: Local wound care in the diabetic, *Clin Podiatr Med Surg* 4:413–418, 1987.
14. Nolan CM, Beaty HN, Bagdade JD: Further characterization of the impaired bacteriocidal function of granulocytes in patients with poorly controlled diabetes, *Diabetes* 27:889–894, 1978.
15. American Diabetes Association: Bedside glucose monitoring in hospitals, *Diabetes Care* 9:89, 1986.
16. American Diabetes Association: Position statement on urine glucose and ketone determinations, *Diabetes Care* 14(suppl 2):39–40, 1991.
17. Larsen ML, Horder M, Mogensen EF: Effect of long-term monitoring of glycosylated hemoglobin levels in IDDM, *N Engl J Med* 323:1021–1025, 1990.

18. Boden G et al: Monitoring metabolic control in diabetic outpatients with glycosylated Hgb, *Ann Intern Med* 92:357–360, 1980.

19. Schade DS et al: Intensive insulin therapy, *Princeton: Excerpta Medica,* 1983, pp 194–223.

20. Shagan BP: Does anyone here know how to make insulin work backwards? Why sliding scale insulin coverage doesn't work, *Pract Diabetiolog* 9:1–4, 1990.

21. Holman RC, Herron CA, Sinnock P: Epidemiologic characteristics of mortality from diabetes with acidosis or coma, United States, 1970–1978, *Am J Public Health* 73:1169–1173, 1983.

22. Peters AL, Davidson MD: Acute complications of diabetes mellitus, *Int Med* 13:30–46, 1992.

23. Rossini AA, Hare JW: How to control the blood glucose level in the surgical diabetic patient, *Arch Surg* 111:945–949, 1976.

24. Alberti KGMM: Diabetes and surgery. In Rifkin H, Porte D, editors: *Diabetes mellitus theory and practice,* New York, 1990, Elsevier.

25. Watts NB et al: Postoperative management of diabetes mellitus: steady state glucose control with bedside algorithm for insulin adjustment, *Diabetes Care* 10:722–728, 1987.

26. Alberti KGMM, Gill GV, Elliott MJ: Insulin delivery during surgery in the diabetic patient, *Diabetes Care* 5(suppl 1): 65–76, 1982.

27. Bild DE et al: Lower extremity amputation in people with diabetes epidemiology and prevention, *Diabetes Care* 12:24–31, 1989.

28. Gay EC et al: Smokers with IDDM experience excess morbidity, *Diabetes Care* 15:947–952, 1992.

29. Harkonen S, Kjellstrand CM: Exacerbation of diabetic renal failure following intravenous pyelography, *Am J Med* 63:939–946, 1977.

30. Schwab SJ et al: Contrast nephrotoxicity: a randomized controlled trial of nonionic and an ionic radiographic contrast agent, *N Engl J Med* 320:149–153, 1989.

31. Ewing DJ, Campbell IW, Clarke BF: The natural history of diabetic autonomic neuropathy, *Q J Med* 49:95–108, 1980.

32. Goldner MG: The fate of the second leg in the diabetic amputee, *Diabetes* 9:100–103, 1960.

33. Larsen K, Christiansen JS, Ebskov B: Prevention and treatment of ulcerations of the foot in unilaterally amputated diabetic patients, *Acta Orthop Scand* 53:481–485, 1982.

34. Gibbons G, Eliopolis G: Infection of the diabetic foot. In Kozak G, editor: *Management of diabetic foot problems,* Philadelphia, 1984, WB Saunders.

35. Smith D, Weinberger M, Katz B: A controlled trial to increase office visits and reduce hospitalizations of diabetic patients, *J Gen Int Med* 2:232–38, 1987.

36. American Diabetes Association: Foot care in patients with diabetes mellitus, *Diabetes Care* 14(suppl 2):18–19, 1991.

37. National Diabetes Advisory Board: The prevention and treatment of five complications of diabetes: a guide for primary care practitioners. HHS Publication No. 83–8392, Atlanta, 1983, Centers for Disease Control.

38. Edmonds ME et al: Improved survival of the diabetic foot: the role of the specialized foot clinic, *Q J Med* 232:763–771, 1986.

15 _____ Microbiology and Antimicrobial Therapy of Diabetic Foot Infections

Patricia Herrera, M.D.

Paul O'Keefe, M.D.

The management of diabetic foot infections requires systemic antimicrobial therapy, in addition to surgery. Faced with an enormous array of antibiotics, clinicians must be familiar with the microorganisms involved in foot infections and the spectrum of the available drugs. Numerous reports have detailed the typical flora contained in foot infections. These reports emphasize the mixed nature of the infections with less attention given to the clinical features of the various types of infections. Bacteriologic results are not correlated with the clinical infection type. We will present a simple approach that will allow clinicians to predict the patients who have infections caused by a single pathogen versus infections with the more complex mixed flora.

This chapter will be organized into sections. The first will present the clinical approach noted above. The discussion will include a review of the typical bacteriology of single pathogen and then mixed infections. A second section will cover the aspects of specimen collection and transport. Finally, we will discuss the antimicrobial agents with emphasis given to those agents that are useful to treat foot infections in diabetics.

CLINICAL APPROACH TO AND MICROBIOLOGY OF DIABETIC FOOT INFECTIONS: CELLULITIS AND MIXED INFECTIONS

Careful examination of a diabetic patient with a foot infection will often provide clues about the microbial organisms causing the infection. Foot infections can present as cellulitis, gangrene, rapidly progressing necrotizing cellulitis, with or without fasciitis, or osteomyelitis. Signs indicative of infection such as warmth, erythema, and swelling are often seen. Tenderness is not a good indicator of infection in diabetics because the frequent coexistent neuropathy precludes the sensation of pain even if there is significant inflammation. When present, ulcers should be thoroughly evaluated for the existence of sinus tracts. Gas produced by anaerobic organisms may be noted by the presence of crepitus as the gas moves through the tissue when pressure is applied. It is also important to look for evidence of tinea pedis, which can cause mild skin breakdown and thus serve as the point of origin for a foot infection.

Cellulitis.—Uncomplicated or simple cellulitis is a soft-tissue infection in which there is no obvious portal of entry such as an ulcer or ischemic toe. Fever and pain are often present, and the affected area is warm, erythematous, and sometimes tender. Erysipelas is a specific type of cellulitis caused by *Streptococcus pyogenes* (group A streptococcus). It is characterized by bright red erythema and a palpable border of induration demarcating involved tissue from uninvolved tissue.

Case 1

A 45-year-old man with a five-year history of diet-controlled diabetes presents with a history of fever and pain in the left foot and leg for one day. He noted pain on the dorsum of his foot in the afternoon of the preceding day. That evening the area was red when he removed his shoe. The following morning when he felt feverish and noted that the red area had spread to just above the ankle, he came to his physician's office. On examination his temperature was 39° C. The dorsum of the foot was bright red with a palpable, well-demarcated border just above the ankle. There were no ulcers or open lesions on the foot, the pulses were good, and sensation was intact. A Gram stain of a sample aspirated from the erythematous border after injection of saline disclosed few polymorphonuclear leukocytes and chains of gram-positive cocci.

This patient has erysipelas. As mentioned previously, this infection is usually caused by group A streptococcus. With this and other types of simple cellulitis, infection is usually caused by a single organism. In most patients, gram-positive cocci, especially group A streptococci and *Staphylococcus aureus* cause cellulitis. In diabetics with lower-extremity infections, *Staphylococcus aureus* and coagulase negative staphylococci are isolated in approximately two thirds of patients in whom only a single organism is isolated.[1] Diabetic patients have a higher rate of colonization of the anterior nares and associated skin colonization with *Staphylococcus aureus*.[2] It has been postulated that

this increased rate of colonization is a likely factor that predisposes diabetics to infections with this organism. Of the other gram-positive cocci, group A streptococcus is the most common cause of cellulitis, but other β-hemolytic streptococci including groups B, C, and G are occasionally found.[3] Rare causes of cellulitis include *Streptococcus pneumoniae,* enteric gram-negative bacilli (*E. coli,* serratia, proteus), and *Pseudomonas aeruginosa.*

Cellulitis may advance rapidly but more often presents as an indolent local infection that may slowly spread to contiguous structures. If not effectively treated, it may involve deeper structures including tendons, joint capsules, and bone.[1]

The cause of cellulitis may be determined from blood cultures or from material aspirated from the subcutaneous tissues under the advancing border or leading edge of the erythema. This procedure is accomplished with a syringe containing 1 cc of nonbacteriostatic saline and an 18- or 20-gauge needle. The saline is injected into the subcutaneous tissue, and the tissue fluid is aspirated back into the syringe. The syringe is sent to the microbiology laboratory where the few drops can be divided for gram stain and culture. Yield from this procedure varies in published reports but is often quite low. One study recovered organisms in only 5% of patients.[4] Uman and Kumin, however, isolated an organism from all seven of the patients on whom they attempted the procedure.[5] Others report recovery rates between these two extremes.[6-8] Swab cultures from the surface are not useful. Occasionally, fluid will weep from the surface or broken vesicles, or bullae will be encountered. Here again, cultures are not useful because the moist surfaces will be colonized with organisms other than the true pathogen. Even with aggressive attempts to determine the cause of simple cellulitis, recovery of organisms has been disappointing. Combining blood cultures, leading-edge aspirates, and skin biopsies, one prospective study documented recovery of a pathogen in less than one third of cases.[9]

Managing cellulitis consists of immobilization, elevation of the foot, and appropriate antibiotics. Only lesions characterized by rapid spread, tense or hard swelling, necrosis of tissue, or extreme toxicity require surgical debridement. In these situations, surgical decompression and debridement of necrotic tissue may be lifesaving. Given the low yield of cultures in simple cellulitis, antimicrobial therapy is often empiric and is based on predicted bacteriology of these single pathogen infections. We would recommend initiation of therapy with a β-Lactam or other antibiotic with activity against gram-positive cocci including *Staphylococcus aureus*. Specific antibiotic therapy will be discussed in a later section.

Mixed Infections.—Whereas simple cellulitis is usually caused by a single pathogen, the mixed infections, as the term implies, are caused by several organisms. Because of the more complex microflora, they must be recognized so that antimicrobial therapy aimed at several different pathogens can be selected.

The hallmark of the mixed infection in a diabetic foot is the presence of an open lesion, usually a trophic ulcer, or an area of ischemic necrosis or gangrene that precedes the infection. The infection begins in the area of the lesion, is usually characterized by erythema and the appearance of foul-smelling drainage, and often progresses slowly. However, when the infection reaches the deeper tissue spaces with accumulation of pus, rapid spread and extreme systemic toxicity may develop.

Other features of mixed infections are necrosis of the soft tissues and invasion of bone. Thus surgical debridement—often extensive—is required in almost all of the cases.

Case 2

A 75-year-old man with a 20-year history of insulin-dependent diabetes mellitus was admitted to the Foot Service with swelling, erythema, and pain in the right foot. For several years he had had a plantar ulcer over the first right metatarsal head, which was managed with monthly debridement of callus and a shoe that redistributed foot pressure. Three months before, he had undergone a triple coronary bypass complicated by a sternal wound infection requiring 4 weeks of postoperative hospitalization. He was sent to a rehabilitation facility where he was up and walking, but his foot care was neglected. One week before admission he noted a foul smell from the foot, and 2 days before admission the dorsum of the foot became red and swollen. He had a shaking chill on the morning of admission and felt feverish. When examined, his temperature was 39.5° C, pulse was 98, and blood pressure was 160/90. The foot was bright red to the ankle. The forefoot was swollen and fluctuant, and pus dripped from the ulcer when pressure was applied to the dorsum of the foot. An x-ray examination of the foot disclosed soft tissue swelling of the entire forefoot, small bubbles of gas, and erosion of the heads of the first and second metatarsals. Gram stain of the pus obtained by aspiration from the pus-filled space yielded gram-positive cocci in chains and clusters, gram-positive rods, and at least three different morphologies of gram-negative rods. Blood cultures grew group B streptococcus.

This patient has a mixed infection characterized by a preexisting trophic ulcer, indolent onset with foul smell as the only noted sign, but development of rapid spread and toxicity. Gram stain suggests a mixed infection with both fecal flora and staphylococcus species. The x-ray documents the presence of bone erosion, which indicates that the infection has been present for enough time to invade and destroy bone before it became apparent to the patient or his caretakers. The clinical signs and presentation of these mixed infections have been detailed in previous chapters. Surgical management has also been discussed. A summary of the studies detailing the bacteriology of these infections follows.

Numerous reports have documented the polymicrobial nature of this infection. It should be stated that the published reports, detailing the bacteriology of diabetic foot infection, have emphasized the more chronic, complex infections complicating ulcer or ischemia. Simple cellulitis, usually caused by a single organism does not provide an accessible source of material for culture and is usually not included in these published studies.

In an early report from investigators known for meticulous bacteriologic technique, Louie et al[10] described the microbiology of 20 diabetic foot ulcers. The ulcers were cultured after debridement and scraping. The investigators found an average of 5.8 organisms per specimen. They cultured anaerobic bacteria from 19 of the 20 foot ulcers. The most frequently isolated anaerobes in their study were bacteroides species and peptococci. The predominant aerobic and facultative bacteria were proteus species, enterococci, *Staphylococcus aureus,* and *E. coli.* The high isolation rate of *Bacteroides fragilis* in Louie's study, when compared with reports published later, may reflect the anaerobic taxonomy prevalent at the time. Since then, many bacteroides have been reclassified to different species and some have even moved to different genera.[11]

A more recent study by Wheat et al[12] provides results of cultures from 54 diabetic foot infections. The most commonly isolated organisms in these mixed infections include *Staphylococcus aureus,* coagulase negative staphylococci, enterococci, and a variety of enterobacteriaceae. The more commonly isolated anaerobes were peptostreptococcus species and bacteroides species.

Sapico et al[13] reports on the microbiologic results of 32 infected diabetic feet. Although they isolated only aerobes in six patients and only anaerobes in one patient they noted that most of the infections were indeed polymicrobial with aerobic and anaerobic organisms involved. They found 4 to 8 species in each patient. The most frequently isolated organisms were bacteroides species, anaerobic streptococci, group D streptococci, clostridium species, and proteus species.

Yet another study by Borrero and Rossini evaluated the bacteriology of 100 consecutive diabetic foot infections.[14] Deep-tissue cultures revealed 301 aerobes and 240 anaerobes. A mean of five bacterial isolates was obtained with an average of three aerobes and two anaerobes per culture. The more commonly isolated organisms in this study included group D streptococci, coagulase negative staphylococci, *Proteus mirabilis, Peptococcus magnus,* and bacteroides species.

Besides the more commonly isolated organisms, one may also encounter unusual organisms that cause diabetic foot infections. Konugres, Goldstein, and Wallace describe three cases in which *Eikenella corrodens,* as part of mixed cultures, was one of the causes of osteomyelitis in diabetic foot infections.[15] *Eikenella corrodens* is a facultative gram-negative rod usually found in the mouth and upper respiratory tract. The organism is slow growing. Infections with this pathogen follow an indolent course. In addition, direct extension to adjacent bone is frequently seen. *Eikenella corrodens* is usually sensitive to ampicillin, penicillin, and second and third generation cephalosporins.[16,17]

Many other reports document the polymicrobial nature of this infection. The results of the studies previously described are summarized in Table 15–1. Note that certain organisms occur with some predictable frequency, and thus should be included when deciding on antimicrobial therapy until culture results are available. Among the gram-positive cocci, aero-

TABLE 15–1.

Bacteriology of Mixed Diabetic Foot Infections: Summary of Isolates From Four Studies

Study Number of cultures	Wheat 54	Louie 20	Sapico 32	Borrero 100
Aerobes				
Staphylococcus aureus	20	7	8	33
Coagulase negative staphylococcus	17	6	3	30
Group B streptococcus	11		5	25
Enterococcus	15	9	13	45
Other aerobic streptococci	12	7	8	15
Proteus sp	12	11	10	56
E. coli	5	6	5	33
Klebsiella sp	6	4	4	24
Pseudomonas aeruginosa	4	4	55	
Other gram negative bacilli	13	4	17	30
Anaerobes				
Bacteroides fragilis	2	9	6	51
Other bacteroides sp	15	8	16	52
Anaerobic streptococci	30	2	8	22
Clostridium sp	3	7	11	18

bic streptococci, especially group B streptococcus, enterococci, and other group D streptococci, *Staphylococcus aureus* and coagulase-negative staphylococci are all frequently isolated. The aerobic and facultative gram-negative bacilli include *Proteus mirabilis, E. coli,* and less commonly pseudomonas species. Important anaerobes include the anaerobic streptococci, fecal bacteroides species, and a large number of species of clostridium. In general, empiric therapy should cover these previously mentioned organisms until cultures have returned. Suggestions for therapeutic regimens will follow in a later section (Table 15–2).

As mentioned earlier, gas produced by anaerobic organisms may be noted by the presence of crepitus on physical examination. When gas production is noted in the evaluation of a soft tissue infection in a diabetic patient, one need not assume that the patient has gas gangrene or even that the gas is produced by clostridial species. Gas gangrene is a medical and surgical emergency associated with extreme systemic toxicity and rapid development of hemolytic anemia and jaundice. It requires immediate and extensive debridement. It can be diagnosed by observing the large gram-positive rods on gram stain of a specimen obtained by needle aspiration of the involved tissue.

Other infections associated with soft-tissue gas may be either indolent or rapidly progressive. The latter may also be associated with severe systemic toxicity and require urgent surgical debridement. When either indolent or rapidly progressive infections are caused by gas-forming bacteria, a gram stain of a needle-aspirated specimen will immediately help determine if gas gangrene is present and whether or not the infection is mixed. It is imperative to diagnose these infections correctly because their treatment and prognosis differ greatly. The other anaerobic organisms that have been associated with soft tissue gas on physical examination or x-ray include peptostreptococci, peptococci, and bacteroides species.[18,19] In addition, gas production has been observed in infections with aerobic organisms. *E. coli* and other facultative bacteria have been associated with gas production.[20]

Air may also be noted in the absence of gas-forming organisms when there is

TABLE 15–2.

Antimicrobial Regimens for Cellulitis and Mixed Diabetic Foot Infections

	Mild	Moderate/Severe
Cellulitis (Single organism)	Cephalexin Dicloxacillin	Cefazolin Oxacillin Nafcillin If penicillin-allergic: erythromycin clindamycin
Mixed	Augmentin Ciprofloxacin (+/−Metronidazole)	Single drug therapy: Unasyn cefoxitin cefotetan ceftizoxime timentin imipenem
Mixed		Combination therapy or penicillin allergy: clindamycin or metronidazole and aminoglycoside aminoglycoside not indicated: clindamycin or metronidazole and aztreonam enterococcus isolated: add ampicillin or vancomycin

an ulcer with a sinus tract reaching the deeper tissues, after surgery with entrapped air, or when there is an open wound. In these settings ambient air has entered either through the sinus opening or as a result of the surgery.

SPECIMEN COLLECTION AND TRANSPORT

Collecting, transporting, and laboratory processing of specimens are critical to the selection of proper antibiotics in the treatment of diabetic foot infections. Several methods for obtaining specimens have been advocated. These include swab cultures, needle aspiration, curettage, and deep-tissue cultures.

The technique for aspiration of the leading edge of a simple cellulitis using nonbacteriostatic saline has been described. Aspiration of pyogenic and other deep-tissue infections, especially those in-

volving gas, is very useful and has a significantly higher yield than leading-edge aspirates. The aspiration should be done through intact skin that has been cleaned and disinfected with isopropyl alcohol or povidone iodine rather than through the heavily colonized open lesion or sinus tract. The needle should be directed toward areas of crepitus or fluctuance, but even a blind puncture into the center of an infected area may often yield sufficient material for culture. Any liquid or pus should be left in the syringe. After the needle has been removed or its tip placed within a rubber stopper, the syringe should be sent to the microbiology laboratory for gram stain and culture. Be careful about needlestick injuries if this technique is used. If the air has been expelled from the syringe, anaerobes will survive in the capped syringe for a prolonged period of time.[21] A specimen of pus in a capped syringe is the most reliable specimen for recovery of anaerobic bacteria from purulent material. We suggest that a protocol for collecting and transporting specimens be developed in conjunction with the microbiology laboratory.

Specimens obtained by curettage are more sensitive and specific than swab specimens. First the surface is decontaminated with a saline-soaked gauze followed by povidone-iodine or isopropyl alcohol. Then the superficial exudate is debrided using sterile instruments. With a scalpel blade, tissue from the base and edges of the ulcer should be scraped, and these specimens are then submitted for culture.[1] Sapico et al[13] note that cultures obtained by curettage of the base of the ulcer correlate better with results of deep tissue culture than those obtained by needle aspiration or swabs of the ulcers.

Bony specimens should be submitted for culture at the time of surgical debridement. Care should be taken to avoid sampling bone that is in contact with the ulcerated area and thus may be contaminated. On the other hand, one should choose bone that appears infected, rather than healthy-appearing bone, to ensure that the culture result is representative of the bone infection. In the presence of adjacent soft tissue infection, it is difficult to obtain a specimen of bone that does not contact the surrounding pus.[12] Although not all components of the infected soft tissue may be present in bone, the bone and soft tissue are part of the same infectious process. When planning therapy, we would recommend that all isolates from the bone specimen be considered.

Deep-tissue cultures are most effectively obtained at the time of open surgical debridement. To avoid contamination of the culture, collect specimens of pus, infected tissue, or bone that have been uncovered during the dissection, rather than specimens in contact with the external environment. Amputated tissue that is not contiguous with open lesions or sinus tracts is also excellent for culture and useful if postoperative antibiotic ther-

apy to treat the residual infection is necessary.

Swab cultures obtained from the surface of an ulceration are unreliable. The surface is heavily colonized with many species of bacteria that may or may not be present in the deeper, infected tissue. Thus the culture results include the colonizers with or without the true pathogens. Superficial culture results have been found to be identical to deep specimens in only 20% of the cases.[12,22]

Regardless of the type of specimen submitted, it should be transported as rapidly as possible to ensure the highest yield of anaerobic microorganisms. When exposed to oxygen, many anaerobes rapidly lose viability and will not be recovered from cultures.

In settings where the syringe itself cannot be used to transport the specimen, specialized transport systems must be used. For liquid specimens or swabs, tubes fitted with tight rubber stoppers and containing oxygen-free gas, and often a small amount of soft agar in the bottom, are used. Prereduced, anaerobically sterilized (PRAS) transport medium is preferable. For low-volume liquid specimens (less than 2 mL) a small volume of nonnutritive broth with an anaerobic indicator will allow easier retrieval of the specimen from the tube. For larger volumes, the oxygen-free tube without the broth can be used.[21]

Specimens on a swab are inferior to liquid or tissue specimens because of lower bacterial yield. With certain cultures, liquid or tissue is not available and a swab must be used. For anaerobic cultures, only commercially available, oxygen-free swabs should be used. If a specimen is obtained on a swab, it should immediately be placed into an anaerobic transport system. The Hungate stopper consisting of a rubber diaphragm within a plastic screw cap can be used for swab specimens by removing the screw cap, inserting the swab into the semisolid media located in the bottom of the tube, and tightly replacing the cap. Using the same tube, aspirated liquid specimens can be injected through the diaphragm. Again, air must be expelled from the syringe before injecting into the medium-containing tube.

Swabs are also problematic because they desiccate, causing bacteria to adhere to the cotton, thereby decreasing the yield of bacteria. In the microbiology laboratory, some of the trapped bacteria can be liberated if the swab is first moistened with prereduced broth prior to inoculation of culture plates. If possible this should be done in an anaerobic environment.

Our institution uses the BBL Port-A-Cul specimen collection and transport products (BBL Microbiology Systems; Cockeysville, Md.). The Port-A-Cul tubes and vials contain a reduced transport medium that helps maintain anaerobiosis. Agar in the medium inhibits the diffusion of oxygen after a specimen on a swab has been inserted. The system includes a resazurin indicator to signify the presence of oxygen in the medium. If the indicator remains colorless, laboratory personnel can determine that the anaerobic environment has been maintained. With swab specimens the screw cap is removed and the swab is inserted into the soft agar medium to approximately 5 mm from the bottom of the tube. The shaft of one swab is broken, after which the cap is quickly replaced and tightened.

The Port-A-Cul vials can be used for liquid specimens. These vials should remain closed at all times. A rubber stopper is exposed by removing the central portion of the aluminum cap. The stopper is disinfected and any air is expelled from the syringe and needle. The needle is then pushed through the stopper and the liquid slowly injected on top of the agar. The specimen should then be taken to the laboratory in a timely fashion.

Anaerobic cultures of tissue specimens are best collected in oxygen-free transport tubes or vials containing PRAS

media to keep the tissue moist. Larger tissue specimens should be placed in sterile Petri dishes or specimen containers. The Petri dish or container should contain gauze dampened with sterile nonbacteriostatic saline to prevent desiccation. The cover should be left loose to allow gas exchange when placed in an anaerobic environment. The container should then be placed into a commercially available pouch containing a gas mixture containing hydrogen which will quickly generate an oxygen-free environment.[21]

In the absence of a tissue-transport system such as the one described previously, tissue or bone specimens should be placed in sterile containers. The container should be brought directly to the microbiology laboratory and the specimen processed immediately in an anaerobic environment.

Obtaining cultures for aerobic processing only is less difficult because there is no need to avoid oxygen. Samples can be obtained on swabs or by aspiration. It is best to hand deliver specimens to the microbiology laboratory to obtain results more efficiently and rapidly and thus significantly impact patient care.

OSTEOMYELITIS

Osteomyelitis can be either an acute or chronic infection of bone. It may be secondary to a hematogenous infection, to a contiguous focus of infection, or to peripheral vascular disease. Osteomyelitis secondary to a contiguous focus of infection is the most common type and occurs as a complication of infected diabetic foot ulcers—particularly if peripheral neuropathy is present. Early diagnosis of this condition is imperative if favorable outcome of therapy is expected.

The course of osteomyelitis secondary to a contiguous focus of infection is usually indolent. Although low-grade fever and local inflammation may be present, these findings are often absent. Therefore the diagnosis may not be readily apparent.

Diagnosis of Osteomyelitis.—The diagnosis of osteomyelitis is made on the basis of appearance on imaging procedures or by histologic analysis and culture of a specimen of bone. Although several imaging procedures are available to help diagnose osteomyelitis, each has certain limitations.

A bone infection is characterized by local bony destruction and new bone formation. On x-ray, patchy bone destruction along with periosteal reaction and ill-defined bone margins may be noted. The patchy bone destruction is also seen with osteopathy, roentgenological changes commonly seen in feet of patients with neuropathy. However, that seen in osteopathy tends to involve the bone diffusely whereas destructive changes of osteomyelitis are usually focal and limited to the area under the infected surface. Furthermore, the lytic bone lesion that characterizes x-rays of osteomyelitis is not apparent until approximately 30% to 50% of the bone mineral has been removed,[23] and thus bone x-rays are insensitive in the diagnosis of early osteomyelitis.

Computed tomography (CT) may be useful in noting bony changes in osteomyelitis. Its utility is limited to certain bones such as the sternum and the long bones. In the foot the sensitivity of the CT scan is limited because of the small amount of soft tissue adjacent to the bone.[24]

The three-phase technetium bone scan has a sensitivity of 70% to 100% in aiding the diagnosis of osteomyelitis.[25] Typically the late-phase scan shows increased uptake localized to the infected bone. Limitations of this technique include its dependence on adequate blood flow to demonstrate the increased uptake—a condition often absent in the lower extremities of diabetics.

Leukocytes taken from the patient, la-beled with Indium-111 and reinjected, have been shown to localize to areas of infection. This test has been evaluated in osteomyelitis and has shown promise in diabetics. Some authors have raised concern about the difficulty in distinguishing infection in bone from infection in adjacent soft tissue. One widely quoted study evaluating several techniques in the diagnosis of osteomyelitis in diabetic feet showed the 24 hour Indium-111 labeled leukocyte scan to be the most sensitive when compared with a plain x-ray, triple-phase bone scan, and 4-hour leukocyte scan.[26]

A variation of the Indium-111 labeled leukocyte scan is the newer procedure using Indium-111 labeled immunoglobulin. Use of Indium-111 labeled immunoglobulin in the diagnosis of infections was first described in 1988.[27] Using immunoglobulin instead of labeled leukocytes simplifies the otherwise tedious and time-consuming techniques required for WBC labeling.[28] In initial studies, labeled immunoglobulin was used to diagnose soft tissue, intraabdominal, and vascular infections.[29,30] In 1990, Oyen et al used this technique to detect bone and joint infections.[31] They studied 29 bone and joint infections in 25 patients. Indium-111 immunoglobulin G identified all 29 acute and chronic sites of infection. The investigators commented that both the site and the extent of infection can be evaluated with this technique.

Microbiology of Osteomyelitis.— Definitive identification of the cause is made by percutaneous needle biopsy or open biopsy of the suspected bone. The specimens of bone should be sent for histological analysis and culture.

More than one organism is usually recovered from osteomyelitis secondary to a contiguous focus of infection, reflecting the polymicrobial nature of these infections. *Staphylococcus aureus* is frequently found as are coagulase-negative staphylococci. The latter are often pathogenic in postsurgical infections. Gram-negative bacilli including proteus, pseudomonas, and klebsiella are also commonly found in these mixed infections. The role of anaerobic bacteria as a cause of osteomyelitis in the foot of diabetics is less well established, perhaps because detailed bacteriology from these lesions has not been published. On the other hand, the importance of anaerobes in other types of osteomyelitis is well established.[32] We believe that anaerobes are as important in osteomyelitis as they are in the diabetic foot infections that are limited to the soft tissues. However, the literature is lacking in this area. Proper collection, transport, and culture of specimens of bone obtained from these lesions must include procedures allowing recovery of these fastidious pathogens.

Therapy of Diabetic Osteomyelitis.—Following diagnostic evaluation including biopsy of suspected osteomyelitis in the diabetic foot, complete surgical debridement of necrotic bone and soft tissue should be undertaken. The importance of surgical intervention in the therapy of osteomyelitis must be stressed given the futility of medical therapy in the presence of gangrene or severe ischemia. Poor blood flow limits delivery of systemically administered antibiotics to the site of infection but also may limit wound healing after debridement. Thus the preoperative evaluation of blood flow as described in other chapters of this book is also emphasized.

After debridement, antibiotic therapy should be started. Choice of antibiotics can be guided by gram stain and culture results. Although most experts recommend 4 weeks of intravenous antibiotics or 4 to 8 weeks of intravenous followed by oral antibiotics for acute or chronic osteomyelitis respectively, opinions on duration of therapy or route of administration are quite variable and consensus is lacking. Numerous regimens have been used with variable success. In patients with chronic osteomyelitis not necessarily involving the foot, Black et al evaluated treatment with short-course intravenous antibiotics (mean duration of intravenous therapy 3.6 days) followed by oral therapy (mean 43 days). They noted that 18 of 21 patients had no clinical signs of recurrence.[33]

Other studies have evaluated oral therapy alone in the treatment of acute and chronic osteomyelitis. Ciprofloxacin has been one of the most frequently studied orally administered drugs. Giamarellou et al studied samples of bone to determine the achievable levels of ciprofloxacin.[34] They found that mean levels in bone exceeded 1 μg/mL when a dose of 750 mg was given to patients with osteomyelitis. Gentry and Rodriguez reported on 31 patients treated with oral ciprofloxacin compared to 28 patients treated with systemic broad spectrum antibiotics. They noted a 33% failure rate in the ciprofloxacin group whereas 31% in the intravenous group failed therapy.[35]

In another report, Gentry et al compared an oral medication, ofloxacin, with parenterally administered cefazolin or ceftazidime. Successful responses up to 18 months after completion of therapy were reported in 14 of 19 (74%) orally treated patients versus 12 of 14 (86%) patients treated parenterally.[36] These differences were not significant.

Although quinolones have been found to be successful in the therapy of osteomyelitis, relapse of infection has been noted. Dellamonica et al. followed 39 patients with chronic osteomyelitis who were treated with either pefloxacin, ofloxacin, or ciprofloxacin. Duration of therapy ranged from 3 to 6 months with follow up of 2 to 5 years. Organisms isolated included *Staphylococcus aureus, Staphylococcus epidermidis, E. coli* and *Pseudomonas aeruginosa.* Nine failures were noted, six of which were in infections caused by *Staphylococcus aureus*.[37] These reports emphasize the importance of long term follow-up after treatment of osteomyelitis.

Using antibiotic-impregnated cement or polymethyl-methacrylate beads in the therapy of osteomyelitis has been advocated by some authors.[38,39] Antibiotic-impregnated beads provide increased local concentration of the drugs along with slow continuous local delivery. The beads release 5% of the antibiotic within the first 24 hours. A sustained elution follows in which progressively decreasing amounts are released over weeks to months.[40] The beads are placed after, and not in place of, debridement and cannot be used as a substitute for necessary debridement or systemic antibiotics.

Several antibiotics have been incorporated into the beads. Heat-stable antibiotics should be used to withstand the exothermic reaction that occurs as the polymethylmethacrylate cement polymerizes. The antibiotics should also be highly water soluble so that rapid elution from the matrix will occur. Antibiotics that have been successfully used include the aminoglycosides: gentamycin and tobramycin; and vancomycin; erythromycin; and clindamycin.[41] Cephalosporins have also been used, but they do not withstand heat as well as the aminoglycosides and their long-term stability at room or body temperature is far less. They do diffuse well from the polymer. Penicillins are also unstable and are difficult to incorporate into the beads in large enough concentrations to achieve adequate levels.

These antibiotic-impregnated polymers have been used in the therapy of osteomyelitis complicating diabetic foot infections. After aggressive debridement the material is fashioned into the appropriate shape and placed into the debrided area where it serves as a spacer (Fig 15–1).[42] These materials cannot be used in wounds that are left open; there must be sufficient soft tissue to close the wound for

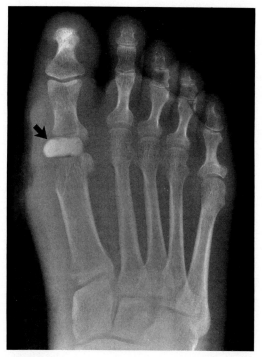

FIG 15–1.
Post operative x-ray of foot after debridement of 1st metatarsal head and proximal phalanx. *Arrow* points to antibiotic-containing polymethylmethacrylate spacer. (Courtesy of Rodney M. Stuck, D.P.M.)

the spacer to be effective. At times, however, a fibrinous granulomatous reaction develops and surrounds the antibiotic-containing polymer. This may limit the amount of antibiotic reaching the surrounding tissue (personal communication, Rodney M. Stuck, D.P.M.). Although antibiotic impregnated beads may have a role in the treatment of bone infections in the feet of diabetics, they cannot substitute for adequate debridement and systemic antimicrobial therapy.

ANTIMICROBIAL THERAPY OF DIABETIC FOOT INFECTION

Management of foot infection in the diabetic requires a comprehensive approach. With these infections, favorable outcome requires aggressive local care, appropriate antibiotics, and surgical intervention when needed. All aspects including optimal diabetic management and management of other underlying diseases including hypertension, heart disease, and particularly peripheral vascular disease will affect the outcome. Debridement of necrotic tissue, drainage of pus, and daily dressing changes will facilitate healing.

Antibiotic therapy should be based on predicted bacteriology while awaiting cultures. Gram stain of a deep-tissue specimen may help choose the initial therapy. It is important to realize, however, that the gram stain does have limitations. Unless results of the gram stain are unequivocal, such as might be seen with an abscess caused by *Staphylococcus aureus*, we recommend using other clinical features of the infection in addition to the gram stain to select empiric antibiotic therapy. Examples of these features include history of an open lesion, presence of odor, or gas in the tissue.

When treating a simple cellulitis in a diabetic, therapy should focus on gram-positive cocci, particularly *Staphylococcus aureus* and beta hemolytic streptococci. Oral therapy should be reserved for patients who are afebrile and have no signs of systemic toxicity, i.e., chills or hypotension. In addition, infection characterized by rapid spread and swelling, which may indicate underlying abscess, should be treated with parenteral drugs. First-generation cephalosporins such as cefazolin or cephalexin, or antistaphylococcal penicillins such as nafcillin, oxacillin, or dicloxacillin would be appropriate. Second- and third-generation cephalosporins are less active against staphylococci and streptococci. Therefore they should not be used for uncomplicated cellulitis.

In complicated foot infections, i.e., those originating from an ulcer, other types of open lesion or an ischemic foot, one must assume that the infection is mixed, containing both fecal bacteria and organisms from the skin. Thus a broad-spectrum antibiotic with activity against aerobic gram-negative bacilli, *Bacteroides fragilis* and staphylococci, or combination therapy should be selected. When results of cultures are available, the therapy can be altered to cover the specific isolates.

The choices for single-agent therapy of complicated foot infections include the β-Lactam/β-Lactamase inhibitor combinations, second- and third-generation cephalosporins with activity against anaerobes, and the very broad spectrum carbapenem, imipenem. Each of these choices will be discussed in the paragraphs that follow.

The β-Lactam/β-Lactamase inhibitor compounds combine a β-Lactam antibiotic such as ampicillin or ticarcillin with an inhibitor of the bacterial β-Lactamase enzyme such as clavulanic acid or sulbactam. β-Lactamases are enzymes that inactivate β-Lactam antibiotics such as penicillin, ampicillin, or ticarcillin. The inhibitor compounds irreversibly bind to the β-Lactamase enzyme so that it cannot inactivate the β-Lactam drug. There are numerous β-Lactamase enzymes produced by bacteria, but only certain of the β-Lactamases are inhibited by clavulanic acid or sulbactam. For example, the enzymes commonly produced by *Staphylococcus aureus, Klebsiella pneumoniae,* and *Bacteroides fragilis* are usually inhibited, whereas β-Lactamases produced by *Pseudomonas aeruginosa* and by hospital-acquired strains of enterobacter and serratia are not.[43]

The commercially available compounds include ampicillin + sulbactam, Unasyn, and ticarcillin + clavulanic acid, Timentin, both of which are formulated for parenteral use only. Amoxicillin + clavulanic acid, Augmentin, is available for oral use only. All three have good activity against gram-positive cocci including *Staphylococcus aureus* resistant to penicillin, but are not active against methicillin-resistant *Staphylo-*

coccus aureus or methicillin-resistant coagulase negative staphylococci. They inhibit many of the gram-negative β-Lactamases and are thus suitable in infections involving *E. coli*, klebsiella, and many proteus species. They have superior activity against anaerobes including *Bacteroides fragilis*. In treatment of infections with *Pseudomonas aeruginosa* and other gram-negative bacilli that produce β-Lactamases that are not inhibited, only ticarcillin + clavulanic acid that has intrinsic activity against these gram-negative pathogens should be used.

The choice of one of these agents as empiric therapy before culture results are available should take epidemiologic circumstances into account. Ampicillin + sulbactam can be used for new onset, untreated infections, whereas ticarcillin + clavulanic acid might be considered in previously treated patients or when the infection has developed in the hospital. In all cases, susceptibility results of the aerobic isolates should be reviewed and therapy changed if resistance is documented.

Of the cephalosporins, the second-generation agents, cefoxitin and cefotetan, and the third-generation drug, ceftizoxime, are most useful in mixed lower-extremity infections. All three are active against most organisms isolated from diabetic foot infections including aerobic gram-negative and gram-positive bacteria as well as the anaerobes including *Bacteroides fragilis*. Among the cephalosporins that have demonstrated efficacy when used as single agents in the treatment of diabetic foot infections, the largest experience has been with cefoxitin. It can be used as a single agent if pseudomonas and enterobacter species are not of concern. Cefotetan, another second-generation cephalosporin, has a similar activity profile as well as clinical experience.[44] Among the third-generation cephalosporins, only ceftizoxime has reliable activity against penicillin-resistant bacteroides species. It has superior activity against enteric gram-negative bacilli when compared with cefoxitin, but, like cefoxitin, it is not active against pseudomonas species.

None of the cephalosporins are active against enterococci in vitro. However, the clinical studies using cefoxitin, cefotetan, or ceftizoxime have documented successful treatment even when enterococcus is isolated.[45-47] We recommend that clinicians exercise caution when using these agents in the treatment of infections containing enterococci. If response is not adequate, repeat the cultures. If large numbers of enterococci are recovered in repeat culture, add ampicillin or vancomycin.

Imipenem, a carbapenem, has a very broad spectrum and covers all of the likely pathogens. It is expensive and should be used as a single agent only in patients who are seriously ill or have organisms recovered in culture that require its use. One must be aware that patients allergic to penicillin may be allergic to imipenem. Therefore do not use imipenem in penicillin-allergic patients. Higher doses of imipenem or the high blood levels seen in patients with renal insufficiency may predispose patients to develop seizures.[48]

Recently, oral therapy with fluoroquinolone antibiotics has been advocated for treatment of diabetic foot infections, including osteomyelitis. Ciprofloxacin, a quinolone carboxylic acid compound, has an extended spectrum of activity and good oral absorption. Peterson et al used oral ciprofloxacin to treat foot infections in 48 patients with peripheral vascular disease, 46 of whom had diabetes mellitus.[49] At 1 year follow-up, 60% were considered to have had a successful outcome in that they required neither continued antibiotic therapy nor amputation. Peterson et al. compared these results with those from a previous study comparing parenteral cefoxitin with ceftizoxime in which the 1-year successful outcome was 28% with cefoxitin and 36% with ceftizoxime and amputation rates were 44% and 36% respectively.[50] Paradoxically, ciprofloxacin lacks *in vitro* activity against anaerobic bacteria including *Bacteroides fragilis* yet has proved to be effective in this and other clinical trials. We would consider using ciprofloxacin in stable patients with mixed infections, even those containing anaerobic bacteria. However, high dosage, 750 mg twice daily, and close follow-up is mandatory. Adding oral metronidazole to ciprofloxacin will provide anaerobic coverage if physicians are particularly concerned about anaerobic bacteria or if the clinical response to ciprofloxacin is not adequate.

Another fluoroquinolone, ofloxacin, has also been evaluated in the treatment of foot infections in the diabetic. Although the numbers are small—12 patients studied of whom 6 had diabetes—favorable results were reported.[51] Tissue levels of ofloxacin were measured and shown to be satisfactory. More information with ofloxacin and other fluoroquinolones is necessary before these promising agents can be recommended.

Many physicians favor combination therapy in the treatment of mixed infections involving fecal anaerobes, especially in seriously ill patients. Also, in patients allergic to penicillins or cephalosporins, avoidance of β-Lactam/β-Lactamase inhibitor combinations, cephalosporins, and imipenem is advisable. The combination regimens typically combine an aminoglycoside such as gentamicin or tobramycin, which have excellent activity against aerobic gram-negative bacilli including *Pseudomonas aeruginosa,* with an antianaerobic drug such as clindamycin or metronidazole. These regimens effectively treat diabetic foot infections and are widely used. Nephrotoxcity occurs in up to 25% of aminoglycoside recipients although clinically significant nephrotoxicity is less frequent.[52] Thus renal function and blood levels must be monitored in patients receiving aminoglycosides, and dosage must be adjusted in patients with re-

nal insufficiency. Metronidazole and clindamycin are less toxic, but patients on clindamycin should be observed for diarrhea and colitis. Patients on clindamycin are more likely to experience *Clostridium difficile*-associated colitis with attack rates ranging from 1 in 10 to 1 in 10,000 patients treated when compared to patients on any other antibiotic.[53]

Two other compounds, vancomycin and aztreonam, are being frequently used as part of double- or triple-combination regimens in the treatment of mixed infections. Vancomycin is effective against nearly all aerobic and anaerobic gram-positive organisms. Its spectrum includes methicillin-resistant *Staphylococcus aureus* and methicillin-resistant coagulase-negative staphylococci, enterococci and clostridia species. It is sometimes added to the broad spectrum β-Lactam agents to cover methicillin-resistant staphylococci and enterococci or as a third agent to the aminoglycoside containing regimens for the aforementioned added coverage. Vancomycin is ototoxic and nephrotoxic, but its nephrotoxicity is less than that of the aminoglycosides. Vancomycin elimination is by the kidney, therefore, in patients with impaired renal function, dosage adjustment is imperative.

Aztreonam is the only β-Lactam antibiotic of the monobactam class that is commercially available. It is active against aerobic gram-negative bacilli including *Pseudomonas aeruginosa,* but it has no activity against gram-positive cocci or anaerobic bacteria. In combination regimens it has been substituted for aminoglycosides in patients at higher risk for nephrotoxicity, such as the elderly. Immunologic cross-reactivity between penicillins and aztreonam does not occur so that aztreonam can be used in penicillin-allergic patients.

The preceding information is summarized in the form of our recommendations (see Table 15–2). For simple cellulitis, therapy should cover *Staphylococcus aureus* and group A streptococcus. Mild infections can be treated with oral agents such as dicloxacillin or cephalexin. More serious infections should be treated parenterally either with nafcillin or oxacillin or with the first-generation cephalosporin, cefazolin. Penicillin-allergic patients can be treated with erythromycin or clindamycin.

For mixed infections, therapy should cover organisms associated with skin and fecal contamination. Mild infections can be treated with amoxicillin and clavulanic acid or ciprofloxacin with or without metronidazole added to the latter. Moderate to serious infections can be treated with single, broad-spectrum agents such as ampicillin and sulbactam, cefoxitin, cefotetan, ceftizoxime, ticarcillin and clavulanic acid or imipenem. Combination therapy with an aminoglycoside plus clindamycin or metronidazole is also recommended. Ampicillin or vancomycin might be added to either single or combination therapy to cover enterococci or methicillin-resistant staphylococci (vancomycin only). Finally, aztreonam may be substituted for the aminoglycoside in combination therapy when nephrotoxicity has occurred or is likely to occur. We must also emphasize that adequate surgical debridement is required for effective treatment in most mixed infections.

REFERENCES

1. Lipsky B, Pecoraro R, Wheat L: The diabetic foot. Soft tissue and bone infection, *Infect Dis Clin North Am* 4(3):409–432, 1990.
2. Jones EW et al: A microbiological study of diabetic foot lesions, *Diabetic Med* 2:213–215, 1984.
3. Baddour LM, Bisno AL: Non-group A beta-hemolytic streptococcal cellulitis. Association with venous and lymphatic compromise, *Am J Med* 79:155, 1985.
4. Goldgeier M: The microbial evaluation of acute cellulitis, *Cutis* 31:649–655, 1983.
5. Uman S, Kunin C: Needle aspiration in the diagnosis of soft tissue infections, *Arch Intern Med* 135:959–961, 1975.
6. Ginsberg M: Cellulitis: analysis of 101 cases and review of literature, *South Med J* 74:530–533, 1981.
7. Fleisher G, Ludwig S: Cellulitis: a prospective study, *Ann Emerg Med* 9:246–248, 1980.
8. Liles D, Dall L: Needle aspiration for diagnosis of cellulitis, *Cutis* 36:63–64, 1985.
9. Hook E et al: Microbiologic evaluation of cutaneous cellulitis in adults, *Arch Intern Med* 186:295–297, 1986.
10. Louie T et al: Aerobic and anaerobic bacteria in diabetic foot ulcers, *Ann Intern Med* 85:461–463, 1976.
11. Shah H, Collins D: Prevotella, a new genus to include bacteroides melaninogenicus and related species formerly classified in the genus bacteroides, *Int J System Bacteriol* 40(2):205–208, 1990.
12. Wheat L et al: Diabetic foot infections. Bacteriologic analysis, *Arch Intern Med* 146:1935–1940, 1986.
13. Sapico F et al: The infected foot of the diabetic patient: quantitative microbiology and analysis of clinical features, *Rev Infect Dis* 6:171–176, 1984.
14. Borrero E, Rossini M: Bacteriology of 100 consecutive diabetic foot infections and in vitro susceptibility to ampicillin/sulbactam versus cefoxitin, *J Vasc Dis* 16:357–361, 1992.
15. Konugres G, Goldstein E, Wallace S. Eikenella corrodens as a cause of osteomyelitis in the feet of diabetic patients. *J Bone Joint Surg* 69:940–941, 1987.
16. Goldstein EJ et al: Susceptibility of Eikenella corrodens to newer and older quinolines, *Antimicrob Agents Chemother* 30:172–173, 1986.
17. Goldstein EJ, Gombert ME, Agyare EO: Susceptibility of Eikenella corrodens to newer beta-lactamase antibiotics, *Antimicrob Agents Chemother* 18:832–833, 1980.
18. Vo N, Watson S, Bryant L: Infections of the lower extremities due to gas forming and nongas-forming organisms, *South Med J* 79:1493–1495, 1986.
19. Wills M, Reece M: Non-clostridial gas in-

fections in diabetes mellitus, *Br Med J* 2:566–568, 1960.

20. Markantone S et al: Nonclostridial gas gangrene, *J Foot Surg* 28:213–216, 1989.

21. Edelstein M: Laboratory diagnosis of anaerobic infections in humans. In Finegold SM, editor: *Anaerobic infections in humans,* New York, 1989, Academic Press.

22. Sharp C, Bessman A, Wagner F: Microbiology of superficial and deep tissues in infected diabetic gangrene, *Surg Gynecol Obstet* 149:217–219, 1979.

23. Norden C: Osteomyelitis. In Mandell G, editor: *Principles and practice of infectious diseases,* ed 3, New York, 1990, Churchill Livingstone.

24. Azouz E: Computed tomography in bone and joint infections, *J Can Assoc Radiol* 32:102–106, 1981.

25. Handmaker H, Leonards R: The bone scan in inflammatory osseous disease, *Semin Nucl Med* 6:95–105, 1976.

26. Newman L et al: Unsuspected osteomyelitis in diabetic foot ulcers, *JAMA* 266(9):1246–1251, 1991.

27. Fischman AJ et al: Detection of acute inflammation with 111-indium labeled non-specific polyclonal IgG, *Semin Nucl Med* 18:335–344, 1988.

28. Thakur ML et al: Indium-111 labeled autologous leukocytes in man, *J Nucl Med* 18:1014–1021, 1977.

29. Rubin RH et al: In-111 labeled non-specific immunoglobulin scanning in the detection of focal infection, *N Engl J Med* 321:935, 1989.

30. LaMuraglia GM et al: Utility of Indium-111 labeled human immunoglobulin G scan for the detection of focal vascular graft infection, *J Vasc Surg* 10:20–28, 1989.

31. Oyen WJG et al: Scintigraphic detection of bone and joint infections with Indium-111-labeled non-specific polyclonal human immunoglobulin G, *J Nucl Med* 31:403–412, 1990.

32. Raff M, Melo J: Anaerobic osteomyelitis, *Medicine* 57:83–103, 1978.

33. Black J et al: Oral antimicrobial therapy for adults with osteomyelitis or septic arthritis, *J Infect Dis* 155(5):968–972, 1987.

34. Giamarellou H et al: Experience with ciprofloxacin in the treatment of various infections caused mainly by pseudomonas aeruginosa, *Drugs Exp Clin Res* 11:351–356, 1985.

35. Gentry LO, Rodriquez GG: Oral ciprofloxacin compared with parenteral antibiotics in the treatment of osteomyelitis, *Antimicrob Agents Chemother* 34(1):40–43, 1990.

36. Gentry L, Rodriguez-Gomez G: Ofloxacin versus parenteral therapy for chronic osteomyelitis, *Antimicrob Agents Chemother* 35(3):538–541, 1991.

37. Dellamonica P et al: Evaluation of pefloxacin, ofloxacin, and ciprofloxacin in the treatment of thirty nine cases of chronic osteomyelitis, *Eur J Clin Microbiol Infect Dis* 8(12):1024–1030, 1989.

38. Seligson D: Antibiotic-impregnated beads in orthopedic infectious problems, *Kentucky Med Assoc* 82:25–29, 1984.

39. Bayston R, Milner RDG: The sustained release of antimicrobial drugs from bone cement, *J Bone Joint Surg* 64B:460–464, 1982.

40. Henry SL et al: Antibiotic impregnated beads, *Orthop Rev* 20(3):242–247, 1991.

41. Popham GJ et al: Antibiotic impregnated beads part II: Factors in antibiotic selection, *Orthop Rev* 20(4):331–337, 1991.

42. Marcinko D: Gentamicin-impregnated PMMA beads: An introduction and review, *J Foot Surg* 24(2):116–121, 1985.

43. Jones RN: In vitro evaluation of aminopenicillin-beta-lactamase inhibitor combinations, *Drugs* 36(suppl 7):17–26, 1988.

44. Fass RJ: Comparative in vitro activities of third generation cephalosporins, *Arch Intern Med* 143:1743–1745, 1983.

45. Tally FP et al: Randomized prospective study comparing moxolactam and cefoxitin with or without tobramycin for treatment of serious surgical infections, *Antimicrob Agents Chemother* 29:244–249, 1986.

46. Wexler HM, Finegold SM: In vitro activity of cefotetan compared with that of other antimicrobial agents against anaerobic bacteria, *Antimicrob Agents Chemother* 32:601–604, 1988.

47. Fu KP, Neu HC: Antimicrobial activity

of ceftizoxime, a β-lactamase stable cephalosporin, *Antimicrob Agents Chemother* 17:583–590, 1980.

48. Calandra GB et al: Safety and tolerance comparison of imipenem-cilastin to cephalothin and cefazolin, *J Antimicrob Chemother* 12(suppl D):125–131, 1983.

49. Peterson L et al: Therapy of lower extremity infection with ciprofloxacin in patients with diabetes mellitus, peripheral vascular disease, or both, *Am J Med* 86:801–807, 1989.

50. Hughes CE et al: Treatment and long-term follow-up of diabetic or ischemic foot infections: a randomized prospective, double-blind trial of cefoxitin vs. ceftizoxime, *Clin Ther* 10(suppl A):36–49, 1987.

51. Desplaces N, Acar JF: New quinolones in the treatment of joint and bone infections, *Rev Infect Dis* 10(suppl 1):179–183, 1988.

52. Smith CR et al: Double blind comparison of the nephrotoxicity and auditory toxicity of gentamicin and tobramycin, *N Engl J Med* 302:106, 1980.

53. Bartlett JG et al: Antibiotic-associated pseudomembranous colitis due to toxin-producing clostridia, *N Engl J Med* 298:531–534, 1978.

16 _____ Surgery in the Infected Foot

Ronald Sage, D.P.M.

Prevention should be the mainstay of any diabetic foot care program. However, certain factors virtually assure us that pedal complications of diabetes will persist in spite of our best preventative efforts. For example, undiagnosed diabetics may present a foot infection as their first evidence of disease. Or, diabetic neuropathic patients who perceive no pain in their feet may find it difficult to believe that a potential for serious foot problems exists. As a result, they may not recognize the need for conscientious foot care. Even highly motivated patients are not always able to comply with ideal recommendations for foot wear, activity levels, and routine care. Poorly motivated patients who take little responsibility for their care are likely to suffer numerous complications in the feet and other parts of the body.

Because of all these factors, serious foot infections are likely to persist in spite of our best efforts at preventative care and patient education. Infections that lead to necrosis of tissue, abscess formation, invasion of bone, or gross suppuration are frequently uncontrollable by noninvasive means. Incision and drainage, debridement, fascial plane decompression, and amputation are surgical steps that may be required to control such conditions. The purpose of this chapter is to discuss the indications, techniques, and the associated perioperative management of patients requiring these procedures.

Medical authorities have long recognized the need for surgery to drain an abscess, wherever its location. Abscess of the foot is no exception.[1] With a severely infected foot, drainage of abscess formation is a primary consideration and should be accomplished expeditiously. Even pulselessness is not a contraindication to incision and drainage. If revascularization is necessary to save the limb, it cannot be safely accomplished until the acute infection is stabilized by using appropriate antibiotic coverage and accomplishing drainage of infected fascial planes or compartments.[2] Other efforts at ulcer care and wound healing are also unlikely to succeed if infection is not controlled.

PATHOGENESIS OF INFECTION

Foot infections in diabetics occur the same way as in nondiabetics. The only difference is the progression of infection, which is likely to be more rapid and extensive because of neuropathy, poor circulation, and an immunocompromised state associated with diabetes. Penetrating, or abrasive trauma, web space infection, and paronychias are all common conditions leading to loss of skin integrity and bacterial contamination of deep tissues.[3] Neuropathic ulcerations, which are painless to the patient, result from tissue necrosis. This necrosis is associated with prolonged pressure sufficient to cause ischemia, or from intermittent, repetitive pressure leading to progressive autolysis of tissue, as described by Bauman, Girling, and Brand.[4] Such painless lesions frequently go unnoticed or unattended until progressive contamination leads to obvious infection.

Early infection may be reversible by host defenses or with appropriate medical therapy. If unresolved, local infection can progress to cellulitis, which is a diffuse, acute soft tissue inflammation with little or no suppuration. These diffuse tissue reactions do not require surgical drainage. If they are known to arise from a specific focus of necrotic tissue, or abscess formation, that area should be drained. Local infection, with or without cellulitis, can extend to the bone, leading to osteomyelitis. This infection is frequently not reversible without excision of the infected bone. Cellulitis or osteomyelitis can become suppurative as bacteria multiply and tissue damage extends. Bacteria may enter the blood stream via direct extension, through venous channels, or lymphatic drainage causing bacteremia. Generalized sepsis occurs when pathogenic bacteria are present in the circulation in sufficient numbers to release endotoxins and produce cellular damage sufficient to cause systemic illness.

There is a serious potential for systemic illness associated with diabetic foot infection. Leibovici et al. reported on a series of 124 diabetic patients who developed bacteremia in 1991. Of these patients, 14% developed this condition as a complication of an extremity infection.[5] It is therefore essential to stabilize foot infection by medical means. It may also be necessary to surgically treat abscess formation, necrotic tissue, and fascial plane infection to save the limb. Revascularization or closure of soft tissue defects are unlikely to succeed unless you first resolve the infection.

INDICATIONS FOR SURGICAL INTERVENTION

General Considerations

Patients who are being treated for foot infection must be stabilized, from both a metabolic and cardiovascular perspective, especially if they will undergo aggressive surgical intervention.[6] Patients should be evaluated for significant hyperglycemia and electrolyte imbalance. Specialists in internal medicine should be consulted for help in correcting any abnormalities. Patients at risk for cardiovascular complications may require cardiology clearance before the operation. If bacteremia or generalized sepsis is present, an infectious disease specialist may help choose appropriate empiric antibiotics until definitive culture results can be obtained.

Although not emergent, nutritional assessment should also be made by obtaining serum albumin levels and total lymphocyte counts. For healing to be successful, significant nutritional deficiency will need to be corrected.[7] Adequate calories need to be provided to avoid loss of protein stores. Oral supplementation should be ordered in consultation with dietary service. The nutrition support team should be consulted in cases of serious malnutrition that may require parenteral hyperalimentation.

Superficial Debridement

The presence of necrotic, or nonviable, skin is an indication for superficial debridement, especially in cases where underlying abscess or ulceration is suspected. Surrounding cellulitis should increase the clinician's suspicion of underlying infection. Significant hyperkeratotic or eczematous tissue surrounding an ulcerative lesion should be debrided to viable noninfected tissue according to American Diabetes Association guidelines.[8] This type of superficial debridement can be readily accomplished in an ambulatory setting. The affected foot should be cleansed. An antiseptic solution may be applied to the area of ulceration and surrounding keratotic or necrotic tissue. Then the abnormal tissue can be cut away using a tissue-cutting forceps or scalpel. The debridement should be carried to viable tissue, taking care to prevent significant damage that might result in extension of the ulcer or necrosis. If a necrotic dry eschar is present without surrounding cellulitis, this may be cleansed and left to demarcate and slough.

Superficial debridement is adequate only in cases that present no evidence of extension to bone or deep abscess formation (Fig 16–1). The most common example of a lesion or abscess requiring only superficial debridement is that found in association with a chronic digital corn, or plantar keratosis. In such cases, considerable keratotic buildup is noted around a chronic pressure point on a toe or beneath a metatarsal head. There is frequent hemorrhaging into the deeper layers of the callus. Fluid may accumulate, which forms a superficial abscess. If left

untreated, the condition may form a deep abscess. On debridement, fluid, pus, or blood may be encountered. However, once the surrounding keratotic tissue is thoroughly debrided, viable tissue should be present at the base of the lesion. There should be no evidence of deep extension. If there is, the physician should consider a more extensive incision and drainage in the operating room.

Take a culture if fluid or pus is encountered. Broad spectrum oral antibiotics should be started if cellulitis is present. Definitive antibiotics may be prescribed when culture results have been obtained if the patient does not respond to the treatment. Hospital admission for parenteral antibiotics is necessary if the cellulitis is ascending more than 2 to 3 cm proximal to the source of infection. Ad-

B

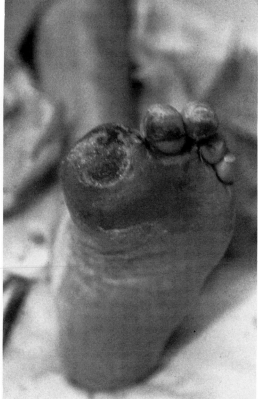

A

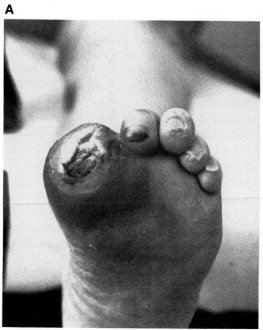

FIG 16–1.
A, Grade I ulcer requiring only superficial debridement. **B,** after debridement.

mission is also appropriate if the patient's temperature is over 100° F, or if the infection may be causing significant hyperglycemia. Inadequate response to outpatient care may also necessitate hospitalization. Sterile dressings should be applied to the wound. The affected foot should be cleansed and new dressings regularly applied. Weight-bearing should be reduced to allow healing to occur.

Incision and Drainage of Abscess Formation

The classic manifestations of an abscess are the following: redness, swelling, tenderness, and heat. Tissues frequently appear under tension. There is often a palpable fluctuance. An abscess can develop if there is no portal of entry, but this is unusual in the diabetic foot. Usually an ulcerated keratosis, blister, puncture, or some other defect in the tissue that probably gave rise to the abscess formation will be apparent. An abscess formation may arise from an infected interdigital corn, such as those commonly seen in the fourth interdigital space, but are easily missed if not closely looked for. A foot abscess may appear as a localized dorsal swelling or as a fluctuant mass that is obvious on the plantar surface. Occasionally an abscess may extend from dorsal to plantar surrounding a metatarsal phalangeal joint or in an intermetatarsal space. An abscess that has penetrated a fascial plane can easily extend proximally in the foot or up the leg along the lines of any associated tendon sheath. Once an abscess has been identified, it should be incised and thoroughly drained.[1] Superficial lesions can be drained by debridement as previously described (Fig 16–2). Deeper infections may require more extensive surgical intervention, which will be described later in this chapter.

A clinical distinction must be made between an abscess formation and cellulitis. Cellulitis is merely a diffuse inflammation of tissue surrounding a focus of infection. It lacks a clear area of liquefaction or accumulation of pus. This condition requires only antibiotic management unless an obvious abscess develops. Incision of a cellulitic area before pus develops may be counterproductive, and the incision may even lead to the spread of infection or necrosis.[1]

Debridement of Deep Infection or Necrosis

It is fairly obvious when a deep infection or fascial plane abscess is present. The patient is likely to be running a fever, and glucose control may have deteriorated. A portal of entry, such as an infected ulcer or obvious web space infection, is usually present. There may be purulent drainage emanating from such a portal. The affected fascial compartment is swollen, red, and tender.[3] To put it simply, the patient and the extremity look sick.

If there is a significant amount of pus, which would cause a physician to suspect that an abscess is present, the pus must be surgically drained. Any necrotic or nonviable tissue associated with abscess or infection should also be debrided.[2, 6, 7] The seriousness of such an infection helps determine if a hospital admission is necessary. Although incision and drainage to compress an acute infection may be initiated at the bedside, thorough drainage, debridement, and exploration of the affected fascial compartments usually require an operating room. As with any infection, deep cultures should be obtained. Empiric antibiotics should be initiated after a consultation with an infectious disease physician. Definitive antibiotic therapy can be prescribed after laboratory studies are available.

Amputation

In general, amputations are performed because of congenital deformity, tumors,

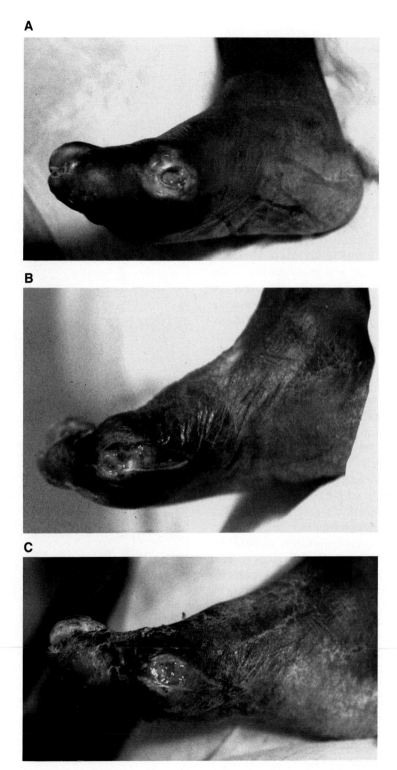

FIG 16–2.
A, Grade III ulcer with deep abscess. **B,** after incision and drainage demonstrating extent of abscess formation.
C, drainage site granulated and contracting.

trauma, or infection and gangrene. Infection or gangrene leading to amputation are most commonly encountered in the diabetic or dysvascular foot. Specific criteria for amputation in these feet may include the following: uncontrollable infection, intractable pain, necrosis of bone or tendon, or prolonged treatment disability leading to muscle wasting and atrophy. These indications may be applied in considering either partial foot amputation, or below- or above-knee amputations.[9, 10]

Uncontrollable Infection.—The first priority in caring for any diabetic or ischemic infection is to stabilize the acute phase.[2] Appropriate antibiotic coverage and the completion of adequate drainage and debridement are essential first steps. If high fever and suppuration persist in spite of these measures, open amputation may be necessary to resolve the infection.

Anaerobic infections with necrotizing fascitis may require aggressive high amputation. These infections are unmistakable in appearance and odor (Fig 16–3). The patient is seriously ill and at high risk for septic shock. The extremity is tense, erythematous, and sometimes cyanotic. Black, putrid, necrotic tissue may be present at the infection's original site. Gas may be noted ascending fascial planes on x-ray. Serious consideration should be given to high amputation in such a situation to avoid fulminant septic shock.

Uncontrollable infection may take on a more chronic form in the patient who develops osteomyelitis secondary to chronic ulceration. Although such situations are rarely life-threatening, they do present a major disability. The lesion constantly drains. Acute flareups of cellulitis will occur unless a meticulous program of daily home care and periodic debridement is maintained. Such lesions may interfere with diabetes control. If a cure is not possible, amputation of the involved part should be considered, weighing the potential disability of the amputation against

A

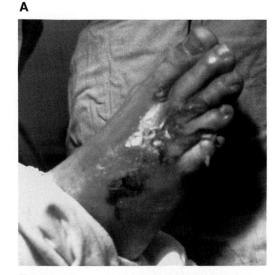

B

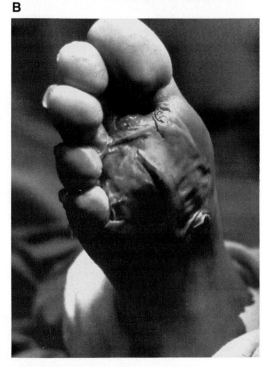

FIG 16–3.
A, dorsal view of foot with extensive mixed infection abscess requiring amputation. **B,** plantar view of same foot.

the disability of the condition. For example, removal of the hallux may be considered preferable to living with a chronic osteomyelitis of the phalanx. On the other hand, long-term wound management may be preferable to below-knee amputation for the patient with chronic osteomyelitis of the ankle.

Intractable Pain.—Ischemic ulcerations or gangrene may result in severe pain. The pain begins as occasional claudication and ultimately leads to night pain, which is relieved only by narcotic analgesics and maintaining the extremity in dependency. Symptoms may localize only to a single toe. If the symptoms involve the entire extremity, the feasibility of revascularization should be considered. If surgery is not possible, there is little hope for relieving this type of pain.

In cases of severe, intractable ischemic pain, the patients are rarely community ambulators. As such, even through, or above-the-knee amputations result in little additional disability. Patients with severe ischemic pain frequently experience an improvement in the quality of life following amputation.

Necrosis of Bone or Tendon.—Extensive deep ulceration may progress to a level where bone or tendon are exposed. Unless the circulation is good, infection is completely controlled, and meticulous local wound care is carried out, these tissues are likely to become necrotic. Granulation, and hence wound contraction, cannot take place over dead bone or tendon. Small areas of such necrosis may be debrided. However, if the necrosis is extensive, and debridement is likely to leave the part useless, amputation should be considered.

Digital ulcerations exposing and necrosing the extensor tendons or phalanges are examples when toe amputations should be considered. Patients with exposed and necrotic fifth metatarsal phalangeal joints may also be helped by a fifth

ray resection (Fig 16–4). Extensive necrosis of tarsal bones and associated soft tissue structures may also require amputation to obtain a healed extremity.

Muscle Wasting.—Elimination of pressure is essential in ulcer care. Whether the lesion is secondary to intermittent pressure encountered in every day walking or the result of chronic pressure on the heel during prolonged bed rest, healing will not take place unless the pressure is eliminated. Pressure will impede granulation and epithelialization and cause extension of necrosis.[4]

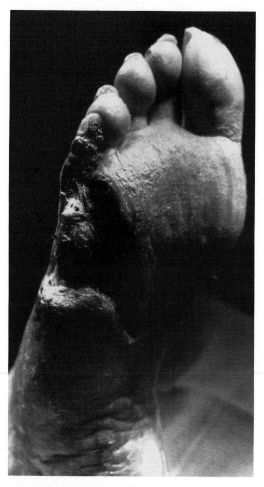

FIG 16–4.
Necrotic fifth metatarsal phalangeal joint requiring ray resection.

Bed rest, wheelchair confinement, and even unilateral non-weight-bearing, prescribed to facilitate healing, result in varying degrees of disuse. As this disuse is prolonged, the usual consequences of muscle atrophy and osteoporosis are inevitable. The question then arises if continued ulcer care and possible limb salvage are preferable to amputation and rapid rehabilitation. If immobilization proceeds for such a long time that significant muscle wasting occurs because of disuse, serious consideration should be given to amputation and prosthesis training. This should be considered as a rehabilitative step, rather than a failure of treatment. This is especially true in cases where severe foot deformity is present and may lead to reulceration once weight-bearing is resumed. Taken in this context, muscle wasting and atrophy may become considerations for amputation in the diabetic ulcer patient.

PREOPERATIVE ASSESSMENT

Foot Evaluation

Physical Examination.—A good evaluation starts with a history and physical exam. The details of the patient's diabetes and medical history are essential for planning treatment and appropriate consultations. The history of the foot condition and the events leading up to the presentation may give an indication of the type of infection present and the duration and likelihood of deep or bone infection. Inspection and palpation of the foot alone can lead the physician to a diagnosis of abscess requiring incision and drainage. Palpation for pulses may be difficult because of swelling associated with infection. However, it is frequently valuable to palpate the pulses of the contralateral extremity to determine if significant vascular disease is present. It is rare for one

foot to be well perfused and the other to be markedly less vascular.

Wagner's grading system for diabetic feet is useful for expressing the severity of a diabetic foot ulcer or infection.[9] Grade 0 feet present no evidence of ulcer or infection. Grade 1 ulcers are superficial lesions, but suggest full thickness erosions of the epidermis; the dimensions of these, and all, lesions should be noted. Grade 2 ulcers may simply be considered deeper lesions that have not yet penetrated to bone or a fascial plane. Grade 3 ulcers extend to bone, or have invaded a fascial plane and may be associated with abscess formation. Osteomyelitis is very likely. Such lesions, almost by definition, represent surgical problems because infected bone needs to be debrided and deep abscesses need to be drained. Grade 4 feet have gangrene of the forefoot, frequently requiring debridement or amputation. Grade 5 implies gangrene of the entire foot that will likely require high amputation.

Medical Imaging.—Various imaging techniques are valuable in the assessment of the infected foot. The surgeon should use imaging techniques as a road map to point out the pathologic condition that requires debridement or drainage. Plain radiographs can help identify bone destruction and gas in the soft tissues. Although frequently associated with anaerobic infection, gas is usually seen with any type of penetrating soft tissue infection arising from an ulceration and may be indicative of abscess formation. Certainly, the physician's belief that surgical intervention may be necessary should be strengthened by the identification of gas in the soft tissues. Bone destruction seen on plain films or a computerized tomography scan (CT) may indicate osteomyelitis, but questionable cases may be resolved by nuclear imaging techniques such as bone scanning or leukocyte Indium scanning. Magnetic resonance imaging (MRI) may help evaluate for osteomyelitis, Charcot foot, or deep abscess formation in questionable cases.[8, 13] Because sophisticated imaging techniques are expensive, they should not be ordered routinely unless the diganosis, or need for surgery, cannot be estabished by physical exam or plain radiographs alone. See Chapter 10 in this book for more details regarding medical imaging.

Circulatory evaluation.—Circulatory evaluation starts with physical examination of the overall skin texture, hair growth, temperature, and pulses. Noninvasive studies may include Doppler examination. Wagner has suggested that Doppler evaluation of arterial pressure in the foot is prognostic for satisfactory healing when the foot pressure is 45% or more of the brachial artery pressure.[9] Although not infallible, this test is often used and may be important in identifying patients who have significant vascular disease.[8]

Recently, measuring transcutaneous oxygen pressure has been shown to be effective in predicting healing of a foot or amputation wound. Wyss et al[11] and Malone[12] have shown that tissue PO_2 levels greater than 30 mm Hg are consistent with healing at various levels of amputation. This test is usually available through the pulmonary service at many hospitals.

Circulatory evaluation done prior to surgical intervention for infection is useful as a prognostic indicator for healing. This evaluation can also identify patients who may require revascularization after the acute infection is stabilized.[2] Poor perfusion should not be considered a contraindication to debridement or drainage of an acute infection, nor should emergent surgery be delayed for invasive vascular studies. In general, revascularization would follow stabilization of acute infection. However, if doubt exists about the quality of the patient's vascular supply, peripheral vascular consultation is always appropriate. Other information about vascular involvement may be found in earlier chapters in this text.

Medical Considerations

In planning appropriate consultation for perioperative medical care, the podiatric surgeon should be aware of the evaluation of physical status completed by the anesthesiologist before surgery. Class 1 patients have no medical problems, other than the pathologic condition associated with the surgery; no diabetic patients will fit this category. Class 2 patients have a stable, chronic medical problem that is well controlled, such as stable diabetes. Class 3 patients are more seriously ill, with unstable medical problems, and are more likely to need intensive, or at least close, medical supervision in the perioperative period. Class 4 patients are very seriously ill, perhaps at risk for septic shock, or other major cardiovascular complications and definitely require intensive perioperative care. Class 5 patients are not expected to survive surgery or the perioperative period.[14] The surgeon should ensure that appropriate medical consultation, clearance, and follow-up have been obtained to provide for the perioperative medical care of a diabetic patient who will undergo surgery for an infected foot.

Glucose control should be optimized, and fluid imbalance corrected if possible, before taking the patient to surgery. Evaluation of serum glucose and electrolytes should be ordered. IV fluids should be started and appropriate administration of insulin initiated based on consultation with an internist or the anesthesiologist. A routine chest x-ray and ECG should be obtained.

Other considerations that may not affect the initial decision to operate, but do affect healing, are nutritional, renal and immune status. Serum albumin should be measured and ideally be maintained at 3.5 mg/dl to facilitate wound healing. Total lymphocyte count, which should be 1500, can also be measured to assess nutrition.[17] Hypoalbuminemia leading to wound failure can come from a number of different causes. These include chronic malnutrition, liver disease, and frequently, renal disease. Patients with significant renal disease can lose large amounts of protein through the urine, and thus develop a negative nitrogen balance, which impairs normal wound healing. Unfortunately, this is often difficult to correct. Loading the patient with dietary protein may aggravate renal disease, and is therefore not recommended. Significant hypoalbuminemia should be brought to the attention of a medical consultant for management. An excellent source of assistance in dealing with these problems can be the hospital nutrition support team.

Severe renal disease may ultimately be treated by kidney transplant. Patients who have undergone such transplants are treated with medications to suppress rejection, such as prednisone, cyclosporine, or imuran.[18] These are immune suppressive medications that may alter the host's resistance to infection and possibly complicate attempts at limb salvage. Because these medications cannot be withdrawn, the presence of immune compromise must be considered for the overall treatment plan. It may be more prudent to accept a below-the-knee amputation rather than risk major sepsis in a transplant patient.

Thorough medical assessment is essential for the patient about to have surgery for a diabetic foot infection. This is important to ensure appropriate management of the diabetes and other medical risk factors, as well as to facilitate wound healing.

SURGICAL TECHNIQUES

Incision and Drainage of Infected Fascial Planes

The presence of pus within a fascial plane of the foot constitutes an abscess and must be drained.[1] These infections may arise from the web space; however, usually they arise from a neuropathic ulceration. Occasionally they arise from a puncture wound.[19] Inspection, palpation, radiographs, or other imaging techniques should indicate the course of the abscess and the compartments involved. The author usually initiates the incision over the abscess itself and extends the incision along the appropriate course. For example, an abscess originating from ulceration of the first metatarsal head would be drained by starting the incision at the ulcer and extending along the medial plantar space as far proximally as would be necessary to drain all purulent matter. The distal and proximal ends of the incision should be carefully inspected to ensure that pus is not tracking beyond the margins of the incision. If such drainage is encountered, the incision would need to be extended. The suspicious compartment or tendon sheath may be compressed from a point well above the infection and milked toward the wound. If purulent material is extruded, the suspicious compartment should be opened further.

Once the abscess has been opened adequately, the wound base and margins should be inspected for obviously necrotic tissue. The necrotic tissue should be debrided to healthy, viable margins. The wound should then be thoroughly irrigated with saline or an antibiotic solution. It should take on a clean, viable appearance if the pus has been adequately drained and appropriate debridement has been accomplished. The wound is then packed open with fluffy gauze dressing material and covered with gauze roll. Such wounds are usually left open to fill in by second intention (Fig 16–5).

A

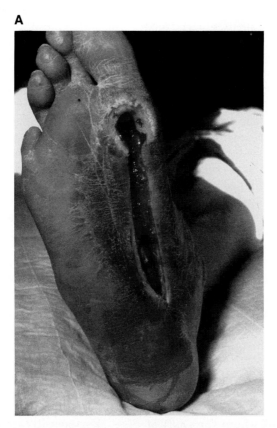

B

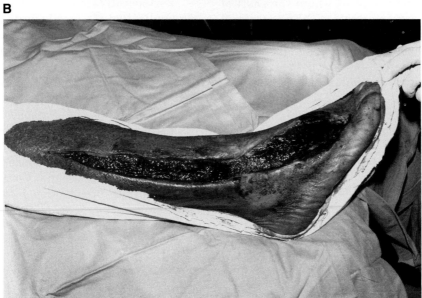

FIG 16–5.
A, open wound following incision and drainage of abductor halluces abscess. **B,** open granulating wound following incision and drainage of extensor digitorum longus abscess, ready for grafting.

Toe Amputation[20]

Toe amputation is frequently performed through the base of the proximal phalanx. This is left in place to maintain intrinsic muscle stability around the metatarsal phalangeal joint. Furthermore, resection at the proximal metaphysis allows for closure over raw cancellous bone, which is an area that is better vascularized than the cartilage of the metatarsal head.

Skin incisions are made with medial and lateral flaps fashioned around the base of the digit. The toe thus becomes the center of a wedge, with an apex directed dorsally and plantarly. In situations where infection appears to extend beyond the base of the toe, this allows for easy proximal extension of the incision to facilitate drainage. The fishmouth incision, which produces dorsal and plantar flaps, is appropriate only when the surgeon is convinced of the localization of the infection distal to the operative site.

Once the skin is incised, the incision is carried directly to bone. Using a periosteal elevator, soft tissues are removed from the point where the shaft of the phalanx intersects with the proximal metaphysis. At this point, the bone is cut using a bone cutter or power instrumentation, as needed. The toe is then removed by severing any remaining soft tissue attachments.

Considerable care should be taken during the incision to ensure that the skin edges are not skived or excessively manipulated. Any remnants of nonviable tissue should be gently debrided. The wound is then thoroughly irrrigated with saline or an antibiotic solution. The skin may be closed, usually without need for deep sutures, if there is not proximal ascending infection. Simple interrupted sutures are preferred.

Amputation through the base of the phalanx keeps soft tissue dissection to a minimum. Considerable retraction and sharp dissection are necessary to disarticulate a toe at the metatarsal phalan-geal joint. Because this manipulation can be detrimental to healing in a compromised patient, it should be avoided.

It frequently becomes necessary, however, to amputate proximal to the bases of the proximal phalanx. This is due to inadequate viability of the proximal skin. In such situations, construction of dorsal and plantar flaps is inappropriate. The medial and lateral flaps are fashioned as previously described. Once the metatarsal phalangeal joint is exposed, the skin edges are retracted and collateral ligaments and tendons are severed to release the digit. The author routinely resects the articular cartilage from the distal end of the metatarsal to close over cancellous bone. Closure over relatively avascular cartilage may impair healing. All roughened areas of bone are rasped and rongeured smooth. The bone is resected proximally enough to allow closure of the skin edges without excessive tension. Deep closure is performed with absorbable sutures as needed. The skin is closed with simple interrupted nylon sutures.

Postoperative management consists of the application of a sterile dressing in the operating room, which is removed 48 hours after surgery. The wound is inspected. If drainage persists, a betadine dressing may be applied. If the wound is dry, dry gauze is sufficient. Sutures are generally kept in about 2 weeks, although the surgeon is cautioned against premature removal. The sutures can stay in for 3 to 4 weeks if there are concerns about the stability of the wound. Conventional or appropriate prescription foot wear is then allowed.

Ray Resection[21]

Ray resection is defined as amputation of a digit and most, or all, of its associated metatarsal. This is an excellent procedure for drainage of an acute infection. It is usually performed in the presence of either abscess or osteomyelitis of a toe and its metatarsalphalangeal joint. Extensive necrosis of skin, soft tissue, or bone in the involved digit may necessitate ray resection to obtain adequate viable skin for closure. Ray resection is often necessary when local infection extends proximally, either along the dorsum of the foot, or through the plantar fascial planes. The procedure allows complete drainage from top to bottom along a longitudinal plane, such as flexor or extensor tendon sheaths.

Although the procedure may be performed as a definitive operation, the surgeon must remember that it carries a high risk of transfer lesion and subsequent reulceration of adjacent metatarsal heads. If another significant metatarsalphalangeal deformity is present in the foot that may lead to later reulceration, provisions

should me made for careful follow-up care following the ray resection (Fig 16–6). It may even be advisable to consider alternative procedures such as pan-metatarsal head resection, or midfoot amputation as the final, definitive operation. However, open ray resection is appropriate and useful as a preliminary drainage procedure for an infection surrounding a metatarsal head.

The procedure is initiated by a longitudinal incision along the shaft of the involved metatarsal extending from the proximal two thirds of the bone to the metatarsal phalangeal joint. Then the incision should diverge smoothly around the base of the toe to fashion medial and lateral flaps. The two converging incisions should form a V plantarly, encompassing

FIG 16–6.
Healed ray resection developing new transfer ulceration.

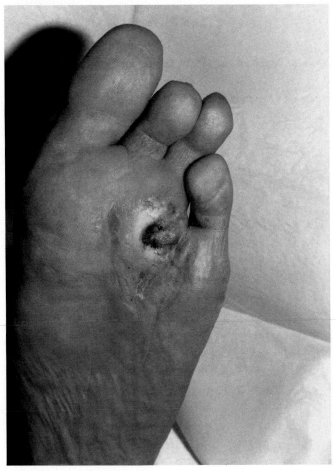

any metatarsal head ulceration present (Fig 16–7,A). The incision is then deepened, and hemorrhaging vessels should be clamped and cauterized. If an abscess is encountered, this is thoroughly drained using sharp and blunt dissection. Any evidence of proximal ascending abscess necessitates the proximal extension of the incision to ensure that all purulent material is thoroughly drained. The toe is disarticulated at the joint. The metatarsal shaft is exposed proximally and resected using either bone cutting forceps or power instrumentation (Fig 16–7,B).

The wound must be inspected for any residual abscess formation. Pus can extend along any of the tendon sheaths or plantar fascial planes. Any suspicious areas should be probed and opened if necessary. Residual nonviable tissue should be debrided. This includes loose lengths of tendon or left-over joint capsules. Take care to avoid violating adjacent, nonin-

fected joints. If infection has tracked medially or laterally to adjacent joints, these must be opened and debrided.

Copious irrigation should be performed with a physiologic solution such as normal saline. When this irrigation is complete the wound should look clean and viable (Fig 16–7,C). If spaces or pockets that might accumulate infectious material are left, a drain should be placed in the wound. The wound itself is left open and packed with gauze. A compression dressing is then applied, avoiding constriction of the remaining toes.

The wound is inspected in 24 to 48 hours. If adequate drainage was obtained during the procedure, there should be marked clinical improvement of any surrounding cellulitis. Wet-to-dry saline dressings or whirlpool with dressing change is provided twice daily. Although using soaks or whirlpool is decried by some, they are used routinely in open foot

A

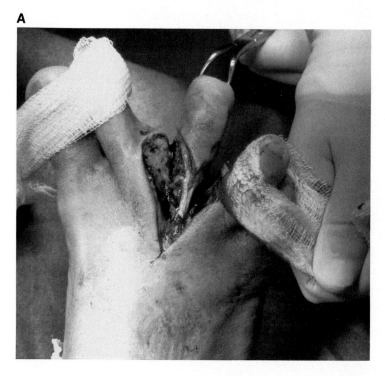

FIG 16–7.
A, initial approach to ray resection. **B,** metatarsal exposed prior to resection. Note abnormal appearance of bone. **C,** clean wound at completion of resection.

B

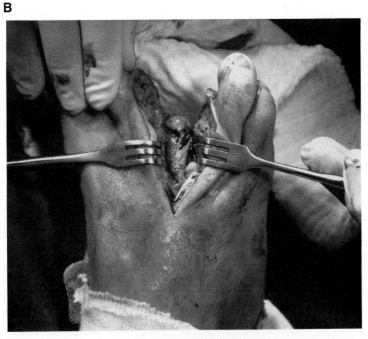

C

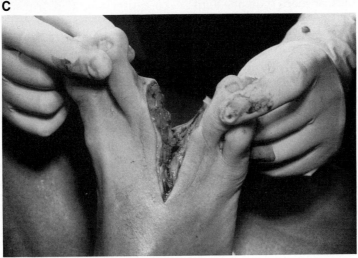

FIG 16–7 (cont'd).

wounds at our institution by orthopedic, podiatric, and vascular services. The treatment is administered at physiologic temperatures under close supervision of physical therapists. We have noted significant benefits of improved drainage of infection and wound cleansing when using this modality.

Once the wound is clean, delayed primary closure may be considered in approximately 1 week. Or the wound may be left to heal by second intention, which usually takes 6 to 8 weeks in nutritionally competent, well vascularized patients. Early closure may lead to new abscess formation, and it is the author's preference to allow secondary closure to take place.

Ray resection runs the risk of transfer ulceration if left as the definitive surgical treatment for diabetic foot infection. Therefore, conscientious local follow-up care is essential. Monthly palliative care may be indicated. In-lay depth shoes with appropriate accommodative insoles should be prescribed. The patient must be warned about transfer ulceration, and educated about appropriate care for the diabetic foot.

Open Midfoot Amputation

Midfoot amputation may be indicated for extensive gangrene or infections of the toes and forefoot.[7, 9, 22] Amputation of a single toe, or ray, becomes inadequate when extensive infection that is affecting multiple tissue planes, or more than one digit or metatarsal is present. In such cases, which would be defined as grade 4 feet by Wagner, amputation of the entire forefoot becomes appropriate. This allows for drainage of all the compartments of the foot, both dorsal and plantar. It also eliminates all of the rays in cases where metatarsal phalangeal joint destruction is extending transversely.

When an open amputation is performed through the metatarsal bases, it is called the transmetatarsal amputation. If the procedure is accomplished by disarticulation at the metatarsal-tarsal joints, it is termed the LisFranc amputation. If infection has extended even more proximally, disarticulation may be done at the midtarsal joint; this type of amputation is known as a Chopart amputation. When done in the presence of infection, each of these procedures should be left open. Efforts should be made to preserve a long plantar flap, if this has not been destroyed by infection or gangrene to facilitate later closure, and weight-bearing. At times, the open midfoot procedure may serve only as an incision and drainage procedure in anticipation of a Syme amputation (ankle disarticulation).

In each case, a dorsal transverse incision is carried to bone near the region of planned amputation across the entire top of the foot. Major vessels should be clamped and ligated. Smaller vessels may be cauterized. If a transmetatarsal amputation is to be performed, the bases may be exposed and osteotomized. Otherwise, the appropriate joints are incised for disarticulation. An incision is then carried distally along the plantar aspect of the foot toward the sulcus. The sulcus is incised, if possible, or the incision is carried across the bottom of the foot proximal to any ulcerated or destroyed tissue and parallel to the sulcus. The incision is then curved back proximally to meet the other side of the dorsal transverse incision. Soft tissues are dissected from the plantar side

FIG 16–8.
Midfoot disarticulation demonstrating dorsal incision and plantar flap prior to closure.

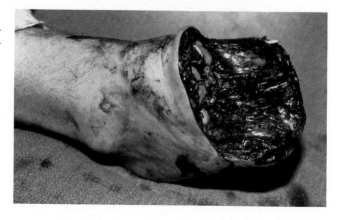

of the bones distal to the disarticulation, and the foot is detached from the plantar flap (Fig 16–8).

The proximal tendon sheaths and fascial planes should be gently compressed from above the infection. If pus appears, the sheaths and fascial planes may need to be opened to further facilitate drainage. At times, significant fascial plane infection that involves the anterior, posterior, or peroneal muscle groups may be discovered. This can be identified by noting pus oozing into the wound from one or more of these muscle sheaths. In many cases, the limb can still be saved if the affected compartment is incised, irrigated thoroughly with saline or an antibiotic solution, and appropriate drains are placed.[7] Once fasciotomy has been performed, an ingress tube should be placed into the wound, and an egress tube should be attached to a suction apparatus (Fig 16–9). Again, the wounds should be inspected in 24 to 48 hours. If no further purulent drainage is noted through the suction apparatus, remove the system and initiate local wound care. If drainage persists, leave the system in for another day. If drainage still persists or if systemic signs of sepsis are not improving, further incision and drainage, or amputation, may be indicated.

Once the acute infection has been stabilized, make plans for closure. These may include delayed primary closure of viable plantar flap, or a more definitive amputation, such as Symes procedure. Leg wounds may usually be left to fill in secondarily. Final plans should take into consideration the likelihood for ambulation, the usefulness of the proposed stump, and the capacity for healing.

Partial Calcanectomy

Occasionally, large heel defects may be encountered as a result of prolonged bed rest or local heel injury. If deep abscess forms, or osteomyelitis of the calcaneus

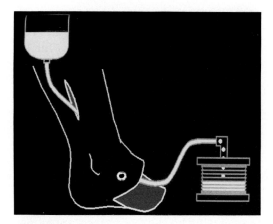

FIG 16–9.
Suction irrigation system for open transmetatarsal amputation and incision and drainage of compartment.

develops, operative intervention becomes necessary to drain or debride infected bone and soft tissue. Patients with significant loss of heel skin often require a below-the-knee amputation because of their inability to obtain a durable closure. However, a partial calcanectomy, which removes up to three fourths of the calcaneus, allows mobilization of a large amount of skin from the medial and lateral sides of the heel. This may facilitate primary or secondary closure in feet that otherwise might not be saved.[23, 24, 25]

The surgical approach should be tailored to fit the size and shape of the ulcer. Ideally, two converging semielliptical incisions should be fashioned around the ulcer, extending longitudinally over the Achilles tendon proximally, and pointing to the toes plantarly and distally. The intervening wedge of skin and ulceration are excised, opening up the back of the heel like a book. A sufficient amount of calcaneus is resected to mobilize enough skin to loosely approximate the edges. There is no need to enter either the subtalar or calcaneal cuboid joints. Usually, resecting the posterior and inferior one half of the heel bone is sufficient. The Achilles tendon, which was detached earlier, should be sewn into the periosteum of the remaining dorsal surface of the calcaneus. Generally, the wound is left open to fill in by second intention (Fig 16–10).

Once healed, the patient may walk on durable plantar skin. If a deformity is present that causes difficulty walking or shoe fitting, a thermoplastic in-shoe ankle foot orthosis can be prescribed with a soft filler to accommodate the heel defect.

METHODS OF CLOSURE

Open Wound Management

In operating on the foot to treat infection, the major goal is to establish drainage of an abscess or purulent material. Premature closure of an infected fascial plane may lead to reformation of an abscess. Therefore, open wound management that allows secondary closure to take place is appropriate in these situations. Healing will take place in an open, partial foot amputation if the infection has been controlled, if there is adequate blood flow, and adequate nutrition is maintained.[7, 21]

Following surgery, the wound is packed with a loose gauze application. If the wound was producing significant moist necrosis or pus, the gauze may be soaked with betadine to facilitate drying of this undesirable material. The betadine should be discontinued in favor of saline when the purulent drainage is eliminated. A compressive gauze dressing is applied

A

B

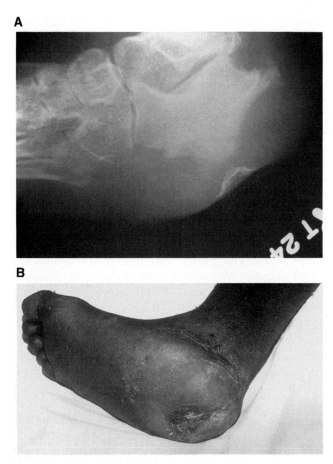

FIG 16–10.
A, resected bone from posterior one half of calcaneus for chronic heel ulcer. **B,** healed foot after partial calcanectomy.

over the packing. The dressing should be sufficient to maintain hemostasis, but not so constrictive that it will compromise blood flow to the remaining digits. This is left in place for 24 to 48 hours.

After this period of time, the dressing is removed, frequently by pouring saline to facilitate loosening, and the wound is inspected. If there is evidence of persisting infection, or substantial necrosis, further surgery may be indicated. If the wound is clean, wet-to-dry saline dressings are applied twice daily, and strict non-weight-bearing on the affected extremity is enforced. This may require physical therapy for crutch training or instruction in use of a walker. Physical therapy may also be helpful in local wound care. A whirlpool, maintained at body temperature to avoid risk of scalding, is helpful in wound cleansing. The therapist may take an active role in performing superficial cleaning and debridement, maintaining an optimal environment for healing to take place. If, under these circumstances the wound does not appear viable, peripheral vascular consultation should be sought.

If the wound progresses normally, granulation will begin to present itself within a few days. The process of wound contraction follows, taking approximately 6 weeks in a typical ray resection. Strict aseptic dressing changes and non-weight-bearing must be maintained during this time, for successful healing.

Delayed Primary Closure

If the open wound remains clinically clean for approximately 5 to 7 days, delayed primary closure can be used to expedite wound healing. This requires adequate surrounding skin for closure without excessive tension on the wound edges. Tissue cultures may be obtained to ensure that bacterial colonization will not lead to reinfection. However, the appearance of the wound and a normal WBC and sedimentation rate may be more helpful in determining that the patient is clinically free from infection and ready for delayed closure. After taking the patient to the operating room for delayed closure, a sterile dressing is applied, and the wound is cared for just like any other surgical incision. Sutures should be left in as long as is necessary to assure adequate healing has taken place.

Primary Closure

Primary closure following surgery for an abscess or osteomyelitis is rarely indicated. If a contaminated wound is resutured primarily, an abscess is likely to be recreated all over again. Primary closure has only been successful in the author's experience when necrosis or gangrene is extremely well localized quite distal to the incision line. Ideally, the infected or necrotic tissue should be draped off away from the incision line if a primary closure is being contemplated. Following such closure, the patient should be monitored closely. Any hint of postoperative infection should be managed by quickly removing sutures, culturing any drainage, initiating antibiotic therapy, and then treating the surgical site as an open wound. If there is evidence of deeper infection, the patient may need to be returned to the operating room for incision and drainage.

Skin Grafts

Various grafting techniques are available to expedite wound closure. It should be remembered that grafted tissue rarely allows for coverage with the same durability as the skin that was lost. This is particularly important in covering plantar defects in weight-bearing areas. Split thickness grafts covering a heel deficit, for example, are doomed to break down when weight-bearing is resumed.

After operating to control infection, the base of the wound must be in good condition to accept any kind of graft. Ideally, the wound should be well granulated and free from infection. It is difficult to get a graft to "take" over exposed bone or tendon. No graft will be successful over necrotic tissue of any kind. Once the wound base is viable and clean, decisions regarding grafting can be made. All grafts carry the risk of added morbidity. The more complex the graft, the greater the risk of graft failure, infection of the donor site, and medical complications associated with prolonged anesthesia. These risks should be weighed carefully against the advantages of grafting, particularly when open wound management may lead to complete closure, given adequate time. Any type of grafting requires experience to assure success. Plastic surgery consultation is appropriate in complex skin coverage situations, especially if the surgeon who performed the initial debridement procedure does not have extensive experience with grafting techniques. More details about reconstructive techniques are discussed in Chapter 18.

Numerous techniques are available to obtain coverage of soft tissue defects. The simplest is the split thickness skin graft. Using a donor site on the thigh or abdomen, a thin layer of skin is shaved, usually perforated, and applied to the defect. A protective dressing is applied, and the wound is given adequate time to epithelialize. A significant scar is usually left after healing, and may be prone to subsequent breakdown.

Transpositional pedicle flaps can be advanced or rotated from healthy areas to cover a defect. The donor site frequently requires split thickness grafting. Random pattern flaps should be at least as wide as they are long to assure viability. Axial pattern flaps, which are based on a specific arterial axis such as dorsalis pedis or lateral calcaneal artery, may be considerably longer than their width.

A neurovascular free flap may be raised from any one of several typical donor sites and anastomosed to a local blood supply to provide coverage in areas not suitable for split thickness or transpositional grafting. However, the surgery takes considerable technical skill, is very prolonged, and requires intensive aftercare. Patients with significant metabolic defects may be poor candidates for such intervention.

It is the author's preference to allow most wounds to contract by second intention. However, there are situations where alternatives such as primary closure, delayed primary closure, or various grafting techniques can be used. The treatment plan should depend on the surgeon's training and experience, the availability of consultative services, and determining if the benefit to the patient outweighs the associated risks.

CONCLUSION

Operative intervention for diabetic foot infection is generally nonelective. If the foot heals, care must be taken to educate the patient about diabetic foot disorders, and steps should be taken to provide the correct follow-up care. None of the procedures described can be considered a panacea for diabetic foot problems in and of itself.

A review of ray resections at our institutions revealed that at least two thirds of the 28 patients studied had subsequent problems, most of them reulcerations.[21] Transmetatarsal or midfoot amputation patients fared somewhat better, but still reulcerated approximately 25% of the time in long-term follow-up studies.[27] A California study published in 1988 revealed better success with a Syme Amputation.[28] Our own retrospective review of using a Syme amputation revealed significant long-term success. In this study, none of the 31 patients who healed their amputations initially required late revisions in up to 5 years of follow-up.[29] It is obvious from these reviews that these procedures are not remedies for diabetic foot problems. If any part of the foot has been salvaged it remains at risk for further problems and must receive proper long-term podiatric care.

The need for surgical intervention for diabetic foot problems may be reduced by educational and preventative care programs.[30] However, until such programs are universally provided, and patients willingly comply, it is likely that foot ulceration and infection will continue to be a major health problem for diabetic patients, and surgical intervention will be required to treat these patients.[31] The interventions previously described are necessary for treating these patients acutely, but the long-term success of these salvage operations is dependent on a sound, ongoing foot care program.

REFERENCES

1. Hirschmann JV: Localized infections and abscesses. In Braunwald E et al, editors: *Harrison's principles of internal medicine,* ed 11, New York, 1988, McGraw-Hill.
2. Gibbons GW, Eliopoulos GM: Infection in the diabetic foot. In Kozak GP et al, editors: *Management of diabetic foot problems,* Philadelphia, 1984, WB Saunders.
3. Maggiore P, Echols RM: Infections in the diabetic foot. In Jahss MH, editor: *Disorders of the foot and ankle,* Philadelphia, 1991, WB Saunders.
4. Bauman J, Girling J, Brand P: Plantar pressures and trophic ulcerations, *J Bone Joint Surg* 45B:652-673, 1963.
5. Leibovici L et al: Bacteremia in adult diabetic patients, *Diabetes Care,* 14(2):89–94, 1991.
6. Taylor LM, Porter JM: The clinical course of diabetics who require emergent foot surgery because of infection in ischemia, *J Vasc Surg* 6:454–459, 1987.
7. Pinzur MS et al: Limb salvage in infected lower extremity gangrene, *Foot Ankle* 8:212-215, 1988.
8. Foot care in patients with diabetes mellitus, Position statement, *Diabetes Care,* 14(suppl 2):18–19, 1991.
9. Wagner FW: The diabetic foot and amputation of the foot. In Mann RA, editor: *Surgery of the foot,* ed 5, St Louis, 1986, Mosby–Year Book.
10. Levin ME, O'Neal LW: *The diabetic foot,* ed 1, St Louis, 1973, Mosby–Year Book.
11. Wyss CR et al: Transcutaneous oxygen tension as a predictor of success after an amputation, *J Bone Joint Surg,* 70(2):203–207, 1988.
12. Malone JM et al: Prospective comparison of non-invasive techniques for amputation level selection, *Am J Surg* 154:179–184, 1987.
13. Zlatkin MB et al: The diabetic foot, *Radiol Clin North Am* 25:1095–1105, 1987.
14. McDonough JP, Quam SR: General anesthesia. In Levy LA, Hetherington VJ, *Principles and practice of podiatric medicine,* New York, 1990, Churchill-Livingstone.
15. Goldman L: Cardiac risks and complications of non-cardiac surgery, *Ann Intern Med* 98:504–513, 1983.
16. Busick EJ, Kozak GP: Management of diabetes during surgery. In Kozak GP et al, editors: *Management of diabetic foot problems,* Philadelphia, 1984, WB Saunders.
17. Dickhaut SC, Delee JC, Page CP: Nutritional status: importance in predicting wound healing after amputation, *J Bone Joint Surg* 66A:71–75, 1984.
18. Carpenter CB, Lazarus JM: Dialysis and transplantation in the treatment of renal failure. In Braunwald E et al, editors: *Harrison's principles of internal medicine,* New York, 1987, McGraw-Hill.
19. Maggiore P, Echols RM: Infections of the diabetic foot. In Jahss MH, editor: *Disorders of the foot and ankle,* ed 2, Philadelphia, 1991, WB Saunders.
20. Sizer JS, Wheelock FC: Digital amputations in diabetic patients, *Surgery* 72:980–989, 1972.
21. Gianfortune P, Pulla RJ, Sage R: Ray resections in the insensitive or dysvascular foot: a critical review, *J Foot Surg* 24(2):103–107, 1985.
22. Pinzur M et al: Amputations at the mid-

dle level of the foot, *J Bone Joint Surg* 68A:1061–1064, 1986.

23. Gaenslen FJ: Split heel approach in osteomyelitis of the os calcis, *J Bone Joint Surg* 13:759–772, 1931.

24. Crandall RC, Wagner FW: Partial and total calcanectomy, *J Bone Joint Surg* 63A:152–155, 1981.

25. Smith DG et al: Partial calcanectomy for the treatment of large ulcerations of the heel and calcaneal osteomyelitis, *J Bone Joint Surg* 74A:571–576, 1992.

26. McGregor IA: *Fundamental techniques of plastic surgery,* ed 7, New York, 1980, Churchill-Livingstone.

27. Sage R et al: Complications following midfoot amputation in neuropathic and dysvascular feet, *J Am Podiatr Med Assoc* 79(6):277–280, 1989.

28. Jang RS, Burkus JK: Long term follow-up of Syme's amputations for peripheral vascular disease associated with diabetes mellitus, *Foot Ankle,* 9(3):107–110, 1988.

29. Pinzur MS et al: Syme's two-stage amputation in insulin requiring diabetics with gangrene of the forefoot, *Foot Ankle* 11(6):394–396, 1991.

30. Malone JM et al: Prevention of amputation by diabetic education, *Am J Surg* 158:520–524, 1989.

31. Holewski JJ et al: Prevalence of foot pathology and lower extremity complications in a diabetic out-patient clinic, *J Rehabil Res Dev* 26(3):35–44, 1989.

17   Vascular Reconstruction in the Diabetic Patient

Anton N. Sidawy, M.D.

Richard F. Neville, M.D.

In 1987, 6.8 million Americans were known to have diabetes mellitus, with over half of all lower-extremity amputations performed in diabetic patients.[1] Therefore, the primary goal in diabetic lower-extremity care is to heal foot ulcerations and thereby prevent amputations and major disabilities. The etiology of foot lesions in diabetics is multifactorial. Vascular insufficiency, neuropathy, and susceptibility to infection are the major factors contributing to the formation of nonhealing diabetic foot lesions. In this chapter we will discuss major vessel arteriosclerosis in diabetics, indications for vascular reconstruction, perioperative management, and the vascular procedures used to treat these patients.

In addition to diabetes other risk factors contribute to the formation of atherosclerotic disease, including smoking, hypertension, hypercholesterolemia, obesity, and dietary habits. Although there is no evidence that treating diabetes will stop the progression of atherosclerotic disease, controlling other risk factors, especially smoking, is very important in slowing disease progression.[2] Proper foot care is also important to prevent the formation of foot lesions that become difficult to heal in the presence of vascular occlusion and ischemia.

The concept of diabetic small vessel occlusive disease often leads to inappropriate management of diabetic patients with nonhealing foot lesions. The formation of these lesions in the presence of normal palpable foot pulses led to the misconception that diabetic patients have arteriolar and capillary occlusive disease which causes skin ischemia and formation of foot lesions. The review by LoGerfo and Coffman[3] demonstrated that most of these lesions are caused by trauma to the insensate diabetic foot. This is a very important concept in the management of diabetic lesions. Daily foot examination by the diabetic patient, wearing appropriately fitting shoes, and immediately reporting any abnormal finding to the physician are important points in the prevention of foot lesions in diabetic patients. The management of established foot lesions should be directed toward the contributing factors, namely, neuropathy, infection, and vascular insufficiency.

In planning the strategy to improve arterial blood flow using reconstructive surgery, it is important to understand the distribution of peripheral vascular disease in diabetic patients. Although the femoral-popliteal segment is the area most commonly affected in diabetics as in nondiabetics,[4] infragenicular occlusive disease in the anterior tibial, posterior tibial, and peroneal arteries is the classic distribution in these patients.[5] It is not unusual to see patients with ischemic foot lesions having a palpable popliteal pulse with occlusive disease isolated to the infragenicular arteries. This infragenicular arterial occlusive disease is usually isolated

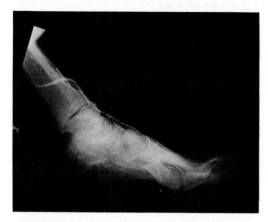

FIG 17–1.
Intraoperative arteriogram of low anterior tibial bypass.
Note the patent blood supply to the foot despite severe
proximal tibial occlusive disease.

to the lower leg, sparing the arterial system in the foot. A study based on arteriography showed no difference in occlusive disease in the arterial system of the foot when diabetics were compared to nondiabetics.[5] This allows for successful vein bypass operations to the foot vessels in diabetics (Fig 17–1).[6]

The presence of diabetes should not prevent the caring physician from managing these patients in the same manner as nondiabetic patients. Antibiotic treatment, drainage and debridement of dead tissue, prevention of trauma, vascular evaluation, and vascular reconstruction, if needed, are the basic principles of management of diabetic foot lesions. Diabetic lesions in the nonischemic foot heal if repetitive trauma is prevented and infection is controlled. In the presence of foot ischemia, the restoration of pulsatile blood flow using vein bypass is necessary to heal the lesion. In this situation diabetic patients show the same propensity to healing as nondiabetics.[7] Infrainguinal vein bypasses in diabetics have patency and limb salvage rates comparable to those performed in nondiabetics despite more bypasses performed for limb salvage in diabetics while more bypasses were done for claudication in the nondiabetic group.[7]

CLINICAL PRESENTATION

The importance of history and physical examination in planning the optimal management of a diabetic foot lesion is paramount. The history provides important information about the indication for vascular intervention. The physical examination determines the extent of foot involvement, infection, and the presence or absence of palpable foot pulses. The presence of palpable foot pulses precludes the need for large vessel revascularization as a prerequisite for healing. In the absence of palpable foot pulses, the noninvasive vascular laboratory examination provides important data that help the surgeon to decide if large vessel reconstruction is necessary for healing.

INDICATIONS

The indications for vascular reconstruction are incapacitating or life-style limiting claudication, rest pain, and tissue loss which includes gangrene and nonhealing ulcers or amputation sites.[8] Claudication should be severely incapacitating and life-style limiting to serve as an indication for vascular reconstruction especially for infragenicular reconstruction. The most common indication for revascularization is limb salvage with signs of pending limb loss, including pain at rest and tissue loss. These findings in addition to the presence of arterial ischemia indicate that the particular limb is threatened and a major amputation is imminent. It is very important in diabetics not to confuse ischemic rest pain with neuropathic pain. Pain due to severe ischemic arterial disease is usually located in the toes and forefoot of the affected limb and is typically described by the patient as burning pain which is worse at night in the recumbent position. This pain improves by placing the foot in the dependent position such as dangling the leg at the side of the bed, standing, or ambulating. If this pain becomes continuous and unrelieved by dependency it indicates that the ischemia is very severe and limb loss is imminent. The severity of ischemic disease in patients with rest pain and tissue loss should be confirmed by noninvasive vascular lab testing. This is important because superficial ulcerations can heal in the presence of moderate ischemia if infection is eradicated and pressure is relieved.

NONINVASIVE CONFIRMATION

Noninvasive vascular studies are used to detect the severity and location of peripheral vascular disease. They help in the screening, diagnosis, and management of patients with peripheral vascular disease. In addition, they are important in the follow-up of vascular bypasses. The most commonly used noninvasive vascular lab studies are Doppler ultrasound and Doppler pressures, ankle/brachial index (ABI), pulse volume recording (PVR), transcutaneous oxygen tension (TcPO$_2$) and photoplethysmography (PPG).

Doppler Ultrasound, Segmental Pressures and Ankle/Brachial Index

Hand-held or stationary Doppler ultrasound with or without the capability of generating wave form tracings is the most widely used device to evaluate ischemia. An experienced examiner can differentiate an acoustically normal from an abnormal Doppler signal. The presence of a Doppler signal indicates that there is blood flow in the examined artery. It does not indicate if this flow is adequate. To determine the adequacy of the flow, segmental Doppler pressure and ABI are measured. The segmental Doppler pressure examination localizes significant vascular occlusion. The presence of a gradient between the thigh pressure and brachial pressure, for example, suggests the

presence of aorta-iliac stenosis or occlusion. To obtain an overall assessment of the blood flow to the foot, the ABI is used. ABI is the ankle pressure divided by the brachial pressure and correlates with the severity of ischemia. In intermittent claudication an ABI of 0.5 to 0.8 is usually obtained. With more severe ischemia as in rest pain or tissue loss the ABI is usually less than 0.5.[9] Ankle pressure and ABI are not without flaws. Noncompressible vessels leading to falsely high ankle pressures were found in the lower extremity of more than 30% of diabetic patients.[10, 11] Therefore, in those patients with signs and symptoms of ischemia and absence of palpable pulses but with high ankle pressures, calcified arteries should be suspected and other noninvasive studies used to determine the adequacy of blood flow.

Pulse Volume Recording

PVR reflects the change of limb volume in response to arterial pulsation. The PVR wave is recorded and its contour and amplitude are studied. Foot pain is most likely ischemic if the amplitude of the wave form at the ankle measures less than 15 mm. Foot ulcers are unlikely to heal if the amplitude is less than 5 mm. These requirements are not different between diabetic and nondiabetic patients.[12]

Transcutaneous Oxygen Tension

The TcPO$_2$ measures the partial pressure of oxygen that diffuses through heated skin.[13] TcPO$_2$ is accurate in predicting healing. Healing is likely if TcPO$_2$ is above 35 to 40 mm Hg and unlikely below 20 to 26 mm Hg. A TcPO$_2$ regional index can be used to account for changes in systemic arterial oxygen tension.[14] To obtain the regional index, the TcPO$_2$ of the foot is divided by the TcPO$_2$ measured at a reference point usually located on the chest. Wounds with a TcPO$_2$ index below 0.4 are unlikely to heal and those with $TcPO_2$ above 0.6 are likely to heal.[15]

Photoplethysmography

PPG uses a diode that emits infrared light into the tissue. The intensity of the light reflected by the cutaneous microcirculation depends on the amount of blood in the microcirculation. This is helpful in the case of calcified arteries where ankle Doppler pressure and ABI are artificially elevated. In addition, PPG can be used to measure toe blood pressure by applying a cuff at the base of the toe and placing the PPG photo cell at the tip of the toe to record skin blood flow during inflation and gradual deflation of the cuff. Using this method, the toe pressure is obtained with the lower limit of normal 50 mm Hg.[16]

PERIOPERATIVE EVALUATION

Preoperative Evaluation

The goal of preoperative evaluation is to identify those patients with a significant risk of perioperative morbidity and mortality. Ideally, preoperative evaluation would diminish the risk to these patients by allowing the safest possible operative intervention. Coronary artery disease is the major cause of complications after vascular reconstruction in the diabetic population, with myocardial infarction accounting for over 50% of perioperative mortality.[17] Cardiovascular risk can impact on the anesthesia method or operative revascularization chosen for each patient.

Initial screening of history and significant risk factors is used to identify patients who require further evaluation with specific cardiovascular testing. However, cardiac symptoms are often latent due to the functional limitations of the diabetic patient. Goldman was first to identify risk factors predictive of increased perioperative risk.[18] Subsequent

multivariate analysis by Eagle resulted in a more useful system that has been prospectively evaluated in vascular patients.[19] Eagle identified five criteria used to prompt additional cardiovascular evaluation including age greater than 70 years, diabetes mellitus requiring treatment, a history of angina or myocardial infarction, ventricular arrythmia requiring treatment, and Q-waves on the ECG.[20] Timing is also important because surgery should be deferred if possible within 3 months of a myocardial infarction, especially if the patient has experienced subsequent congestive heart failure or unstable angina.[21]

Many noninvasive methods to evaluate cardiac function exist, although cardiac catheterization remains the gold standard. The exercise stress test is a common noninvasive test, but often is not useful in the vascular population because these patients cannot ambulate sufficiently to stress their myocardial reserve.[22] Echocardiography measures left ventricular ejection fraction and has been advocated by some groups. However, echocardiography is technician-dependent and the sensitivity and specificity of the test are questionable. Dipyridamole-thallium scans provide a functional assessment of myocardial perfusion. A nuclear scan is obtained after administration of intravenous thallium. Dipyridamole is a coronary vasodilator that causes a vascular steal distal to critical coronary stenoses. Filing defects appear on the thallium scan in areas of underperfused myocardium. The scan is repeated in 4 hours with reperfused areas designated as reversible defects consistent with viable myocardium at risk for ischemia when stressed. This test appears to be an accurate functional test to assess preoperative cardiac risk.[23] Holter monitoring to detect silent myocardial ischemia during normal daily activity has also proved an accurate assessment of perioperative cardiac risk in recent series.[24]

Cardiac catheterization is an invasive assessment of coronary artery anatomy and left ventricular function. Intravenous contrast is injected into the coronary arteries with delineation of critical stenoses. Assessment of function is made by ejection fraction determinations. This is an invasive test with risk to the punctured artery and to renal function from nephrotoxic contrast materials. However, a positive noninvasive test usually prompts a cardiac catheterization prior to therapeutic procedures such as coronary angioplasty or bypass surgery.

Noncardiac complications of vascular procedures involve pulmonary and renal function. Diabetic patients with vascular disease often use tobacco, resulting in pulmonary dysfunction. If there is a clinical history of pulmonary dysfunction, preoperative arterial blood gases and pulmonary function studies should be obtained. Incentive spirometry and pulmonary toilet are beneficial in all patients. Renal insufficiency is a common problem because there often exists a component of diabetic nephropathy exacerbated by the contrast agents used during perioperative arteriography and the hemodynamic changes occurring at surgery. Diabetic vascular patients should have blood urea nitrogen (BUN) and creatinine values monitored before and after any arteriogram and during the perioperative period. Careful hydration should be performed to avoid nephrotoxicity and renal insufficiency. Perioperative stroke can also occur and noninvasive carotid testing should be performed before the operation for any patient with a history of a transient ischemic attack or stroke.

Intraoperative Management

Intraoperative monitoring is especially important in the diabetic vascular patient to maintain adequate perfusion to vital organ systems. Common clinical signs of end-organ perfusion include adequate urine output and specific gravity, cerebral function, and ECG findings of ischemia or dysarrhythmias. Peripheral perfusion may be assessed by examining the extremities for cool skin and cyanosis.

Invasive monitoring is used perioperatively to help maintain adequate perfusion prior to the development of clinical ischemia. Arterial lines are used in most vascular reconstructions allowing continuous monitoring of blood pressure. Central venous pressure is monitored through an indwelling catheter reflecting an approximation of blood volume, venous tone, and right ventricular function. However, central venous pressure may not correlate with left ventricular function in the presence of coronary artery disease or myocardial dysfunction. Left heart performance can be monitored with a Swan-Ganz catheter measuring pulmonary artery diastolic pressure and capillary wedge pressure as a reflection of left ventricular function. This correlation is lost with pulmonary vascular hypertension, mitral stenosis, pulmonary embolization, or superventricular tachycardia. Because left heart catheterization carries a 1% to 3% complication rate, specific indications for such monitoring should be followed.[25] Appropriate indications include ejection fraction less than 30%, clinical risk factors indicative of increased perioperative risk, chronic renal failure, and aortic surgery. In the diabetic vascular patient these indications are often present and most are monitored intraoperatively with a Swan-Ganz catheter. A recent advance in intraoperative monitoring is transesophageal echocardiography. This is a method by which wall motion of the myocardial chambers can be assessed during surgery with changes in intraoperative management stimulated by abnormalities in the myocardial wall motion.[26]

Invasive monitoring can be used to improve perfusion by optimizing cardiac output that is determined by heart rate and stroke volume. Stroke volume is affected by preload, afterload, and myocardial contractility, with preload the most easily manipulated factor. Preload can be determined using a Swan-Ganz catheter and intravascular volume adjusted to attain optimal myocardial function. A preoperative Starling curve of myocardial performance can be constructed by plotting cardiac index against pulmonary capillary wedge pressure. Each individual's optimal pulmonary capillary wedge pressure is useful information during the intraoperative and postoperative period. The Swan-Ganz catheter also allows measurement of mixed venous O_2 saturation, which is a reflection of the oxygen saturation of the blood returning to the right heart. The Fick equation relates oxygen consumption to cardiac output and the arterial venous oxygen difference.[27] Each patient's oxygen consumption can be evaluated from the mixed venous O_2 and cardiac output. Subsequent manipulation of the cardiac output can optimize oxygen delivery to match oxygen consumption.

Postoperative Management

Postoperative care is a continuation of pre- and intraoperative management. Surgical technique and an appropriate operation combined with proper intraoperative hemodynamic management can lead to an uncomplicated postoperative course. In the postoperative period, clinical signs are important to assess renal, cerebral, coronary, and peripheral perfusion. Invasive monitoring is continued for 24 to 72 hours with the realization that 40% of perioperative myocardial infarction occurs 48 hours after the operation.[24] Cardiac output is optimized to maximize oxygen delivery and myocardial stress is minimized to decrease oxygen demand. This involves decreasing respiratory work and treating any fever or infection which is present. The goal of perioperative management in a diabetic vascular patient is the safe completion of a successful operation minimizing cardiac, pulmonary, and renal morbidity and mortality.

VASCULAR RECONSTRUCTION

Once the decision has been made to revascularize a limb based on physical findings and noninvasive vascular studies, an arteriogram is obtained. The preoperative arteriogram is important in selecting the optimal mode of therapy, and, if a bypass is planned the arteriogram identifies appropriate inflow and outflow sites.

1. *Choice of optimal therapy:* Although vascular bypass is the mainstay in the treatment of symptomatic vascular occlusion, other modes of therapy are now available and some of them are highly efficacious. Short areas of significant stenosis can be treated by balloon angioplasty especially if they are located in the iliac artery. Complete occlusion can be recanalized with lytic therapy using urokinase or streptokinase, especially if the occlusion is recent. The underlying arterial stenosis can then be treated with various endovascular procedures, including balloon angioplasty or atherectomy. Long segment occlusions are usually treated by bypass procedures. In addition, the preoperative arteriogram defines inflow lesions which may need to be addressed with endovascular therapy prior to distal infrainguinal bypass.

2. *Determining the type of bypass used:* The preoperative arteriogram defines the points of inflow and outflow for the bypass. It is often difficult to demonstrate distal arteries for possible bypass on the preoperative arteriogram. Several techniques for enhancement of distal vessel opacification are used including intraarterial injection of vasodilators such as papaverine and reserpine, reactive hyperemia, antegrade arteriography, intraar-

terial digital subtraction angiography and proximal occlusion with a balloon while injecting the eye distally.[28] In addition to visualizing distal vessels, injection of vasodilators such as papaverine may unmask a hemodynamically significant stenosis in the aortoiliac segment before originating a bypass distal to the lesion. A more than 15% drop in femoral to brachial pressure ratio after the injection of papaverine in the femoral artery indicates the presence of a hemodynamically significant lesion proximally.[29] The preoperative arteriogram identifies the outflow vessel to receive the bypass. Although the distal anastomosis is preferentially performed to arteries with run-off to the foot, recent reports indicate that bypasses to isolated segments of the tibial and peroneal arteries result in acceptable patency and limb salvage rates.[30]

Endovascular Procedures

In 1964 Dr. Charles Dotter performed the first dilation of an atherosclerotic stenosis by sequentially passing larger catheters through the lesion.[31] Andres Gruntzig then developed the double lumen polyvinyl balloon catheter, greatly increasing the ease and effectiveness of arterial dilation. These advances have led to an explosion of intraluminal devices for the treatment of atherosclerotic lesions (Fig 17–2). Although these devices can be applied percutaneously, they are invasive and should be implemented in appropriate clinical situations by those familiar with the treatment of vascular disease.

Transluminal angioplasty with balloon catheters is the most commonly used endovascular therapeutic procedure. Balloon dilation creates a controlled injury resulting in plaque fracture and separa-

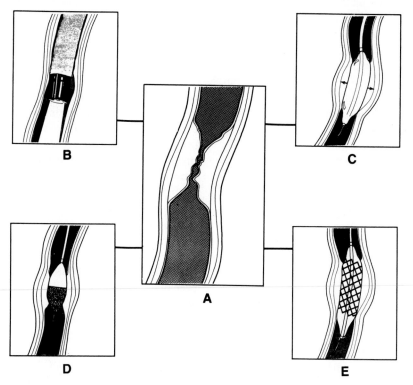

FIG 17–2.
Endovascular procedures. **a,** arterial atheroma; **b,** laser ablation; **c,** balloon angioplasty; **d,** rotational atherectomy; **e,** balloon-mounted stent.

tion from the media of the arterial wall.[32] The media is thus released allowing an increase in the arterial lumen. The controlled injury heals thereby remodeling the lesion into one less obstructive of arterial flow. The role of plaque compression by the balloon accounts for only 5% of angioplasty's effect.

Balloon angioplasty has been performed in the aorta, iliac, femoral, and tibial arteries with varied success. Difficulty in objective interpretation of the data arises from lack of uniform reporting standards, variability of indications and patient populations, exclusion of initial failures from follow-up, and different methods used to evaluate therapeutic success. In the aortoiliac system the effectiveness of balloon angioplasty approximates that of surgical reconstruction for the appropriate lesion. Aortoiliac angioplasty results in patency rates of 90% at 1 year and 70% at 5 years, which is comparable to surgical results of 95% and 87%, respectively.[33] Clinical series of femoral-popliteal angioplasty report 75% one year patency with 45% five year patency.[33, 34] These results are slightly less than those reported with femoral-popliteal bypass. The results of infrapopliteal angioplasty are significantly inferior to surgical revascularization. One-year patency after tibial angioplasty is approximately 45%.[35] This compares to 70% to 90% patency with surgical revascularization.[36]

It becomes obvious that angioplasty is most successful in the aortoiliac system, less so in the femoral-popliteal segment, and least in the tibial arteries. Favorable lesions for angioplasty include focal stenoses or short occlusions as opposed to diffuse disease or chronic, total occlusions beyond 5 to 7 cm. Patients with claudication have better success with angioplasty than do those treated for limb salvage.[33] The major complications of balloon angioplasty are acute thrombosis and restenosis. Early failure occurring within 1

month indicates an ineffective initial dilatation, which is prominent with eccentric lesions. Late restenosis occurs due to myointimal hyperplasia and accelerated atherosclerosis, the same processes that plague surgical revascularization.[37]

Many catheter-based devices have been developed to improve balloon angioplasty and decrease the restenosis rate. The first group of such devices involved thermal angioplasty. Lasers (NdYag, argon), electricity, and radiofrequency were used to generate thermal energy by heating catheter tips of various configurations. After initial enthusiasm, disadvantages quickly became obvious. Thermal energy was not selective and insufficient for true plaque ablation. Thermal systems were ineffective against calcified lesions and actually caused arterial vasospasm, thrombosis, and chronic damage secondary to the thermal energy. Clinically, thermal angioplasty was inferior to balloon angioplasty in the aortoiliac system with decreased patency reported as early as 9 months after the procedure.[38]

Other laser angioplasty systems applied direct laser energy (argon hybrid probe, excimer, and pulsed-dye lasers) to take advantage of selective absorption by the plaque and precise ablation with minimal effects on surrounding normal tissue. However, clinical trials demonstrated an inability to control the laser energy resulting in arterial perforations, early occlusions, and no benefit as compared to balloon angioplasty. Although these lasers could cross occlusions longer than 5 cm, restenosis was unaffected by the direct laser systems.[38] The search continues for the ideal laser angioplasty system involving efficient ablation of variable composition atheroma, minimal damage to surrounding tissue, and decreased restenosis. The energy must be transmitted through flexible optical fibers and be cost effective.

Atherectomy catheters were developed to debulk atherosclerotic lesions without balloon dilatation. The Kensey catheter and Auth rotoblator mounted a rotating cam tip and diamond-covered brass burr, respectively, at the end of a flexible catheter.[39, 40] Theoretically, as the catheter rotated at 1,000,000 rpm atheroma would be preferentially destroyed and leave the normal arterial wall intact. Clinical use with these catheters resulted in initial failures, perforation, embolization, and destruction of the intima with hemorrhage into the media. Neither device solved the problem of reocclusion and restenosis. The Simpson atherocath consisted of a rotational blade in a cylindrical housing with a balloon opposite the opening in the housing.[41] After positioning across the lesion, the balloon was inflated and the rotational blade advanced, shaving the atheroma into the cylindrical housing. Theoretically, this catheter would debulk the atherosclerotic lesion leaving a smooth luminal surface without the need for balloon dilatation. However, this atherectomy catheter was time consuming, ineffective against total occlusions and diffuse disease, and did not solve the problem of restenosis. This device made a major contribution to the study of atherosclerotic lesions by retrieving tissue for histologic study.

Intravascular stents are expandable coils placed in the artery to increase the effectiveness of angioplasty. Stents can tack down intimal flaps raised by balloon dilation and provide support against the elastic recoil which may play a role in restenosis. The Palmaz stent recently released by the Federal Drug Administration (FDA) for clinical use is an articulated, metallic stent deployed by dilation on a standard balloon catheter.[42] Other stents include various coils and mesh work patterns which are either self expanding on release or are deployed on a balloon catheter. The initial clinical work with intravascular stents points to a possible role for stents after acute occlusions, with a possible reduction in restenosis in fibroplastic lesions such as graft stenosis.

The role of endovascular imaging systems such as angioscopy and intravascular ultrasound in the treatment of occlusive arterial disease is yet to be defined. Intravascular ultrasound consists of a transducer in the tip of a flexible catheter which is inserted into a vessel to deliver cross-sectional images of the lumen and vessel wall. Plaque composition and the exact dimensions of stenosis can be measured and used to guide endovascular treatment.[43] Angioscopy involves a flexible fiberoptic catheter attached to a camera which transmits and reproduces an image on a video monitor. Irrigation is required to clear the vessel of blood, allowing an image to be obtained. Angioscopy has been used for evaluation of anastomotic sites, thromboembolectomy, carotid endarterectomy, and as a method of vein preparation with in situ vein bypass.[44]

Endovascular techniques should be considered an adjunct to the treatment of peripheral vascular disease in the diabetic population. Transluminal angioplasty should be included as a standard option in the treatment modalities available to the diabetic patient with vascular disease, although diabetics have a higher reocclusion rate after angioplasty.[45] Other devices should be considered experimental at this time and used in the context of approved clinical protocols to collect objective data. Despite the initial wave of enthusiasm for these "minimally-invasive" devices, critical appraisal is required to achieve proper device application in appropriate clinical situations and continue to advance technical refinements.

INFLOW PROCEDURES

Inflow procedures address occlusive disease in the aorta and iliac arteries of symptomatic limbs. Symptomatic aorto-iliac disease is manifested as claudication in the calf with extension to the thigh and buttock area. Rest pain and tissue loss are unusual with isolated aortoiliac disease because significant collaterals develop maintaining distal perfusion. Limb-threatening ischemia, rest pain, and tissue loss occur when multilevel occlusive disease involves a combined distribution of aortoiliac and infrainguinal disease. Claudication and rest pain may be relieved by treatment of the inflow problem, however, tissue loss may require the addition of a distal revascularization. The Leriche syndrome is a classic symptom complex of aortoiliac disease involving hip and thigh claudication, impotence, and absent femoral pulses.[46] Impotence occurs as flow to the internal pudendal artery is decreased, causing insufficient flow for erectile function. Indications for treatment of inflow disease include disabling claudication, rest pain, or tissue loss.

Aortobifemoral Bypass

The standard treatment for diffuse aortoiliac disease is aortobifemoral bypass (Fig 17–3). Unilateral aortofemoral bypasses are performed; however, aortoiliac disease is commonly bilateral, mandating bilateral reconstruction. The magnitude of the operation is such that repeat operation for progression of contralateral disease is best avoided. The operation involves placing a synthetic graft from the infrarenal abdominal aorta to each femoral artery. The most commonly used grafts are made of Dacron in a knitted or woven fashion and polytetrafluoroethylene (PTFE). Opinions differ about which graft material is best, and the choice is determined by the preference of the surgeon.

The bypass is performed through a transabdominal (midline or transverse) or retroperitoneal (flank) approach. After the aorta is exposed, tunnels are created in a retroperitoneal position under the inguinal ligament and into the groin. The

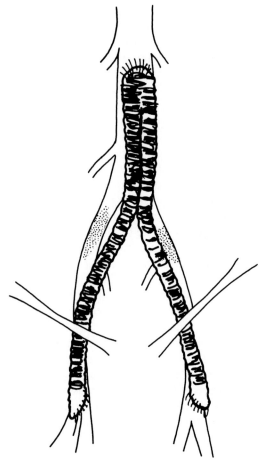

FIG 17–3.
Aortobifemoral bypass.

patient is then anticoagulated with heparin. The aorta must be controlled proximally and distally with vascular clamps to halt blood flow and allow the bypass to be performed. The diabetic aorta is often heavily calcified, which requires careful application of vascular clamps. The proximal anastomosis is performed in an end-to-side or end-to-end configuration. An end-to-side anastomosis maintains flow through the native aorta to patent arteries such as the internal iliac arteries and the inferior mesenteric artery which supplies the pelvis and hind gut. The end-to-end configuration is best for patients who have complete aortic occlusion or will not suffer from decreased forward flow through their native aorta. Each limb of the graft is placed through the retroperitoneal tunnel already created along the anatomic course of the native arteries. The distal graft limbs are anastomosed to the common femoral arteries unless there is disease at the orifice of the profunda femoris. In this case the distal graft is used as a patch to open the profunda femoris orifice. This is done because of the importance of maintaining flow through the profunda femoris, which is an artery supplying the thigh musculature and a source of collateral flow to the lower leg. Prior to the completion of each anastomosis, loose atheromatous debris and thrombus are flushed out to prevent distal embolization.

Results of aortobifemoral bypass are excellent with 100% immediate patency, and 5- and 10-year patency greater than 80% and 75%, respectively.[47] Diabetics have patency comparable to nondiabetic patients, although diabetics suffer higher mortality in long-term follow-up and have an increased number of subsequent distal revascularizations.[48] Postoperatively, patients return to normal function with more than 80% of patients symptom free after 5 years and half of those who previously have not worked due to ischemic symptoms returning to employment.[49] Operative mortality rates are below 5%. Recognized complications include colonic ischemia, retrograde ejaculation, graft thrombosis, graft infection, and hemorrhage as well as the previously mentioned cardiopulmonary and renal problems.

Endarterectomy

Arterial endarterectomy is one of the first procedures used to treat aortoiliac occlusive disease. Endarterectomy involves proximal and distal control with the artery opened through a longitudinal arteriotomy. The atherosclerotic plaque is removed from the arterial wall by separation of the plane between the plaque and the outer media or adventitia. The procedure was used extensively prior to the development of vascular graft materials but currently has a limited role in the treatment of aortoiliac occlusive disease. Bypass grafting and transluminal angioplasty have largely replaced endarterectomy as primary therapy for aortoiliac disease. The technique remains useful for focal atherosclerotic lesions and is confined to iliac artery or terminal aortic focal stenosis in combination with a bypass procedure.

Iliofemoral Bypass

In the patient with unilateral inflow occlusive disease an iliofemoral bypass is an excellent option, especially for patients who are at increased risk for an abdominal aortic procedure. The operation is performed through a flank approach and a retroperitoneal dissection. The bypass extends from the common iliac artery to the femoral artery using an 8 mm Dacron or PTFE graft (Fig 17–4). The graft is tunneled in an anatomic position in the retroperitoneum and brought under the inguinal ligament into the groin for anastomosis to the femoral artery. A cross-femoral graft can be constructed in patients with bilateral iliac disease. Results are excellent with 5-year patency reported between 75% and 90%.[50]

Extra-Anatomic Procedures

Extraanatomic bypasses do not follow the normal anatomic course of the arterial tree. These operations are performed when the risk of an anatomical procedure is excessive due to the patient's medical condition or infected tissue planes. The procedures can be performed using regional and/or local anesthesia minimizing the cardiopulmonary risk of a general anesthetic and intubation. Examples of extraanatomic procedures include femoral-femoral and axillofemoral bypass.

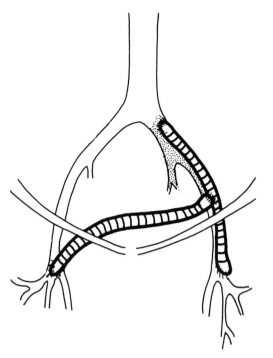

FIG 17–4.
Retroperitoneal iliobifemoral bypass.

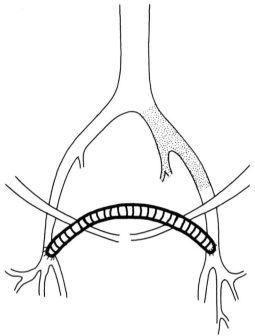

FIG 17–5.
Cross-femoral bypass.

Femoral-femoral bypass is appropriate for unilateral aortoiliac disease in a patient considered a poor operative risk for an intraabdominal procedure. The bypass requires a contralateral femoral artery with normal blood flow. Blood is routed from the femoral artery with sufficient flow to the femoral artery on the symptomatic side with an 8 mm externally reinforced PTFE graft (Fig 17–5). The graft is placed through a subcutaneous tunnel in a suprapubic position on the anterior abdominal wall in a C configuration. Patency rates for crossover femoral-femoral bypass are 60% to 80% at 5 years.[51] Progression of disease in the donor iliac artery can occur, however, it is relatively uncommon.

Axillofemoral bypass is performed in patients with aortic or bilateral iliac disease who are at high risk for an intraabdominal procedure. The proximal anastomosis is performed at the first portion of the axillary artery. This artery can be exposed with minimal dissection inferior to the midportion of the clavicle. Externally reinforced PTFE is tunneled in a subcutaneous position along the anterior axillary line to the ipsilateral femoral artery. A femoral-femoral bypass can be added using the graft as an inflow source to the contralateral femoral artery, forming a functional axillobifemoral revascularization with improved 5-year patency as compared to unilateral axillofemoral grafts (Fig 17–6).[52] Patency rates in axillofemoral bypasses are 70% at 5 years but are inferior to those of aortofemoral, iliofemoral, and femorofemoral bypasses. Thrombectomy can be performed to salvage failed grafts.[52]

OUTFLOW PROCEDURES

Endarterectomy

Endarterectomy was a commonly performed operation for lower-extremity re-

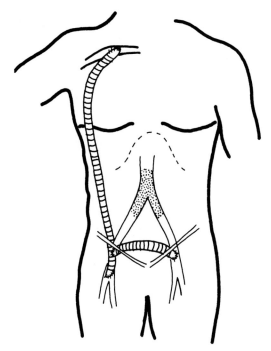

FIG 17–6.
Axillobifemoral bypass.

vascularization. Open or closed endarterectomy techniques were used to restore patency to entire superficial femoral or popliteal artery segments. The results of long segment endarterectomies, however, were not satisfactory and this procedure fell into disfavor after the emergence of autogenous vein bypass, which offered 5-year patency rates of 72% compared to 32% for long segment endarterectomy.[53] Therefore, an autogenous vein bypass became a more appealing alternative for management of long segment occlusions. Short segment or "segmental" endarterectomy resulted in better patency and was recommended as an alternative to femoral popliteal bypass in localized lesions of the femoral artery especially if the saphenous vein is not adequate.[54] Segmental endarterectomy maintains the patency of an artery delaying or obviating the need for bypass. Hence endarterectomy of a significant lesion of the superficial femoral artery at Hunter's canal offers an alter-

native to femoral popliteal bypass with patency rates of 57% at 7 years.[55]

Using preoperative arteriographic guidance and knowledge of arterial superficial anatomy, the area of the occlusive lesion is localized along the course of the artery. The artery is dissected free and isolated. After adequate heparinization, an arteriotomy is started in a soft area of the arterial wall and continued through the area of occlusion to a short distance beyond the lesion. The endarterectomy is started in a plane that splits the media of the artery; in this location the vascular wall easily separates. Usually the endarterectomy is terminated by cutting both ends of the plaque well beyond the occlusive area. The remaining plaque is secured to the arterial wall using fine vascular sutures especially at the distal end to prevent flap formation and subsequent thrombosis. Since atherosclerotic disease usually extends well beyond the area of the occlusion, very seldom "feathering" of the plaque is possible to remove the occlusive lesion. The arteriotomy area can be closed with a patch using autogenous vein or prosthetic material such as PTFE or Dacron. An endarterectomized segment of the occluded superficial femoral artery can also be used to patch common femoral and profunda femoris endarterectomy sites.

Profundaplasty

The common femoral artery divides into two major branches: the superficial femoral and the profunda femoris arteries. The profunda originates from the posterolateral aspect of the femoral artery and runs posteriorly and caudad. It gives rise to very important branches which supply the thigh and interconnect to form a collateral network which eventually connects with collaterals of the popliteal artery. Therefore the profunda femoris artery is an important carrier of collateral flow to the lower limb after superficial femoral artery occlusion.[56]

Atherosclerotic disease of the profunda follows a typical distribution involving the origin of this vessel with possible extension to its first branch, the lateral circumflex artery. However, in a small number of patients, especially diabetics, the disease extends into the distal profunda.[57] Because the atherosclerotic disease of the profunda is usually in its origin, it lends itself to segmental endarterectomy and patch angioplasty. Patch angioplasty of the profunda artery is called profundaplasty. Profundaplasty can be done alone or in conjunction with inflow procedures such as aortofemoral, axillofemoral, or iliofemoral bypasses.[56, 58] When inflow procedures are done in the presence of superficial femoral artery occlusion, widening the origin of the profunda femoris artery using profundaplasty is important to maintain the patency of these bypasses and to supply adequate blood flow to the lower extremity via the profunda and its collaterals.

Profundaplasty can also be performed in conjunction with infrainguinal bypasses, especially if the profunda stenosis is not very significant and profundaplasty is not expected to relieve the symptoms if done alone. Less commonly, profundaplasty can be performed alone in symptomatic patients in whom infrainguinal bypasses are not feasible or adequate patency is not expected due to unsatisfactory autogenous vein or the absence of a suitable outflow artery for the distal anastomosis.[59]

Profundaplasty begins with the dissection of the common, superficial, and profunda femoris arteries. The profunda dissection is carried distally until the consistency of the artery softens, which indicates the end of the atherosclerotic lesion. The arteriotomy is started on the anterior aspect of the common femoral artery and is carried down the profunda until a normal arterial wall is encountered and the end of the atherosclerotic plaque is delineated. A patch is used to close the arteriotomy and widen the lumen of the artery in that area. The patch material used is either autogenous vein, an endarterectomized segment of occluded superficial femoral artery, or prosthetic material. The profundaplasty can be done with or without endarterectomy of the atherosclerotic plaque.

The best results of profundaplasty are obtained when the profunda stenosis is severe, usually in patients with patent popliteal artery and adequate run off to the foot. In addition, patent profunda is important in lowering the level of amputation; 100% of limbs amputated below the knee had patent profunda, whereas only 11% of limbs with thrombosed profunda had below-the-knee amputation.[60]

Infrainguinal Bypasses

Infrainguinal bypasses aim to restore circulation to the popliteal, anterior tibial, posterior tibial, peroneal, pedal, or plantar arteries. Although the indications for infrainguinal revascularization follow the general indications for lower-limb revascularization, bypasses to the infragenicular arteries are seldom performed for claudication. This is especially true in diabetics where the vast majority of these bypasses are performed for limb-threatening situations such as rest pain and tissue loss.[61] In each bypass three important factors need to be determined: the inflow artery, the outflow artery, and the conduit.

1. *The inflow artery:* The most commonly used inflow artery for infrainguinal bypasses is the common femoral artery. For a long time the use of the superficial femoral or popliteal arteries for inflow was avoided because the superficial femoral artery was thought to be readily affected by the atherosclerotic process, thereby limiting the longevity of bypasses originating distal to the common femoral artery. However, various investigators reported excellent patency rates in infra-

genicular bypasses using the superficial femoral and popliteal arteries as inflow (Fig 17–7).[62–64] In comparing the limb salvage rates of bypasses originating from the superficial femoral and popliteal arteries to those originating from the common femoral artery we found that the patency rates and limb salvage rates of the former bypasses were more favorable.[64] In addition, the use of tibial and peroneal arteries as inflow vessels was also found to be favorable and offered good patency rates.[65] Seemingly, shorter bypasses result in better patency and limb salvage rates.[66] It is very important to remember, however, that the inflow of the bypass should not originate distal to a hemodynamically significant lesion. If the preoperative arteriogram demonstrates a he-

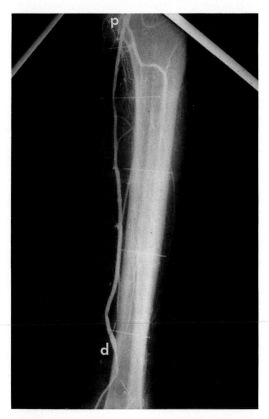

FIG 17–7.
Popliteal-posterior tibial bypass using in situ saphenous vein graft. *p,* proximal anastomosis; *d,* distal anastomosis.

modynamically significant proximal stenosis, it should be treated or the bypass should originate proximal to it.

2. *The outflow artery:* The preoperative arteriogram is very important in selecting the most suitable outflow vessel for bypass. Infrainguinal bypasses can be performed to the popliteal, anterior tibial, posterior tibial, peroneal, pedal, or plantar arteries.

The popliteal artery.—The patency and limb salvage rates of bypasses performed to the popliteal artery (femoral popliteal bypass) above the knee are better than those performed to the below-knee popliteal segment if prosthetic material is used as the conduit. In addition, autogenous saphenous vein (ASV) is superior to PTFE material in bypasses placed to the below-knee popliteal artery (76% for ASV vs 54% for PTFE).[67] This difference becomes significant after 2½ years of observation.

The better the runoff to the foot, the better the results of this bypass. However, acceptable patency rates were reported when popliteal bypasses were performed to an isolated popliteal segment lacking runoff to the foot when autogenous venous material was used for conduit indicating that isolated popliteal artery may have enough runoff via collaterals.[68, 69]

The popliteal artery is approached medially in its above- or below-knee position. The subcutaneous tissue and fat are sharply incised and the deep fascia opened. The artery, accompanied by the popliteal vein (in the below-knee segment it is surrounded by a pair of veins), is carefully dissected to prevent vascular injury, and isolated with vessel loops or umbilical tapes. The lateral approach to the popliteal artery can be used in situations where medial scarring or infection makes the medial approach unadvisable.

The tibial and peroneal arteries.— Bypasses to the tibial and peroneal arteries (tibio-peroneal bypasses) are primarily used for limb salvage in patients with rest pain or tissue loss. They are commonly performed bypasses in diabetics due to the typical distribution of diabetic atherosclerotic vascular disease in the tibio-peroneal location. Autogenous vein is the conduit of choice in the infrapopliteal location. Prosthetic grafts should only be used as a last resort after all autogenous vein sources have been exhausted because the limb salvage rate for prosthetic bypasses to infrapopliteal arteries was significantly worse than those for ASV.[67]

Although the peroneal artery is more difficult to dissect and does not directly continue to the foot, connecting with the plantar arch via terminal branches, the peroneal artery offers the same limb salvage rates as bypasses performed to the anterior or posterior tibial arteries. In a retrospective review of 78 tibioperoneal vein bypasses performed on 75 patients the 5-year limb salvage rates were 80%, 78%, and 81% for the peroneal, anterior tibial, and posterior tibial, respectively, with an overall mortality rate of 2%.[64] This excellent limb salvage rate reflects the value of tibial reconstruction. None of the 78 grafts failed after 12 months of follow-up. Of the bypasses failing in the first month, all limbs required major amputation. Of the eight bypasses failing in the next 11 months, only three required major amputation (38%). Therefore, if an open wound heals before the failure of a bypass, a major amputation can be avoided. Although it is preferable to perform distal bypasses to tibial and peroneal arteries with good runoff to the foot, recent reports of bypasses to isolated tibial artery segments were very favorable.[30]

The anterior tibial artery is approached via an incision placed in the anterior compartment of the leg lateral to the tibia. The deep fascia is incised longitudinally between the tibialis anterior and the extensor digitorum longus muscles. The bellies of these two muscles are bluntly separated and the dissection is carried deeper until the anterior tibial vascular bundle is found. In the lower third of the leg, this artery is located in a more superficial plane covered only by the skin, the deep fascia and the extensor retinaculae. The saphenous vein is harvested via a separate incision.

To perform the distal anastomosis, the vein is passed in a subcutaneous tunnel or through the interosseous membrane. The posterior tibial and peroneal arteries are located in the posterior compartment of the leg and they can be approached via the medial incision made for saphenous vein harvest. The incision is deepened, anterior or posterior to the saphenous vein, in the subcutaneous tissue, and the attachment of the soleus muscle to the tibia is incised and the posterior compartment entered. Bluntly, a plane is developed by displacing the belly of the soleus muscle posteriorly. The first vascular bundle encountered is the posterior tibial. The peroneal vascular bundle is found deeper and lateral to the posterior tibial.

The peroneal artery moves laterally as it progresses down in the leg, so a lateral approach to this artery is advisable in patients with large legs when a distal peroneal bypass is contemplated. In the distal third of the leg, a longitudinal incision is made in the skin over the fibula. The bone is cleared from the muscular insertions using a periosteal elevator and a 5 to 10 cm segment of the bone is resected to expose the peroneal vascular bundle. Control of these arteries, especially if diseased, is crucial. Fine silastic vessel loops or intraluminal occluders can be used. The use of a thigh tourniquet is recommended to control blood flow to the leg during the performance of the distal anastomosis. In that situation, only the anterior aspect of these arteries needs to be dissected, and the circumferential dissection for placement of vessel loops is avoided due to the lack of back bleeding when the tourniquet is inflated.[70] The anastomosis is done with fine vascular sutures (7-0 Prolene) using magnification.

The dorsalis pedis and plantar arteries.—Bypasses to these arteries are now commonly performed to heal foot lesions and obtain limb salvage. Multiple reports indicate excellent patency and limb salvage rates. It is easy to approach the dorsalis pedis artery on the dorsum of the foot just lateral to the tendon of the extensor hallucis longus which crosses the artery in a lateral to medial direction. The medial and lateral plantar arteries are approached as described by Ascer and Veith.[71] Depending on the location of the saphenous vein in the inframalleolar region, a tunnel may or may not be needed to pass the end of the vein from its harvest incision to the incision used for the dissection of these arteries. If a tunnel is needed the subcutaneous route is used.

The results obtained with dorsalis pedis bypass in diabetics are very favorable, with a limb salvage rate of 87%,[72] while those reported for plantar bypasses are also favorable.[71]

3. *The conduit:* The conduit of choice for infrainguinal bypasses is the autogenous vein. The most commonly used vein is the greater saphenous vein. Other autogenous vein sources include the arm vein and lesser saphenous vein. There are many ways a vein can be prepared for use in the infrainguinal position (Fig 17–8).

a. *The reversed vein method:* Any vein including the greater saphenous can be prepared using this method. The vein is harvested by ligating its branches and by completely removing it from its bed to be used as a free graft. The vein is reversed so its valves do not interfere with blood flow; therefore, the vein's distal end is used for construction of the proximal anastomosis and its proximal end is used for the distal anastomoses.

b. *The in-situ greater saphenous vein method:* This method can only be used in

preparing the greater saphenous vein for an infrainguinal bypass. Leather and his colleagues[73] popularized the concept of in-situ bypass, which is performed by ligating the branches of the vein and disrupting its valves while keeping the vein in its site. The proximal vein end is used for the proximal anastomosis and distal vein is used for the distal anastomosis so a better size match is obtained between the ends of the vein and the inflow and outflow arteries. The disruption of the valves can be done blindly or under direct vision. After preparation of the greater saphenous vein, either the proximal anastomosis is performed between the proximal end of the vein and the inflow artery to distend its proximal portion down to its first competent valve,[74] or the same effect is obtained by irrigating the proximal end of the vein by papaverine-containing fluid. The prograde distention of the vein allows the localization of its first valve, which can be blindly disrupted by introducing a valvulotome or a valve cutter via its branches or its distal end. With the introduction of the angioscope the same methods can be used under direct vision by introducing the angioscope in the proximal end of the vein before constructing the inflow anastomosis and introducing the valve disruption instrument from the distal end of the vein.[75] This method can be done either by completely unroofing the vein, leaving it exposed but kept in its bed, or by leaving the overlying skin intact except in areas where branches are to be ligated. The location of the branches is determined by marking the skin in areas where branches are seen back bleeding during angioscopic guided valvulotomy.

c. *The translocated vein method:* Any vein, including the greater saphenous, can be prepared using this method. The vein is completely harvested from its bed, its branches tied, its valves disrupted and used in nonreversed prograde fashion. This method can be used when a vein needs to be placed in a remote area from

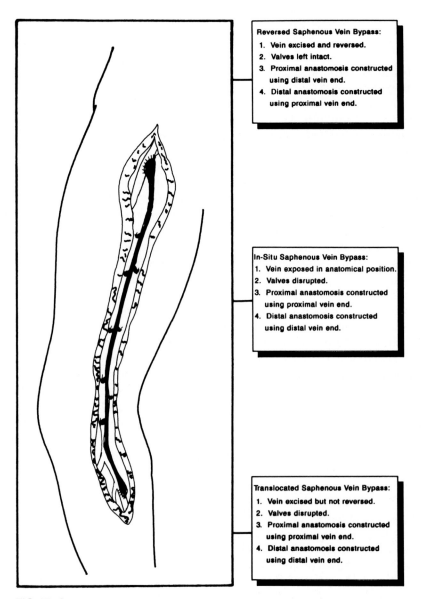

FIG 17–8.
Methods of autogenous vein preparation.

its site as placing an arm or lesser saphenous vein as an infrainguinal bypass or a thigh vein in a popliteal distal bypass position. This method allows a better size match between the ends of the vein and the inflow and outflow arteries.

The patency and limb salvage rates of different vein bypass methods are comparable. So the surgeon should use a familiar method with which he or she is able to obtain good results.

Arm veins can also be used for infrainguinal bypasses. The cephalic vein from the wrist up to the shoulder area can be harvested for that method. If the cephalic vein in the forearm is not adequate due to its small size, then the cephalic-antecubital-basilic complex could be harvested in one segment. When this vein complex is stretched out it will be composed of two segments: one nonreversed larger diameter segment that consists of the basilic vein and another reversed smaller diameter cephalic vein segment. In this setup the larger end is used for proximal anastomosis and its valves are disrupted using the valvulotome, and the smaller end is used for the distal anastomosis.[76]

The lesser saphenous vein can also be used for infrainguinal bypasses. This vein is approached either by placing the patient prone on the operating room table, the vein harvested, the patient moved to the supine position, and the bypass completed; or it can be approached medially through the same incision used for greater saphenous vein harvest by developing the flap posteriorly.[77] The patency rate of arm vein and lesser saphenous vein bypasses is favorable and is better than those of prosthetic material, such as PTFE or Da-

cron, which has limited patency and limb salvage rate to the infrapopliteal vessels. Therefore, their use should be avoided if possible.[67]

At the end of every infrainguinal bypass procedure an intraoperative arteriogram is performed.[78] This arteriogram evaluates the distal anastomosis, the distal vasculature, and the presence of competent valves and arteriovenous fistulae in an in situ bypass graft. If any problem is found on the operative arteriogram, it should be corrected while in the operating room to obtain optimum results (Fig 17–9 A, B).

In conclusion, aggressive vascular evaluation of the diabetic patient suffering from foot lesion is paramount. If indicated, vascular reconstruction should be performed to enhance healing and decrease the incidence of major-limb amputation, which returns these patients to an active and productive life.

A   **B**

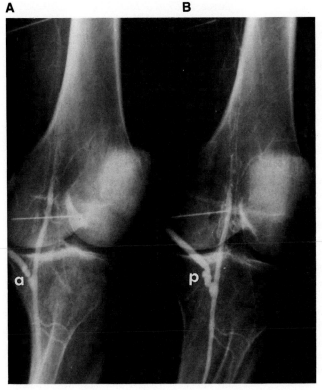

FIG 17–9.
A, intraoperative arteriogram of femoral popliteal in situ vein bypass. Note the constriction at the heel of the popliteal anastomosis *(a).* **B,** intraoperative arteriogram of the same bypass after placement of autogenous vein patch *(p)* to widen the anastomotic constriction.

REFERENCES

1. Centers for Disease Control: Prevalence and incidence of diabetes mellitus— United States, 1980–87, *MMWR* 39:809–812, 1990.
2. Juergens JL, Baker NW, Hines EA: Arteriosclerosis obliterans: review of 520 cases with special reference to pathogenic and prognostic factors, *Circulation* 71:429, 1960.
3. LoGerfo FW, Coffman JD: Vascular and microvascular disease of the foot in diabetes, *N Engl J Med* 311:1615–1619, 1984.
4. Strandness DE, Priest RE, Gibbons GE: Combined clinical and pathologic study of diabetic and nondiabetic with severe vascular disease, *Circulation* 36:83–91, 1967.
5. Menzoian JO et al: Symptomatology and anatomic patterns of peripheral vascular disease: differing impact of smoking and diabetes, *Ann Vasc Surg* 3:224–228, 1989.
6. Pomposelli FB et al: A flexible approach to infrapopliteal vein grafts in patients with diabetes mellitus, *Arch Surg* 161:724–729, 1991.
7. Rosenblatt MS et al: Lower extremity vein graft reconstruction: results in diabetic and non-diabetic patients, *Surg Gynecol Obstet* 171:331, 1990.
8. Kempczinski RF, Bernhard VM: Management of chronic ischemia of the lower extremities: introduction and general considerations. In Rutherford RB, editor: *Vascular surgery,* Philadelphia, 1989, WB Saunders.
9. Jager KA et al: Non-invasive assessment of upper and lower extremity ischemia. In Bergan JJ, Yao JST, editors: *Evaluation and treatment of upper and lower extremity circulatory disorders,* Orlando, Fla, 1984, Grune & Stratton.
10. Christensen T, Neubauer B: Increased arterial wall stiffness and thickness in medium-sized arteries in patients with insulin-dependent diabetes mellitus, *Acta Radiol* 29:299, 1988.
11. Gibbons GW, Wheelock FC: Problems in the non-invasive evaluation of the peripheral circulation in the diabetic, *Prct Card* 8:115, 1982.
12. Raines JK et al: Vascular laboratory criteria for the management of peripheral vascular disease of the lower extremities, *Surgery* 79:21, 1976.
13. Clark LC: Monitor and control of blood and tissue oxygen tensions, *Trans Am Soc Artif Intern Organs* 2:41, 1956.
14. White RA et al: Non-invasive evaluation of peripheral vascular disease using transcutaneous oxygen tension. *Am J Surg* 144:68, 1982.
15. Hauser CJ, Shoemaker WC: Use of transcutaneous Po_2 regional perfusion index to quantify tissue perfusion in peripheral vascular disease, *Ann Surg* 197:337, 1983.
16. Vincent DG et al: Non-invasive assessment of toe systolic pressures with special reference to diabetes mellitus, *J Cardiovasc Surg* 24:22, 1983.
17. Partamian JO, Bradley RF: Acute myocardial infarction in 258 cases of diabetes. Immediate mortality and five year survival, *N Engl J Med* 273:455–461, 1965.
18. Goldman L et al: Multifactorial index of cardiac risk in noncardiac surgical procedures, *N Engl J Med* 297:845–850, 1977.
19. Cambria RP et al: The impact of selective use of dypyridamole-thallium scans and surgical factors on the current morbidity of aortic surgery, *J Vasc Surg* 15:43–51, 1992.
20. Eagle KA et al: Combining clinical and thallium data optimizes preoperative assessment of cardiac risk before major vascular surgery, *Ann Intern Med* 110:859–866, 1989.
21. Rao T, Jacobs KH, El-Etr A: Reinfarction following anesthesia in patients with myocardial infarction, *Anesthesiology* 59:499–505, 1983.
22. Jamieson WR et al: Influence of ischemic heart disease on early and late mortality after surgery for peripheral occlusive vascular disease, *Circulation* 66:92I–97I, 1982.
23. Eagle KA et al: Dipyridamole-thallium scanning in patients undergoing vascular surgery, *JAMA* 257:2185–2189, 1987.
24. Raby KE et al: Detection and significance of intraoperative and postoperative myocardial ischemia in peripheral vascular surgery. *JAMA* 268:222–227, 1992.

25. Sise MJ et al: Complications of the flow-directed pulmonary catheter: a prospective analysis in 219 patients, *Crit Care Med* 9:315–318, 1981.

26. Eisenberg MJ et al: Monitoring for myocardial ischemia during noncardiac surgery, *JAMA* 268:210–216, 1992.

27. Robertson JM, Buckberg GD: Cardiovascular monitoring and perioperative management of the vascular surgery patient. In Moore WD, editor: *Vascular surgery,* Philadelphia, 1986, WB Saunders.

28. Kadir S: Arteriography of the lower extremity vessels. In Kadir S, editor: *Diagnostic angiography,* Philadelphia, 1986, WB Saunders.

29. Flanigan DP et al: Aortofemoral or femoropopliteal revascularization? A prospective evaluation of the papaverine test, *J Vasc Surg* 1:215–223, 1984.

30. Belkin M et al: Clinical and hemodynamic results of bypass to isolated tibial artery segments for ischemic ulceration of the foot, *Am J Surg* 164:281–285, 1992.

31. Dotter CT, Judkins MP: Transluminal treatment of arteriosclerotic obstruction: description of a new technique and a preliminary report of its application, *Circulation* 30:654–670, 1974.

32. Zarins CK, Glagov S: Histopathology of plaque dilatation and remodeling following balloon angioplasty. In Moore W, Ahn S, editors: *Endovascular surgery,* Philadelphia, 1989, WB Saunders.

33. Johnston KW: Factors that influence the outcome of aortoiliac and femoropopliteal percutaneous transluminal angioplasty, *Surg Clin North Am* 72(4):843–850, 1992.

34. Gallino A et al: Percutaneous transluminal angioplasty of the lower limbs—five year follow-up, *Circulation* 70:619–623, 1984.

35. Schwarten DE, Cutcliff WB: Arterial occlusive disease below the knee: treatment with percutaneous transluminal angioplasty performed with low profile catheters and steerable guide wires, *Radiology* 169:71–74, 1988.

36. Rutherford RB et al: Factors affecting the patency of infrainguinal bypass, *J Vasc Surg* 8:236–246, 1988.

37. Ip JH, Fuster V, Badimon L: Syndromes of accelerated atherosclerosis: role of vascular injury and smooth muscle proliferation, *J Am Coll Cardiol* 15:1667–1687, 1990.

38. Self SB, Seeger JM: Laser angioplasty, *Surg Clin North Am* 72(4):851–868, 1992.

39. Kensey KR et al: Recanalization of obstructed arteries with a flexible, rotating tip catheter, *Radiology* 165:387–389, 1987.

40. Ahn SS et al: Removal of focal atheromatous lesions by angioscopically guided high-speed rotary atherectomy, *J Vasc Surg* 7(2):292–300, 1988.

41. Simpson JB et al: Transluminal atherectomy for occlusive peripheral vascular disease, *Am J Card* 61:96–101, 1988.

42. Palmaz JC et al: Placement of balloon expandable stents in iliac arteries—first 171 patients, *Radiology* 174:969–975, 1990.

43. Neville RF et al: Intravascular ultrasonography: validation studies and preliminary intraoperative observations, *J Vasc Surg* 13(2):274–283, 1991.

44. White GH: Angioscopy, *Surg Clin North Am* 72(4):791–821, 1992.

45. Spence RK et al: Long-term results of transluminal angioplasty of the iliac and femoral arteries, *Arch Surg* 116:1377–1386, 1981.

46. Leriche R, Morel A: The syndrome of thrombotic obliteration of the aortic bifurcation, *Ann Surg* 127:193, 1948.

47. Crawford ES et al: Aortoiliac occlusive disease: factors influencing survival and function following reconstructive operation over a twenty-five year period, *Surgery* 90:1055, 1981.

48. Bartlett FF, Gibbons GW, Wheelock FC: Aortic reconstruction for occlusive disease: comparable results in diabetics, *Arch Surg* 121:1150, 1986.

49. Waters KJ, Prud G: Return to work after aortofemoral bypass surgery, *Br Med J* 2:556, 1977.

50. Sidawy AN et al: Retroperitoneal inflow procedures for aorto-iliac occlusive vascular disease, *Arch Surg* 120:794–796, 1985.

51. Brief DK et al: Crossover, femoro-femoral grafts followed up five years or more, *Arch Surg* 110:1294, 1975.

52. LoGerfo FW et al: A comparison of the late patency rates of axillobilateral femoral and axillounilateral femoral grafts, *Surgery* 81:33, 1977.

53. Darling CR, Linton RR: Durability of femoropopliteal reconstructions, *Am Surg* 123:472, 1972.

54. Glutelius JR, Kreindler S, Luke JC: Comparative evaluation of autogenous vein bypass graft and endarterectomy in superficial femoral artery reconstruction, *Surgery* 57:28, 1965.

55. Ouriel K, Smith CR, DeWeese JA: Endarterectomy for localized lesions of the superficial femoral artery at the adductor canal, *J Vasc Surg* 3:531, 1986.

56. Bernhard VM, Militello JM, Geringer AM: Repair of the profunda femoris artery, *Am J Surg* 127:676, 1974.

57. King TA, DePalma RG, Rhodes GR: Diabetes mellitus and atherosclerotic involvement of the profunda femoris artery, *Surg Gynecol Obstet* 159:553, 1984.

58. Pearce WH, Kempczinski RF: Extended autogenous profundaplasty and aortofemoral grafting: an alternative to synchronous distal bypass, *J Vasc Surg* 1:415–418, 1984.

59. Graham AM, Gewertz BL, Zarins CK: Efficacy of isolated profundaplasty, *Can J Surg* 29:330, 1986.

60. Towne JB et al: Profundaplasty in perspective: limitations in long term management of limb ischemia, *Surgery* 90:1037, 1981.

61. Rosenblatt MS et al: Lower extremity vein graft reconstruction: results in diabetic and non-diabetic patients, *Surg Gynecol Obstet* 171:331–335, 1990.

62. Veith FJ et al: Superficial femoral and popliteal arteries as inflow sites for distal bypasses, *Surgery* 90:980–990, 1981.

63. Schuler JJ et al: Early experience with popliteal to infrapopliteal bypass for limb salvage, *Arch Surg* 118:472–476, 1983.

64. Sidawy AN et al: Effect of inflow and outflow sites on the results of tibioperoneal vein grafts, *Am J Surg* 152:211–214, 1986.

65. Veith FJ et al: Tibiotibial vein bypass grafts: a new operation for limb salvage, *J Vasc Surg* 2:552–557, 1985.

66. Ascer E et al: Short vein grafts: a superior option for arterial reconstructions to poor or compromised outflow tracts. *J Vasc Surg* 7:370–378, 1988.

67. Veith FJ et al: Six-year prospective multicenter randomized comparison of autologous saphenous vein and expanded polytetrafluoroethylene grafts in infrainguinal arterial reconstructions, *J Vasc Surg* 3:104–114, 1986.

68. Mannick JA et al: Success of bypass vein grafts in patients with isolated popliteal artery segments, *Surgery* 61:17–25, 1967.

69. Corson JD et al: Comparative analysis of vein and prosthetic bypass grafts to the isolated popliteal artery, *Surgery* 91:448–451, 1982.

70. Bernhard VM, Boren CH, Towne JB: Pneumatic tourniquets: a substitute for vascular clamps in distal bypass surgery, *Surgery* 87:709, 1980.

71. Ascer E, Veith FJ, Gupta AK: Bypasses to plantar arteries and other tibial branches: an extended approach to limb salvage, *J Vasc Surg* 8:434–441, 1988.

72. Pomposelli FB et al: Efficacy of the dorsal pedal bypass for limb salvage in diabetic patients: short-term observation, *J Vasc Surg* 11:745–752, 1990.

73. Leather RP, Shah DM, Karmody AM: Infrapopliteal arterial bypass for limb salvage: increased patency and utilization of the saphenous vein "in-situ," *Surgery* 90:1001–1009, 1981.

74. LoGerfo FW, Sidawy AN, Quist WC: A technique for prevention of spasm in in-situ vein grafts, *Contemp Surg* 28:75, 1986.

75. Miller A et al: Angioscopically directed valvulotomy: a new valvulotome and technique, *J Vasc Surg* 13:813–821, 1991.

76. Logerfo FW, Paniszyn C, Menzoian JO: A new arm vein graft for distal bypass, *J Vasc Surg* 5:889–891, 1987.

77. Chang BB et al: The lesser saphenous vein: an underappreciated source of autogenous vein, *J Vasc Surg* 15:152–157, 1992.

78. Liebman PR et al: Intraoperative arteriography in femoropopliteal and femorotibial bypass grafts, *Arch Surg* 116:1019–1021, 1981.

18

Christopher E. Attinger, M.D.

Use of Soft Tissue Techniques for Salvage of the Diabetic Foot

The functional goal of treating the diabetic foot ulcer should be to salvage as much of the foot as possible. Four goals must be achieved: minimize the energy that the diabetic has to expend ambulating, maximize the surface area over which the ambulating weight is distributed, optimize the biomechanics of the remaining foot, and avoid the psychologic depression that accompanies a major amputation. To achieve this goal, one has to be familiar with the wide range of soft tissue salvage techniques now available and be able to choose the optimal one under different circumstances. One also has to understand the effect that the various operations and amputations have on the biomechanics of the foot to avoid reulceration.

When considering soft tissue reconstruction, one always needs to go through a decision tree,[1] evaluating options from the simplest to most complex reconstructive technique: (1) allow the ulcer to heal by secondary intention; (2) close the wound primarily; (3) apply a split-thickness or full-thickness skin graft; (4) use a local fascial, fasciocutaneous, muscle, or musculocutaneous flap, or (5) use a microvascular free flap transfer. The choice depends on the ulcer location, the new biomechanics of the reconstructed foot, and the patient's health.

SECONDARY INTENTION CLOSURE

Wound closure by secondary intention[2, 3] consists of allowing the ulcer to heal by itself. The process occurs when granulation tissue (the product of angiogenesis and collagen deposition) fills in the defect, the wound edges contract, and the wound finally epithelializes. The process requires careful wound care and can take 8 to 12 weeks. The time can be somewhat shortened by the expensive addition of topical growth factors.[4] With or without growth factor, the resultant scar from secondary intention can be hyperkeratotic (Fig 18–1) and may require a lifetime of care so that it does not become the focus for a new ulcer. However, the process does not require an operation and is the process of choice for the medically ill patient.

For the wound to close, a hospitable environment has to exist in which there is adequate blood supply, normal tissue exists at the base of the wound, and the wound is not infected. To ensure that adequate blood supply exists to the area, refer to the chapter on revascularization. When debriding, ensure that all eschar, nonviable tissue and debris have been removed and that only healthy normal-looking tissue remains (the presence of clotted venules at the edge mandate further debridement). To "sterilize" the wound (< 100,000 bacteria/g of tissue), debriding plus either topical antibiotics only or top-

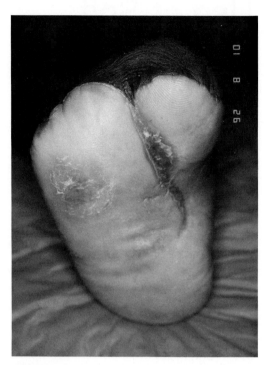

FIG 18–1.
Hyperkeratosis from a wound allowed to heal by secondary intention.

ical and systemic antibiotics may be required.

Once the wound is clean and noninfected, caring for it thereafter should be done gently: "Do not place anything on it that one would not put on one's eye." The use of hydrogen peroxide, 1% Dakin's solution, povidone-iodine, and chlorhexidine[5] should be discouraged. If a topical antibiotic is required, it should control local bacteria while allowing the wound to heal. Silver sulfadiazine[6] used two or three times daily not only controls gram-negative and gram-positive bacteria but also stimulates epithelialization.

The local environment then has to be optimized so that collagen deposition, angiogenesis, epithelialization, and wound contracture can rapidly ensue. The wound has to stay hydrated, oxygenated, under adequate temperature, and with provisions for adequate waste removal.[7, 8] Occlusive, Hydrogel, composite polymeric,

and hydrocolloid dressings all were designed to provide such an environment.[9] In addition, these dressings tend to decrease the pain for reasons that are poorly understood. One can also add filler products (gels, powders, beads, granules, or pastes) to the wound to help absorb the exudate from heavily secreting wounds while keeping the environment clean.

PRIMARY CLOSURE

Primary closure is the direct apposition of wound edges with stitches so that the wound is covered by normal tissue. One has to be sure that the wound itself is clean and that the wound edges have no cellulitis or induration. The edges themselves must be able to come together without excessive tension (a 4-0 nylon should be able to hold the wound together without breaking). It is preferable in closing an open wound to minimize the amount of deep stitches because the latter can potentiate subsequent infection. The least reactive absorbable stitch (e.g., PDS, Dexon, or Vicril) is best.[10]

When closing the skin, it is best to use a simple nylon stitch and *evert* the edges. It is critical to place both stitches at equal depth and ensure that more tissue is encompassed at the bottom of the stitch than at the top by using an Erlenmeyer flask configuration (Fig 18–2). As the scar matures, it goes from a ridge to a flat scar (vs. going from flat to a depression when good eversion is not initially achieved). Accurate apposition also prevents a vertically uneven scar, which can be the source of hyperkeratosis and future breakdown. If it is difficult to achieve good accurate eversion with a simple stitch, one can use a vertical mattress stitch as an aid. Horizontal mattress stitches are to be discouraged because they cause too much ischemia of the enclosed skin edge. For an excellent and very early illustrated book on basic surgical technique, refer to Milton T. Edgerton's[11] book the *Art of Surgical Technique*.

SKIN GRAFT

Skin grafting is harvesting epidermis with a varying thickness of accompanying dermis and placing it on a recipient base. A split-thickness skin graft includes epidermis and a portion of dermis. The more dermis included, the thicker the graft (Fig 18–3). A full-thickness graft includes epidermis and all of the dermis.

The anatomy of the skin is such that the dermis represents 95% of the skin thickness and epidermis only 5%. The dermis contains sebaceous glands and is otherwise relatively acellular. It is made up principally of collagen and elastin. The subcutaneous tissue contains the sweat glands and hair follicles. The blood supply arises from a vascular network that lies on top of fascia and sends vertical branches up through the subcutaneous tissue and dermis. The vessel arborise along the way and terminate as capillary buds between dermal papillae. The thinner the graft (i.e., the more superficial the dermis is harvested), the larger the number of vessels that are transected.

Preparation of Recipient Site

For a graft to be successful, it is important that the recipient site be noninfected and well vascularized. To sterilize a potential recipient site, one must perform radical surgical debridement of all necrotic tissue. Appropriate antibiotics have to be administered to get rid of any surrounding cellulitis. The bacterial count of the recipient bed should be less than 100,000/g of tissue before successful grafting can be undertaken.[12] Topical sulfadiazine (Sylvadine) applied three times daily to the wound will sterilize its surface[6] without harming the healing tissue. More expen-

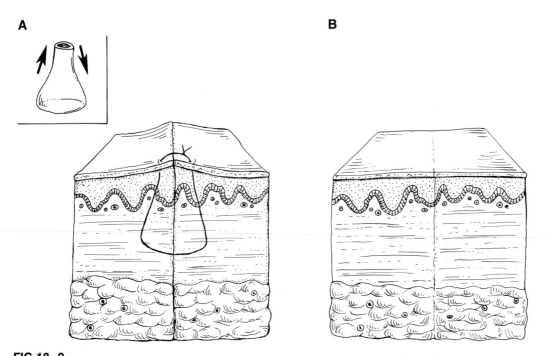

FIG 18–2.
A, an Erlenmeyer flask configuration for placement of the suture assures that both edges of the wound evert. **B,** after healing, the wound is flat.

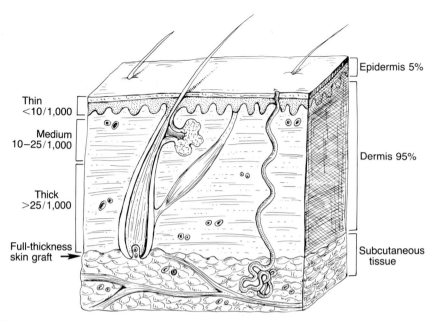

FIG 18-3.
Increasing thicknesses of a split-thickness skin graft incorporate increasing amounts of dermis. A full-thickness skin graft includes the entire dermis.

sive biologic dressings (pig skin or amniotic membrane) changed every 24 hours will do the same.[13] It is important to remember that granulation tissue contains bacteria in its interstices and as such needs to be *removed* at the time of grafting.

The recipient bed must be sufficiently vascular to accept a skin graft. The presence of red granulation tissue, pH at 7.4,[14] transcutaneous oxygen tension level greater than 40 mm Hg, and epithelialization at the border of the granulation tissue suggest that sufficient blood supply exists. Although the granulation tissue has to be removed before grafting, the blood supply that supported it before its removal will do the same to the new skin graft. One cannot graft on denuded cortical bone or tendon; intact periosteum and paratenon are required. However, if the exposed tendon or bone is less than 0.5 cm wide, surrounding tissue will provide enough support to allow the skin graft over it to survive. Otherwise more extensive soft tissue coverage is needed before

grafting is possible. For fresh wounds, a skin graft should take well on muscle or fascia. If only fat is present, one should delay grafting until granulation tissue has formed over it.

Split-Thickness Skin Graft

The thinner the graft harvested, the higher the chances of its take. This may be in part because of the higher number of transected blood vessels through which primary revascularization can be established.[15] The thinner the graft is, the more it will shrink as it heals because the decreased amount of dermis is less effective in inhibiting secondary contraction.[16] In contrast, full-thickness dermis is believed to prevent contraction by inhibiting both myofibroblast proliferation[17] and prolylhydroxylase activity[18] (an important enzyme in collagen synthesis). The thinner the graft, the greater the chance for hyperpigmentation.[19] Finally, the thinner the graft, the more susceptible it is to trauma[20] because of the absence of anchoring rete pegs and the loss of lubricating sebaceous glands.

Appropriate donor sites for split-thickness skin grafts include thighs and buttocks (Fig 18–4). Care should be used to harvest the graft from a location where it will be hidden by a normal bathing suit. If a small piece is needed and one wants to limit aesthetic donor morbidity, a *thin* graft from the instep may be appropriate. We usually harvest skin at a thickness of $^{15}/_{1,000}$ in.

Although older techniques exist to harvest skin, we have found that either the Zimmer air-driven dermatome or the electrically driven Padgett dermatome are the easiest to operate and most reliable (Fig 18–5). One has to set the desired width of the graft by placing the correct width guard (5, 8, or 10 cm). The thickness is set (usually $^{15}/_{1,000}$ in.) and checked by introducing a no. 15 blade between the cutting blade and base. The donor site is prepped after being shaved. Its surface is then lubricated with mineral oil, and the area to be grafted is placed under moving tension using a tongue blade. The dermatome is set in motion and approaches the donor site much like a plane landing. Constant pressure is maintained, and when sufficient skin is harvested, the dermatome is lifted off of the donor site. The skin graft is then stored in a saline solution–soaked cotton gauze.

The donor site bleeding can be minimized by placing topical thrombin or a dilute concentration of epinephrine (1: 200,000) on the donor site. One can dress

A

B

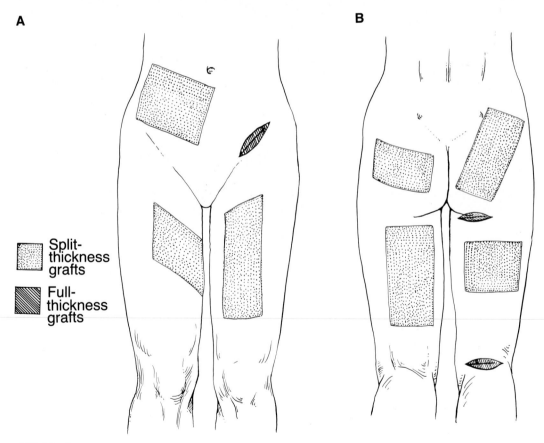

Split-thickness grafts

Full-thickness grafts

FIG 18–4.
Anterior (**A**) and posterior (**B**) views of split- and full-thickness skin graft donor sites for the foot.

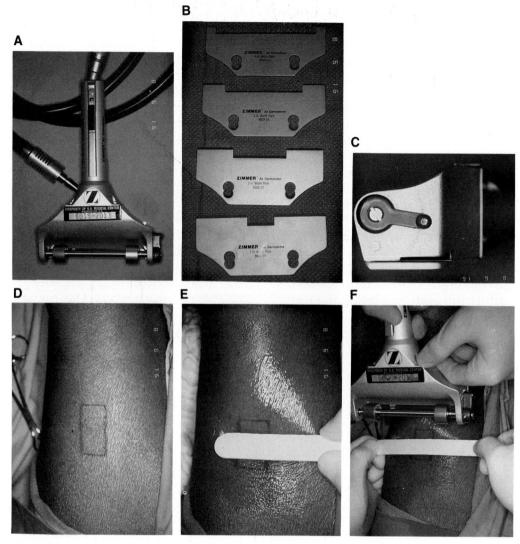

FIG 18–5.
A, Zimmer dermatone. **B,** various blade widths. **C,** setting of depth of cut (¹⁵/₁,₀₀₀ in.). **D,** exact marking of the donor piece. **E,** lubricating the donor site with mineral oil. **F,** harvesting the skin graft.

it with Xeroform or scarlet red and treat the site with repeated heat lamp treatments lasting 20 minutes at a time to dry out the site. One then trims the nonattached covering daily until it falls off. This dressing is labor intensive and painful. One can also use an occlusive dressing (Opsite or Tegaderm) or a semipermeable dressing such as BioBrane. These dressings have the advantage of minimizing the donor site pain and speeding up the epithelialization of the donor site.[8] One, however, has to be careful that the fluid that collects under the dressing does not become infected, which in turn would slow down the reepithelialization of the donor site.

Improved adherence of the graft and control of the bleeding at the just prepared recipient site are achieved by spraying topical thrombin on the site before grafting.[21] If the bleeding at the recipient site cannot be adequately controlled to prevent potential hematoma, it is best to dress it sterilely and place the graft back on the donor site. One can then return in 24 to 48 hours to place the graft on the recipient site.

One then has to decide whether to mesh (Fig 18–6) the harvested skin graft or not before placing it on the recipient site. The advantage of meshing is that hematomas or seromas cannot build up because any fluid created leaks out between the graft interstices. Unless skin is in short supply, there is no advantage to meshing at a ratio greater than 1½ to 1 or to stretching the mesh far apart. The only advantage to not meshing is that the resultant crisscross pattern of the healed graft is avoided.

Insetting the graft has to be done carefully. It is usually inset loosely and tacked into place by a running 5-0 Chromic stitch along its periphery. Stay or bolster sutures are strategically placed around the graft to hold the bolster down. The bolster is built by first placing Xeroform and then

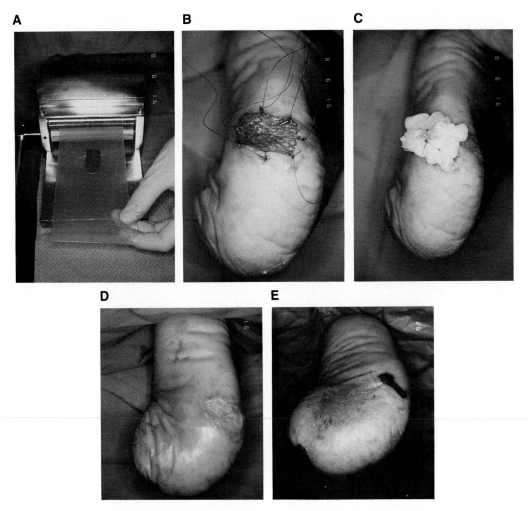

FIG 18–6.
A, meshing the skin graft. **B,** the skin graft with bolster stitches (4-0 nylon). **C,** tying the bolster with Xeroform and wet cotton over the skin graft. **D,** preoperative defect. **E,** postoperative healed split-thickness skin graft.

normal saline solution–soaked cotton. The water is forced out of the cotton by tying down the bolster stitches. This allows the skin graft to conform exactly to the recipient site. The foot and lower leg should then be placed in a posterior splint to prevent motion and resultant shearing. A gentle Ace wrap holds it all together.

Physiologic Phases in Skin Graft Take

The biologic steps for graft survival begin with a *plasmatic imbibation phase* that lasts 48 hours. The graft is ischemic during this time, passively taking up fluid while the underlying bed proliferates. There are diverging opinions as to whether actual nutrition of the graft occurs.[22, 23] Although split-thickness skin grafts can tolerate this ischemia for up to 5 days, full-thickness skin grafts can do so for only 3 days.[24] Therefore, a graft threatened by an underlying hematoma can be salvaged if the clot is removed before the graft's tolerance for ischemia is exceeded. Evacuation of the hematoma reestablishes contact so that revascularization of the graft can proceed.

The *inosculatory and capillary growth phase* starts after 48 hours when capillary budding from the recipient bed makes contact with the graft vessels. One theory suggests that an anastomosis occurs between host and recipient vessels.[25] Another suggests that the graft is revascularized by an ingrowth of vessels arising from the recipient bed.[26] In this model the graft vessels serve as nonviable conduits for the new vessels to grow into at a rate of 5 μm/hour.[27] A third and less popular theory suggests that both processes contribute to revascularization of the graft.[28] Circulation actually occurs between the fourth and seventh day. The flow is initially all toward the graft whether the anastomoses are to arteries or veins. Venous outflow drainage develops by day 6.[29] Lymphatic drainage is established by day

6, and the graft is able to drain the accumulated fluid by day 9.[30]

The graft on an extremity should be kept elevated for 7 to 10 days until venous drainage is fully established and graft venous stasis can be avoided. A meshed graft can first be examined at 7 days, by which time it should have taken. Of course, it should be examined sooner if one is worried about potential infection. However, if the graft is unmeshed, it is important to examine it at 48 hours to ensure that there is no fluid collection between the graft and its bed inhibiting revascularization. As previously mentioned, if the collection exists, it should be aspirated with a needle.

Full-Thickness Skin Graft

The best donor sites for full-thickness skin grafts are flexor surfaces such as the groin, the antecubital fossa, and the popliteal fossa (see Fig 18–4). The harvesting site can be closed primarily and leaves a thin linear scar. An accurate pattern of the recipient site is made and then encompassed within a lenticular pattern, where a length/width ratio of at least 4:1 (this ratio ensures that no dog ears are created when the wound is closed). That lenticular pattern is then drawn out with the long axis along Langer's skin lines (i.e., parallel to the flexor crease). The recipient pattern is first cut out and the fat trimmed from its underside with a sharp scissors. It will shrink up to 40% of its existing size because of the elastin within the dermis. It is then stored in a normal saline solution–soaked sponge. The remaining lenticular pattern is then excised, and the skin edges are undermined and closed with interrupted deep dermal stitch and a running superficial dermal stitch.

The stored graft is then placed on the recipient site and sewn into place with a running 5-0 Chromic. It stretches back out to its original size as it is sewn in place.

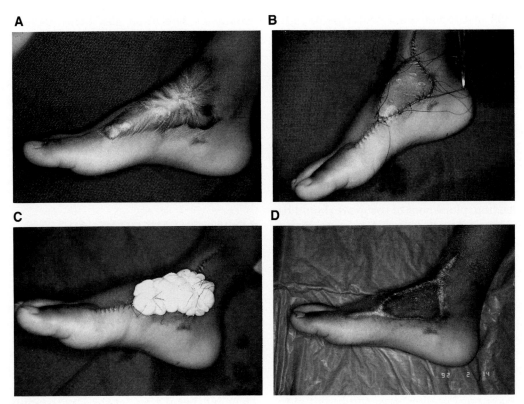

FIG 18–7.
A, hypertrophic scar on a burned foot. **B,** scar excised and covered by a full-thickness skin graft from the groin. **C,** full-thickness skin graft, bolstered with Xe-roform and wet cotton. **D,** healed full-thickness skin graft.

It is important to place several small perforations in the full-thickness graft to allow fluid to escape if a seroma or hematoma should form. Then 4-0 nylon stay sutures are strategically placed along the edges and tied tightly over a Xeroform and soaked wet cotton bolster (Fig 18–7). This ensures excellent coaptation of the graft on recipient site by helping prevent hematoma, seroma, or shearing.

It is more difficult to achieve 100% take with a full-thickness graft because the revascularization is more tenuous. Primary revascularization can be interrupted if the initial contact between the graft and the underlying dermis is disturbed by hematoma, shear, seroma, and so forth. That portion of the graft not revascularized by primary revasculariza-tion (day 4–7 after skin graft) must then receive its blood supply via a slower process involving neovascularization. The process is triggered by the anaerobic metabolism of the skin graft itself, releasing vasoactive substances to stimulate capillary growth. The prolonged ischemia the skin graft faces causes an initial loss of the epidermis and capillary dermis, which then are replaced by a thin capillary dermis and attenuated epidermis.[31] The resulting graft is smooth, fibrotic, and tight with a silvery sheen.[32]

If the full-thickness graft takes primarily, there is no contraction of the wound. The lubrication of the skin is normal, and there is no change in skin color or texture. The neurotization that occurs reflects that of the underlying bed and returns in the following order: pain, light touch, and temperature. Sensory recovery starts at 4 weeks and can take up to 1 to 2 years to complete.[33]

Complications of Skin Grafting

Hematoma is the most common cause of graft failure. It prevents the capillary buds from the underlying bed to make contact with the skin graft. For this reason it is suggested that if there is excessive bleeding, placement of the graft should be delayed 24 to 48 hours. A useful adjunct is the use of topical thrombin, which not only helps stop the bleeding but also acts as a glue to hold the graft in place.

Infection[34] is the second most frequent cause of graft failure. The key is to graft *only* when the recipient bed has been debrided to normal tissue and is relatively sterile (< 100,000 bacterial colonies/g of tissue[35]). The presence of bacteria[36] (especially β-hemolytic *Streptococcus* or *Pseudomonas*) can be lethal to the graft. They produce a high level of proteolytic enzymes and plasmin, which dissolve the fibrin that holds the graft to the recipient bed.

Seroma also leads to graft failure and is more prominent in areas where a confluence of lymphatic channels meet: groin or axilla. Meshing the graft in those areas can be very helpful. Atraumatic tissue handling will likewise minimize the amount of necrotic tissue left behind. A bolster dressing is also helpful.

Shearing from movement of the underlying bed detaches the graft. It is therefore important to immobilize the graft on the bed and prevent movement of the underlying bed by splinting the leg. If one uses a bolster, it is important that the pressure on the graft does not exceed 30 mm Hg or else blood flow to the graft will be compromised. By the same token, it is important to keep the foot elevated so that the venous hydrostatic pressure does not inhibit outflow from the just revascular-

ized graft. Elevation also helps decrease the edema, which inhibits oxygen diffusion and nutrition. Bodenham and Watson,[37] however, have been able to ambulate their venous stasis patients after 48 hours by using a combination of stitching the graft in and applying continual pressure to it with a foam rubber splint and Ace wrap. This would not work in a vascularly compromised or recent distally revascularized extremity.

LOCAL CUTANEOUS FLAPS

A random skin flap whose design was based on a length/width ratio is an outmoded concept implying a lack of knowledge of cutaneous blood flow. The accepted ratios of length to width were 3:1 in the face, 2:1 on the trunk, and 1:1 on the extremity. This was the principle that guided flap design this century until Milton[38] in 1970 wrote a landmark paper showing that it was not the length/width ratio but the presence of an artery at the base of a flap that determined its success. The rediscovery and refinements by Taylor et al.[39] of the Manchot[40] (1889) and Solomon[41, 42] (1939) treatises on cutaneous and muscle blood flow have enabled surgeons to design flaps based on anatomic principles. That knowledge, combined with the expanded use of the delay principle,[43] now enables surgeons to design complex flaps with the full confidence that they will survive.

The basic local flaps will be reviewed, including rotation, transposition, and advancement flaps. It is important to keep the vascular and cutaneous anatomy[44] of the foot in mind so that the base of the designed flap is optimally vascularized. The preoperative and interoperative use of the Doppler[45] helps ensure that the flap is indeed well vascularized. It enables one to determine whether the flow to a particular area of the foot is antegrade or retrograde (the flow can be redirected because of an occlusion of either the anterior tibialis or posterior tibialis). It also can determine that 12%[46] of patients who have no connection between the dorsalis pedis artery and lateral plantar artery and the 10% who are without a dorsalis pedis artery. Thus, the inexcusable loss of a flap because of the wrong orientation of the base of the flap can be avoided.

ANATOMIC PRINCIPLES OF SKIN FLAPS

A defined area of skin can receive blood from one of three principle sources: directly from a cutaneous artery, from musculocutaneous perforating arteries, or from fasciocutaneous arteries. Those specific cutaneous territories supplied by an artery are called angiosomes.[47] Angiosomes are connected to one another by choke vessels that open up when blood flow to a single angiosome is compromised. An angiosome will thus be able to carry a neighboring angiosome. However, it will not carry the angiosome beyond the neighboring one unless a delay procedure is employed. This gives sufficient time for two sets of choke vessels to open up[48, 49] so that the distal angiosome can now survive. The veins that drain that same territory are called venosomes.[50] Venosomes are linked by valveless oscillating veins that allow redirection of flow when the normal drainage has been interrupted. The oscillating veins are located in the same area as the choke vessels, and therefore angiosomes and venosomes overlap and indeed together comprise an angiotome.

Direct cutaneous arteries run in subcutaneous fat parallel to the skin. They are usually accompanied by two venae commitantes, veins that drain the area supplied by the cutaneous artery. Because these flaps have a direct blood supply, they have a far larger length/width ratio than traditional random flaps. They are tradi-

tionally known as *axial pattern flaps* and can be used as a *pedicled flap* (i.e., the flap at its base is dissected free of all but the tissue surrounding the feeding artery and veins, which then gives the flap added mobility), as an *island flap* (where the vascular pedicle is dissected completely free for a certain length and the flap is then transferred to a local site separate from the donor site while the pedicle is buried under the intervening tissue), or as a *free flap* (where the pedicle is totally detached and then hooked up by microsurgery to recipient vessels anywhere on the body). The most famous direct cutaneous flap is the forehead flap based on the supratrochlear vessel, and it has been used for more than 3,000 years for nasal reconstruction. The foot has three such flaps: the dorsalis pedis flap, the lateral calcaneal flap, and the filleted toe or first web space island flap.

Musculocutaneous flaps consist of muscle, fascia, subcutaneous fat, and skin. The muscle receives its blood supply according to one of the five patterns as defined by Mathes and Nahai.[51] The patterns (Fig 18–8) include type I (one vascular pedicle), type II (one dominant vascular pedicle entering at or near the origin, with minor pedicles entering the muscle belly), type III (two major vascular pedicles from separate regional arteries), type IV (segmental minor vascular pedicles along the entire length of the muscle), and type V (one dominant vascular pedicle at the origin with several smaller secondary segmental pedicles at the insertion). The skin is more likely to receive blood from musculocutaneous perforators if the muscle is broad rather than thin. The skin paddle obviously must overly the muscle and, without delay, can extend to only a few cm beyond the edge of the muscle. Although the abductor hallucis longus (type II), abductor digiti quinti (type II), and flexor digiti minimi (type II) have overlying skin paddles, these are relatively narrow and cause significant donor de-

Type I   Type II   Type III   Type IV   Type V

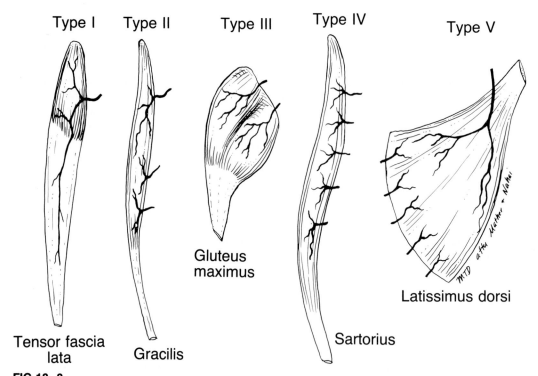

Gluteus
maximus

Latissimus dorsi

Tensor fascia
lata   Gracilis   Sartorius

FIG 18–8.
The five muscle types defined by pattern of vascular supply. (Adapted from Mathes SJ, Nahai F: *Clinical* *applications for muscle and musculocutaneous flaps.* St Louis, 1982, Mosby. Used by permission.)

fects if harvested as a unit. In the foot it is usually preferable to harvest the muscle without the overlying skin paddle and then skin graft the muscle.

The fasciocutaneous system is the chief source of blood supply to the skin. It arises from a major regional artery as perforators that pass along the fascia between muscle bellies and then fan out at the level of the deep fascia. There they form a plexus that gives rise to vessels that rise through the subcutaneous tissue to the overlying dermis. Classical examples include the fasciocutaneous systems that arise along the long axis of the three arteries of the leg: anterior tibial artery, posterior tibial artery, and peroneal artery. A classical fasciocutaneous flap of lower leg is the posterior tibial flap based on fasciocutaneous perforators from the posterior tibial artery.

Once the blood supply to the flap is established, it is important to ensure that it not be compromised by extensive tension, kinking of the pedicle, external pressure, hematoma, infection, or decreased systemic flow because of vasospasm or decreased cardiac output. Tension can best be seen if a white area develops anywhere along the flap as it is inset. Kinking of the pedicle usually affects venous return first and occurs when the flap is sharply angulated. External pressure can develop from tight external bandages or poor positioning. Hematoma causes damage not only by a volume effect but also because of the free radicals that it releases. Infection likewise can be disastrous because the inflammatory response causes edema, which leads to compromised blood flow and tissue destruction.

It is therefore important to preplan the flap exactly. Knowing the vascular anatomy of the foot and its skin allows the safe design of flaps based on anatomic principles. The term *random flap* with its obligate 1:1 length/width ratio in the foot is a flap based on unknown vascular anatomy. *Axial pattern flaps* have identifiable blood flow at their base and have a length/width ratio that depends on the angiosome that the artery serves. These flaps must be preplanned using a Doppler, and they can be extended beyond their angiosomes using delay principles.

LOCAL FLAPS

Local flaps are adjacent to the defect and are either rotated on a pivot point or are advanced forward from their base[52] to cover the defect. They include at a minimum the epidermis, dermis, and subcutaneous tissue. They can include the underlying fascia, muscle, or both. The donor site is either closed primarily or skin grafted. It is important to carefully preplan the flap by determining the size of the defect after debridement and using a slightly larger pattern to plan the chosen flap. When the pattern is moved from its base to cover the defect, it is important

that the flap move without tension. If the dimension of the flap is larger than 1:1, a Doppler has to be used to make sure that sufficient blood supply exists at its base. Atraumatic technique is a must when one is dissecting the flap (bipolar cautery, sharp dissection rather than cautery dissection, grasping flap with skin hooks rather than pickups) and insetting it (half buried horizontal mattress with nonreactive suture).

FLAPS THAT ROTATE AROUND A PIVOT POINT

These flaps[53] rotate around a single pivot point and as a result need to be planned carefully so as to avoid excessive tension along the radius of the arc of rotation. The *rotation flap* (Fig 18–9) is designed when a pie-shaped triangle defect is created to remove a lesion or preexistent defect. The base of the triangle lies along the circumference of a semicircular flap that is drawn so that it can be rotated into the defect. To see whether excessive tension will oc-

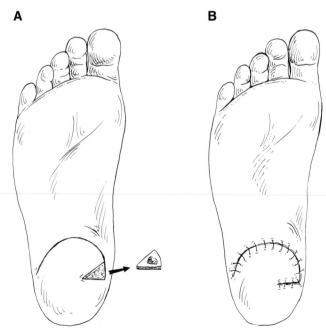

A, **B**

FIG 18–9.
A, rotation flap designed to cover a defect. **B,** flap rotated to repair a heel defect.

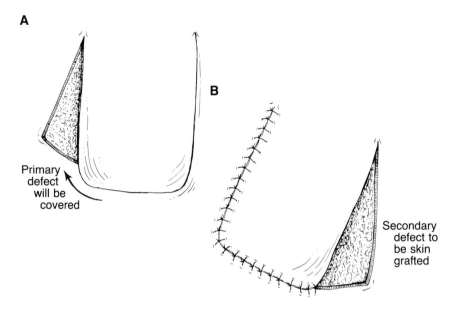

FIG 18–10.
A, transposition flap designed. **B,** the flap rotated into position and the defect covered with a split-thickness skin graft.

cur, a trial pattern with gauze is rotated into position. The flap is then cut and includes skin and subcutaneous tissue. If vascular anatomic considerations dictate, it can include fascia, muscle, or both. If despite planning the tension is too great, it can be released with a back cut toward the center of the circle. However, then the base of the flap is narrowed, and the tip viability may be at jeopardy. To avoid this, it is wise to Doppler the base of the flap before cutting it to ensure that perforators exist and will not be threatened if a back cut is needed. When the flap is rotated into position, the outer circumference is longer than the inner, and a dog ear may exist at the pivot point. It should be excised away from the flap so as not to compromise the flap.[54]

Transposition flaps (Fig 18–10) are rectangular with rounded edges and can be rotated up to 90 degrees. The end of the flap has to be longer than the distance between the pivot point and the edge of the defect so that when the flap is rotated it can fit in exactly. Preplanning with gauze is the key to avoid excessive ten-

sion. It is wise to ensure that perforators exist at the base of the flap especially if the length is to exceed 1:1. The donor site can usually be closed primarily. Otherwise it requires skin grafting without bolster stitches (they may cause extensive tension to the flap).

The Limberg flap[56] (Fig 18–11) is another transposition flap that depends on the looseness of adjacent tissue. It is used when the defect is a rhomboid with angles of 60 and 120 degrees. The sides of the flap are the same length as that of a rhomboid limb, and the flap is oriented so that it will swing 60 degrees to fill the defect. Thus, four possible flaps are possible with each design. Before cutting, it is important to pinch the skin with the thumb and forefinger to ensure that the skin is loose enough to rotate into the defect. When dissecting, it is important to ensure that the edges of the rhomboid are likewise slightly undermined. This flap is useful on the dorsum of the foot but has little role on the sole of the foot.

Z-plasty[57] is a type of rotation flap used extensively to both lengthen existing scars and reorient them along lines of minimal tension (Fig 18–12). The key is to have *loose* skin around the existing scar. The Z-plasty consists of three limbs of equal length in the shape of a Z. The angle between the limbs can vary from 30 to 90 degrees, and the wider the angle, the more the theoretical gain in length.[58] Clinically 60 degrees has been found to be most useful and yields a theoretical 75% gain in length. The actual gain is anywhere from 28% to 45% less than calculated.[58] The length of the center limb also determines the amount of length gained, and the longer it is, the larger the gain. The theoretical gain in length is the difference between the long and short diagonal (Fig 18–13), and the combination of wider angle and longer limb yields the greatest gain in length.

The center limb changes its orientation 90 degrees after the flaps are rotated. It is important to reorient the new central limb along the lines of minimal tension so

that as it heals there will be minimal tension on it and hence less propensity for hypertrophic scarring and contracture. The lines of minimal tension lie perpendicular to the line of pull of underlying muscle or tendons and are parallel to wrinkles.[59] Although the resulting scar is three times the length of the original scar, the central limb, now along the lines of minimal tension, should barely be visible.

Although a longer length can be gained with long limbs, this may be impractical in the foot where insufficient tissue may exist. A single large Z-plasty may be cosmetically unacceptable. For both reasons, it is important to be able to do multiple small Z-plasties along an existing scar. A variation on the multiple sequential Z-plasty is the four-flap Z-plasty.[60] One designs a 90-degree/90-degree Z-plasty and then subdivides each 90-degree limb into two 45-degree triangles. The repositioning of the four triangles permits a gain in length of up to 124%.

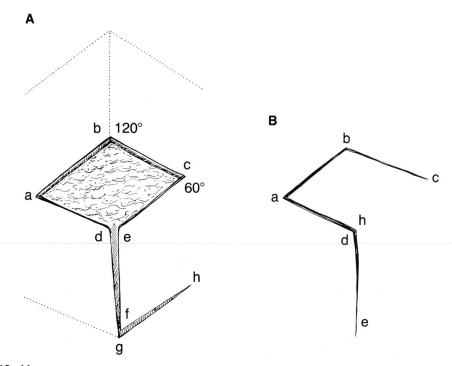

FIG 18–11.
A, four possible designs of the Limberg flap. **B,** the inferior right Limberg flap rotated into position.

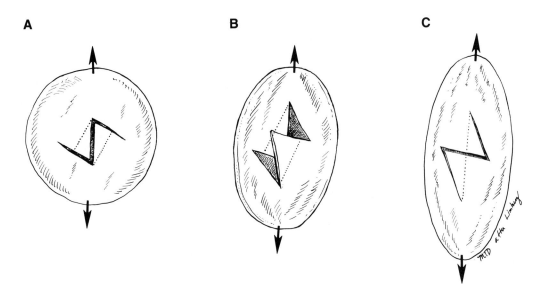

FIG 18–12.
A, Z-plasty central limb has to be lengthened, and thus two additional limbs of equal length are designed. **B,** triangles created are juxtaposed. **C,** gain in length is along the initial central limb, although the new central limb is now at 90 degrees from its initial position.

This four-flap Z-plasty is extremely useful in webspace contractures.

Use of Z-plasty has to be tempered with surgical judgment because often the desired gain in length is unobtainable because the surrounding tissue is not mobile enough for Z-plasty. Z-plasty works well to relieve scar contractures that cross flexor creases (Fig 18–14). They work well in areas of burn scar, although there is a 20% chance of tip necrosis. One can decrease this risk by widening the distal limb of the Z by curving the limbs of the incision and by securing the limbs in their new position using skin tapes rather than sutures.[61] Z-plasties are also useful in releasing congenital annular or circular scars. These should be done in two stages, with half the circumference being completed at each sitting.[62, 63]

An *interpolation flap* has a soft tissue pedicle with a distal skin island that is rotated into a defect that is close to but not adjacent to the donor site. If the pedicle is to be buried underneath the skin between the donor and recipient site, a tunnel is created and the bridge deepithe-lialized. If the bridge is to lie over the skin, it should be tubed so that the pedicle's undersurface is protected from infection or desiccation. At 10 to 14 days, the pedicle is separated from the flap and can be returned to the donor site. Indeed, from 1916 to the late 1970s, this was the principal way in which flaps were transferred from one part of the body to another.

An *island flap* is a specialized interpolation flap where the only link between the cutaneous flap and its bed is the neurovascular bundle (Fig 18–15). Littler[64] first used this flap in 1955 to give sensation to an insensate thumb by taking an island flap from the fourth digit and transferring to the thumb. This type of flap can be very useful in the foot because one can create an island flap based on the digital vessels,[65] the lateral calcaneal artery,[66] or the dorsalis pedis artery.[67] An island flap is clearly a very elegant way to transfer a flap because the results are aesthetic and can be very functional. The donor site can be closed either primarily or with a skin graft.

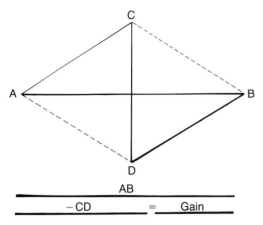

$$\frac{AB}{-CD} = \text{Gain}$$

FIG 18–13.
The estimated gain in length from a Z-plasty is
$AB - CD$ = gain in length. The actual length gained
is approximately one third less of the theoretical value.

ADVANCEMENT FLAPS

Advancement flaps (Fig 18–16) are moved directly forward to fill a defect without rotation or lateral movement. A rectangle of skin is dissected out and includes at a minimum skin and subcutaneous tissue. The flap is advanced into the defect, thereby creating a folding of the tissue at both ends of its base. Those folds (Burow's triangles) are removed so that the skin can be sutured together without causing any irregularities in the contour. It is best to excise those triangles in such a way as not to compromise the width of the flap. It is also important that the tension on the flap is adjusted so that there is no blanched area when it is in its new position. One should wait 15 minutes to

A

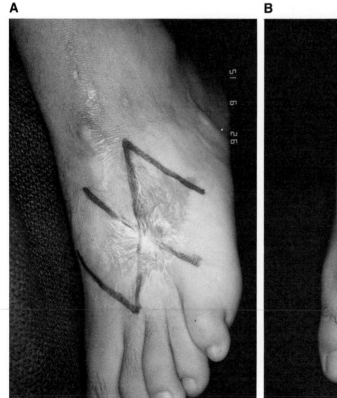

B

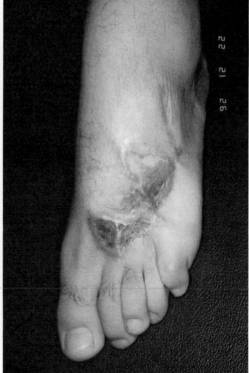

FIG 18–14.
A, burn scar on dorsum of foot causing hyperextension of metatarsophalangeal joint with planned double Z-plasty drawn in. **B,** the healed Z-plasty (required an additional small full-thickness skin graft distally to completely cover the defect after scar release).

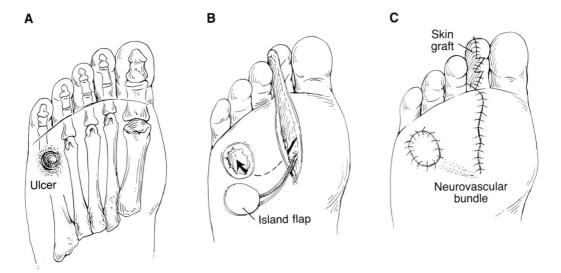

FIG 18–15.
A, plantar defect over fifth MTP. **B,** island flap based on the fibular neurovascular bundle of the second toe. **C,** island flap in place with the pedicle buried and the donor site skin grafted.

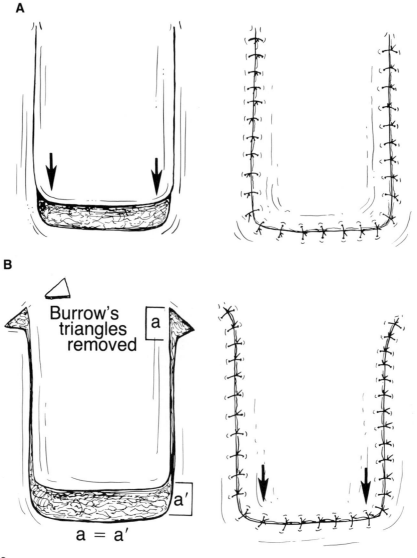

FIG 18–16.
A, flap advanced directly. **B,** resultant proximal dog ears removed so that advanced flap inserts smoothly.

allow for normal skin relaxation before judging whether the new position of the flap is too tight.

A V-Y flap (Fig 18–17) is a V-shaped flap whose sides are advanced, creating a Y when the incisions are closed. The V-Y flap is very useful in the forefoot, where it is used to close the defect from a metatarsal head ulcer.[68] It is important to realize that the advancement is limited to 1 to 2 cm forward motion in the foot. Therefore, if the defect is larger, double

V-Y flaps (see Fig 18–30) can be used to close defects up to 3 to 4 cm wide. This is more useful in the midfoot or hindfoot.

LOCAL MUSCLE AND MUSCULOCUTANEOUS FLAPS

One can transfer a simple muscle or muscle with overlying soft tissue to cover a soft tissue defect. It is obviously critical to know both the anatomic blood supply to

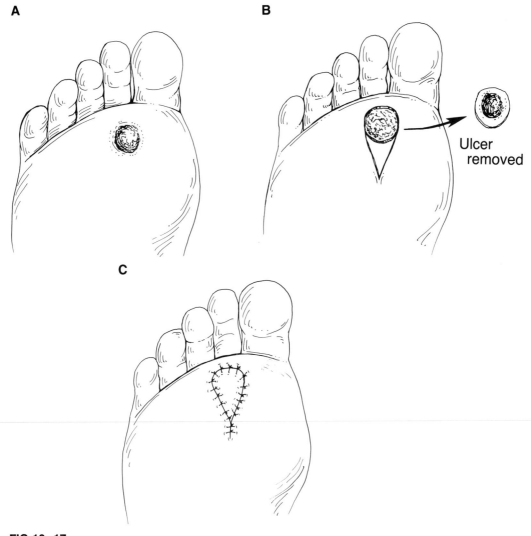

FIG 18–17.
A, ulcer over second MTP. **B,** V-Y flap planned to fill existent defect. **C,** V-Y flap advanced and defect closed. Note that donor site closed primarily as well.

the muscle and that of the overlying skin. It is also important to assess whether atherosclerotic disease has altered the normal pattern of blood flow and adjust the plan accordingly. One then has to be able to judge whether the planned arc of rotation will allow the flap to adequately fill the defect. The distal end of the rotated muscle is usually small and narrow, and the flap planning should take this into account. If the defect is one of skin with underlying tissue, and arterial supply to the skin overlying the planned muscle flap is not dependable, it is preferable to transfer the muscle without skin and skin graft the muscle. This allows one to close the donor defect without skin grafting.

Abductor Digiti Minimi Flap

The abductor digiti minimi flap (Fig 18–18) is a muscle flap used to fill defects of the lateral ankle joint or skin.[69] The blood supply from the lateral plantar artery enters the muscle medially near its origin at lateral tuberosity of the calcaneus. A minor pedicle is found entering the muscle more distally. The muscle then tapers out

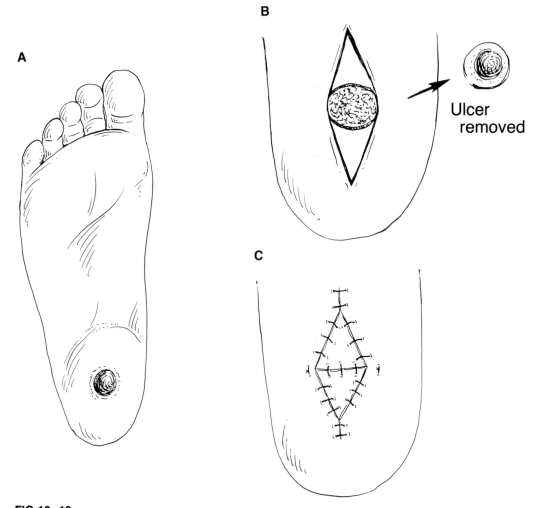

FIG 18–18.
A, large heel ulcer. **B,** double V-Y flaps planned after excision of ulcer. **C,** both V-Y flaps advanced to close the defect.

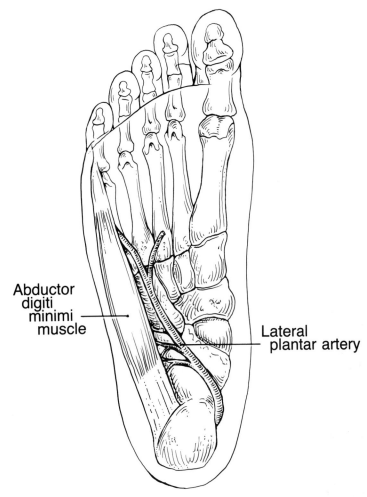

FIG 18–19.
Abductor digiti minimi flap.

to a tendon at the base of the fifth meta-tarsal, where it then goes on to insert to the lateral proximal phalanx of the fifth digit. The muscle can be dissected out via a lateral incision along the line where the sole meets the dorsum of the foot. It can then be dissected out and rotated posteriorly into the soft tissue[70] or bony defect without discernible functional loss.

Abductor Hallucis Brevis Muscle Flap

The abductor hallucis brevis muscle (Fig 18–19) is the medial posterior foot and ankle counterpart to the abductor digiti

minimi for the lateral foot and ankle defects. The muscle arises from the medial calcaneal tubercle and inserts on the medial proximal phalanx of the hallux. The blood supply is from the medial plantar artery and supplies two arteries to the muscle: one proximal and one in the midportion of the muscle. It is important to ensure that the posterior branch is the main branch[71] so that the flap can be based on it. By placing a microvascular occlusive clamp on the distal branch and observing the muscle, one can determine whether the blood flow from the posterior branch is sufficient to allow the muscle to survive on it alone. Proximally it is sometimes fused to the flexor digitorum brevis muscle. It becomes tendinous proximal to the first metatarsophalangeal (MCT) joint. By approaching it from medial to lateral and by detaching the muscle at its distal tendinous junction, one can easily dissect the muscle. It can be freed up from its origin for added mobility.

The flexor hallucis brevis muscle, which lies medial to the abductor, can be harvested with the abductor hallucis if more bulk is needed. It should be split along its tendon and the medial half of the

muscle used. Ger[70] believes that there is no morbidity as long as the flexor hallucis longus muscle is intact.

Flexor Digitorum Brevis Muscle Flap

The flexor digitorum brevis muscle[72] (Fig 18–20) should be considered only in the well-vascularized nondiabetic foot. The use of this muscle flap is not recommended in diabetics because its harvesting may weaken the bony midfoot arch and thus help precipitate Charcot's changes there. It originates from the medial calcaneal tu-

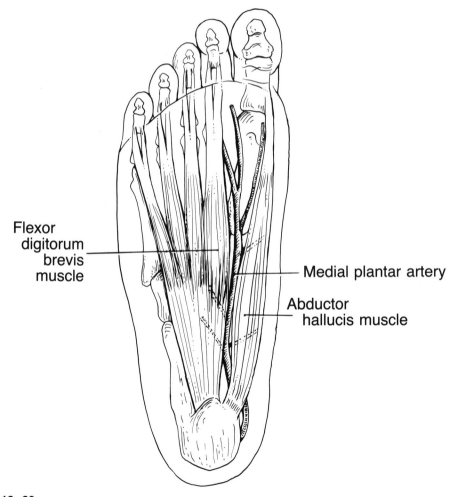

Flexor digitorum brevis muscle

Medial plantar artery

Abductor hallucis muscle

FIG 18–20.
Abductor hallucis minimi flap; flexor digitorum brevis flap (with *only* the medial plantar vascular contribution shown).

bercle and the plantar aponeurosis and splits into four tendons at the metatarsalphalangeal joint to then insert on either side of the proximal middle phalanges. Although the blood supply originates proximally from both the medial and lateral plantar artery, the latter is the principal blood supply. The flap should be dissected via a midline plantar incision, and the plantar fascia should be spared if the foot is to bear weight. It should be detached distally from its tendons and then folded back on itself to cover heel defects. An extra centimeter can be gained if the plantar origin is detached as well. Sensibility can be added to the flap if it is dissected with the overlying fascia and skin.[73]

FASCIOCUTANEOUS FLAPS

These flaps receive their blood supply either directly or via perforators that rise to the surface along fascial septae between muscle bellies. The advantage of these flaps is that they are thin and pliable and reliable. They are used to cover exposed bone or tendon but usually not to fill a large dead space. They are not as useful as muscle in treating osteomyelitis because the blood flow per centimeter squared is threefold to fivefold less.

Direct Cutaneous Blood Supply

Dorsalis Pedis Flap

The dorsalis pedis cutaneous flap (Fig 18–21) is a direct skin flap in the foot. It was first described by O'Brien and Shanmugan[74] in 1973, used as a pedicled and island flap by McCraw and Furlow[75] in 1975, and used as a free flap by Leeb et al.[76] in 1977. Its advantage is that it is thin and can be used as a sensory flap if the superficial peroneal nerve is incorporated with it. The planning and dissection of the flap have to be meticulous to avoid

distal tissue necrosis and minimize the donor defect.

The potential flap territory (10 by 12 cm) overlies the artery, which extends from the extensor retinaculum to the proximal first interosseous space. The territory extends medially and laterally to the dorsal skin's juncture with the sole. However, its distal extent is far less reliable because the first dorsal interossei may receive its blood supply from the plantar metatarsal arteries. Before one considers using this flap as either a free or a pedicled flap, it is imperative to know: Is the dorsalis pedis arterial flow antegrade or retrograde? Which vascular system supplies the first dorsal metatarsal artery? Is the anterior branch of the peroneal artery dominant? If the distal portion of the flap is supplied by the vascular blood supply from the sole of the foot, a delay[77] of that portion of the flap should be done to avoid distal flap necrosis.

The dorsalis pedis flap should be used only in well-vascularized patients as a second resort because of donor site morbidity. The donor site is best handled with a full-thickness skin graft from the groin. The flap should be used only as a pedicled flap in a patient who cannot undergo a free fasciocutaneous flap transfer. It is excellent in covering medial and lateral malleolar defects (Fig 18–22).

Filet of Toe Flap

The filet of toe flap (Fig 18–23) has to be chosen carefully because a toe is being sacrificed. It has the advantage of having the same characteristics as that of the sole that it is filling, and as sensate flap as the rest of the sole. It can be rotated locally[78] or carried on its neurovascular bundle[79, 80] for more proximal placement. The dissection of the flap is best done by making a dorsal incision along the extensor tendon and removing the phalangeal bones without disturbing the flexor tendon sheath and its accompanying two neurovascular

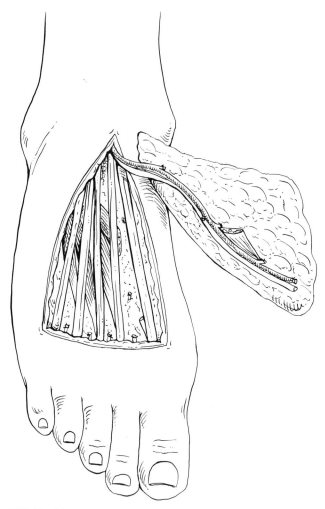

FIG 18–21.
Dorsalis pedis arterial cutaneous flap.

bundles that lie deep and lateral to the tendon. Attempts should be made to preserve the proximal portion of the proximal phalanx to avoid entering the metatarsophalangeal (MTP) joint, thus keeping the capsule with its tendinous attachments intact. The flap is made more pliable by removing the flexor tendon and extensors. The volar plates can be carefully removed by splitting them in the middle and dissecting them off from medial to lateral. The distal tuft can be splayed out by making radial cuts along the side of the septae. The flap should be inlaid without tension and with care so that the skin edge does not invaginate because this will lead to skin depressions that are difficult to keep clean.

Fasciocutaneous Flaps

Lateral Calcaneal Artery Fasciocutaneous Flap

The lateral calcaneal artery flap[81] (Fig 18–24) derives its blood supply from the calcaneal branch of the peroneal artery. The artery is accompanied by one or two venae commitantes and lies anterior to the achilles tendon. It arises deep to the peroneals, starts its downward course relatively superficially at the upper lateral malleolus, and then becomes deeper as it reaches the fascia overlying the extensor retinaculum. The artery then branches, with one end continuing downward and the other going toward the proximal fifth metatarsal. Within the flap is both the lesser saphenous vein and sural nerve (anterior to and parallel to the artery).

To dissect the flap, one must Doppler out the artery along its full length. The artery should lie along the midaxis of the flap, which allows for an 8 by 4 cm vertical flap to be harvested. To make the flap longer, one can extend the distal incisions along either side of the bifurcated artery toward the proximal fifth metatarsal. This extends the flap by up to 6 cm and allows for coverage of heel defects[82] (Fig 18–25). Because the vascular supply to the extended flap is sometimes questionable, it is best to check tip perfusion interoperatively using fluorescein. If the viability is questionable, the dissection is stopped,

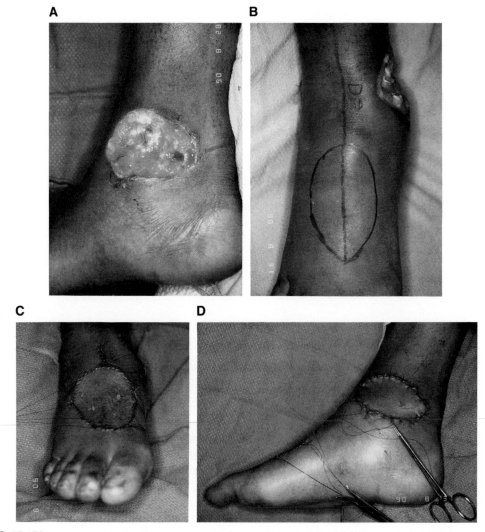

FIG 18–22.
A, preoperative lateral ankle defect. **B,** dorsalis pedis flap drawn out. **C,** dorsum of foot donor site covered with a full-thickness skin graft from the groin. **D,** dorsalis pedis pedicled flap sewn into defect.

A

B

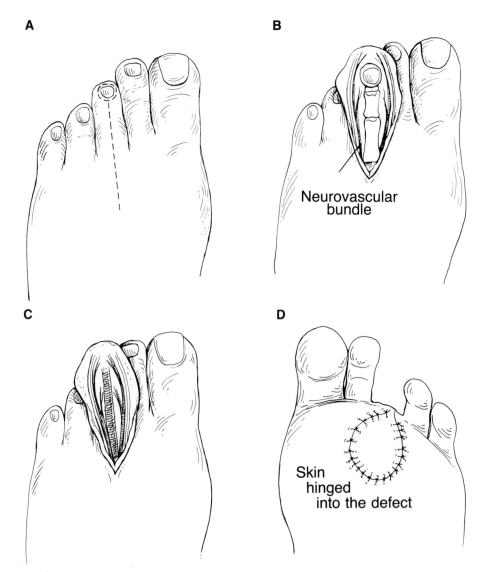

C

D

FIG 18–23.
A, dorsal incision removing the entire nail bed and nail fold. **B,** the phalangeal bones exposed before removal (the metatarsophalangeal joint is left intact). **C,** the flap after removal of the phalangeal bones with both neu-rovascular bundles intact. **D,** the flap is sewn into the defect at the base of the third metatarsophalangeal joint.

and the flap is delayed for 5 to 7 days. Obviously the donor site will require skin grafting. When one is harvesting the flap, it is advisable to start with the lateral incision down to periosteum and then dissect up retrograde (otherwise it is easy to go too superficially and transect the vascular pedicle).

Plantar Flaps
The blood supply to the sole of the foot is supplied by the medial and lateral plantar branches of the posterior tibialis artery. The lateral plantar artery gives off a branch that pierces the proximal attachment of the flexor digitorum brevis and then extends posteriorly and laterally

to supply the heel. The principal cutaneous blood supply thereafter comes from perforators that arise along either side of the flexor digitorum brevis and pierce the plantar fascia. They then supply the overlying skin. The lateral plantar artery turns medially at Lisfranc's joint to join the dorsal circulation via the deep perforator at the proximal lateral first metatarsal. The common digital arteries arise from the distal lateral plantar artery.

The lateral plantar flap can be based either proximally or distally, depending on the defect and the connection of the

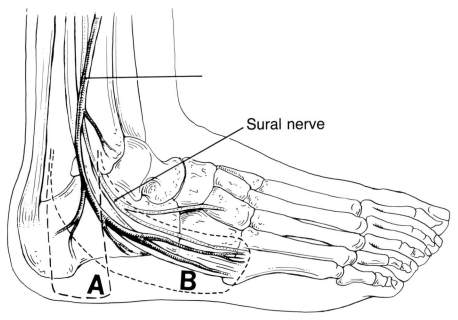

FIG 18–24.
A, posterior calcaneal flap. *B,* extended calcaneal flap to reach heel defects.

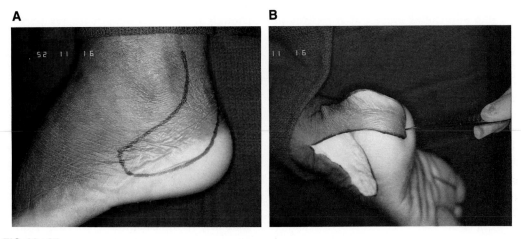

FIG 18–25.
Designed dissection of an extended calcaneal flap showing its capability of covering proximal heel defects.

plantar artery with the dorsalis pedis. If based proximally, the flap is used to fill heel defects. One then has to ensure a patent system between the dorsal and plantar circulation or else the blood supply to the digits can be compromised. The flap need only include the perforators, plantar fascia, and lateral plantar artery, although it has classically included the flexor digitorum brevis.[83] It is rotated from lateral to medial and posteriorly while the donor site is skin grafted. This is a flap fraught with danger because it requires extensive dissection that can compromise the blood supply to the forefoot.

The medial sole flap[84] is based on a cutaneous branch of the medial plantar artery and is designed over a non-weight-bearing portion of the sole. The medial plantar runs along between the flexor digitorum brevis and abductor hallucis. It provides blood to the overlying skin via a direct cutaneous branch that takes off at its origin and lies above the fascia. It carries with it the medial plantar nerve that gives off cutaneous branches for sensation to the overlying skin. The flap is dissected from distal to proximal, and the medial plantaris artery has to be tied off distal to the cutaneous perforator so that there can be a greater arc of rotation to the flap. The abductor hallucis can be included to give the flap additional bulk, but it is best to leave it in place so that the skin graft over the donor site has a better chance of taking. A neurosensory flap[85] that measures 5 by 6 cm can be dissected and used to cover heel defects. The donor site is skin grafted. The dissection and risk of vascular compromise is far less than that of the lateral plantar flap, thus making it a much more viable option.

MICROSURGERY

The advent of microsurgery and free flaps have revolutionized our ability to cover soft tissue defects. Free flaps can include fasciocutaneous, musculocutaneous, osteocutaneous, and osteomusculocutaneous flaps. In good microsurgical centers they can be performed with a 95% or better degree of confidence.[86] The donor site does not include the foot, and the donor morbidity can be minimal. However, the free flap has to have adequate inflow through one of the three distal arteries, preferably the distal posterior tibial or dorsalis pedis artery. If the flow to the foot is inadequate because of trifurcation atherosclerotic disease, the foot needs to be revascularized via an in situ graft to a distal artery, which can go as far as the dorsalis pedis or plantar arteries. It is also important to ensure that there is adequate venous drainage by using Doppler visualization of the deep and superficial veins in question.

The free flap anastomosis, whenever possible, should always be done end to side (end-to-side patency rates are superior to end-to-end patency rates) so that the distal blood flow is not compromised.[87] It is best to ensure that the free flap pedicle be of adequate length so no intervening vein graft is needed. The patency rate drops precipitously if an interposition vein graft is required. Perioperative anticoagulation using either aspirin, Dextran 40, or heparin is useful to preserve patency, although it is not a substitute for perfect technique. For a more thorough discussion of microsurgical technique, the reader is referred to three recent excellent texts on the subject.[88–90]

We now have the ability to specifically tailor each free flap to the particular defect so that the rebuilt foot ends up with a *normal* soft tissue envelope. This means that the foot should not have bulky excessive tissue that can break down.

For the dorsum of the foot, we prefer to use fasciocutaneous free flaps from either the parascapular area, the radial forearm, the lateral arm, or the temporalis fascia with split-thickness skin graft. The advantages of these flaps are that they can be innervated, are thin, have minimum donor morbidity, and have very reliable vascular pedicles. For the sole of the foot, we rely on muscle flaps with split-thickness skin grafts because they seem to hold up better over time, provided that the patient has adequate orthotics. The muscle flap we rely on the most are the last two to three slips of serratus muscle. This flap has no donor morbidity, can be very large, can be innervated, and has a long pedicle. Excellent backup flaps include the gracilis flap, the latissimus dorsi flap, and the rectus abdominus flap. Of these three, only the gracilis muscle has minimal donor site morbidity and can be harvested from the ipsilateral leg. However the flap itself is relatively small and has a short pedicle.

Should osteocutaneous flaps be required, the flap of choice is the contralateral fibular flap. One can replace up to two metatarsals and provide thin skin coverage. Should the vascular supply to the contralateral leg be inadequate, a second choice would include the radial forearm osteocutaneous free flap or the parascapular osteocutaneous free flap. The advantage of using vascularized bone is that the risk of infection is diminished, and the bony union is more rapid and reliable. It enables one to preserve the foot architecture without resorting to biomechanically inferior amputations.

SOFT TISSUE COVERAGE BY AREA

Whenever a soft tissue defect is evaluated, it is important to ensure that the bony framework is biomechanically optimal. Not correcting an obvious bony malalignment or performing a poorly designed amputation will threaten whatever soft tissue repair is chosen. The residual bony skeleton dictates the soft tissue repair chosen. This requires an intimate knowledge of foot biomechanics in general and

the biomechanically optimal amputation at each level. Of course, the more the foot skeleton is preserved, the more the pressure of ambulation is dissipated over the whole foot.

It is important to fully understand the state of the foot's vascular supply, namely, ankle-brachial indexes, toe pressures, pulse Doppler waveforms, and transcutaneous oxygen tension. Is the flow to the dorsum of the foot antegrade or retrograde? Does the foot need a bypass before soft tissue reconstruction?

The mode of soft tissue reconstruction chosen and the bony architecture remaining depend on the patient's medical condition, the vascular supply to the foot, and the sensory supply to the foot. One has to determine whether the patient is a candidate for a long microvascular reconstruction (6–10 hours) or whether the patient can tolerate only an ankle block. This determines whether a shorter, less biomechanically optimal amputation is chosen over a less radical amputation that requires microvascular coverage.

The decision tree for the soft tissue coverage requires consideration of the simplest to the most complex: secondary intention, primary closure, skin graft, local flap, and microvascular free flap. Much dissection in the foot is to be avoided because it may disrupt an already fragile blood supply. Rapid primary healing avoids the hyperkeratosis seen with secondary intention healing. Thus, often the simplest procedure turns out to be the technically most complex, namely, a microvascular free flap.

Dorsum of Foot

If the tendons are covered by at least paratenon and the bone by periosteum, the simplest procedure is a full-thickness skin graft or split-thickness skin graft (Figs 18–26 and 18–27). Otherwise, one has to use local or free flaps to protect the tendons, bone, and neurovascular bundle.

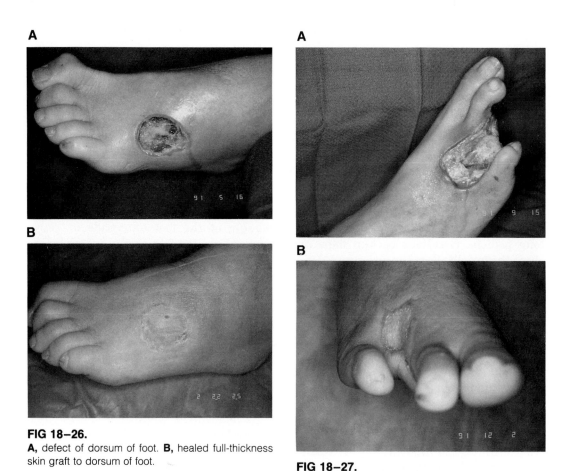

FIG 18–26.
A, defect of dorsum of foot. **B,** healed full-thickness skin graft to dorsum of foot.

FIG 18–27.
A, defect on dorsum of foot s/p amputation of third and fourth toe. **B,** healed status post split-thickness skin graft. Note amount of contraction in the wound.

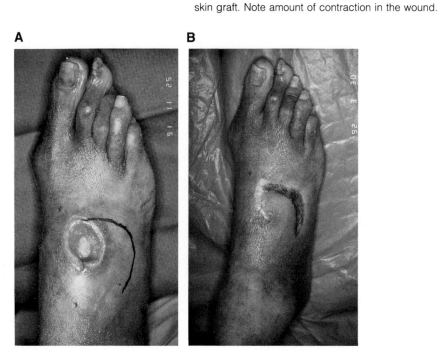

FIG 18–28.
A, open defect over Lyfranc's joint with a rotation flap drawn in. **B,** the wound healed 1 year later. Note that a split-thickness skin graft was used to cover the donor site.

Local flaps include rotation flaps (Fig 18–28), advancement flaps, dorsalis pedis flap, and extensor digitorum brevis flap with split-thickness skin graft. Local flaps should be planned with a Doppler to ensure that the appropriate antegrade/retrograde flow exists at the base of the flap when it is cut. If a free flap is chosen, it should be fasciocutaneous, thin, and innervated (Fig 18–29). The patient's habitus dictates where the donor site would be. One obviously wants the thinnest possible flap so that the foot resumes a normal configuration. A free flap frees one from the constraint of limited local soft tissue availability so that one can be more generous with the debridement of scarred tissue and preparation of the recipient bed.

Forefoot (Sole)

Adequate padding is essential, and thus secondary intention, primary closure, filet of toe (Fig 18–30), and V-Y advancement flaps are ideal. If a transmetatarsal amputation is to be done because more than two toes are gone and a side of the foot has a large soft tissue defect, the healthy remaining toes should be filleted and used

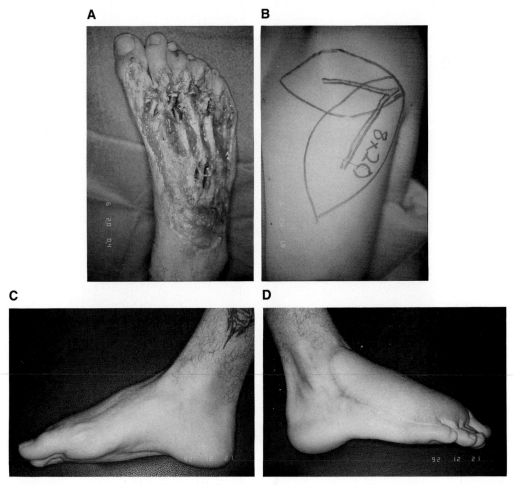

FIG 18–29.
A, degloved foot with exposed metatarsals and metatarsophalangeal joints. **B,** parascapular fasciocutaneous free flap (8 by 20 cm) planned. **C** and **D,** the foot 2 years status post repair.

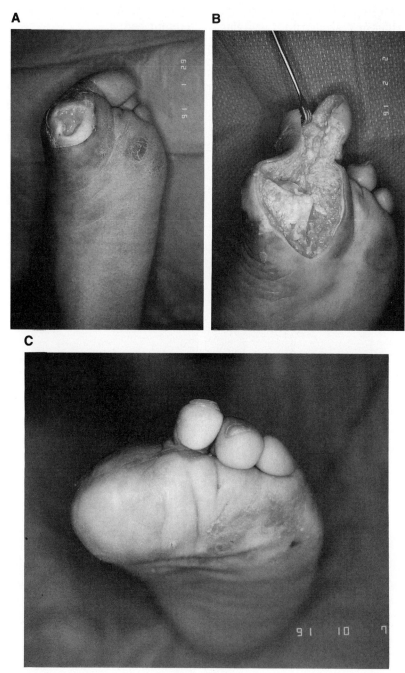

FIG 18–30.
A, first metatarsophalangeal ulcer. **B,** filet of first toe. **C,** healed foot.

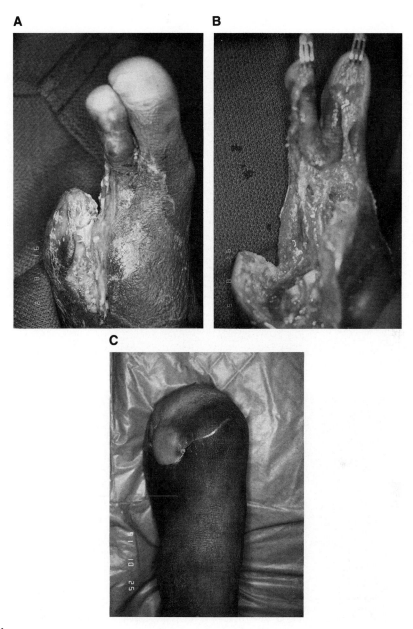

FIG 18–31.
A, defect in a patient with chronic renal failure and adult-onset diabetes mellitus with amputated third, fourth, and fifth toes. **B,** filet of first and second toes. **C,** healed transmetatarsal amputation.

to preserve length (Fig 18–31). Because a transmetatarsal amputation is such a good option, there is usually enough soft tissue to avoid using a free flap. However, the latter should be considered to preserve length.

Midfoot (Sole)

If the defect is on the non-weight-bearing aspect of the foot, a split-thickness skin graft is the easiest (Fig 18–32). Secondary intention and local flaps, including V-Y advancement (Fig 18–33) flaps, are useful

A   B   C

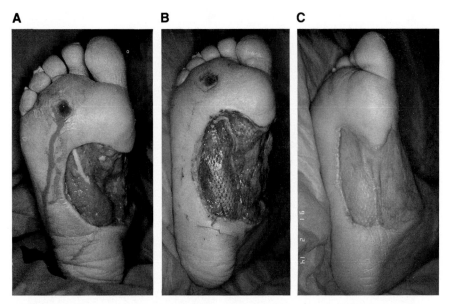

FIG 18–32.
A, open defect midfoot instep. **B,** split-thickness skin graft 5 days postoperatively. **C,** healed split-thickness skin graft over midfoot.

A   B   C

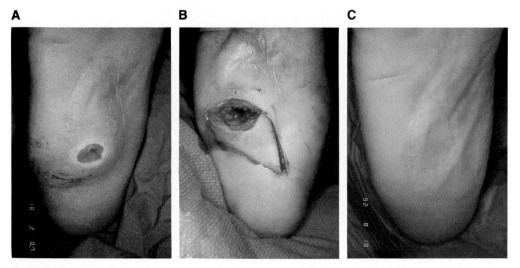

FIG 18–33.
A, recurrent ulcer in the midfoot of a Charcot foot. **B,** V-Y designed over a previously healed double V-Y flap (bone exostosis removed). **C,** healed flap.

for small defects. Larger defects are best treated with either medial plantaris fasciocutaneous island flaps, local muscle flaps with split-thickness skin graft, or free muscle flaps covered with split-thickness skin graft (Fig 18–34).

Hindfoot (Sole)

Other than V-Y flaps (Fig 18–35) for small defects, local flaps are usually to be discouraged because the dissection is too extensive, the flap never quite reaches to where it should, and prolonged hospital-

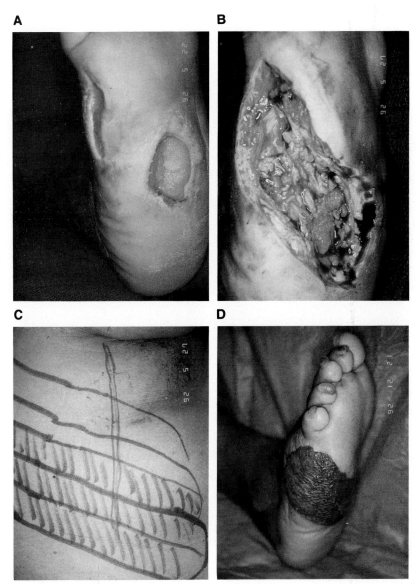

FIG 18–34.
A, midfoot defect in a diabetic foot. **B,** debridement wound. **C,** serratus muscle donor site. **D,** healed ser- ratus free flap with split-thickness skin graft.

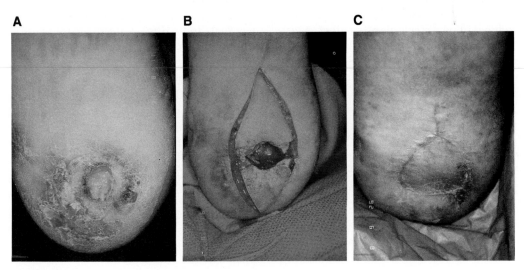

FIG 18–35.
A, heel defect. **B,** double V-Y flap. **C,** healed flap.

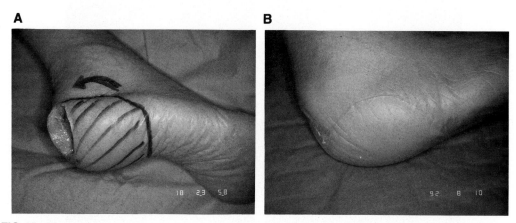

FIG 18–36.
A, rotation flap designed to cover heel defect after partial calcanectomy. **B,** healed flap after a 4-month course of wound care.

ization from wound complications result (Fig 18–36). Free musculocutaneous flaps with skin graft (Figs 18–37 and 18–38) are optimal, provided they are well tailored and orthotics are available afterward. For Chopart's amputations, flaps preserving the blood supply can be designed to achieve adequate coverage (Fig 18–39).

Ankle

Skin grafts work extremely well on the Achilles tendon (Fig 18–40) but are less than ideal on the malleoli. For the ankle joint and for malleolar defects, local flaps are ideal. The muscle flaps (abductor digiti minimi, abductor hallucis) are ideal for osteomyelitis in and around the ankle joint if the skin defect is small (Fig 18–41). Fasciocutaneous flaps that work well include the lateral calcaneal arterial flap (Fig 18–42), local medial malleolar flaps based on perforators of the posterior tibial artery, and the dorsalis pedis flap. The usual caveats concerning maintenance of blood flow obviously have to be respected. Donor sites have to be skin grafted. Free flaps in this area can be either fasciocutaneous or muscle with skin graft (Fig 18–43) but must be of minimal bulk to be functional.

CONCLUSION

Soft tissue repair of the diabetic foot requires close cooperation between the bone surgeon, infectious disease specialist, diabetologist, and, most important, the podiatrist who will provide care for the patient postoperatively. Although the soft tissue techniques just described provide the tools to heal most of the patients without infection and avoid below-knee amputation, they do not prevent an unacceptably high recurrent ulcer rate approaching 50%. The key is in designing the best biomechanical amputation and providing the correct shoe thereafter to ensure optimal redistribution of weight during gait. How to accomplish this is the most exciting and unknown part in the management of diabetic foot ulcers.

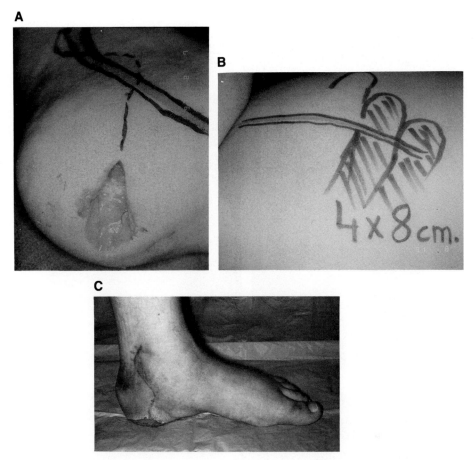

FIG 18–37.
A, chronic 8-year ulcer over heel with posterior tibial receptor vessels drawn in. **B,** serratus muscle free flap donor site. **C,** healed foot.

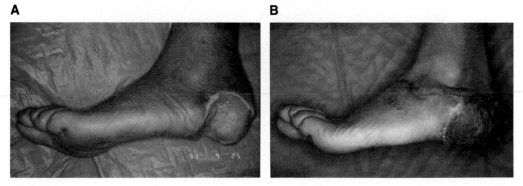

FIG 18–38.
A, heel defect, including entire sole. **B,** healed status post latissimus dorsi free flap with split-thickness skin graft.

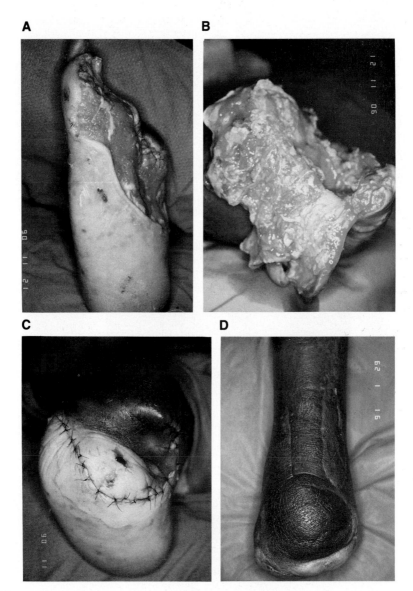

FIG 18–39.
A, open forefoot after anterior tibialis revascularization using in situ vein graft. **B,** filleted forefoot and midfoot. **C,** inset flap. **D,** healed flap.

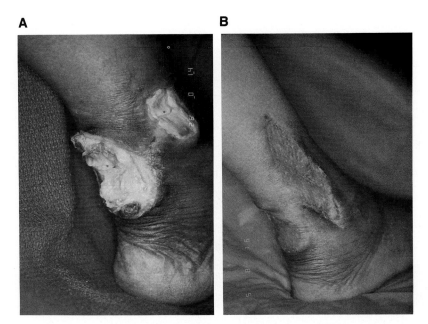

FIG 18–40.
A, necrotic Achilles tendon in a diabetic. **B,** healed tendon after multiple debridements and split-thickness skin graft.

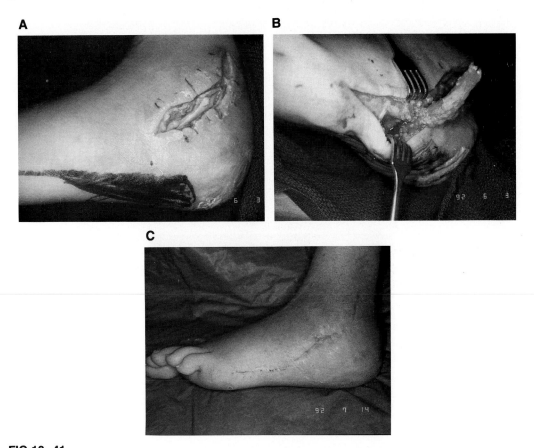

FIG 18–41.
A, defect of the lateral malleolus involving ankle joint with the abductor digiti minimi muscle flap drawn out.
B, harvested abductor digiti minimi muscle flap.
C, healed wound.

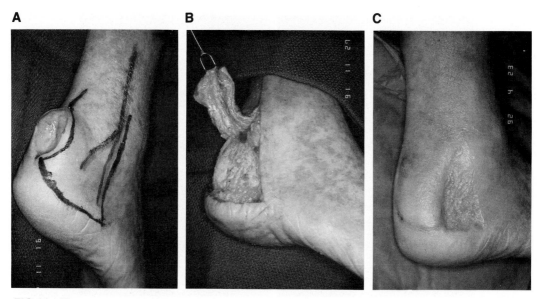

FIG 18–42.
A, Achilles tendon defect. **B,** harvested posterior calcaneal flap. **C,** healed wound with skin-grafted donor site.

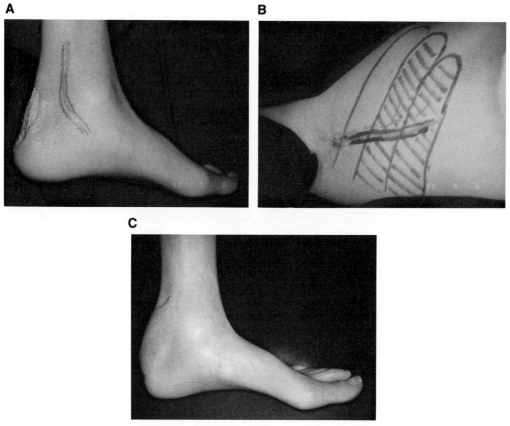

FIG 18–43.
A, Achilles tendon defect. **B,** serratus muscle free flap donor site. **C,** healed with split-thickness skin graft.

REFERENCES

1. Mathes SJ, Nahai F: *Clinical applications for muscle and musculocutaneous flaps,* St Louis, 1982, Mosby–Year Book.
2. Peacock EE: *Wound repair,* ed 3. Philadelphia, 1984, WB Sauders.
3. Hunt TK et al: *Soft and hard tissue repair: Biological and clinical aspects,* New York, 1984, Praeger.
4. Knighton DR et al: Classification and treatment of chronic nonhealing wounds. Successful treatment with autologous platelet-derived growth factors (PDWHF), *Ann Surg* 204:322, 1986.
5. Alvarez O, Rozint J, Wiseman D: Moist environment of healing: Matching the dressing to the wound. In *Wounds: A compendium of clinical research and practice,* April 1988, vol 22, issue 3, pp 1–12.
6. Kucan JO et al: Comparison of silver sulfadiazine, povidone-iodine, and physiological saline in the treatment of chronic pressure ulcers, *J Am Geriatr Soc* 29:232, 1981.
7. Mertz PM: Intervention: The dressing effects on wound healing. In Eaglestein WH, editor: *New directions in wound healing.* ER Sqibb, 1990.
8. Ryan TJ, editor: *An environment for healing: the role for occlusion,* International Congress and Symposium Series, London, 1985, Royal Society of Medicine.
9. Katz S, McGinley K, Leyden JJ: Semipermeable occlusive dressings. Effects of growth of pathogenic bacteria and reepithelialization of superficial wounds, *Arch Dermatol* 122:58, 1986.
10. Edlich RF et al: Physical and chemical configuration of sutures in the development of surgical infection, *Ann Surg* 177:679–687, 1973.
11. Edgerton MT, Milton T: *The art of surgical technique,* Baltimore, 1988, Williams & Wilkins.
12. Krizek TJ, Robson MC: The evolution of quantitative bacteriology in wound management, *Am J Surg* 130:579, 1975.
13. Salisbury RE, Caines R, McCarthy LR: Comparison of the bacterial cleaning effects of different biologic dressings on granulating wounds following thermal injury, *Plast Reconstr Surg* 66:596, 1980.
14. Ye RC: The relationship of pH of the granulation tissue and the take of the graft, *Plast Reconstr Surg* 19:213, 1957.
15. Zoltan J: Transplantationlehre, In *Handbuch der Plastichen Chirugie,* Berlin, 1965, Walter de Gruyter, pp 1–244.
16. Rudolph R: The effect of skin graft preparation on wound contracture, *Surg Gynecol Obstet* 142:49, 1976.
17. Rudolph R: Inhibition of myofibroblast by skin grafts, *Plast Reconstr Surg* 63:473, 1979.
18. Bertolami CN, Donoff RB: The effect of skin grafting upon prolylhydroxylase and hyaluronidase activities in mammalian wound repair, *J Surg Res* 27:359, 1979.
19. Mir Y, Mir L: The problem of pigmentation in the cutaneous graft, *Br J Plast Surg* 14:303, 1961.
20. Rudolph R, Klein L: Healing process in skin grafts, *Surg Gynecol Obstet* 136:641, 1973.
21. Burleson R, Eiseman B: Nature of bond between partial thickness skin and wound granulation, *Am Surg* 177:181, 1973.
22. Coverse JM, Uhlshlschmid GK, Ballantyne DL: Plasmatic circulation in skin grafts, *Plast Reconstr Surg* 43:495, 1969.
23. Hinshaw JR, Miller ER: Histology of healing split thickness, full thickness autogenous skin grafts and donor sites, *Arch Surg* 91:658, 1965.
24. Peer LA, Walker JC: The behavior of autogenous human tissue grafts, *Plast Reconstr Surg* 7:6, 1951.
25. Clemmesen T: The early circulation in split thickness grafts, *Acta Chir Scand* 124:11, 1962.
26. Converse JM, Ballantyne DL Jr: Distribution of diphosphopyridine nucleotide diaphorase in rat skin autografts and homografts, *Plast Reconstr Surg* 30:415, 1962.
27. Zarem HA, Zweifach BW, McGehee JM: Development of microcirculation in full thickness autogenous skin grafts in mice, *Am J Physiol* 212:1081, 1967.
28. Smahel J: The healing of skin grafts, *Clin Plast Surg* 4:409, 1977.
29. Birch J, Branemark PI: The vascularization of a free full thickness skin graft, a

vital microscopic study, *Scand J Plast Reconstr* 3:1, 1969.

30. Mcgregor IA, Conway H: Development of lymph flow from autografts and homografts of skin, *Transplant Bull* 3:46, 1956.

31. Gloor M, Ludwig G: Revascularization of free full thickness skin autografts, *Arch Dermatol Forsch* 246:211, 1973.

32. Kelton PL, Philip L: Principles of skin grafts. In *Selected reading in plastic surgery,* Dallas, Texas, Baylor University Medical Center, August 1990, Vol 6.

33. Waris T et al: Regeneration of cold, warmth, and heat sensibility in human skin grafts, *Br J Plast Surg* 42:576, 1989.

34. Flowers R: Unexpected postoperative problems in skin grafting, *Surg Clin North Am* 50:439, 1970.

35. Robson MC, Krizek TJ: Predicting skin graft survival, *Arch Plast Surg* 22:479, 1989.

36. Teh BT: Why do skin grafts fail? *Plast Reconstr Surg* 63:323, 1979.

37. Bodenham DC, Watson R: The early ambulation of patients with lower limb grafts, *Br J Plast Surg* 24:20, 1971.

38. Milton SH: Pedicled skin flaps: The fallacy of the length-width ratio, *Br J Surg* 57:502, 1970.

39. Taylor GI, Palmer JH, McManamny D: The vascular territories of the body (angiosomes) and their clinical application. In McCarthy JG, editor: *Plastic surgery,* Philadelphia, 1990, WB Saunders.

40. Manchot C: *The cutaneous arteries of the human body,* [translated by Ristic J & Morain WD]. New York, 1983, Springer Verlag.

41. Salmon M: *Arteres de la Peau,* Paris, 1936, Masson et Cie.

42. Salmon M: *Arteres des muscles des membres et du tronc,* Paris, 1936, Masson et Cie.

43. Hooper JE: Pedicle flaps: an overview. In Krizek TS, Hooper JE, editors: *Symposium on basic science in plastic surgery,* vol 15, St Louis, 1976, Mosby–Year Book.

44. Cormack GC, Lamberty GH: *The arterial anatomy of skin flaps,* New York, 1986, Churchill Livingstone.

45. Taylor GI, McCarten G, Doyle M: The use of the Doppler probe for planning flaps: Anatomical study and clinical application. *Br J Plast Surg* 43:1, 1990.

46. Huber JF: The arterial network supplying the dorsum of the foot, *Anatomical Record* 80:373, 1941.

47. Taylor GI, Palmer JH: The vascular territories (angiosomes) of the body: Experimental studies and clinical applications, *Br J Plast Surg* 43:1, 1990.

48. Callegari PR, Taylor GI, Caddy CM et al: An anatomic review of the delay phenomenon: I. Experimental studies, *Plast Reconstr Surg* 89:397, 1992.

49. Taylor GI, Corlett RJ, Caddy CM et al: An anatomic review of the delay phenomenon: II. Clinical applications, *Plast Reconstr Surg* 89:408, 1992.

50. Taylor GI, Caddy CM, Watterson PA et al: The venous territories (venosomes) of the human body: Experimental study and clinical implications, *Plast Reconstr Surg* 86:185, 1990.

51. Mathes SJ, Nahai F: Classification of the vascular anatomy of muscles: Experimental and clinical correlation, *Plast Reconstr Surg* 67:177–187, 1981.

52. Jankauskas S, Cohen IK, Grabb WC: The techniques of plastic surgery. In Smith JW, Aston SJ, editors: *Grabb and Smith's plastic surgery,* ed 4, Boston, 1991, Little, Brown & Co.

53. Imre J: Lidplastic—und plastische operationen. In *Den weichteile des gesichts.* Budapest, 1928, Studium Verlag.

54. Jackson IT: *Local flaps in head and neck reconstruction,* St Louis, 1985, Mosby–Year Book.

55. Limberg AA: *Mathematical principles of the local plastic procedures on the surface of the human body,* Leningrad, 1946, Government Publishing House for Medical Literature.

56. Horner W: Clinical report on the surgical department of Philadelphia Hospital for the month of May, June, July 1837, *Am J Med Sci* 21:105, 1837.

57. McCregor IA: The theoretical basis of Z-Plasty, *Br J Plast Surg* 9:256, 1957.

58. Furnas DW, Fischer GW: The Z-plasty: Biomechanics and mathematics, *Br J Plast Surg* 24:144, 1971.

59. Kraissl CJ: The selection of appropriate lines for elective surgical incisions, *Plast Reconstr Surg* 8:1, 1951.

60. Woolf RM, Broadbent TR: The four-flap Z-Plasty, *Plast Reconstr Surg* 49:48, 1972.

61. Wilkenson TS, Rybka RJ: Experimental study of prevention of tip necrosis in ischemic Z-plasties, *Plast Reconstr Surg* 47:37, 1971.

62. Stevensons TW: Release of circular contricting scars by Z flaps, *Plast Reconstr Surg* 1:39, 1946.

63. Dingman RO: Some application of the Z-Plasty procedure, *Plast Reconstr Surg* 16:246, 1955.

64. Littler JW: Neurovascular pedicle method of digital transposition for reconstruction of the thumb, *Plast Reconstr Surg* 12:303, 1955.

65. Littler JW: Principles of reconstructive surgery of the hand. In Converse JM, editor: *Reconstructive plastic surgery*, vol 4, Philadelphia, 1964, WB Saunders, pp 1636–1639.

66. Grabb WC, Argenta LC: The lateral calcaneal artery skin flap, *Plast Reconstr Surg* 68:723, 1981.

67. McCraw JB, Furlow LT: The dorsalis pedis arterialized flap, *Plast Reconstr Surg* 55:177, 1975.

68. Colen LB, Repogle SL, Mathes SJ: The V-Y plantar flap for reconstruction of the forefoot, *Plast Reconstr Surg* 81:220, 1988.

69. Ger R: The surgical management of ulcers of the heel, *Surg Gynecol Obstet* 140:909, 1975.

70. Ger R: The management of chronic ulcers of the dorsum of the foot by muscle transposition and free skin grafting, *Br J Plast Surg* 29:199, 1976.

71. McCraw JB: Selection of alternative local flaps in the leg and foot, *Clin Plast Surg* 6:227, 1979.

72. Hartrampf CR Jr, Scheflan M, Bostwick J III: The flexor digitorum brevis muscle island pedicle flap: A new dimension in heel reconstruction, *Plast Reconstr Surg* 66:264, 1980.

73. Scheflan M, Nahai F, Hartrampf CR Jr: Surgical management of heel ulcers—a comprehensive approach, *Ann Plast Surg* 7:385, 1981.

74. O'Brien B, McLeod AM, Shanmugan M: Experimental transfer of composite free flaps with microvascular anastamoses, *Aust N Z J Surg* 43:285–288, 1973.

75. McCraw JB, Furlow LT Jr: The dorsalis pedis arterialized flap: A clinical study, *Plast Reconstr Surg* 55:177–185, 1975.

76. Leeb D, Ben-Hur N, Mazzarella L: Reconstruction of the floor of the mouth with a dorsalis pedis flap, *Plast Reconstr Surg* 59:379–381, 1977.

77. May JW: Letters to the editor, *Plast Reconstr Surg* 59:909, 1977.

78. Emmet AJJ: The filleted toe flap, *Br J Plast Surg* 29:19, 1976.

79. Snyder GB, Edgerton MT: The principle of island neurovascular flap in the management of ulcerated anaesthetic weight-bearing areas of the lower extremity, *Plast Reconstr Surg* 36:518, 1965.

80. Buncke HJ, Colen LB: An island flap from the first web space of the foot to cover plantar ulcers, *Br J Plast Surg* 33:242, 1980.

81. Grabb WC, Argenta LC: The lateral calcaneal artery flap (the lateral calcaneal artery, lesser saphenous vein and sural nerve skin flap), *Plast Reconstr Surg* 68:723, 1981.

82. Yanai A, Park S, Iwao T et al: Reconstruction of a skin defect of the posterior heel by a lateral calcaneal flap, *Plast Reconstr Surg* 75:642–646, 1985.

83. Reiffel RS, McCarthy JG: Coverage of heel and sole defects: a new subfascial arterialized flap, *Plast Reconstr Surg* 66:250–260, 1980.

84. Shanahan RE, Gingrass RP: Medial plantar sensory flap for coverage of heel defects, *Plast Reconstr Surg* 64:295, 1979.

85. Harrison DH, Morgan BDG: The instep island flap to resurface plantar defects, *Br J Plast Surg* 34:315, 1981.

86. Acland RD: *Microsurgery practice manual,* Louisville, Ky, 1977, University of Louisville Microsurgery Laboratory, Price Institute of Surgical Research, Department of Surgery, Health Sciences Center.

87. Godina M: Preferential use of end to side arterial anastomoses in free flap transfers, *Plast Reconstr Surg* 64:673, 1979.

88. Buncke HJ: *Microsurgery: Transplantation-replantation,* Philadelphia, 1991, Lea & Febiger.

89. O'Brien B, Morrison WA: *Reconstructive microsurgery,* New York, 1987, Churchill Livingstone.

90. Shaw WW, Hildalgo DA: *Microsurgery in trauma.* Mount Kisco, NY, 1987, Futura.

19 — Hyperbaric Oxygen Therapy in Diabetic Foot Infections

Jean Gordon, M.D.

Problems involving the foot pose many potentially major complications for persons with diabetes. These problems and their subsequent complications are costly in money and in time spent for hospitalization and rehabilitation. Foot problems are responsible for more hospitalizations than any other diabetic complication.[1,2] Approximately $200 million are spent each year to treat diabetic foot infections.[5] Diabetic persons are five times more likely than the general population to develop gangrene as a complication of diabetes foot infection and 15% of these individuals go on to require amputations.[1-3] Limb loss is the most feared complication of diabetes, because more than 60% of diabetics with amputation of 1 leg will not be alive in 5 years.[2,3]

PREDISPOSING CAUSES

Foot problems in the diabetic occur as a result of malfunction of three systems: the nervous system, the vascular system, and the immune system.[1-3,5,13] Problems of the nervous system include autonomic system dysfunction, loss of sensation, and motor nerve destruction.[1]

The Nervous System

Autonomic Nerve Dysfunction
Autonomic nerve dysfunction can lead to a decrease in sweating, causing dry,

cracked skin that provides a portal for bacteria to enter and cause infection. Secondly, the flare reaction that normally occurs in response to injury is inhibited, leading to impaired delivery of blood to the injured area. Thirdly, in contrast, destruction of sympathetic nerves may mimic autosympathectomy, leading to increased blood flow that contributes to bony absorption and development of Charcot foot.[1,5]

Loss of Sensation

Loss of protective sensation can lead to serious complications. Unnoticed relatively minor trauma from foreign bodies, shoe abnormalities, or bony foot prominences can cause skin injury secondary to local ischemia. These minor injuries can then develop into full thickness ulcers. Once formed, these ulcers remain painless and may eventually become infected—the most frequent presenting complaint.[1,3,5]

Motor Nerve Dysfunction

Motor nerve dysfunction causes foot deformity leading to development of new pressure points. Ultimately, ulcers and infection occur at these sites.[1,3,5]

The Vascular System

Vascular abnormalities in diabetics involve both the large and small blood vessels.[1, 13] Large vessel disease and the resultant ischemia are a well-known cause of local painful ulcerations, primarily of the toes. Small vessel disease includes, but is not limited to, capillary basement membrane thickening that can lead to decreased diffusion of oxygen and other nutrients into the tissues.

The Immune System

Diabetics have an increased susceptibility to infection because of certain immune system abnormalities. They have deficiencies in white cell diapedesis, adherence, and chemotaxis, which are thought to be influenced by an increase in plasma ketoacid concentration. Hyperglycemia causes defective white cell phagocytosis and promotes the growth of bacteria.[3, 5] Angiopathy, which leads to hypoxia, inhibits white blood cell (WBC) killing of bacteria by reducing the formation of superoxide radicals. Angiopathy also impairs the delivery of antibiotics, antibodies, and granulocytes to the affected site.[4, 5] These problems increase the risk of developing infections and contribute to delayed healing.

MECHANISMS OF INFECTION

Most diabetic foot infections occur as a result of some sort of trauma.[3, 5] *Blisters* usually are due to improperly fitting footwear and lead to separation of the superficial layers of the skin and accumulation of fluid. Skin breakdown allows bacteria to enter and infection supervenes. *Abrasions* leave the deeper layers of the skin unprotected by the horny outer layer and the risk of infection subsequently increases. *Ulcers* may result from extension of abrasions or breakdown over pressure points. *Calluses* and *corns* are excess growth of tough, horny skin. In an attempt to remove them, the patient may inadvertently introduce bacteria to deeper layers

of skin and thereby promote infection. Infection may also be introduced via puncture wounds, fissures, or from crush or degloving injuries.[3, 5]

TYPES OF INFECTIONS

Infections of the diabetic foot may range from minor, asymptomatic fungal infections to severe limb or life-threatening disorders.[5] We will address only the most serious infections here, although one must be diligent not to dismiss an apparently serious problem as a minor one. An example of this is a patient who presents with a small ulcer and bead of pus, but who may have underlying extensive soft tissue destruction.

Foot infections that develop include neuropathic ulcers, deep plantar abscesses, and cellulitis/necrotizing soft tissue infections.[5] They are usually polymicrobial, (*Staphylococcus aureus*, *Streptococcus* spp., gram negative species and anaerobes are frequently isolated), and require complex and prolonged management.

Neuropathic Ulcers

Neuropathic ulcers are most often located on the plantar surface and do not have *primary* ischemia as a prominent risk factor. They arise from skin breakdown over a preexisting callus. A crater develops centrally and an indolent infection develops beginning in the superficial skin and soft tissues. If not aggressively treated, it progresses to a more inflammatory process involving the tendons and joints and may eventually develop into septic arthritis and osteomyelitis.

Abscesses of the Deep Plantar Space

Abscesses of the deep plantar space can involve any or all of the deep compartments: the medial, central, and lateral compartments. The medial compartment contains the muscles associated with the big toe: the abductor hallucis, hallucis brevis, and flexor hallucis longus. The central compartment contains the flexor digitorum brevis, the quadratus plantae, peroneus longus, tibialis posterior, lumbricalis interossei, and adductor hallucis. The lateral compartment contains the muscles associated with the fifth toe: abductor digiti quinti, flexor digiti quinti brevi, and adductors to the fifth toe. Infections of these deep compartments (primarily the central compartment) account for 25% of all above the knee (AKA) and below the knee (BKA) amputations in diabetics.[5]

Necrotizing Infections

Necrotizing infections occur mostly in the loose tissues of the dorsum of the foot. The foot may become erythematous and swollen—a simple cellulitis. This situation is often complicated by systemic symptoms of fever, hyperglycemia, and ketoacidosis. Simple cellulitis may progress rapidly to a necrotizing infection if there is local vascular insufficiency and inadequate collateral circulation.[2, 5]

COMPLICATIONS OF FOOT INFECTIONS IN DIABETICS

Diabetics, as previously mentioned, have more severe infections than the general population. These severe infections induce disturbances of nitrogen balance which lead to increased gluconeogenesis, immobilization of fatty acids, hyperglycemia, and acidosis.[5]

Small vessels in the area adjacent to infected tissue commonly become occluded by thrombus. In a normal foot, this is limited to the margins of the infection, but in the diabetic the occlusive process becomes exaggerated, leading to increased areas of necrosis. Multiple, partial, and complete

occlusions can lead to almost complete cessation of blood flow and resultant tissue hypoxia. Tissue hypoxia increases the risk of infection and delays wound healing.[4, 5, 10, 17, 18]

WOUND HEALING

For successful wound healing to occur, a complex series of local and systemic factors must take place. It involves recognition of injury, which then stimulates the accumulation of clotting factors and circulating cells—platelets, polymorphonuclear leukocytes (PMNs), and macrophages. Then, the next phases of healing are initiated. These cells remove dead and dying tissue and foreign bodies. The cells also release growth factors that act locally and systemically to attract other inflammatory cells and initiate collagen repair. There must also be adequate circulation to bring oxygen, nutrients, and the necessary inflammatory cells, as well as to remove toxic wastes.[4] The fibroblast is also integral in wound healing.

Platelets are a source of thromboplastin (TA_2), prostaglandin (PG), and platelet-derived growth factor (PDGF). TA_2, PG, and PDGF stimulate angiogenesis, fibroblast growth, and collagen synthesis. TA_2 is a powerful vasoconstrictor (reduces wound edema) and PG mediates pain and vascular permeability. Fibroblasts synthesize collagen—an important part of tissue restoration and continuity. PMNs participate in wound healing by ingesting and killing bacteria. Macrophages produce chemotactic, angiogenic, mitogenic, and collagen stimulating factors.[4, 25, 26]

EFFECTS OF DIABETES ON WOUND HEALING

As has been shown in animal studies, there is decreased wound strength and wound collagen in diabetics.[19, 42] At about

8 hours after injury, there is a decrease in wound capillaries, fibroblasts, polymorphonuclear leukocytes, and collagen, and an increase in edema in subjects with diabetes.[4, 22, 23, 42] Platelets demonstrate an increase in aggregation in diabetes, inhibiting their action. PGDF enhances healing, therefore any lack or malfunction would have an adverse effect on healing.[4, 24] Studies of fibroblast activity in diabetics have not consistently been demonstrated,[28] but a high molecular substance found in the serum of diabetic animals does inhibit collagen formation in culture.[29] This may be the cause of apparent decreased wound collagen noted in diabetics. In diabetics, PMNs have been found to demonstrate decreased phagocytosis and killing,[33] decreased chemotaxis,[30] decreased adhesiveness,[31] and a decreased respiratory burst.[32] These dysfunctions are most important when there is infection present. Most studies involving macrophage function are inconclusive, but there is a suggestion of decreased effectiveness.[25, 26] All these effects are primarily due to a lack of insulin.

THE EFFECT OF OXYGEN ON WOUND HEALING AND INFECTION

Any injury, inflammation, or repair requires an appropriate increase in metabolic activity. This metabolic response includes increased oxygen demand. Because most injuries to the tissues also involve the microcirculation, and oxygen delivery is limited by diffusion distances, these increased demands are placed in environments that are significantly hypoxic.[6] Low oxygen concentration leads to decreased rates of fibroblast and epithelial cell reproduction as well as collagen synthesis.[6, 7, 17, 43–45]

Phagocytic leukocytes (PMNs), are the first and most important line of defense against tissue infection. Normally, PMNs move to the site of injury and infection and ingest and kill bacteria.[11, 17] Bacterial killing involve two phases—degranulation and oxidative. The oxidative phase depends on the availability of molecular oxygen, which is converted to high energy radicals such as superoxides, hydroxyls, and peroxides for bacterial killing. Loss of killing ability occurs at tissue oxygen concentrations below 30 mm Hg.[11] High oxygen concentrations (such as those that exist under hyperbaric conditions) can act as an antibiotic by impairing anaerobic bacterial metabolism. These conditions also act synergistically with some antibiotics (sulfonamides, aminoglycosides), resulting in a five- to tenfold increase in the antibiotics' activity level.

Delivery of oxygen to tissues is limited by diffusion distances; therefore, increasing such delivery is vital in wound healing. Oxygen delivery can be increased by improving circulation and/or increasing the tissue oxygen concentration (TOC). TOC can be increased by breathing 100% oxygen with the use of a mask. This increase, however, is offset by the increased work of breathing and venous pooling,[13] which limits practical clinical application. Hyperbaric oxygen therapy (HBOT) is the ideal way to increase tissue oxygen concentration. HBOT involves placing the patient into a one-person chamber (monoplace, Fig 19–1), which is pressurized with 100% oxygen, or into a multiplace chamber, which is pressurized with air while the patient breathes 100% oxygen by using a head tent or tightly fitting mask. The optimal TOC for wound healing is 50 to 100 mm Hg.[10] HBOT at 2 to 2.5 absolute atmospheres (ATA) for 1 to 2 hours on a daily basis has been proven to produce such TOCs.[10] This elevation of TOC is also found for several hours after treatment is completed. This length and frequency of treatment corresponds to the

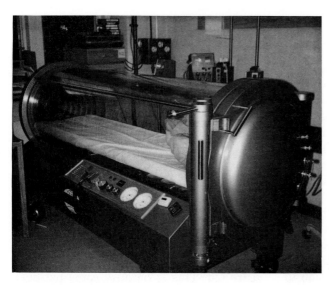

FIG 19–1.
Sechrist monoplace hyperbaric chamber treats a single patient at a time.

cell cycle of fibroblasts (~24 hours) and cell mitosis (1 hour).[1, 21, 27, 33–36] HBOT is not a primary treatment option but serves as an important adjuvant to appropriate wound debridement, dressing changes, and antibiotic therapy.[44]

EFFECTS OF HYPERBARIC OXYGEN THERAPY

Hyperbaric oxygen therapy increases tissue oxygen delivery; there are also other effects that positively affect wound healing. The primary effects of HBOT include a tenfold increase in dissolved oxygen, which increases the diffusion distance up to three times the normal distance. Hyperbaric oxygen conditions also cause some drying of tissues that may be beneficial in actively draining wounds. Secondary effects include vasoconstriction (reduced edema formation), neovascularization, increased fibroblast growth, increased WBC oxidative killing, synergism of antibiotics, increased osteoclastic activity (necessary for bone remodeling and growth), and increased red cell deformity (allows improved flow in restricted spaces).[6, 37, 38]

COMPLICATIONS OF HYPERBARIC OXYGEN THERAPY

Barotrauma is the most common side effect of HBOT. Barotrauma is damage to tissues from contraction or expansion of enclosed spaces. The ears, sinuses, lungs, and dental caries are the most commonly involved. Most of these can be prevented by adequate patient education and premedication.

Confinement anxiety, especially with monoplace chambers, is not uncommon. This is usually averted or managed with tranquilizers, diversions (TV), and relaxation techniques. Oxygen toxicity seizures are a commonly voiced concern. Most reported cases occur above 3 ATA and in patients with uncorrected acidosis, vitamin E deficiency, and poorly controlled seizure disorders. Drugs that lower the seizure threshold also increase the risk.

There have also been some reported cases of increased myopia (especially in diabetics). The mechanism is uncertain but is usually reversible within days of the completion of a course of treatment.[36, 39]

PATIENT SELECTION AND TREATMENT

A hyperbaric medicine consultation can be carried out at the bed side of hospitalized patients or as an outpatient in the office or hyperbaric unit. Apprehension is often high because this modality may be unfamiliar; therefore, patient education emphasizing that HBOT enables patients to safely breathe high concentrations of oxygen is warranted.[20]

A detailed medical history must be obtained to determine if the patient has a condition in which hyperbaric oxygen therapy is effective and to find any conditions that may be a contraindication to its use. A chest radiograph and any available pulmonary function tests should be reviewed by the consulting hyperbaric physician. The pulmonary status is of particular importance because the act of compression and decompression have a direct effect on the lungs. Patients who have an unvented pneumothorax, for example, or who have a significant risk of developing one (e.g., chronic obstructive pulmonary disease or asthma) might develop a tension pneumothorax on decompression. This is a condition with life-threatening potential. These patients should have a pulmonary medicine consultation before hyperbaric treatment begins.[20]

A thorough cardiac history and physical are also necessary. Patients who have borderline congestive heart failure may develop frank pulmonary edema from stress, heat, or confinement anxiety in the chamber.[20]

Air equilibration of the ears and sinuses is important for patient comfort. Most patients can easily be taught to clear their ears, but if they are unable to do so, nasal or oral decongestants may be necessary. Obstacles to patients clearing their ears include inability to learn, eustachian tube abnormalities, allergic rhinitis, or nasal polyps. A few of these patients may need myringotomy to treat middle ear pressure build-up.

A baseline ophthalmology examination is recommended for any patient with diabetes, with a history of head and neck radiation, with a history of cataracts, who is on chronic steroid therapy, or is over 50 years old. This is because some patients who undergo prolonged hyperbaric oxygen treatment develop a reversible myopia.

Once these criteria have been met, the decision to refer a patient for HBOT should begin with a peripheral vascular evaluation.[18] Palpation and Doppler evaluation of pedal pulses, ankle-brachial pressure determination, and angiography may be needed to evaluate the level of vascular occlusion.[45] When results indicate severe large vessel occlusion that is amenable to revascularization, it should be carried out primarily. If results of testing are borderline or questionable, transcutaneous tissue oxygen measurements (TCO_2) (Fig 19–2) over the skin adjacent to the wound site can help determine if increased oxygen delivery to the foot can be accomplished.[18] TCO_2 values less than 30 mm Hg usually heal poorly even under hyperbaric conditions, although there are

FIG 19–2.
Transcutaneous oxygen monitor (Radiometer, model TCM3).

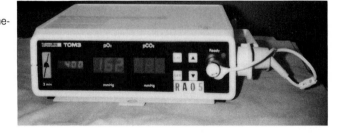

some anecdotal reports of response to HBOT in recalcitrant cases.

Diabetics who have wounds that do not respond to standard treatments or with severe infections should be referred to a physician or specialist trained and experienced in the administration of HBOT. Before treatment is begun, the consulting physician must determine, through medical history, physical, and ancillary evaluation, if the patient's condition is amenable to HBOT and if there are any coexisting conditions that may represent contraindications to therapy.

Once the patient has been deemed a suitable candidate for hyperbaric oxygen therapy, written consent is obtained. For each dive the patient is required to have no flammable objects on the body. Therefore, all flammable cosmetic products (e.g., shampoo, hairspray, perfume) and clothing must be removed before treatment begins. The patient is required to wear all-cotton gowns during each dive. Treatment schedules involve hyperbaric oxygen at 2.0 to 2.5 ATA of pressure for 60 to 120 minutes per treatment. Relatively simple wounds can be healed completely with once-a-day treatments, and on average, require 6 to 8 weeks of therapy. Complicated wounds may require longer treatment schedules, and in the case of severe life-threatening wounds, twice-a-day treatments may be necessary. The usual maximum number of treatments for one wound problem is 100, or approximately 17 weeks. After this length of time, the costs of HBOT may outweigh its benefits, and the risks of toxic side effects increase. This does not, however, prevent reinstitution of hyperbaric oxygen treatment for new wound problems that occur.

SUMMARY

Diabetes causes many potentially major foot infections. Recovery from these con-

ditions is complicated by hypoxia and other impaired healing responses. If not addressed aggressively, these infections may lead to limb loss, alteration of lifestyle, and early death. Prevention of infection is the best means to prevent these consequences. However, when infection does occur, aggressive wound debridement, dressing changes, and antibiotic therapy are the first line of treatment.

In those cases where severe infections exist (e.g., necrotizing tissue infections), complications develop, or healing is significantly delayed due to wound hypoxia and edema, hyperbaric oxygen therapy is a proven and effective adjuvant to achieve wound healing.

REFERENCES

1. Blair VP III, Drury DA, Levin ME: Diabetic foot care. In Bergman M, Sicard GA, editors: *Surgical management of the diabetic patient,* New York, 1991, Raven Press.
2. Butler B, Jules KT, Trepal MJ: Diabetic foot management. In Bergman, Sicard, editors: *Surgical management of the diabetic patient,* New York, 1991, Raven Press.
3. Sapico FL, Bessman AN: Diabetic foot infections. In Frykberg, editor: *The high risk foot in diabetes,* New York, 1991, Churchill Livingstone.
4. Goodson WH III. Wound healing in diabetes. In Bergman, Sicard, editors: *Surgical management of the diabetic patient,* New York, 1991, Raven Press.
5. Penn I: The diabetic foot: infections. In Sammarco, editor: *The foot in diabetes,* Philadelphia, 1991, Lea & Febiger.
6. Hunt TK, Niinikoski J, Zegerfeldt B: Role of oxygen in repair processes, *Acta Chir Scand* 138:109–110, 1972.
7. Niinikoski J: Oxygen and wound healing, *Clin Plast Surg* 3:361–374, 1977.
8. Jain KK: The history of hyperbaric medicine. In *Textbook of hyperbaric medicine,* Lewiston, NY, 1990, Hogrefe and Huber.

9. Jain KK: Physical, physiological, and biochemical aspects of hyperbaric oxygenation. In *Textbook of hyperbaric medicine,* Lewiston, NY, 1990, Hogrefe and Huber.

10. Jain KK: Hyperbaric oxygen therapy in wound healing. In *Textbook of hyperbaric medicine,* Lewiston, NY, 1990, Hogrefe and Huber.

11. Jain KK: Hyperbaric oxygen therapy in infections. In *Textbook of hyperbaric medicine,* Lewiston, NY, 1990, Hogrefe and Huber.

12. Gorman DF: Oxygen therapy in the diabetic foot. In Frykberg RG, editor: *The high risk foot in diabetes,* New York, 1991, Churchill Livingstone.

13. Davis JC: The use of adjuvant hyperbaric oxygen therapy in treatment of the diabetic foot, *Clin Podiatr Med Surg* 2:429–437, 1987.

14. Sheffield PJ: Tissue oxygen measurements. In Davis JC, Hunt TK, editors: *Problem wounds—the role of oxygen,* New York, 1988, Elsevier.

15. Grim PS et al: Hyperbaric oxygen therapy, *JAMA* 263:2216–2220, 1990.

16. Preface. In Davis JC, Hunt TK, editors: *Problem wounds—the role of oxygen,* New York, 1988, Elsevier.

17. Rabkin JM, Hunt TK: Infection and oxygen. In Davis JC, Hunt TK, editors: *Problem wounds—the role of oxygen,* New York, 1988, Elsevier.

18. Davis JC, Buckley CJ, Barr P-O: Compromised soft tissue wounds: Correction of wound hypoxia. In Davis JC, Hunt TK, editors: *Problem wounds—the role of oxygen,* New York, 1988, Elsevier.

19. Davis JC: Local management of problem wounds. In Davis JC, Hunt TK, editors: *Problem wounds—the role of oxygen,* New York, 1988, Elsevier.

20. Davis JC, Dunn JM, Heimbach RO: Hyperbaric medicine: patient selection, treatment procedures and side-effects. In Davis JC, Hunt TK, editors: *Problem wounds—the role of oxygen,* New York, 1988, Elsevier.

21. Cohn GH: Hyperbaric oxygen therapy, *Postgrad Med* 79;2:89–92, 1986.

22. Mustard JF, Packham MA: Platelets and diabetes mellitus, *N Engl J Med* 311:665–667, 1984.

23. Trovati M et al: Insulin directly reduces platelet sensitivity to aggregating agents. Studies in vitro and in vivo, *Diabetes* 37:469–473, 1988.

24. Grotenhorst GR et al: Stimulation of granulation tissue formation by platelet-derived growth factor in normal and diabetic rats, *J Clin Invest* 76:2323–2329, 1985.

25. Jones CA, Seifert MF, Dixit PK: Macrophage migration inhibition in experimental diabetes, *Proc Soc Exp Biol Med* 29:298–304, 1980.

26. van Rees EP, Voorbij HAM, Dijkstra CD: Neonatal development of lymphoid organs and specific immune responses *in situ* in diabetes-prone BB rats, *Immunology* 65:880–883, 1988.

27. Hunt TK, Pai MP: The effect of varying ambient oxygen tensions on wound metabolism and collagen syntheses, *Surg Gynecol Obst* 135:561–567, 1972.

28. Rowe DW et al: Abnormalities in proliferation and protein synthesis in skin fibroblast cultures from patients with diabetes mellitus, *Diabetes* 26:284–290, 1977.

29. Spanheimer RG: Direct inhibition of collagen production *in vitro* by diabetic rat serum, *Metabolism* 37:479–485, 1988.

30. Mowatt AG, Baum J: Chemotaxis of polymorphonuclear leukocytes from patients with diabetes mellitus, *N Engl J Med* 284:621–627, 1971.

31. Bagdade JD, Walters E: Impaired granulocyte adherence in mildly diabetic patients. Effects of their nondiabetic first-degree relatives, *Diabetes* 29:309–311, 1980.

32. Nielson CP, Hindson DA: Inhibition of polymorphonuclear leukocyte respiratory burst by elevated glucose concentrations in vitro, *Diabetes* 38:1031–1035, 1989.

33. Niinikoski J, Hunt TK, Zegerfeldt B: Oxygen supply in healing tissue, *Am J Surg* 123:247–252, 1972.

34. Remensnyder JP, Majno G: Oxygen gradients in healing wounds, *Am J Pathol* 52:301–308, 1968.

35. Silvers IA: Local and systemic factors which affect the proliferation of fibroblasts. In Kulonen E, Pikkarainen J, editors: *The biology of fibroblast,* New York, 1973, Academic Press.

36. Sheffield PJ, Dunn JM: Continuous monitoring of tissue oxygen tension during hyperbaric oxygen therapy. In Smith G, editor: *Proceedings of the 6th international congress on hyperbaric medicine,* Aberdeen, Scotland, 1977, Aberdeen Press.

37. Strauss MB et al: *Hyperbaric oxygen therapy in emergency medicine,* 1990.

38. Strauss MB: Mechanisms of HBO. In *Orientation course in hyperbaric medicine—Manual,* Long Beach Memorial Hospital, 1990, Long Beach, CA.

39. Lyne AJ: Ocular effects of hyperbaric oxygen, *Trans Ophthal Soc UK* 42:593–599, 1977.

40. Goodson WH III, Hunt TK: Studies of wound healing in experimental diabetes mellitus, *J Surg Res* 22:221–227, 1977.

41. Lundgren C, Sandberg N: Influence of hyperbaric oxygen on the tensile strength of healing skin wounds. In Ledingham IM, editor: *Hyperbaric oxygenation. Proceedings of the Second International Congress,* London, 1965, Livingstone.

42. Lundgren C, Zederfeldt B: Influence of low oxygen pressure on wound healing. *Acta Chir Scand* 135:55, 1969.

43. Uitto J, Prockop DJ: Synthesis and secretion of underhydroxylated procollagen at various temperatures by cells subject to temporary anoxia, *Biochem Biophys Res Comm* 60:414, 1974.

44. Undersea and Hyperbaric Medical Society: Enhancement of healing in selected problem wounds. In *Hyperbaric oxygen therapy: A committee report,* Bethesda, Maryland, 1989.

45. Kindwall EP, Goldmann RW: *Hyperbaric medicine procedures,* Milwaukee, 1984, St Luke's Hospital.

20 Growth Factors and Repair of Acute and Chronic Wounds

David R. Knighton, M.D.

Vance D. Fiegel, B.S.

The process of normal wound healing results when an interplay between the various cell types found in the wound space and their capacity to both produce and respond to an array of growth factors occurs in a timely fashion. These growth factors affect cellular migration, proliferation, extracellular matrix production, enzyme activity, and the production of additional growth factors. The repair process is largely regulated by locally acting growth factors.

The objective of this chapter is to briefly review the process of wound repair, with emphasis on the roles played by locally acting growth factors. The clinical usefulness of growth factors requires that they be part of an overall wound care program. The details of such a program are discussed in this chapter.

MORPHOLOGY OF NORMAL WOUND REPAIR

Cutaneous wounds can be divided into three major categories: (1) partial thickness, (2) full thickness, and (3) complex wounds (Fig 20–1).[1] A partial thickness wound describes a defect that removes the most superficial part of the skin, the epidermis, leaving the lower layers largely intact. This is accomplished by migration of keratinocytes from the edge of the wound and from the hair follicles and sweat glands.[2]

In full thickness wounds, both the epidermis and dermis are lost, uncovering the subcutaneous tissue, fascia, or muscle. To repair this type of wound, vascularized connective tissue grows from the wound edge.[3, 4] Fibroblasts begin to migrate into the wound space from connective tissue at the wound edge within 24 hours. As they move, fibroblasts produce matrix molecules (collagen and glycosaminoglycans), which form an extracellular matrix. Capillary buds are seen in the perfused microcirculation at the wound edge by 48 hours after wounding. These buds grow into the wound space and provide a new capillary network for the wound connective tissue.

Fibroblast proliferation and migration and capillary growth continue as a unit until the wound space is completely filled with new tissue. The newly formed granulation tissue is then covered with epithelium. Full thickness wounds also close by contraction, which occurs through cellular forces pulling the edges of the wound toward its center.

A complex wound penetrates to tendons, ligaments, bones, and internal organs. These wounds also heal by granulation tissue formation and epithelization, but when tendons and ligaments are injured and then reapproximated surgically, they tend to fuse into the mass of granulation tissue which closes the remainder of the wound.[4]

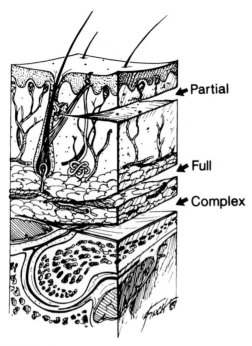

FIG 20–1.
Cross-sectional diagram of the dermis and underlying connective tissue indicating the depth at which partial, full, and complex wounds occur. (From Knighton DR, Fiegel VD, Doucette MM: *Chronic wound care: a clinical source book for healthcare professionals,* King of Prussia, PA, 1990, Health Management Publications, Inc. Used by permission.)

GROWTH FACTORS AND REPAIR

The cellular activities associated with wound repair are regulated by locally acting growth factors (Fig 20–2). These biomolecules, usually small polypeptides, stimulate cell proliferation, movement, and biosynthetic activity. They can act as paracrine (produced by one cell type to act on another in the local area) or autocrine (produced by a cell acting on itself) factors. This is a rapidly changing field, and new growth factors with potential roles in wound repair are continually being isolated and characterized.

Locally acting growth factors can be grouped into three large categories: (1) mitogens, which signal cells to proliferate; (2) chemoattractants, which stimulate cellular migration; and (3) transforming growth factors, which alter the phenotypic state of the cell.

Mitogens can be divided into competence and progression factors. For cells to divide, they must be stimulated to progress from the resting state to a state of readiness to replicate deoxyribonucleic acid (DNA) and divide (Fig 20–3). Competence factors stimulate cells to make this transformation. Progression through the division cycle requires the presence of progression factors.[5] Platelet derived growth factor (PDGF) and epidermal growth factor (EGF) are examples of competence factors. Known progression factors include insulin-like growth factor (IGF-1) and the other somatomedins.

Chemoattractants can be divided into chemotactic factors and chemokinetic factors. Chemotactic factors work through cell surface receptors which, on reaching one side of a cell in higher concentrations than the other, cause the target cell to move in a given direction. Examples of chemotactic factors are C5a, a chemoattractant for neutrophils, and PDGF, a chemoattractant for fibroblasts.[6, 7] Chemokinetic factors increase the rate of cell migration, but not in a directional manner.[8] An example of chemokinesis is the effect of albumin on neutrophil migration.[9] Many growth factors act as both mitogens and chemoattractants, depending on concentration and target cell.

The most studied transforming growth factor is transforming growth factor β (TGF-β). TGF-β is reported to have a variety of activities, dependent on the cell type affected and the microenvironment in which it is acting.[10] In certain concentrations, it inhibits fibroblast division and stimulates increased production of matrix molecules (collagen and glycosaminoglycans). It also induces the production of PDGF in certain cells. Transforming growth factor α (TGF-α) shares considerable homology with EGF, binds to the same receptor, and evokes many of the same responses as EGF.[11]

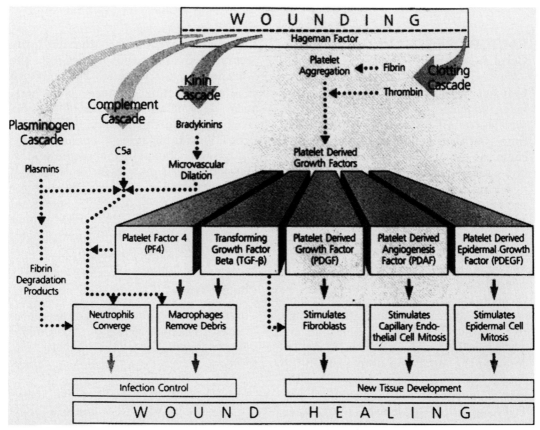

FIG 20–2.
Wounding unleashes a series of events culminating in the accumulation of inflammatory cells and growth factors in the wound. This results in stimulation of cell division leading to new tissue formation and eventual healing of the wound. (From Knighton DR, Fiegel VD, Doucette MM: *Chronic wound care: a clinical source book for healthcare professionals,* King of Prussia, PA, 1990, Health Management Publications, Inc. Used by permission.)

CELL CYCLE

FIG 20–3.
Schematic diagram depicting the cell cycle. In response to PDGF and EGF, cells at resting state (G_0) are stimulated to a state of readiness to replicate DNA and divide (G_1). (From Knighton DR, Fiegel VD: The diabetic foot, ed 5, 1993, St Louis, Mosby–Year Book. Used by permission.)

GROWTH IN SIZE

G_2

DNA REPLICATION

MITOSIS

CELL DEATH

G_1

G_0

FACTORS REGULATING COLLAGEN SYNTHESIS

Collagen production by fibroblasts provides the molecular structure which gives tensile strength to the healing wound. The time course of collagen deposition, biochemical details of collagen production, and interplay between synthesis and lysis in wound repair are all well known. The regulatory mechanisms controlling the rate of collagen production, type of collagen produced, and proportion of collagen in the extracellular matrix are largely unknown. The role of growth factors in the regulation of wound healing collagen synthesis is closely linked to fibroblast biology. Growth factors such as PDGF which regulate fibroblast proliferation and migration affect collagen synthesis by increasing the number of fibroblasts in the wound.[12] Growth factors also affect the rate of collagen synthesis per fibroblast. TGF-β significantly increases the collagen production/cell as well as stimulating an increase in RNA levels for type I, III, and V collagen.[13, 14]

GROWTH FACTORS AND CHRONIC WOUND REPAIR

Chronic nonhealing wound repair is a complex and dynamic process involving the effects of ischemia, infection, repeated trauma or pressure, and/or medications which interfere with the process of normal repair. These processes change over time depending on the therapeutic intervention and the patient's compliance with the intervention. To determine the effect of a particular intervention, such as growth factor administration, on wound repair requires careful monitoring of the state of ischemia, infection, trauma, and the patient's compliance, along with the wound repair endpoints, including infection control, granulation tissue formation, and epithelialization. At present, the most completely studied and used growth factors in chronic foot wounds are the naturally occurring mix of growth factors from the α-granule of the platelet. This mixture of growth factors, protease inhibitors, and matrix molecules is called platelet-derived wound healing formula (PDWHF). PDWHF contains at least five locally acting growth factors from α-granulates: platelet-derived growth factor (PDGF),[15] platelet-derived angiogenesis factor (PDAF),[16] platelet-derived epidermal growth factor (PDEGF),[17] transforming growth factor-beta (TGF-β),[18] and platelet factor 4 (PF4).[15]

Clinical Trials

Three separate clinical trials have documented the effectiveness of this comprehensive approach to the diabetic foot ulcer.

1. Retrospective study of 88 diabetic patients with 124 plantar and metatarsal head ulcers.[19]
2. Prospectively randomized double-blind, placebo-controlled trial of PDWHF where diabetic patients comprised roughly half of the patients.[20]
3. Two limb-salvage studies. One on patients recommended for amputation[21] and a second study where a panel of experts on amputation studied case reviews to determine the severity of the wound and predict whether amputation was necessary.

The retrospective study examined 88 diabetic patients with 124 plantar and metatarsal head ulcers.[19] Their wounds were in existence for an average duration of 30 weeks. Forms of treatment during this time included dressings (72%), soaks (69%), oral antibiotics (52%), debridement (46%), intravenous antibiotics (31%), topical creams (30%), peroxide (28%), and whirlpool (20%). None of the wounds healed with these treatment modalities.

The patients were then admitted to the Outpatient Wound Healing and Limb Salvage Clinic.

On admission to the clinic, the average wound volume was 11,996 cu mm. The average glycosylated hemoglobin was 8.9 (normal is 3.4 to 6.1). Besides neuropathy, 24% of the limbs were ischemic, as evidenced by $TcPO_2$. Limbs with $TcPO_2 < 30$mm Hg were considered ischemic. The average wound grade according to the Wound Care Center (WCC) Wound Grading System was 3, which is a full thickness ulcer that involves tendon, bone, ligament, and joint. Of the ulcers, 26% also had abscess and/or osteomyelitis.

The patients then participated in a comprehensive wound management program. Twenty-four percent of the limbs were revascularized, 75% of the wounds were surgically debrided, and all of the patients (100%) treated the wounds topically with PDWHF for an average of 65 days. The outcome of this treatment protocol was that 115 (93%) of the 124 wounds achieved 100% epithelialization in an average of 7.8 weeks. The wounds were followed for 12 months and there was no breakdown during that time.

Double-Blind, Randomized, Crossover, Placebo-Controlled Trial

To test the independent efficacy of PDWHF, a double-blind, crossover, placebo-controlled trial was performed.[20] A total of 32 patients were randomized into treatment and control groups. All patients received standard wound care as previously described. The placebo was the platelet buffer combined with microcrystalline collagen without platelet α-granule release products. Patients randomized to the control group had blood drawn and the PDWHF stored for use after the crossover period. Both groups were treated for 8 weeks and then the placebo patients were crossed over to the positive arm of the study, treatment with PDWHF.

When the patient populations in each group were analyzed and wounds graded using the wound grading system, the two groups were matched except for the area measurement. Patients randomized to the control group had a higher area measure than controls due to two patients with very large wounds.

A total of 13 patients finished the positive arm and 11 patients finished the control arm. In the positive arm, 17 out of 21 total wounds achieved 100% epithelization in an average of 8.6 weeks. In the placebo group of 11 patients, 2 out of 13 wounds (15%) healed during the initial 8 weeks of placebo treatment, and 11 of 13 wounds (85%) failed to heal in 8 weeks and were crossed over to the positive group. After crossover, all 11 nonhealed wounds achieved 100% epithelization in an average of 7.1 weeks. When analyzed statistically, there is a high degree ($p \leq = .0002$) of significance between the two groups.

Limb Salvage Study

Many of the patients referred to the clinic have limbs at risk of amputation due to ischemic nonhealing wounds. We retrospectively studied 24 of these patients to determine if treatment in the clinic under defined protocols with the use of PDWHF resulted in limb salvage.[21]

Patients were studied if they had ischemic nonhealing extremity ulcers that required amputation according to their referring physician. Recommended amputations at the transmetatarsal level (TMA) or higher were included. Minor amputations of the toes were not included. Success was defined as 100% epithelialization of the wound, progressive epithelial maturation, and the ability to tolerate limited weight-bearing.

The patients ranged in age from 28 to 80 years, with 9 patients (38%) 65 years or older. The primary diagnosis was diabetic mellitus in 21 patients (88%), atherosclerotic peripheral vascular disease in

2 patients (8%), and rheumatoid arthritis in 1 patient (4%). All patients over the age of 65 had diabetes mellitus.

Eleven patients had a total of 15 prior amputations, 7 patients had a total of 10 prior vascular procedures, and 6 of these 7 patients had vascular reconstructions in the limb that was now threatened.

The referring physician recommended below-the-knee amputation (BKA) in 18 patients, TMA in 5 patients, and a ray amputation in 1 patient (this patient was included because he needed a BKA on our evaluation).

The patients had a total of 26 ulcers. The mean duration of conventional unsuccessful therapy was 26 weeks, with a range of 3 to 43 weeks.

Regarding other factors, 46% (11 of 24) of the patients smoked and 21% (5 of 24) were on steroids (4 for renal transplantation and 1 for severe rheumatoid arthritis).

Arteriograms were performed in 13 of 24 patients (54%), 11 of 24 patients (45%) underwent vascular reconstruction, and 20 of 24 patients (83%) had operative wound debridement before beginning PDWHF therapy.

The patients were followed for an average of 15 months, with a range of 7 to 29 months. Follow-up data were obtained from the patients' last clinic visit or phone conversation.

Of the 24 patients, 4 (17%) required amputation. Two patients' wounds did not heal. One required an above-the-knee amputation (AKA), the other a BKA. The other two patients' wounds were healing. One had a clotted vascular bypass resulting in amputation, and the other developed necrotizing soft tissue infection from walking on a plantar surface ulcer; both required BKA.

In all, 19 of 24 patients (79%) healed 21 of 26 wounds. Two patients' wounds recurred after healing; one of these patients' wounds healed a second time by the end of the study. Two patients were still

healing at the end of the study, leaving a total of 18 of 24 patients (75%) healed with 20 to 26 wounds (77%) healed. Most important, 17 of 18 patients who healed are ambulatory, with one healed patient unable to ambulate because of a previous stroke. The 2 patients who were still healing are on restricted ambulation. Of the 4 amputees, 2 ambulate on prostheses and 2 are nonambulatory.

A second study on amputation prevention involved an independent review panel composed of an orthopedic surgeon, a vascular surgeon, and an endocrinologist. They conducted a blinded retrospective review of 71 diabetic patients with a total of 124 wounds on 81 limbs. Based on their expertise, the review panel classified the wounds' severity and identified the limbs' risk for amputation. Their judgement was compared to the actual outcome.

The review panel predicted 65 (80%) of the limbs would be salvaged and 16 (20%) would be amputated. The actual outcome was that 75 (93%) of the limbs were salvaged and 6 (7%) were amputated ($p < 0.005$). This study demonstrated that the combination of aggressive revascularization and debridement, infection control, and unweighting of plantar ulcers, along with the use of PDWHF, were effective in amputation prevention.

CONCLUSION

Growth factors play a pivotal role in normal wound repair. Currently available data suggest that their role in the care of diabetic ulcers will be to complement aggressive wound care, which includes wound excision, revascularization, infection control, and protection.

Acknowledgment

The authors thank Ms. Joyce Reha for the preparation and editing of this manuscript.

REFERENCES

1. Maibach HI, Rovee DT: In *Epidermal wound healing,* St Louis, 1972, Mosby–Year Book.
2. Pang SC, Daniels WH, Buck RC: Epidermal migration during the healing of suction blisters in rat skin: a scanning and transmission electron microscopic study, *Am J Anat* 153:177–191, 1978.
3. Clark RAF: Cutaneous tissue repair: basic biologic considerations, *J Am Acad Dermatol* 13:701–725, 1985.
4. Hunt TK: In *Wound healing and wound infection: theory and surgical practice,* New York, 1980, Appleton-Century-Crofts.
5. Deuel TF: Polypeptide growth factors: roles in normal and abnormal cell growth, *Ann Rev Cell Biol* 3:443–492, 1987
6. Snyderman R, Phillips J, Mergenhagen SE: Polymorphonuclear leukocyte chemotactic activity in rabbit serum and guinea pig serum treated with immune complexes: evidence for C5a as the major chemotactic factor, *Infect Immunol* 1:521–525, 1970.
7. Seppa H et al: Platelet-derived growth factor is chemotactic for fibroblasts, *J Cell Biol* 92:584–588, 1982.
8. Wilkinson PC: Chemotaxis and chemokinesis: confusion about definitions, *J Immunol Methods* 110:143–144, 1988.
9. Wilkinson PC, Allan RB: Assay systems for measuring leukocyte locomotion: an overview. In Gallin JI, Quie PG, editors: *Leukocyte chemotaxis: methods, physiology and clinical implications,* New York, 1978, Raven Press.
10. Sporn MB et al: Some recent advances in the chemistry and biology of transforming growth factor-beta, *J Cell Biol* 105:1039–1045, 1987.
11. Massague J: Epidermal growth factor-like transforming growth factor: isolation, chemical characterization, and potentiation by other transforming factors from feline sarcoma virus transformed rat cells, *J Biol Chem* 258:13606–13620, 1983.
12. Grotendorst GR et al: Stimulation of granulation tissue formation by platelet-derived growth factor in normal and diabetic rats, *J Clin Invest* 76:2323–2329, 1985.
13. Ignotz R, Massague J: Transforming growth factor-β stimulates the expression of fibronectin and collagen and their incorporation into the extracellular matrix, *J Biol Chem* 261:4337–4345, 1986.
14. Ignotz R, Endo T, Massague J: Regulation of fibronectin and type I collagen mRNA levels by transforming growth factor β, *J Biol Chem* 262:6443–6446, 1987.
15. Kaplan KL et al: Platelet alpha-granule proteins: studies on release and subcellular localization, *Blood* 53:604–618, 1979.
16. Michaeli D, Hunt TK, Knighton DR: The role of platelets in wound healing: demonstration of angiogenic activity. In Hunt TK, Heppenstall RB, Pines E, Rouee D, editors: *Soft and hard tissue repair: biological and clinical aspects,* New York, 1984, Praeger.
17. Oka Y, Orth DN: Human plasma epidermal growth factor/beta-urogastrone is associated with blood platelets, *J Clin Invest* 72:249–259, 1983.
18. Assoian RK, Sporn MB: Type-beta transforming growth factor in human platelets: release during platelet degranulation and action on vascular smooth muscle cells, *J Cell Biol* 102:1217–1223, 1986.
19. Fylling CP, Knighton DR, Gordinier R: The use of a comprehensive wound care protocol including topical growth factor therapy in treatment of diabetic plantar ulcers. The 13th International Diabetes Federation Congress Satellite Symposium on Diabetic Neuropathy, Singapore, November 16-18, 1988.
20. Knighton DR et al: Stimulation of repair in chronic nonhealing cutaneous ulcers: prospectively randomized blinded trial using platelet-derived wound healing formula, *Surg Gynecol Obstet* 170:56–60, 1990.
21. Knighton DR et al: Amputation prevention in an independently reviewed at-risk population using a comprehensive protocol and platelet-derived wound healing formula, *Am J Surg* 160(5):466–471, 1990.

21 _____ Overview of Wound Care Management

Richard M. Jay, D.P.M.

Stephen D. Lasday, D.P.M.

Karen K. Charland, M.S.N., R.N.

At some time in their careers, all primary care, family practice, and podiatric physicians will encounter diabetic patients. The diabetic patient presenting to the physician brings with him or her a very involved group of conditions that lead to breakdown of the skin and deeper tissues. Neuropathy, in combination with angiopathy, gives the treating clinician a significant challenge in attempting to heal wounds of the diabetic foot. In addition, the nephropathy that has undoubtedly occurred results in the accumulation of metabolic waste and toxins in the circulation and skin, further hindering the process by which wounds heal.[1]

The neuropathy is perhaps the most dangerous complication that will occur because it cuts off the primary communication between the lower extremity and the central nervous system. The patients get no pain signals from the insensate foot, and they go through an incredible amount of denial regarding the impending seriousness of their condition. This denial should be considered another complication of diabetes because it is a very real entity that the treating physician must take into account when treating this category of patient.

These wounds are difficult to treat because even when properly managed, these wounds may not heal as well as expected. And when they do, it is often temporary if not properly maintained. Ulceration in a nearby location can be a common frustration to both patient and physician. The care of the diabetic is best managed by a team of experts familiar with long term patterns of ulceration and wound healing as it occurs in the diabetic patient. This chapter will attempt to provide an orderly approach to the identification of susceptible patients, prevention, and treatment from the point of view of a team approach.

ASSESSMENT

The etiology of the presenting wound must first be assessed so that appropriate management may be instituted. There are many conditions that will produce both painful and neuropathic ulcers, and to make matters more difficult, they often present in combination. Ulcers resulting from venous stasis are common, and they often occur in diabetics and in the obese. Venous wounds are approached from the standpoint of compression, using inflation boots to sequentially move the edema back into the circulation from the extracellular space. Patients with peripheral arterial vascular disease do not always have painful ulcers, as is classically described. Nonetheless, whether painful or anesthetic, arterial ulcers must first have the arterial tree restored before local treatment can be truly be effective.[2] Neuropathy can be seen in association with dry and wet gangrene. Mal perforans ulcers should not be assumed to be the result of long-standing diabetes. Alcoholism, especially in the urban population, is also a frequent cause of distal neuropathy. Trauma, such as spinal cord injury, can also result in total or partial loss of sensation. Other etiologies such as collagen vascular disease or burns should not be ruled out. For example, a patient presented to our institution with a gangrenous right great toe. He related no significant medical history. He did mention that he was seen by a podiatrist for removal of an infected ingrown toenail about 2 weeks previous to coming to our emergency room. Having no clinically evident peripheral vascular disease aside from his localized well demarcated gangrene, the first assumption made was that the other podiatrist had used epinephrine in the local anesthetic. On physical exam, however, a discoid facial rash and alopecia led us to suspect lupus, with a vascular manifestation in the foot. Antinuclear antibody testing confirmed our diagnosis. This illustrates the need to be aware of underlying disease that can manifest itself in ways that allow wounds to form and become chronic in nature.

HISTORY AND PHYSICAL

At our wound center, a thorough history and physical (H & P) are performed on every patient by a team of physicians and nurses specializing in wound care. The object is to use as many resources as possible to understand a patient's past medical history. In addition, the wound is evaluated and measured in length, width, and depth, and wound deficit volume is calculated. The patients all fill out a questionnaire in which they list their medical history, specific wound history, and previous treatments they may have had to heal the wound. A list of allergies and medications is also supplied by the patient. Social history is an important factor as well. Nicotine and alcohol history are commonly obtained in a routine history and physical, but we always include the patient's caffeine use history as well. Caffeine isn't always considered a social drug, but its effect on wound healing in the vascularly compromised patient can be very deleterious.

The patient's height, weight, and appetite are included in our interview, as their daily habits are something that can be altered through education. The need for adequate patient education cannot be stressed enough. As health care givers, we can only see the patient for a limited amount of time, even if it is several times a week. Dietary and weight-bearing status are things that fall within the patient's responsibility, and in the long term probably have a greater impact on wound healing than anything else that a medical professional can do.

Past medical history is, of course, something that needs to be included in every H & P. Previous surgical history is equally imperative. It is the rare patient that comes to our center without previous treatment. If this treatment has included vascular reconstruction or surgery specific to the wound, such as plastic or osseous reconstruction, this knowledge is an integral part of the treatment plan. The underlying goal in obtaining the H&P is to determine why an ulcer does not heal. This is aided by obtaining a specific wound history for each wound that the patient has. A wound will not form without inciting factors, and these inciting factors are not always local to the site of injury. For example, many of our patients have chronic obstructive pulmonary disease (COPD), which will yield a local hypoxia at the injury site that will contribute to delayed healing.[3] The patient's cardiac status must also be taken into account, as heart failure leading to venous congestion is a distinct problematic entity that must be taken into account.[4] Nutritional status must be maintained during wound healing as well. Whether a deficit manifests as an intake deficiency, or as a loss in the form of vomiting or diarrhea, the local environment of the wound will suffer. Because the patient is directly responsible for self management between visits, some idea of the mental status should be ascertained. If the patient cannot take care of himself or herself, then a home care nursing service must be involved to do daily (or more frequent) dressing changes and other care.

WOUND HISTORY

The specific history aimed at the wound itself is a crucial aspect of our history. The initial incident that allowed the wound to form can be from a wide variety of causes. Trauma is the obvious cause in an otherwise healthy person. This can be in the form of laceration or bruise, to a foreign body, occult or otherwise. Previous surgery is another common cause of the chronic wound. Wound dehiscence or failed secondary intention closure is an uncommon surgical complication that can be a common source of the chronic wound.[5] In the diabetic or otherwise neuropathic patient, the mal perforans ulcer cannot be overlooked, and it is the most common type of wound that we see.

The previous modalities that were attempted on the patient are important to ascertain why they did or did not work. The use of systemic medications and their allergies should be inquired into, as should those of topical preparations. Protective devices such as orthoses or splints may have been used. If not used properly they can cause iatrogenic wounds to form in other areas. If this has happened in the past, the clinician should be aware of it. The use of total contact casts or regular casts should be part of the interview as

well. Patient's compliance can often be hindered with long-term casting, despite its necessity.

Debridements that have been performed in the past will often result in altered anatomy, especially if osseous reconstruction or resection was involved in the surgery. Postdebridement, any antibiosis that was used, whether prophylactic or therapeutic, should be on record, as well as its effectiveness. If there was a need for therapeutic antibiosis, inquiry should be made regarding the patient's clinical course. Many wound patients are immunocompromised to some extent, and they will not exhibit usual signs of infection or responses to treatment. Culture results and clinical response to treatment should be documented. Specific inquiry should be made into the most recent antibiotic given, its duration, and its effectiveness.

Because these patients are chronic wound formers, many times they recur or break down in other locations, as previously mentioned. Understanding the pattern of skin breakdown, its etiology, and recurrence scenario will assist in creating a treatment plan.[2]

The physical exam should begin with a general overview of the patient. General aspects of the patient can be assessed on entering the treatment room, such as whether the person is pathologically obese and the patient's attention to personal hygiene, which can be a sign of his or her self image and a predictor of the patient's compliance. A patient's current state of ambulation and dependence on devices or wheelchairs can also be assessed.

WOUND EXAM

A quick observation on their mental status should also be a part of the examination for patients with a chronic wound. This need not be a psychiatric overview, but their alertness and ability to remember and follow directions should be known. Their motor function and coordination must be taken into account, as a component of their gait pattern. Just as motor abnormalities will contribute to the formation of a wound and prevent a wound from healing, deficits in sensorium will allow the early stages of wound healing to progress.[6] In the bulk of our patients, this sensory exam, along with a vascular assessment, is the core of the exam. Vibratory sense is the earliest of senses to be lost in the diabetic state. This can be easily assessed with the use of a 128-cycle tuning fork. When the fork is struck and held against bony prominences, the patient should be able to feel the vibration for about 20 seconds. The clinician should start distally, at bony prominences such as the tips of the toes, the apex of hammered digits, prominences of bunion deformities, and head proximally to Lis-Franc's joint, and the malleoli and tibial crest. One should also test areas of ulceration, such as a plantar Charcot breakdown.

Proprioceptive and sharp-dull discrimination are vital to a wound free foot, and these senses are invariably lost in the diabetic or otherwise neuropathic patient. The test for proprioception is one of the simplest tests that can be done without instrumentation, yet it is often performed incorrectly so that the examiner is not getting a true appreciation of the patient's true proprioceptive sense. The examiner should place his or her thumb and forefinger on the medial and lateral aspect of the hallux. After taking the digit through a gentle range of motion, the examiner should ask the patient the location of the digit in space (up or down) while the patient's eyes are closed. This test is too often performed without taking care to place the examiner's hand properly. If the examiner's finger and thumb are located in a dorsal and plantar fashion, pressure is induced on the skin with changing forces and direction through the range of motion. As a result, the patient may be

able, for example, to feel the slightly increased pressure of the thumb on the dorsal aspect of the toe and say that the toe is down. Proprioception has not been tested here; the patient uses pressure sense to give an answer, and if the examiner is not aware of this, an inadequate survey of the patient's sensorium will result. Sharp-dull discrimination loss will, of course, allow a patient to step on a pin or nail while thinking it is perhaps just the fold of a sock in his or her shoe. For a description of this technique, see Chapter 2. Extremities should be tested bilaterally at similar levels, as is the case with all of the testing mentioned in this chapter.

Light touch is the primary sense that will allow the patient to sense and prevent areas of impending breakdown. When this is lost, ulceration is inevitable. Therefore, quantifying the pressure sense in a patient's foot is crucial to the exam. The optimal piece of instrumentation to quantify light touch sensation in a pinpoint distribution adequate for awareness of impending breakdown is the Semmes-Weinstein filament. This is a nylon probe that is calibrated so that, when pressed against the patient's skin, it will buckle at 10 grams of linear pressure.[6] This is the amount of pressure necessary for protective sensation. Therefore, if the probe buckles without the patient being able to feel it against the skin, then the patient is at significant risk for the development of neuropathic wounds. This is an effective test for an instrument smaller than a ballpoint pen. It should be noted that the Semmes-Weinstein filament can be obtained from the Hansen's Disease Center in Carville, Louisiana, and should be among the equipment used by all wound care professionals.

GENERAL EXAM

The rest of the physical exam should cover the major regions of the body. A cardiac exam should take notice of signs of congestive failure, such as jugular venous distention, peripheral edema, pallor, or cyanosis. Also, incisions should be looked for in case the patient failed to mention previous surgery in the history portion of the interview. One would want to make sure that the incision healed properly, and that the treating team is aware of the extent to which the lower extremity venous system was sacrificed for cardiac vessel grafting. In addition, general cardiac status and history of arrhythmias should be noted in preparation for surgical reconstruction.

The examination of the lungs should take into account the ability of the respiratory system to supply enough oxygen to the blood, so that the oxygen can be taken to the site of wound repair. Lung sounds such as rales or rhonchi should be noted. In addition, a good pulmonary examiner should take a step back, and see the shape of the chest, whether accessory muscles are being recruited to expand the chest size during breathing, and whether there is peripheral cyanosis. It should be determined as to whether cyanosis is pulmonary or cardiac. As always, the extremity surgeon should consult with appropriate specialists who are familiar with the protocol and practices of the wound healing regimen to assist in discovering the etiology of each wound scenario. In this fashion, the team approach will always benefit the patient.

The exam of the arterial system will help determine the cause of the patient's wound. In addition, knowledge of the patient's gait function will allow any postoperative treatment to be geared to encouraging healing and preventing further breakdown. The examination should take into account the general muscular status of the extremity. In neuropathic patients, there is often a motor component to the neuropathy, which will result in wasting of the intrinsic musculature of the foot. In cases of severe wasting, pedal deformity that promotes wound formation will result. Joint disease will also directly cause

pressure that can lead to a wound if severe or even moderate deformity is present. If the joint disease affects gait function, the disease may also indirectly cause pressure leading to wound formation. Previous surgery should be noted in regard to its effect on gait.

The skin should be examined for character, temperature, texture, and general appearance. Lesions and the actual wound should be noted and measured. Rashes and other abnormalities should be examined with the understanding that in the case of surgical intervention the patient has already demonstrated an inability to heal in some capacity. To plan a surgical incision over abnormal skin would be making the surgeon's task increasingly difficult.

WOUND EVALUATION

Evaluating wound characteristics is an extremely important aspect of wound care treatment, however, it is a process where subjective observations can lead to inconsistencies between evaluators. It then becomes difficult to determine true improvements or regressions within the wound. To lend this process more objectivity and consistency, a standard wound care assessment tool has been developed that is used at each patient visit. The highlights of this method will be reviewed. On the initial visit, wound duration in months and exact wound location, including a diagram, are determined and documented on a wound data summary sheet. The wound is graded according to a six grade scale that incorporates thickness of ulcer, involvement of bone, ligament, or joint, and the extent of infection (Table 21–1).[7]

Each wound is measured at every visit for length, width, depth, and undermining, if present, in millimeters. These measurements, compared to those of the previous visit, yield some information regarding healing. However, it is important to remember that a decrease in size

TABLE 21–1.

Wound Grade

Grade	Thickness of Ulcer	Involvement of Tendon, Bone, Ligament, Joint	Infection, Necrosis, Gangrene
1	Partial-dermis & epidermis	None	Minor or none
2	Full-subcutaneous only	None	Minor or none
3	Full	Yes	Minor or none
4	Full	Yes	Abscess and/or osteomyelitis
5	Full	Yes	
6	Full	Yes	Necrotic tissue in wound Gangrene in wound & in surrounding tissue

alone may not necessarily be a reliable indicator of healing. Other wound characteristics must be assessed. These include presence and extent of epithelialization, granulation tissue quantity, color and texture, presence of fibrin, wound discharge, periwound skin, and any exposed bone or tendon. Additional factors that are evaluated include the presence of necrotic tissue, periwound erythema, or edema.[8]

Wound maturity and healing are measured by the percentage of epithelial tissue coverage. A functional assessment scale defines the varying degrees of wound maturity. For example, a wound with a functional assessment score of 1 is defined as less than 100% epithelialized, has wound drainage, and requires a dressing. A functional assessment level of 4 reflects fully cornified, mature skin and is considered a healed and functional wound.[9]

Photographic documentation is obtained at each visit in the form of color slides. This visual account of wound status is extremely helpful when used in conjunction with written documentation (Fig 21–1).

NONINVASIVE VASCULAR TESTING

Before any type of surgical intervention is planned, a battery of tests is ordered for each patient, so that an adequate assessment of their wound status will be known. The initial phase of testing is noninvasive testing of the vascular status of the extremity. Transcutaneous oxygen testing (tcO_2) is performed on various patients. Diabetics and all patients without palpable pedal pulses should receive this test, which can assess relative oxygen tension in the skin under an electrode as compared with a control. A value of less than 30 mm Hg is not conducive to wound healing without arterial reconstruction. In our center, the periwound skin is compared to the skin of the chest wall. In addition, the skin of the dorsum of the foot is compared to the chest wall. These tests are performed with the patient supine and with the extremity elevated.[3,5,10] This test can be ordered as an initial screen, and if values are found to be unacceptable, more detailed testing can then be ordered.

The arterial Doppler is another noninvasive test used extensively in the treatment of the chronic wound. This test is used on patients with no palpable pulses or with unacceptably low tcO_2 levels. The analysis of the waveform studies then gives the involved physicians a qualitative assessment of the peripheral vasculature, as opposed to the tcO_2 study that gives an estimate of gross quantity of vascular supply whether or not an acceptable minimum exists.[4,11]

OTHER VASCULAR TESTING

If the previous two studies do not yield an adequate amount of information regarding the blood supply to the extremity, or if the results are not conducive to proceeding with debridement or amputation, an angiogram should then be ordered. While invasive, the study gives the vascular surgeon a map with which to plan

CLINIC VISIT

Patient Name _____

ID # _____ Date _____

──────────── RECENT MEDICAL INFORMATION ────────────

Any change in medicine? ____ No ____ Yes If yes, list _____
_____

Recent blood transfusion? ____ No ____ Yes If yes, when _____

▲ Hospitalization or surgery since last visit? ____ No ____ Yes If yes, Month _____ Year _____ Where _____
Why? _____

▲ Adverse Reactions ____ No ____ Yes If yes, describe _____
_____

Vital Signs	TPR _____	BP _____	FSBS _____	
▲ Wound Location				
▲ Wound #	#	#	#	#
▲ Wound Width				
▲ Wound Length				
▲ Wound Depth				
▲ Undermining				
▲ % Epithelium				
▲ Functional Assessment Rating	☐1 ☐2 ☐3 ☐4	☐1 ☐2 ☐3 ☐4	☐1 ☐2 ☐3 ☐4	☐1 ☐2 ☐3 ☐4
▲ Debride/Remodel	☐ Yes ☐ No	☐ Yes ☐ No	☐ Yes ☐ No	☐ Yes ☐ No
▲ Compliance	☐ Yes ☐ No	☐ Yes ☐ No	☐ Yes ☐ No	☐ Yes ☐ No
▲ PROCUREN® Prescribed?	Start ____ Cont ____ DC ____	Start ____ Cont ____ DC ____	Start ____ Cont ____ DC ____	Start ____ Cont ____ DC ____
▲ Number of Doses				
▲ If Wound TX Complete Outcome*				

* A = Amputation C = Converted D = Died F = Financial G = Graft H = Healed N = Non-compliance O = Other P = Poor Healing

▲ Grade (If Changed)				
Photo Mag.				
Fibrin	None Mild Mod Mark 0% 1-25% 26-75% 76-100% ☐1 ☐2 ☐3 ☐4	None Mild Mod Mark 0% 1-25% 26-75% 76-100% ☐1 ☐2 ☐3 ☐4	None Mild Mod Mark 0% 1-25% 26-75% 76-100% ☐1 ☐2 ☐3 ☐4	None Mild Mod Mark 0% 1-25% 26-75% 76-100% ☐1 ☐2 ☐3 ☐4
Granulation Tissue Quantity	☐ 1 None Present ☐ 2 Only Base Covered ☐ 3 ≥ Half Filled ☐ 4 Completely Filled	☐ 1 None Present ☐ 2 Only Base Covered ☐ 3 ≥ Half Filled ☐ 4 Completely Filled	☐ 1 None Present ☐ 2 Only Base Covered ☐ 3 ≥ Half Filled ☐ 4 Completely Filled	☐ 1 None Present ☐ 2 Only Base Covered ☐ 3 ≥ Half Filled ☐ 4 Completely Filled
Granulation Tissue Color	☐1 Pale/Gray ☐2 Pink ☐3 Brt Red ☐4 N/A ☐5 Covered w/Epithelium	☐1 Pale/Gray ☐2 Pink ☐3 Brt Red ☐4 N/A ☐5 Covered w/Epithelium	☐1 Pale/Gray ☐2 Pink ☐3 Brt Red ☐4 N/A ☐5 Covered w/Epithelium	☐1 Pale/Gray ☐2 Pink ☐3 Brt Red ☐4 N/A ☐5 Covered w/Epithelium
Granulation Tissue Texture	Spongy Firm N/A ☐1 ☐2 ☐3	Spongy Firm N/A ☐1 ☐2 ☐3	Spongy Firm N/A ☐1 ☐2 ☐3	Spongy Firm N/A ☐1 ☐2 ☐3
Exposed Bone	☐ Yes ☐ No	☐ Yes ☐ No	☐ Yes ☐ No	☐ Yes ☐ No
Exposed Tendon	☐ Yes ☐ No	☐ Yes ☐ No	☐ Yes ☐ No	☐ Yes ☐ No

FIG 21–1.
Clinic visit chart.

the reconstruction. At our institution, angiography can now be performed using the magnetic resonance imaging (MRI) coil with specific settings. This yields a noninvasive form of angiography without any form of injected dye.

VASCULAR INTERVENTION

If these studies do not yield an acceptable picture of the patient's vasculature, then arterial reconstruction is required. While it is major surgery, bypass surgery should be attempted even in situations where long-term patency is not expected. The goal of vascular reconstruction is to raise the tcO$_2$ in the vicinity of the wound to allow for adequate closure of the wound.[3,5,10]

DEBRIDEMENT FOLLOWING BYPASS

Once epithelialization has been achieved, graft patency is not as crucial; the extremity will usually stay viable anyway. Therefore, the rate of patency of lower extremity bypass grafts is lower than the rate of limb salvage.[12,13] As a result, we routinely perform our debridements or amputations in the severely vascularly compromised patient at the time of vascular bypass. Because graft failure may be high in these patients, the importance of immediate local intervention cannot be overstressed. Waiting to see how, if any, improvement occurs before definitive treatment is performed does not make good clinical sense. The graft will never be as patent as immediately following anastomosis. Blood supply will be most abundant following anastomosis. Adequate oxygenation will be most prevalent at this time as well. Therefore, it is prudent to proceed with debridement as quickly as possible, preferably when the patient is still on the table following by-

pass. It is well known that the diabetic suffers from so-called macrovascular disease. If macrovascular repair through angioplasty or bypass surgery is successful, local tcO$_2$ levels surrounding the wound will increase even in the presence of microvascular disease.[10] Even though arterioles may be in a diseased state in the diabetic, if an increase in the blood flow can be achieved, wounds can heal. It should be noted that collateral vessels are usually not adequate in these cases, and vascular reconstruction to the distal vessels should be attempted. In keeping with the concept of team management, a good vascular surgeon should always be a part of the wound care team.

LOCAL WOUND MANAGEMENT

The wound is the reason the patient has presented for care; therefore, it should receive the bulk of attention in the treatment regimen. These patients have lost the first barrier the body has to resist infection: the skin. It then becomes important to determine if infection is present. As part of the history, the physician should determine if fever and chills have been present, and if the patient is currently, or has been, on antibiotic therapy in the past. Patients coming to a wound center are often referred from other clinicians who may have initiated therapy.

WOUNDS—CONTAMINATION AND INFECTION

The extremity should be examined as well, with special attention given to the wound characteristics. The level of edema should be noted, and whether it is of a pitting variety or nonpitting. Induration and brawniness can affect the skin's ability to heal itself as well. Erythema and crepitance must be noted to get an idea of the acuteness of the infection and to what level any cellulitis extends. If there is a great deal of crepitance, aggressive anti-biosis and surgical debridgement should be undertaken. The wound itself should be measured and probed for deep sinus tracts, communication with osseous struc-tures, or breaks in fascial septa. Drainage and how "angry" any purulence looks should also be noted. An assessment of what organisms are involved is a must, but there are some principles of culture taking that need to be addressed. One ax-iom is that all ulcers are superficially col-onized. To swab a superficial ulcer is therefore useless and can give inaccurate results. In the presence of frank drain-ing pus, however, the pus should be cul-tured. Another axiom is that all cultures should be gram stained. When you con-sider that culture results can take more than 48 hours, and a gram stain takes a few minutes and can be performed in the emergency room or in an office setting, the relevance becomes clear. The gram stain will allow the physician to initiate effective therapy immediately, rather

than begin a shotgun type of therapy that may be inadequate and miss dangerous pathogens.

A more effective and accurate method of obtaining a wound culture is to remove any necrotic tissue in the wound, includ-ing the hyperkeratotic border that sur-rounds most chronic wounds, and obtain a culture of the newly debrided deeper tis-sue. On occasion, bone will be exposed, and if soft, gray or otherwise necrotic, this can be sent for culture and biopsy as well (Fig 21–2).

Bone biopsies should not be taken through a contaminated wound; this will yield an inaccurate assessment as to which organisms are actually present in the bone. When the biopsy is performed it should be carried out through an adjacent noncontaminated site. Through a small incision (less than 1 cm) an adequate amount of bone can be collected with the aid of a Craig biopsy needle set of various sizes. Enough bone is harvested to send for pathology and culture with sensitivi-ties.

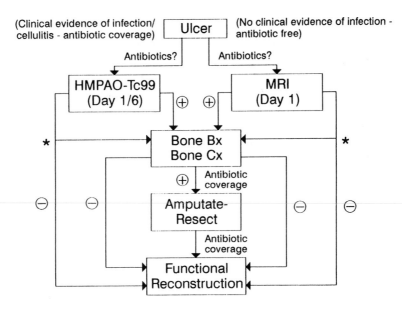

FIG 21–2.
Flow chart of suspected ulcers with underlying osteomyelitis.

If the wound is superficial without undermining, then topical dressings should suffice. At no time should betadine, whether full strength or diluted, be used on wounds. While decidedly toxic to bacterial cells, the betadine is also toxic to fibroblasts, macrophages, and endothelial cells. We have found that it tends to leave the skin indurated after prolonged use, and while it will prevent bacterial infection, it will also hinder a wound's ability to heal itself. Therefore saline wet-to-dry dressings should be used in the presence of superficial wounds that have drainage. Silver sulfadiazine or bacitracin is appropriate where some antibiosis is warranted.

Deeper infections must be treated with antibiotics, of course. If the infection appears to be absolutely limited to the periwound area and is only minimally invasive, then oral antibiotics and close outpatient management are warranted. Most infected chronic wounds are polymicrobial in the diabetic scenario, and broad-spectrum coverage is required. These wounds will often have gram-positive and gram-negative aerobes, as well as anaerobic bacteria. It is important to note that even though culture results show only one bug, the presence of occult organisms in the diabetic is something the astute physician should be aware of. For specific information regarding antibiotic use refer to Chapter 15.

LIMB-THREATENING INFECTION

Patients who are febrile, with cellulitis or signs of invasive illness, are promptly admitted for intravenous antibiotics and surgical debridement where appropriate. Ampicillin/sulbactam is used intravenously to cover the broad spectrum of bacteria seen in a polymicrobial infection. The usual dosage is 3.0 g IV every 6 hours. In the renally compromised, the dosage should be 1.5 g. Ciprofloxacin at 400 mg every 12 hours IV and clindamycin 600 mg every 6 hours are used in the penicillin-allergic patient. In the case of the threatened limb, antibiotic therapy is initiated in the form of vancomycin, an aminoglycoside, and metronidazole. Dosage in this case is dependent on renal function. However, antibiotics alone will not solve the problem in the face of abcess. MRI is useful in this regard, given time. If there is no time for such a study based on the clinical condition of the patient, such as sepsis, high temperature ($>102°F$), or rigors, surgical intervention must be the primary concern.

All necrotic tissue is removed during the debridement, and cultures taken for aerobic, anaerobic, fungal, and mycobacterial culture. Gram's stain should be considered a necessity of surgical debridement. Exposed bone and tendon should be removed. Bone should be resected to good bleeding cancellous bone, while tendons should be resected as proximally as possible. Any tendon left in the wound is an avascular nidus for infection and will allow proximal tracking of the infection.

DEBRIDEMENT

Debridement of nonhealing wounds is of paramount importance. The purpose is to remove heavily contaminated tissue that can potentially invade deeper tissue and create infection. The process of debridement removes necrotic, devitalized tissue which prevents wounds from resisting infection. Any devitalized tissue remaining in a wound enhances infection and further resists healing. The devitalized tissue acts as a medium that encourages bacteria to grow. This tissue inhibits leukocyte phagocytosis, thus allowing more bacteria to thrive.

Deep debridement of necrotic tissue to a strong bleeding surface of bone and muscle with contractile evidence is a must for complete debridement. Wounds in contact with frank purulence should be left opened. As the wound heals it gains resistance to infection and a choice can be made at that time whether to close the wound, with or without a graft, or continue to leave the wound open.

Wounds left open have an increase in vascular permeability. Intravascular fluids leak into the wound. Fibrinogen, one of the protein fluids present in the wound, is not resorbed by the lymphatics and forms into fibrin. The fibrin acts as a coagulum over the wound and incorporates the bacteria. This incorporation prevents it from contact with antibiotics. When the fibrinous coagulum is removed with interval debridement the antibiotic therapy becomes more effective. The repair phase of the wound can continue successfully with the formation of capillary bed and fibrous tissue, yielding a firm granulating bed that is able to resist infection.

POST DEBRIDEMENT

Once the infection is under control, patients are placed on oxygen via nasal cannula to enhance wound healing.[3,5,10] They are also placed at complete bed rest with twice or three times daily dressing changes. When the patients are stable enough to be mobile, they are sent to physical therapy for gait training with no weight to the affected part. This is in the form of complete non-weight-bearing, or partial weight-bearing with modified surgical shoe or total contact cast.

Oral antibiotics are prescribed as previously mentioned, and patients are seen regularly for office debridements. They should change their dressings twice daily at home. It should be noted that in the face of osteomyelitis, patients are placed on 6 weeks of at-home antibiotics based on culture results from debridement. Home infusion nursing is arranged prior to discharge from the hospital.

PLATELET DERIVED GROWTH FACTOR THERAPY

The use of autologous platelet derived growth factors as a wound treatment modality must be approached in a systematic fashion. There are contraindications to the use of growth factors such as malignancy in the wound site, and the concurrent use of specific metabolites or antineoplastic agents. In addition, there must be an adequate platelet count as these growth factors are located within the platelets.

Once it has been determined that the patient is an appropriate candidate for the use of autologous platelet derived growth factors, the patient's blood is drawn for processing. The amount of blood drawn is directly related to the patient's platelet count. For example, a platelet count of 150,000 requires withdrawal of 200 cc of blood, whereas a platelet count of 400,000 requires only 100 cc. This yields approximately 90 days' worth of treatment.

Once the phlebotomy has occurred, the blood is sent to a processing facility. To review the processing briefly, the whole blood is centrifuged, leaving the platelets suspended in plasma. The blood is put in a centrifuge once more, and the platelets are separated from the plasma. The platelets are stimulated to produce the growth factors by the addition of thrombin. This solution is concentrated and combined with a sterile platelet buffer which is dispensed to the patient in single-dose vials of 10 cc each. These vials are frozen to $-30°F$ and are thawed only when they are ready for use.

SUMMARY

The most important aspect of our approach to the wound patient is that of the team. Moreover, the patient is an integral part of the management team. Wounds require 24-hour maintenance, and only the patient can provide that. Our role is that of educator and guide, and to intervene when conditions warrant.

The evaluation and treatment of non-healing wounds have undergone many changes in the past few years. Specialized wound care centers have been developed in which patients with long-standing wounds are evaluated and treated. A multidisciplinary team of health care providers staff these centers, so that each patient can receive comprehensive care in one setting. Data concerning the etiology of non-healing wounds, wound characteristics, and wound-healing rates can be gathered, recorded, and analyzed in the wound care center. The effectiveness of traditional and new treatment methods can be scientifically determined.

Platelet derived wound healing factors (PDWHF) in the treatment of non-healing wounds is one of the newest treatment modalities available. An understanding of the normal process of wound healing and the complex reasons why wounds do not heal is necessary for the development and clinical use of PDWHF.

It is possible to isolate platelets, activate them, and isolate growth factors. Platelets may be obtained from the patient's own blood (autologous PDWHF) or from pooled donor platelets (homologous PDWHF). The growth factor solution is then applied directly to the wound. Wound healing is a complex event involving multiple systems. The reasons why wounds do not heal present even more complicated problems. Usually a combination of pathological conditions, rather than a single factor, interferes with wound healing. No single treatment option can be expected to heal a wound and keep it healed. Each factor preventing the wound healing process must be addressed and altered. These problems require the expertise unique to many specialities and are best treated in the context of a multidisciplinary wound care center.[14]

REFERENCES

1. Fylling CP, Knighton DR: Amputation in the diabetic population: incidence, causes, cost, treatment and prevention, *J Enterostomal Ther* 16:247–255, 1989.
2. Kanzler MH, Gorsulowsky DC, Swanson NA: Basic mechanisms in the healing cutaneous wound, *J Dermatol Surg Oncol* 12:1156–1164, 1984.
3. Knighton DR, Silver IA, Hunt TK: Regulation of wound healing angiogenesis—effect of oxygen gradients and inspired oxygen concentration, *Surgery* 90:262–270, 1981.
4. Sumner DS: Evaluation of venous circulation using the ultrasonic Doppler velocity detector. In Rutherford RB ed: *Vascular surgery,* Philadelphia, 1977, WB Saunders.
5. Niehaus LP, Kallibjian A: Application of transcutaneous oxygen measurement in podiatric surgery, *J Foot Surg* 28(2):124–126, 1989.
6. Bell JA: Light touch-deep pressure testing using Semmes-Weinstein monofilaments. In Hunter JM et al, editors: *Rehabilitation of the hand,* St Louis, 1984, Mosby–Year Book.
7. Knighton DR et al: Classification and treatment of chronic nonhealing wounds: successful treatment with autologous platelet-derived wound healing factors (PDWHF), *Ann Surg* 204:322–330, 1986.
8. Fylling CP: Comprehensive wound management with topical growth factors. *Ostomy Wound Management* 22:62–71, 1989.
9. Knighton DR et al: Stimulation of repair in chronic, nonhealing, cutaneous ulcers using platelet-derived wound healing formula, *Surg Gynecol Obstet* 170:56–60, 1990.
10. Burgess EM et al: Segmental transcutaneous measurements of PO_2 in patients requiring below the knee amputation for peripheral vascular insufficiency, *J Bone Joint Surg* 64(A):378–382, 1982.
11. Karanfilian RG et al: The value of laser Doppler velocimetry and transcutaneous oxygen tension determination in predicting healing of ischemic forefoot ulcer-

ations and amputations in diabetic and nondiabetic patients, *J Vasc Surg* 4:511–516, 1986.

12. Knighton DR, Fylling CP, Doucette MM: Wound healing and amputation in a high risk diabetic population, *Wounds* 1:107–114, 1989.

13. Doucette MM, Fylling CP, Knighton DR: Amputation prevention in a high risk

population through comprehensive wound healing protocol, *Arch Phys Med Rehabil* 70:780–783, 1989.

14. Weingarten MS: The management of the chronic non-healing wound. In *The Graduate Hospital Wound Care Center educational manual,* 1992.

22 Prophylactic Surgery in the Diabetic Foot

Robert Frykberg, D.P.M.
John Giurini, D.P.M.
Geoffrey Habershaw, D.P.M.
Barry Rosenbloom, D.P.M.
James Chrzan, D.P.M.

Elective surgery in the patient with diabetes mellitus has traditionally been viewed with skepticism and apprehension. Even today, patients with foot deformities having the potential to eventually ulcerate are reluctant to undergo corrective procedures because of conventional wisdom precluding any thought of such intervention. Ironically, it is the presence of structural deformities and their progression that pose a potentially greater threat to the health of the diabetic patient than the potential risk of prophylactic foot surgery.

Structural deformity (with attendant biomechanical abnormalities) has been found by numerous authors to be a major predisposing factor to injury and ulceration in the neuropathic foot.[1-8] Hammertoes, plantarly displaced metatarsal heads, and Charcot's deformities are frequently encountered in patients with peripheral neuropathy and result in localized concentrations of pressure. Holewski et al.[2] have demonstrated a 68% incidence of structural deformity in their review of 92 diabetic male patients seen for foot evaluation. Hammertoes and plantar callosities were evident in 32% and 51% of the patients, respectively, whereas a limitation of ankle joint dorsiflexion was present in 63% of the subjects. The prevalence of hammertoe deformities showed a very significant correlation with ulcer or amputation in patients with vascular disease or neuropathy. Borssen et al.[1] reported similar findings in their examination of 380 diabetic patients aged 15 to 50 years living in the county of Umea, Sweden. They too warned that these relatively common deformities could lead to ulceration with the development of neuropathy if left untreated. Cavanagh et al.[3] reported that foot deformity was more likely to predispose neuropathic individuals to ulceration than were alterations in function or variations in body mass. Although neuropathic patients typically have higher than normal plantar forefoot pressures, structural deformities tend to concentrate ground reaction forces over small prominences for extended periods of time. Studies by Boulton et al.[9] and Duckworth et al.[10] have elucidated these findings and revealed that in all cases abnormally high plantar pressures were found under the sites of previous ulceration.

Recent studies indicate the putative role of limited joint mobility in the development of increased plantar pressures and neuropathic plantar ulceration without specifically determining an association with structural deformities.[11-13] However, Masson et al.[14] documented the significance of foot deformities in the causation of elevated pressures in patients with rheumatoid arthritis and diabetes mellitus. Ulceration occurred only in those diabetic patients with neuropathy, emphasizing the roles of both insensitivity and deformity in the pathogenesis of foot lesions.

From the foregoing, it is clear that structural deformities pose an ever-present danger to the diabetic patient. With increasing age and duration of diabetes, the incidence of associated complications such as neuropathy, vascular disease, retinopathy, and nephropathy also increases.[15, 16] These factors have also been found to be significantly associated with an increased prevalence of foot ulcerations or infections when compared with diabetic patients without a history of such foot lesions.[1, 6] It is imperative, therefore, to neutralize the effects of deformity in the foot by conservative measures such as appropriate footwear and accommodative insoles, periodic foot care and evaluation, and ongoing patient education.[7] When these measures fail to control the development of preulcerative or ulcerative lesions, reconstructive foot surgery should be considered. Similarly, when significant deformities exist or develop even in the absence of ulceration or in those patients with a previous history of ulceration, thought must be given to their correction with an eye toward long-term prevention of serious limb-threatening foot lesions. Recognizing the potential for progression of the disease and the inherent morbidity of diabetic foot ulcerations, an aggressive approach to structural deformity is therefore warranted.

In its purest sense, prophylactic surgery refers to surgery performed in an effort to prevent the occurrence of more serious associated disease or pathology. In this regard, prophylactic correction of significant hammertoe or hallux valgus deformities in the diabetic individual can be expected to prevent the eventual development of ulceration by removing or reducing discrete areas of high pressure.[17]

Numerous authors have advocated prophylactic surgery in patients with diabetes, structural deformity, and active or previous history of ulceration.[7, 17, 18–31] These reports, however, are interspersed with or primarily concerned with foot surgery undertaken to promote the healing of recalcitrant plantar ulcers. In this sense, they cannot be truly considered preventive but curative in nature. Often, for instance, a metatarsal head resection will be employed to decompress the underlying osseous structure and thereby promote the healing of a recalcitrant plantar ulcer with or without primary closure of the ulcer.[27, 28, 30] This same procedure can be performed as an isolated operation or as a pan metatarsal head resection to prevent the recurrence of intermittent ulcerations on the sole of the foot.[23] Similar uses are reported for metatarsal neck osteotomies and Keller's arthroplasties for recurrent ulcerations of the great toe.[18–20, 31]

It becomes evident that definitive or nonemergent foot surgery for the diabetic patient encompasses three general categories, as outlined in Table 22–1. *Ablative* procedures are the traditional amputations that diabetic patients were usually relegated to because of the misconception over the presence of "small vessel disease," as put forth by Goldenberg et al.[32] With clarification of the true nature of diabetic foot pathology and the knowledge that there is indeed no "small vessel" atherosclerosis in their feet, diabetic patients are now given equal opportunity for access to reconstructive surgical procedures.[33] Therefore, ablative procedures should be reserved for cases of digital, forefoot, or partial foot gangrene and infection that is otherwise beyond salvage. Using the Wagner classification system,[34] foot lesions graded as 3, 4, or 5 would necessitate amputation of the involved part.

Curative foot surgery encompasses those procedures necessary to engender healing of active recalcitrant or recurrent ulcerations, osteomyelitis, or septic joints

TABLE 22-1.

Foot Surgery Categories

Category	Indications	Type
Ablative	Grade 3, 4, 5	Toe, ray, transmetatarsal amputation, Chopart's, Symes, below-knee amputation, etc.
Curative	Grade 1, 2, 3	Metatarsal head resection, osteotomy, joint resection, sesamoidectomy, Keller's bunionectomy, etc.
Prophylactic/ reconstructive	Grade 0	Metatarsal osteotomy, head resection, sesamoidectomy, digital arthroplasty, bunionectomy, etc.

without resorting to digital or partial foot amputations. Metatarsal head resection, often termed as an "amputation," is considered curative in this regard rather than ablative because the overall integrity and appearance of the foot is maintained. Early reports by Kelly and Coventry[27] in 1958 and others[35, 36] established the efficacy of single metatarsal head resections, joint resections, and toe amputation combined with head resection in curing refractory plantar ulcerations. Recent studies corroborate the ability of such procedures to provide rapid healing of long-standing neuropathic ulcerations even in the presence of moderate peripheral vascular disease.[28, 37]

Panmetatarsal head resection or removal of multiple metatarsal heads for recurrent forefoot lesions has also been met with a high success rate and few recurrences.[23, 25, 38] Sesamoidectomy in the presence of active ulceration has also been demonstrated to be of value in resolving these chronic neuropathic lesions where ray or transmetatarsal amputation would have been traditionally performed.[25, 39] Simple metatarsal osteotomy can provide the same curative results when used in patients without osteomyelitis or joint space involvement.[7, 17, 22]

Prophylactic surgery, synonymously considered *reconstructive* surgery, is performed on grade 0 feet with a prior history of ulceration or with potential for future ulceration. Conditions commonly treated in this manner would be recalcitrant onychocryptosis, significant hammertoe or clawtoe deformities, hallux valgus, prominent metatarsal heads with refractory hyperkeratoses, and midfoot dorsal, medial, or plantar exostoses. All diabetic patients with these deformities should not, however, be immediately considered for prophylactic surgery. Gudas[24] reported on a modest number of elective procedures that resulted in a 31% incidence of complications. This 69% success rate, although unusually low, emphasizes the need for thorough preoperative evaluation and justification for prophylactic correction of foot deformities. Preoperative assessment, as discussed in the following section, should consist of thorough medical, vascular, neurologic, biomechanical, and, if available, plantar pressure evaluations. Conservative treatment in the form of routine podiatric care, orthoses, protective footwear, and patient education always precedes elective surgery and should be considered the mainstay of treatment for the diabetic foot.

Notwithstanding, prophylactic surgery plays an integral role in the overall management of the high risk foot and fulfills the primary goal of prevention of ulceration. Well-conceived, aggressive intervention at the opportune time is therefore recommended to achieve structural improvement and a commensurate reduction in abnormal forces exerted on the foot.

PREOPERATIVE EVALUATION

Optimum medical control is paramount when elective reconstructive procedures on the diabetic patient are considered. Hyperglycemia, not only indicative of impaired glucose homeostasis and attendant abnormalities of insulin utilization, portends other metabolic consequences such as nitrogen wasting, lipolysis, ketogenesis, and gluconeogenesis.[40] These catabolic effects of uncontrolled diabetes are obviously counterproductive to efficient wound healing. In addition to the many complications of diabetes resulting from prolonged hyperglycemia,[15, 41] high blood glucose levels also result in an inefficient immune response to infection highlighted by impaired leukocyte chemotaxis and phagocytosis.[42-45]

Cardiovascular disease is the leading cause of death among people with diabetes and accordingly has a high prevalence in this patient population.[46] Therefore, each patient must undergo a thorough cardiac evaluation for evidence of coronary artery disease, myocardial infarction, valvular heart disease, congestive heart failure, and uncontrolled hypertension.[47] Other manifestations of macrovascular disease, specifically cerebrovascular and peripheral vascular disease, must also be ruled out in those patients with heart disease.[16, 48] Diabetic nephropathy, or glomerulosclerosis, is a serious complication of the disease and can be attributed to microvascular disease.[16, 48] Although mild degrees of renal impairment are fairly common, the incidence of renal failure and end-stage renal disease (ESRD) increases with duration of diabetes.[41] According to

the U.S. Department of Health and Human Services, the incidence of diabetic ESRD has been increasing at about 10% per year since 1983, accounting for 1.5 cases per 1,000 people with diabetes.[46] Aside from protein loss and azotemia, patients with chronic renal failure develop hypertension, left ventricular hypertrophy, anemia, and bleeding diatheses.[47] Such disturbances have obvious deleterious effects on the surgical patient and must be thoroughly assessed and stabilized preoperatively. Although renal insufficiency may contribute to ulcer formation and anecdotally delay healing, Griffiths and Wieman[49] report that in their series patients with renal disease were no less likely to heal than were diabetic patients with normal renal function. Therefore, patients with nephropathy, although requiring more frequent and cautious monitoring, should expect a reasonably good chance of healing their foot wounds, provided that all other parameters for healing are optimized.

The vascular status of the foot is a major consideration in the preoperative evaluation of surgical candidates and will ultimately determine the ability of the foot to heal. Noninvasive arterial testing should be performed on a routine basis and especially for those patients with diminished or absent pulses. Although Wagner[34] has reported that ankle/brachial ratios of approximately 50% are consistent with healing, the unreliability of ankle pressures in the diabetic patient has made digital arterial pressures, digital photoplethysmography recordings, and transcutaneous oxygen tension measurements more informative in this regard.[50-53] In general, digital arterial pressures should be greater than 55 to 60mm Hg,[51, 54, 55] transcutaneous oxygen tension should be more than 40 mm Hg,[50, 56] and digital photoplethysmography should reveal adequate pulsatility and amplitude.[53] Not infrequently, vascular reconstruction may be necessary to provide the optimum perfusion to allow subsequent elective foot surgery. Therefore, preoperative vascular surgery consultations should be freely encouraged, especially in those instances where there is any question of diminished pedal blood flow.

The importance of structural deformity in the causation of diabetic foot ulcerations has already been discussed. Therefore, it is prudent to assess the effects of such deformities on the sole of the foot by means of a variety of devices available that can qualitatively or quantitatively measure foot pressures.[57–59] The Harris mat, optical pedobarograph, Electrodynogram (Langer Electronics Group, Deer Park, N.Y.) and EMED (Novel, USA, Minneapolis, Minn.) systems have been commercially available for such purposes over the last decade, each having its own advantages and disadvantages.[57] A relatively new system, the FSCAN (Tekscan, Boston, Mass.) has promise in this regard because it uses in-shoe technology consisting of thin pressure-sensitive insole sensors that interface with a transducer and personal computer. A recent study reported that the FSCAN could provide reproducible measurements of static and dynamic foot pressures inside the shoe with a variety of displays once the data were acquired.[59] Problems with calibration between separate sensors have been addressed with an updated software version. Regardless of which method is used, potential trouble areas can be ascertained and current or previous sites of ulceration can be critically evaluated. Once corrected, the feet should be reevaluated for documentation of efficacy of the procedure and periodically assessed for changes or appropriateness of footwear therapy.

ANESTHESIA

Because cardiovascular disease is a major concern in most diabetic patients, local,

regional, or spinal anesthesia are preferred over general anesthesia as circumstances permit. Although infected areas cannot be directly blocked, local anesthetic injections proximal to the surgical site can be safely performed to affect a nerve or nerves or segmental block.[22, 60] Lidocaine, 0.5% or 1%, is most frequently used and commonly mixed with 0.5% bupivacaine to provide rapid onset of anesthesia, as well as prolonged duration of action for 6 to 12 hours. The use of epinephrine in digits is still quite controversial and cannot be generally recommended in these patients. However, the vasoconstriction and relative hemostasis afforded make its use in other sites advantageous. Discretion and proper patient selection are necessary when one considers the use of this agent in foot surgery.[22]

Digital blocks are certainly the easiest to perform and can be used in all cases requiring anesthesia of a toe only (e.g., nail surgery, hammertoe correction, distal debridement or amputation). Usually, all four digital nerves must be infiltrated to produce adequate anesthesia of the entire toe. Either a ring block technique (Fig 22–1) or an inverted V block (Fig 22–2) can be employed using a 25-gauge 1½-in. needle on a 3-mL syringe. A total of 3 mL for the great toe and 2 mL for the lesser toes is usually sufficient. When the metatarsophalangeal joint or metatarsal head is to be operated on, a more proximal V block should be done around the distal portion of the involved metatarsal shaft. Bunionectomy procedures usually require a digital block in combination with a circumferential segmental block of the first metatarsal proximal to the metatarsal neck.

Ankle blocks are extremely useful in providing anesthesia to the entire foot when multiple surgical sites must be approached or when incisions traverse multiple nerves such as employed in panmetatarsal head resections or transmetatarsal amputations.[22, 60] Accordingly, the

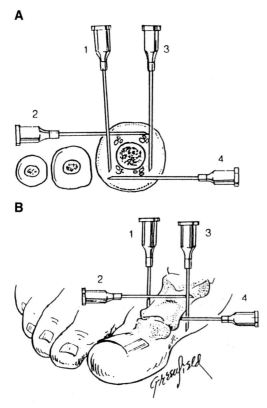

FIG 22–1.
Injection technique for the great toe. **A,** cross-sectional view. **B,** dorsal view. (From Frykberg RG: Podiatric problems in diabetes. In Kozak GP et al, editors: *Management of diabetic foot problems,* Philadelphia, 1984, WB Saunders. Used by permission.)

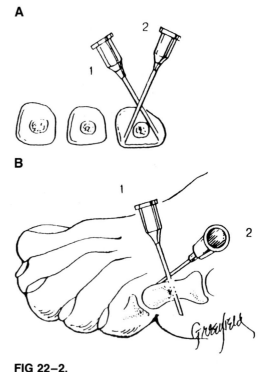

FIG 22–2.
Inverted V block for lesser toes. **A,** cross-sectional view. **B,** dorsal view. (From Frykberg RG: Podiatric problems in diabetes. In Kozak GP et al, editors: *Management of diabetic foot problems,* Philadelphia, 1984, WB Saunders. Used by permission.)

surgeon or anesthesiologist must be familiar with the distribution of both the deep and superficial nerves crossing the ankle and the innervation they provide (Figs 22–3 and 22–4). The two deep nerves, the deep peroneal and the posterior tibial, run adjacent to the dorsalis pedis artery and the posterior tibial artery, respectively. The other four nerves that cross the ankle, starting laterally, are the sural, intermediate dorsal cutaneous, medial dorsal cutaneous, and saphenous nerves. These are all superficial and can be easily blocked with a subcutaneous ring of anesthetic starting behind the lateral malleolus and proceeding across the anterior surface of the ankle to the medial malleolus. The anterior tibial (deep peroneal) nerve is blocked by palpating the dorsalis pedis pulse and injecting around it deep to the fascia, taking care to aspirate before infiltration. The more difficult posterior tibial nerve is similarly located and blocked adjacent to the posterior tibial artery. Ten to 20 mL of anesthetic will usually be required and should be delivered with a 1½-in. 25-gauge needle on a 10-mL syringe.

TOENAIL SURGERY

A number of conditions may cause changes in the growth pattern of the nails. These include changes caused by local disease states, genetic changes, infection, systemic disease, aging, and mechanical instabilities. In and of themselves, many

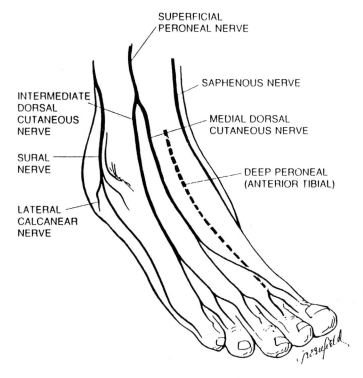

FIG 22–3.
Dorsal nerve supply of the foot. The broken line indicates the position of the deep peroneal (anterior tibial) nerve. (From Frykberg RG: Podiatric problems in diabetes. In Kozak GP et al, editors: *Management of diabetic foot problems,* Philadelphia, 1984, WB Saunders. Used by permission.)

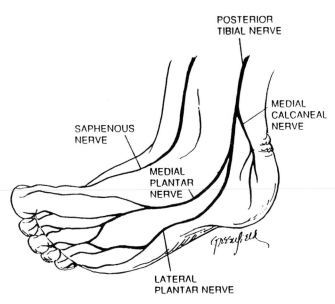

FIG 22–4.
Plantar nerve supply of the foot. (From Frykberg RG: Podiatric problems in diabetes. In Kozak GP et al, editors: *Management of diabetic foot problems,* Philadelphia, 1984, WB Saunders. Used by permission.)

of these changes may not cause severe problems. However, in the diabetic with neuropathy or vascular compromise small changes may lead to limb threatening problems. Once a problem has been identified, a decision to provide either conservative or surgical treatment is necessary. If the nail has undergone a change that will lead to a continued history of recurrent infection, ulceration, or chronic pain, surgical intervention is necessary. The recommendation must be made to permanently remove a portion of the offending nail or the complete nail through partial or total matrixectomy. There are many procedures in the literature describing partial or total matrixectomy, including sharp dissection, chemical cauterization, or laser matrixectomy. It is recommended that surgical procedures in diabetics with peripheral changes involving the sensory or vascular system have sharp procedures performed. Chemical and laser procedures are usually followed by some form of home hydrotherapy, which is generally to be avoided in the diabetic population. The techniques available for performing a partial or total matrixectomy are Frost, Winograd, Suppan, or Zadick procedures.

The indications for using a Frost or Winograd procedure are recurrent infection or pain secondary to a chronic ingrown nail border with or without a hypertrophied nailfold. Anesthesia is obtained by a local infiltrative block at the base of the toe. Hemostasis is obtained by use of a Penrose tourniquet at the base of the toe wrapped in gauze and clamped with a straight hemostat.

Frost Procedure

1. A cut is made using an English nail nipper at the apex of the border deformity. The cut is carried proximally 1 cm past the eponychium.

2. The next incision is made at the proximal end of the first incision at an angle of 80 degrees and carried plantarly 1 to 1.5 cm.
3. A flap is raised using a no. 15 blade. It is placed through the first incision and is worked on the bone proximal to distal undermining the intended flap.
4. A third incision is made using a no. 10 blade. It is carried from the origin of the first incision, distal to proximal, parallel to the first, and joining it at the eponychium.
5. The wedge of tissue is now removed by sharp dissection, with careful attention paid to its attachment at the bone.
6. The bone at the base of the wound and matrix area is rasped with a nasal rasp. Sutures are placed proximally and distally.
7. The tourniquet is released, and a nonadherent dry sterile dressing is placed around the toe.

Winograd Procedure

1. A cut is made using an English nail nipper at the apex of the border deformity. It is carried 1 to 1.5 cm proximal to the eponychium.
2. The cut is deepened along its length to the level of the phalanx with a no. 10 blade.
3. From proximal to distal, a second semielliptical incision is made joining the ends of the first incision and encompassing the marginal nail fold.
4. The wedge of tissue created is then removed, including nail plate, nail bed, nail matrix, and hypertrophic skin fold.
5. The cut is sutured proximally and distally.

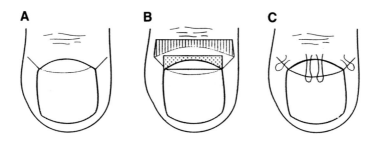

FIG 22–5.
Zadik procedure. **A,** skin incisions at 45 degrees to nail margins. **B,** created skin flap. **C,** skin closure. (From Nicklas BJ: Prophylactic surgery in the diabetic foot. In Frykberg RG, editor: *The high risk foot in diabetes mellitus,* New York, 1991, Churchill Livingstone. Used by permission.)

6. The tourniquet is released, and a dry sterile dressing applied.

Zadik Procedure

The procedure of choice for total matrixectomy is the Zadik procedure. It allows good visualization and is used in lieu of a terminal Symes (Fig 22–5).

1. Remove the entire nail plate.
2. At each border of the eponychium, a 1-cm oblique incision is made extending proximally and plantarly.
3. The flap thus created is reflected proximally, allowing visualization of the nail matrix.
4. A transverse incision is now made at the level of the lunula, the width of the nail bed.
5. The nail matrix is dissected sharply off the phalanx from distal to proximal.
6. The borders are then sutured.
7. The tourniquet is released, and povidone-iodine–soaked nonadherent gauze and a dry sterile dressing are applied.

Postoperatively, the first dressing change for any of these procedures is on the third postoperative day. Sutures are removed at this time. The patient is started on a regimen of twice daily dress-ing changes and wears an open shoe for 2 to 3 weeks. If no problems develop in follow-up on postoperative months 2 and 4, the patient is discharged from the service.

HAMMERTOE DEFORMITIES OF LESSER DIGITS

Digital deformities in the diabetic patient have a number of contributing factors. In excessive pronation, there is an inability of the interossei to stabilize the distal and proximal interphalangeal joints against the metatarsophalangeal joint. In conjunction with this, we see an increase in contracture of the long flexors. This leads to digital contracture. In the supinated or cavus foot, there is an overpull of the long extensors against an unstable distal and proximal interphalangeal joint. There is an increased pull of the long flexor, with resultant mallet or hammertoe deformity.

The contributing factor that exacerbates this in diabetes is peripheral neuropathy with resultant intrinsic muscular wasting. This further leads to destabilization and hammertoe formation. Sensory neuropathy will also increase a diabetic's tendency to grip the toes to the ground for balance with ambulation, resulting in extensor override.

Another contributing factor is osteoarthropathy. Collapse of the arch will put an increased stretch on the long flexors, which are now destabilized through pronation and intrinsic wasting. This also results in hammertoe contractures. These deformities in association with peripheral neuropathy and peripheral vascular disease leads to tissue breakdown when stressed by conventional shoe gear. The question then arises as to what to do and when to do it. The physician must recognize that deformity in and of itself does not necessitate surgical intervention. It is the failure of conservative care to prevent epidermal ulceration that leads to surgical repair of a digital deformity. When faced with a digital deformity that has resulted in a history of recurrent ulcer, first determine whether the deformity is rigid or flexible. If the deformity is rigid, a bony procedure will be necessary in conjunction with release of soft tissue contracture to relieve it. If the deformity is flexible, simple soft tissue release may be all that is necessary to resolve the ulceration.

Flexor Tenotomy

1. Ulcer on digital tip digit is recurrent.
2. Ulcer on proximal or distal interphalangeal joint is recurrent.
3. Deformity is easily reducible.
4. Ulcer is superficial, and there is no osteomyelitis.

Procedure

1. Local anesthesia using appropriate technique.
2. Transverse incision or stab at the level of the flexor crease.
3. Toe held in dorsiflexion.
4. Number 61 Beaver blade used to perform flexor tenotomy.

Postoperatively, dressing should be changed twice weekly, with the digit splinted into position. The patient may return to appropriate footwear (e.g., running shoe or extra-depth shoe) at 1 week.

Distal Symes for Lesser Digits

Indications

1. Ulcer distal toe
2. Probes to bone
3. No systemic symptoms or cellulitis

Procedure

1. Fishmouth incision ellipsing ulcer on the nail, nail bed, nail matrix, or nail plate.
2. Debridement of distal phalanx proximally, removing all osteomyelitic bone back to bleeding base.
3. Wound closed with 4-0 or 5-0 nylon.
4. Digit splinted in corrected position.

Postoperative Care

1. Dressings changed wet to dry two times daily for 2 weeks or until drainage from the incision ceases.
2. Patient ambulates in postoperative or Ipos shoe.
3. Sutures removed at 14 days.
4. Use of conventional shoe gear resumed at 3 to 4 weeks.
5. Appropriate intravenous or oral antibiotics continued until incision is dry and ulcer is closed.

Proximal or Distal Interphalangeal Joint Arthroplasty

Indications

1. Recurrent ulcer on interphalangeal or distal interphalangeal joint.
2. Bone may or may not be involved.
3. Nonreducible deformity.

Procedure for Fixed Deformity Without Ulcer (Fig 22–6)

1. Appropriate digital block with local anesthesia.

2. Central dorsal linear or semiel-liptical incisions.
3. Blunt dissection to the level of the proximal or distal interpha-langeal joint.
4. Transverse tenotomy or capsulot-omy.
5. Freeing the head of the phalanx.
6. Removal of the head of the pha-lanx using double-action bone cutter or oscillating saw.
7. Tendon reapproximated with 3-0 absorbable suture.
8. Cutaneous closure with 4-0 nylon.
9. Digit splinted in correctional po-sition.

Procedure for Fixed Deformity With Ulcer Present

1. Two semielliptical incisions dor-sally, allowing for excision of ulcer.
2. Removal of all infected soft tis-sue.
3. If no osteomyelitis, procedure con-tinued as for fixed deformity without ulcer.
4. If osteomyelitis present, joint re-moved completely proximally and distally to bleeding bone.
5. Wound closed with full-thickness nonabsorbable sutures.
6. Intravenous antibiotics continued until there is no drainage from incision site.

7. Dressing changes wet to dry daily.

Postoperative Care

1. Non-weight-bearing crutches are used until incision is dry.
2. Ambulation in postoperative shoe as appropriate.
3. Removal of sutures at 2 to 3 weeks.
4. Use of conventional shoe gear re-sumed at 4 to 5 weeks.

METATARSAL SURGERY

Various surgical procedures have been de-scribed to treat the mal perforans ulcer beneath the lesser metatarsal heads, many of which are suitable for the treat-ment of intractable plantar keratoses or preulcerative lesions. Although all these are successful in the hands of their re-spective authors, no one report has out-lined the indications for alternative op-erations for ulcers in similar locations but with different presenting characteristics. Our approach affords the surgeon a cer-tain flexibility in that the depth of the ulcer at the time of the operation dictates the choice of procedure and assures that no one procedure be performed in every situation. The superficial ulcer, by defi-nition one that does not extend deep to the level of bone or joint, is treated with an

A   **B**   **C**

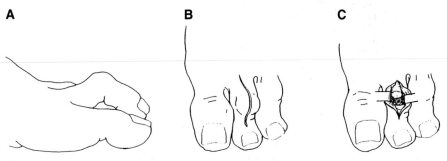

FIG 22–6.
A, isolated hammertoe deformity. **B,** skin incision. **C,** proximal phalangeal head resection. (From Nicklas BJ: Prophylactic surgery in the diabetic foot. In Frykberg RG, editor: *The high risk foot in diabetes mellitus,* New York, 1991, Churchill Livingstone. Used by permis-sion.)

A   **B**   **C**

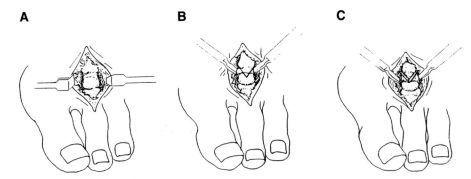

FIG 22–7.
A, exposure of metatarsal head. **B,** V-osteotomy at metaphyseal neck. **C,** distal capital fragment is repositioned or realigned for improved weight distribution. (From Nicklas BJ: Prophylactic surgery in the di- abetic foot. In Frykberg RG, editor: *The high risk foot in diabetes mellitus,* New York, 1991, Churchill Livingstone. Used by permission.)

elevating osteotomy created at the level of the metatarsal neck. This is intended to alleviate the plantar pressure contributing to the development of the ulcer. The advantage of metatarsal osteotomy over metatarsal head resection in cases of superficial neuropathic ulcers is that a tremendous increase in transfer of weight is avoided and the foot that is created is biomechanically more sound. Transfer lesions are encountered less frequently because the osteotomized metatarsal still bears weight. Performance of the osteotomy in diabetic patients does not differ from previously described operations performed in nondiabetic patients. If an ulcer is present at the time of surgery, it must be walled off from the field to prevent cross-contamination. The skin incision is made dorsally, centered over the involved metatarsal. The osteotomy may be performed in a number of varying methods (V, colectomy, osteoclasis), depending on the surgeon's preference (Fig 22–7). This includes the use of power instrumentation or manual instruments. Internal fixation devices are not routinely used. The skin is then closed in standard fashion, again depending on the discretion of the surgeon. Postoperative care optimally requires non-weight-bearing, especially when an ulcer is present.

In some instances, ulcers beneath the fifth metatarsal head may require resection of the metatarsal head (also through a dorsal approach) to promote healing. We have not seen any clinically significant difference between osteotomy and metatarsal head resection of ulcers beneath the fifth metatarsal head. In some cases adjacent metatarsals may need to be elevated, especially in feet in which there is a high likelihood of a transfer ulcer.

In our experience, metatarsal head resection is reserved for deep ulcers that involve bone or joint, including cases of osteomyelitis. This procedure is often done in deference to a ray amputation and enables the toe to be salvaged. Therefore, the foot does not lose as much structural and functional integrity as one in which the toe has been removed.

Our approach to the metatarsal head resection differs from those described in the literature. Because these are feet in which there is direct extension of the ulcer to the level of the bone or joint, the ulcer can be addressed with the incision. Using a plantar approach, the ulcer is excised with a double elliptical incision that completely excises all necrotic tissue along with the ulcer. Through this incision the bone is directly visualized and resected if infected. When undrained sepsis is encountered unexpectedly, the wound is packed open (and closed secondarily after the infection has resolved). After an adequate flush, the clean wound is closed primarily.

A tension-free closure is done along the distal two thirds to three fourths of the incision using full-thickness retention sutures of 3-0 nonabsorbable suture interspersed with simple sutures of 4-0 nylon. Deep absorbable suture is not routinely used. The most proximal aspect of the wound may be packed open for dependent drainage as the patient lays in bed. Exceptions to this rule are those cases in which an ischemic patient or one who has recently undergone vascular reconstruction is operated on. In these cases it is often best to close the entire incision rather than place a packing under tension.

This approach to the metatarsal head resection allows for the rapid healing of ulcers. A great advantage that we have seen after this procedure is that the patient leaves the hospital with a healing wound (essentially an incision) that requires minimal care, which is routinely performed by a family member. Weightbearing must be avoided up to 1 month after this procedure while the sutures are in place, because there is a great risk of wound dehiscence in the immediate postoperative period.

The closure done on the plantar aspect obviates the need for extensive local muscle or fasciocutaneous flaps. These may be occasionally used for soft tissue defects that are quite large and would not seem to respond to local excision with some form of primary closure. It has been our experience, however, that there are very few wounds on the plantar surface that cannot be closed primarily after excision. If necessary, multiple metatarsal heads may be removed through the plantar approach, because the incision may be oriented transversely.

The final procedure that is performed for ulcers involving the lesser metatarsal heads is the panmetatarsal head resection. Originally described for the patient with rheumatoid deformities, Jacobs[26] was the first to describe its usefulness for the patient with the neuropathic foot. After this, Giurini et al.[23] reviewed this procedure in similar patients.

The panmetatarsal head resection may be used as a primary procedure or in cases of salvage for the neuropathic foot. When it is used as a primary procedure, the patient may have a deep ulcer that has created a large soft tissue defect beneath the metatarsal heads or a foot that is reminiscent of the rheumatoid foot with prominent metatarsal heads, clawtoes, and atrophied fat pad. More often than as a primary procedure, the panmetatarsal head resection is used as a salvage operation in those feet that may have had a prior amputation. These are patients who have undergone prior ray resections, have failed prior attempts at metatarsal osteotomies, or have lost the first metatarsophalangeal joint and have developed transfer lesions beneath the remaining metatarsal heads. In addition, patients who are candidates for transmetatarsal amputation are candidates for this procedure.

There are multiple approaches to the panmetatarsal head resection in the neuropathic foot. If there is a superficial lesion, or the lesion is not present at the time of operation (in cases of recurrent ulceration), multiple dorsal incisions are used. Depending on the surgeon's preference, three, four, or five incisions may be used. Care must be taken to avoid creating a narrow bridge on the dorsum between incisions, especially in a patient with underlying arterial insufficiency.

In situations where an ulcer extends to the bone or joint, the ulceration is addressed from the plantar aspect, as described previously with single metatarsal head resections. In these situations, a number of options are available to the surgeon. The ulcer may be addressed plantarly and the remainder of the procedure performed through "clean" dorsal incisions; adjacent metatarsal heads may be resected through the same linear incision; or, finally, all of the metatarsal heads may be resected through a transversely directed incision. This last approach may also be modified to a "T" in which the linear arm is the ulcer excision and the transverse aspect addresses the remaining metatarsal heads.

After the procedure, closure is performed in the usual fashion. For operations that involve a plantar approach, the incision is closed as described in the previous section. Dorsal wounds are closed based on the surgeon's preference. Weight-bearing is not allowed, especially when an ulcer or plantar incision is present.

Technically, the procedure requires that an even parabola be created, with care taken to bevel the distal aspect of the metatarsals from distal-dorsal to proximal-plantar. In the neuropathic foot, a slight discrepancy in the weight-bearing parabola or in plantar spicules left inadvertently may doom the procedure to failure. Also, when this procedure is performed, the first metatarsophalangeal joint must be addressed with either a Keller procedure or a modified Keller-Mayo. Implants are not routinely used in the neuropathic foot. Also, contracted lesser digits may be addressed if necessary.

From a functional standpoint, the panmetatarsal foot is similar to the foot that has undergone transmetatarsal amputation. There are, however, differences between the procedures that make the panmetatarsal head resection a more attractive procedure. First, the function of the long flexors and extensors is not compromised as in the transmetatarsal amputation. Although one might argue that their function is diminished, it is still

present. Overpowering of the inverters or Achilles tendon is not frequently seen, a complication that frequently complicated transmetatarsal amputation. Second, shoeing becomes easier, because the toes are left intact. Again, although the argument may be made that the toes lose their function in gait after resection of the metatarsal heads, they still can be used as a "filler" in a pair of shoes. Finally, the prospect of amputation is a great fear of the diabetic patient. Avoiding amputation is psychologically more appealing to the patient with diabetes.

FIRST RAY SURGERY

All surgical planning in the diabetic patient with an open ulceration begins with evaluation of the ulceration itself. A differentiation must be made between a purely neuropathic ulceration and an ulceration with significant ischemia because this will determine the initial course of treatment. When pedal pulses are absent or ulcers are slow to respond to appropriate conservative care, a full vascular evaluation is warranted. This should begin with arterial noninvasive studies and progress to arteriograms if necessary. Where possible, revascularization of ischemic lesions should be performed before podiatric surgery. A purely neuropathic ulceration with a well-perfused forefoot may be amenable to immediate surgical intervention, provided the acute infectious process is adequately controlled. In addition to a patient's vascular status, the depth of the ulcer, along with all structures involved, should be made before any surgical intervention. Is the ulcer superficial without evidence of bone or joint involvement? Does the ulcer and infection involve the flexor tendon but not the underlying bone, or does the ulcer, in fact, communicate with the joint and bone? This knowledge is critical to selecting the best approach to the ulcer. A superficial ulcer is best approached through a dorsal incision, whereas an infected joint is best approached by ulcer excision and joint resection. This will be discussed in greater detail in subsequent sections. It is also important to determine the full extent of the infection and debride all necrotic tissue preoperatively in an attempt to control the infection. This may require an extensive incision and drainage procedure. It is imperative that the surgeon recognize this preoperatively because failure to do so will most certainly lead to failure of any surgical intervention. The key with any initial debridement is to debride all apparently infected and necrotic tissue but leave sufficient tissue behind so as not to compromise later reconstruction of the wound.

Because of foot mechanics the region of the first ray—hallux and first metatarsophalangeal joint—is one of the more common locations for plantar ulcerations (see Table 22–1). These ulcerations most commonly result from limited motion at the first metatarsophalangeal joint (i.e., hallux limitus or hallux rigidus), leading to compensatory hyperextension of the interphalangeal joint. It is not uncommon to see heavy callus formation with subsequent ulceration at this location. In addition, arthritic changes involving the first metatarsophalangeal joint may also limit joint motion, thus increasing the risk of ulceration. Prior injury or Charcot's joint disease of the first metatarsophalangeal joint will often produce a hallux limitus or rigidus. Excessive pronation is an additional risk factor for chronic ulcerations on the plantar medial aspect of the first metatarsal head or proximal phalangeal base. Finally, progressive metatarsal deformities may develop in these neuropathic patients. Along with sensory neuropathy, many of these patients suffer from a progressive motor neuropathy, which typically affects the intrinsic muscles of the foot. This leads to wasting and weakness of the intrinsic muscles, thus creating destabilization of all metatarsophalangeal joints. Progressive clawing of the digits and plantarflexion deformities of the metatarsals, including the first metatarsal, will develop over time. This will lead to increased focal pressures in these areas. Approximately two sixths of all forefoot pressure is taken up by the first metatarsal, whereas the lesser metatarsals bear one sixth of the body weight each. In the presence of a plantarflexed first ray, these pressures can reach significant levels.

Procedures for Chronic Ulcerations

Interphalangeal Joint Arthroplasty

Ulcerations may develop on either the dorsal or plantar surface of the interphalangeal joint of the hallux. A rigidly contracted digit (hallux hammertoe) may develop irritation from the toebox of a shoe, resulting in a dorsal ulceration in the neuropathic foot. A hallux limitus, either functional or structural, will result in hyperextension of the interphalangeal joint, leading to a direct plantar or a plantar medial ulceration. Finally, abnormal pronation excessively loads the medial aspect of the hallux and first ray such that the patient pivots on the medial condyle of the proximal phalanx. This can result in callus formation and potential ulceration in the presence of sensory neuropathy. One means of reducing the risk of recurrent ulcerations in this area is by restoring motion at the first metacarpophalangeal joint. Hallux interphalangeal joint arthroplasty allows for additional motion and reduces the forces generated at the interphalangeal joint. This allows for eventual resolution of the hyperkeratotic lesion and ulceration. When performed for a medial plantar ulceration, an arthroplasty relieves the intrinsic pressure of the medial condyle and interposes additional soft tissue between the bone and ground, resulting in resolution of the ulceration.

Operative Technique.—The hallux interphalangeal joint arthroplasty can be approached by either a dorsal longitudinal incision or a serpentine incision centered over the interphalangeal joint. We prefer to approach the joint through a serpentine incision because this allows for excellent exposure and minimizes retraction on skin edges. Once the joint is identified, a transverse capsular incision is made exposing the head of the proximal phalanx. A no. 64 blade facilitates release of the medial and lateral collateral ligaments of the interphalangeal joint. The head of the proximal phalanx is next resected just proximal to the articular surface. Wound closure is achieved in typical layered closure. The postoperative care of the foot is dictated by the status of the ulceration. In the presence of an open ulceration, the dressings are changed the next day, and the patient maintains a nonweight-bearing regimen until the ulcer is completely healed. Their activity is advanced gradually, as is their return to shoe gear. If the ulceration is healed at the time of surgery, the dressings are not changed until the third postoperative day. The surgeon and patient would be well served to maintain limited activity for the first 10 to 12 days (e.g., bathroom privileges), although weight-bearing can be allowed in a postoperative shoe. The presence of sensory neuropathy prevents early warning signs of infection, and excessive activity in the early postoperative period can lead to unnecessary complications. Sutures are typically left in place for 2 weeks.

Condylectomy and Exostectomy

Occasionally recurrent ulcerations at the plantar medial aspect of the hallux may occur from a prominent exostosis, or "spur," on the medial condyle of the distal phalanx. This can most often be detected radiographically. The additional pressure caused by this spur can be further accentuated by excessive pronation in the propulsive phase of gait. If such a prominence does exist, surgical resection can be performed.

Operative Technique.—A dorsomedial incision is made directly over the interphalangeal joint. Once the medial condyle of the distal phalanx is identified and freed from the surrounding ligamentous attachments, it is resected using either a small double-action bone cutter or rongeur. Care must be taken not to leave any bony spicules behind, because these can serve as potential pressure points in the future.

Although this procedure is both simple and effective, this may create instability at the level of the interphalangeal joint. Lateral deviation of the hallux or even Charcot-type changes have been seen within the joint itself. It is believed that these changes occur from the unilateral disruption of the medial collateral ligament, leading to uneven wear on the joint. For this reason, we favor the hallux arthroplasty when faced with a plantar medial ulceration.

Keller Bunionectomy

Hallux limitus or hallux rigidus generally results from arthritic changes within the first metatarsophalangeal joint itself. These may occur from prior injury to the joint, as seen in fractures or Charcot's joint type of injuries or from years of ambulation on feet with biomechanical pathology. This lack of dorsiflexory motion at the metatarsophalangeal joint results in a compensatory hyperextension at the interphalangeal joint. A Keller-type procedure, as performed in other cases of hallux rigidus, will restore motion at the first metatarsophalangeal joint, leading to resolution of the ulceration.

Operative Technique.—The surgical approach to the first metatarsophalangeal joint is through a standard dorsomedial incision. Our preferred capsular incision is a U-shaped capsulotomy with the base directed proximally and the flap distally. This will allow for interposition of the distal capsule into the joint space. This will help reduce the dead space created and the shortening that commonly occurs with this procedure. It will also cover the first metatarsal head, preventing bone-on-bone contact between the cut surface of the proximal phalanx and the first metatarsal head. The base of the proximal phalanx is freed from the collateral ligaments and is then resected using power instrumentation (Fig 22–8). Once this is completed, the sesamoids retract proximally. However, in severely arthritic joints or if the sesamoids remain prominent, it is advisable to remove the sesamoids at this time. The distal end of the joint capsule is now interposed across the joint space and sutured to the lateral capsule with 2-0 nonabsorbable suture. The remaining joint capsule is reapproximated with 3-0 nonabsorbable suture. At times it may be advantageous to insert a K wire to maintain the digit in a rectus position. Although this is acceptable in the presence of a healed ulceration, the use of foreign material should be discouraged in the presence of an open ulceration,

because this unnecessarily increases the risk of infection. If a K wire is used in the neuropathic foot, we recommend that it be removed before ambulation. The remainder of the wound is closed in standard layered fashion. As in the previous discussion, the postoperative care is dictated by the degree of ulcer healing at the time of surgery.

In addition to the usual complications of foot surgery, potential complications of this procedure include wound dehiscence, prolonged swelling, hallux extensus, transfer callus or ulceration, and lesser metatarsal stress fracture. Wound dehiscence most commonly occurs as a result of hematoma formation from the cut bone surfaces. Careful dissection and meticulous hemostasis can reduce hematoma formation. Although not absolutely necessary, the use of closed-suction drainage may be advisable. Postoperative edema can be best managed with a mild compressive dressing, elevation of the limb, and limited activity in the early postoperative period. The presence of a hallux extensus postoperatively usually results from not having properly evaluated the extensor hallucis longus tendon preoperatively or intraoperatively. If preoperative or intraoperative evaluation shows the extensor hallucis longus to be tight, it should be lengthened during surgery.

The more significant complications from the Keller arthroplasty is the development of transfer lesions or lesser metatarsal fractures. Because the first metatarsophalangeal joint is a significant weight-bearing structure, its loss will result in transfer of weight and pressure to adjacent structures. This can be manifested by either callus or ulcerations. In some individuals the forces will be so great that stress fractures may occur of either a single metatarsal or multiple metatarsals. Unfortunately, there is no predictive index for the development of these complications. Recently, the F-scan pressure measuring system has been used

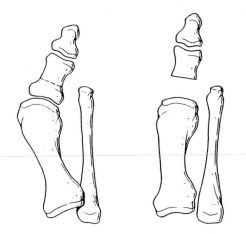

FIG 22–8.
Keller's procedure. (From Nicklas BJ: Prophylactic surgery in the diabetic foot. In Frykberg RG, editor: *The high risk foot in diabetes mellitus*, New York, 1991, Churchill Livingstone. Used by permission.)

to detect abnormal pressures in the diabetic neuropathic foot.[59] Although the technology is new, and the data are not yet analyzed, this may identify those patients at risk of developing such problems so that preventive measures can be taken. As a rule, all these patients should be fitted with soft accommodative orthoses.

Sesamoidectomy

Two factors predispose diabetic patients to the development of ulcerations under the first metatarsal. The first is the amount of weight-bearing forces generated through this area. The second factor that leads to increased risk of ulceration is progressive motor neuropathy. As motor neuropathy progresses, there is denervation of the intrinsic musculature. This leads to instability at the level of the metatarsophalangeal joints, resulting in progressive plantarflexion deformities of the metatarsals. The tibial and fibular sesamoid bones, normally located plantar to the first metatarsal head, play an important role in the normal function of the first metatarsophalangeal joint. However, as the first ray becomes progressively more plantarflexed, the sesamoid bones become more prominent and therefore contribute to the development of sub–first metatarsal ulcerations.

Sesamoid planing procedures have been described for intractable plantar keratoses and chronic ulcerations. These may work well for the treatment of intractable plantar keratoses. However, because motor neuropathy is a progressive disorder, the first metatarsal can be expected to plantarflex further because further muscle weakening occurs. This results in eventual prominence of the sesamoid bones, once again making planing procedures ineffective. Because first metatarsal osteotomies carry increased morbidity and potential for complications, we have been performing sesamoidectomy procedures for resolution of sub–first metatarsal ulcerations. We have found this procedure to be relatively simple with little morbidity for the patient and highly effective in resolving the problem of recurrent ulceration.

The basic indication for this procedure is the presence of a recurrent plantar ulceration directly under the first metatarsal head. A contraindication of this procedure is extension of the ulceration into the joint space. This is diagnostic of osteomyelitis on a clinical basis and requires excision of the involved joint. A relative contraindication of this procedure is the presence of a rigidly plantarflexed first metatarsal, and the surgeon may be advised to perform a first metatarsal osteotomy. This will be discussed in greater detail later in this chapter. We prefer, however, to still perform a sesamoidectomy in these few cases and to perform a first metatarsal osteotomy in those few cases where there is recurrence of the original ulceration.

Operative Technique.—The surgical approach for a sesamoidectomy is through a medial incision at the level of the first metatarsophalangeal joint. This allows for excellent exposure of the tibial sesamoid and adequate exposure of the fibular sesamoid should it be necessary to resect it as well. After a linear capsulotomy, further dissection and excision are facilitated by a no. 64 blade and phalangeal clamp. It is always necessary to excise the tibial sesamoid. Whether to proceed and excise the fibular sesamoid is based on intraoperative evaluation. Once the tibial sesamoid has been excised, if a plantar prominence remains directly underlying the ulcer, it is recommended that the fibular sesamoid be excised as well. This is often necessary when the first metacarpophalangeal joint is in a rectus alignment. In the presence of a severe hallux abductovalgus deformity, the fibular sesamoid is often in the first interspace and therefore does not contribute to the etiology of the ulceration. The fibular sesamoid can be left alone in this case with little risk of recurrence. The postoperative care once again includes a period of non-weight-bearing. Because the incision is made at the juncture of the dorsal and plantar skin, early weight-bearing will cause shearing forces across the incision and potential wound complications. Two potential complications of this procedure are the development of hallux hammertoe and hallux valgus. We have not encountered an increased incidence of hallux valgus; however, we have seen several cases of hallux hammertoe. One important modification to this procedure that we believe reduces the risk of hallux hammertoe development is lengthening of both the extensor and flexor hallucis longus tendons. Since incorporating this modification into the procedure, we have noted a significant reduction in the development of hallux hammertoe. As with any plantar ulceration, return to weight-bearing and full ambulation is dictated by ulcer healing. Ambulation should not be allowed while the ulcer remains open.

First Metatarsal Osteotomy

Although the majority of ulcerations respond well to excision of the sesamoids, a small number will fail to resolve. This most commonly results from the presence of a rigidly plantarflexed first ray. In these cases an osteotomy of the first metatarsal should be considered, either at the level of the surgical neck or metatarsal base. However, because of the increased morbidity of this procedure and the significant complications that may result from this procedure, it is rarely a procedure of first choice. An osteotomy of the first metatarsal requires a prolonged period of non-weight-bearing, as well as immobilization in a cast. In addition, the use of fixation devices, either K wires or screws, is imperative for proper stability of the osteotomy and bone healing. These additional variables, although important to the successful healing of the osteotomy, increase

the risk of postoperative complications. In our experience, the overall success rate of the sesamoidectomy procedure does not warrant the risk of the more involved and morbid procedure as a first choice.

Operative Technique.—An osteotomy of the first metatarsal may be performed either at the surgical neck or at the metatarsal base, just distal to the first metatarsal-medial cuneiform articulation. The decision as to where to place the osteotomy is based on the degree of plantarflexion of the first ray. For moderate degrees of plantarflexion, a distal first metatarsal osteotomy is adequate to elevate the metatarsal head. The surgical approach for a distal osteotomy is similar to that of any bunionectomy. A dorsal longitudinal incision is made centered over the first metatarsophalangeal joint and deepened to the level of the joint capsule. The joint is exposed through a capsulotomy of the surgeon's preference. Once the first metatarsal head is exposed, the periosteum is reflected at the level of the surgical neck. A sagittal saw is used to make a V-osteotomy in a dorsal to plantar direction. Once this is completed, the first metatarsal head is raised and fixated with two crossed 0.045 K wires. The incision is closed in a layered fashion. Although the sensate patient is generally allowed to ambulate on this type of osteotomy, we recommend that the neuropathic diabetic patient be kept non-weight-bearing for a minimum of 4 weeks. Because of absence of protective pain sensation, the neuropathic patient will tend to be overactive and place excessive pressure on the operated foot. This may result in a number of complications, such as excessive swelling and hematoma formation leading to wound dehiscence and possible infection. In addition, the osteotomy may be disrupted, resulting in possible dislocation of the capital fragment and nonunion.

In more severe plantarflexion deformities, the osteotomy is best performed at the base of the first metatarsal. The osteotomy can be created in one of two manners. A dorsiflexing wedge with the base directed dorsally and the apex plantarly can be made approximately 1 cm distal to the first metatarsal-medial cuneiform articulation. All attempts should be made to leave the plantar hinge intact. Two 0.062 K wires are used in a crossed manner for fixation. One K wire is directed from dorsal-medial-proximal to plantar-lateral-distal across the osteotomy. The second K wire is directed from dorsal-lateral-proximal to plantar-medial-distal. Most recently the osteotomy has been modified to allow for fixation with a single 3.5 cortical screw. An oblique osteotomy is created directed in the same manner as mentioned previously. Temporary fixation is achieved with a single 0.062 K wire, which will serve as the pilot hole for the cortical screw. A second K wire is inserted parallel to the first wire. At this time the first wire is removed, and a 3.5 cortical screw is inserted using standard AO technique. Postoperative care requires the use of a non-weight-bearing below-knee cast for a minimum of 8 weeks, followed by a weight-bearing cast for 4 weeks. Certain precautions need to be taken in the application of a cast in the insensate patient. It is advisable that the cast be well padded and that the cast be changed frequently (e.g., every 2 weeks). This will reduce the risk of abrasions and friction blisters.

First Metatarsophalangeal Joint Resection

Up to this point we have been discussing surgery for the superficial recurrent neuropathic ulceration. Implied in this definition is the fact that bony involvement of joint involvement has been actively ruled out. Without evidence of osteomyelitis, either clinical or radiographic, the surgeon should make every effort at saving the underlying bony structures. However, in the case of documented osteomyelitis, the involved structures should be excised to eliminate the focus of infection. The diagnosis of osteomyelitis is made by destructive changes visible on radiographs. In addition, an ulceration with direct communication to bone is sufficient for a clinical diagnosis of osteomyelitis in spite of negative radiographs. Therefore, an ulceration that extends into the first metatarsophalangeal joint or to the first metatarsal head is best treated with resection of that joint.

One is most commonly faced with an open, draining ulceration when osteomyelitis is present. The initial treatment for this ulceration is to gain adequate control of the acute infectious process. This may require an extensive incision and drainage procedure, along with debridement of all infected soft tissue. Once this has been accomplished, consideration is then given to the surgical approach of the infected joint. Although one could certainly approach this from a dorsal incision, we prefer to excise the ulceration and infected tissue to the joint level. The joint resection is then performed from a plantar approach, and the wound is closed, allowing it to heal in a primary fashion. The advantages to this approach are that (1) it allows for primary healing of the wound and ulceration, resulting in faster overall healing; (2) because the wound is allowed to heal by primary intention, there is greater likelihood for healing in the vascularly compromised diabetic patient; and (3) it avoids the need for a second incision on the foot where there has already been demonstrated difficulty in healing an original insult.

Operative Technique.—The plantar incision is planned in such a way that the entire ulceration is excised, as well as any remaining necrotic tissue. In addition, the incision should create enough laxity in the tissues so that the resulting wound can be reapproximated with little to no tension on the skin edges. This generally requires that the length of the incision be three to four times the width at the widest part. This most often corresponds to the location of the ulceration. The incision is made full thickness so that there is no undermining of skin edges, which minimizes dead space. Once the resulting wedge of tissue is adequately excised, it is removed from the operative field, as are all contaminated instruments. The first metatarsophalangeal joint should be readily visible at this stage. If not already free, the first metatarsal head should be freed from all soft tissue attachments. Power instrumentation is used to resect the first metatarsal head proximal to the area of osteomyelitis, ensuring an adequate margin of safety. This is best determined by degree of mineralization of the remaining bone and by adequate bleeding from the remaining proximal end. The sesamoid bones should be excised as well, because there is a high probability they are infected and may serve as a persistent focus of osteomyelitis if left behind. We also advise that the articular cartilage be removed from the base of the proximal phalanx because that is avascular tissue, which has poor resistance to infection. An added benefit to this is that the bleeding cancellous surface will help support granulation tissue. This is best accomplished with a rongeur.

Once all infected tissue has been excised, including bone, the wound is irrigated copiously with the surgeon's choice of irrigant. If a tourniquet was used at the start of the procedure, it should be deflated at this point so that the viability of the remaining tissues can be properly evaluated. Any tissue that does not bleed adequately should be further debrided at this time back to healthy bleeding tissue. Once this has been accomplished, the wound is ready for closure. For closure we prefer to use a combination of 3-0 nonabsorbable nylon sutures in a full-thickness fashion interposed with 5-0 nonabsorbable sutures. We prefer this method of wound closure rather than using deep absorbable

sutures because the addition of this foreign material may serve as a focus of infection. We additionally choose to leave the proximal portion of the incision open so that it can be packed for several days postoperatively. This will allow for adequate drainage of hematoma and other serous material (Fig 22–9).

The postoperative care after this procedure is critical to the successful healing of this wound. The patient is kept at complete bed rest with elevation of the involved foot to help reduce postoperative edema. The dressing and packing are changed daily until all drainage has ceased and there is evidence that the open wound is granulating. The patient is discharged totally non-weight-bearing only after the wound is completely dry. It is of utmost importance that the patient is completely non-weight-bearing for a minimum of 3 weeks. Ambulation earlier than this may result in wound dehiscence or hypertrophic scar formation (Fig 22–10).

Although this procedure is successful in resolving plantar ulcerations, the surgeon and patient must consider several complications. The most obvious is the risk of postoperative infection. This most commonly results from inadequate debridement or resection of infected, necrotic tissue. All efforts must be made at the time of surgery to assess the adequacy of both soft tissue debridement and bony debridement. The surgeon is best advised to remove additional bone if there is any concern regarding the quality of the remaining bone. An additional complication is the development of a transfer callus or ulcer, most commonly to the second metatarsal. We have already discussed the importance of the first metatarsal with regard to weight-bearing forces. It is reasonable to assume that the adjacent metatarsals must accept a greater percentage of pressure once the first metatarsal is excised. The patient must be made aware of this possibility so as to

A

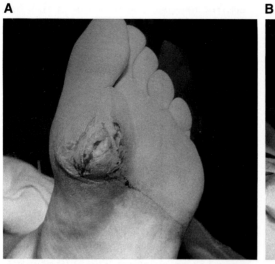

B

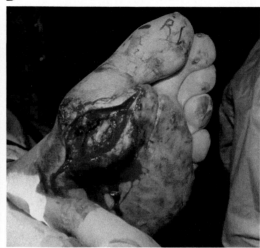

C

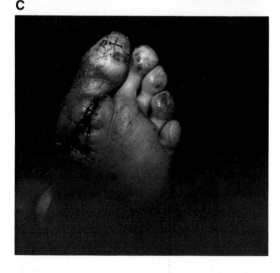

FIG 22–9.
A, plantar ulceration extending into first metacarpo-phalangeal joint. **B,** ulceration is excised in an elliptical manner exposing extensor hallucis longus and first metacarpophalangeal joint capsule. **C,** after excision of all infected tissue and resection of first metacar-pophalangeal joint, wound is closed distally and packed proximally.

avoid any misconceptions postoperatively. Should this occur, we recommend that an isolated metatarsal osteotomy be performed at a later date. In certain isolated cases where the likelihood of a transfer ulcer developing is high, a second metatarsal osteotomy can be performed at the time of the first metatarsophalangeal joint resection. Additional complications of this procedure (i.e., wound dehiscence and hypertrophic scar formation) have already been discussed. Once again, total non-weight-bearing for a minimum of 3 weeks is usually sufficient to avoid these problems.

MIDFOOT SURGERY

One of the more challenging and difficult problems for the foot surgeon is the midfoot whose normal structure has been altered by neuropathic changes of prior ablative surgery, such as first ray amputation. The degree of resulting deformity may range from barely detectable on clinical examination to severe rockerbottom appearance, as commonly seen in classic Charcot's joint disease. The deformity not only may vary in its location but also in the degree of stability, which is influenced by the current stage of the Charcot process. A fully coalesced neuroarthropathy, regardless of location, is often very stable, allowing the patient to ambulate with little difficulty. These may show significant bony prominences, which, if free of ulceration, can and should be managed conservatively with shoe therapy. On the other hand, when there is significant loss of bony substance or there is concomitant involvement of the rearfoot, the foot is severely unstable such that the medial column collapses. This not only results in unsteady ambulation but also leads to focal pressure along the medial aspect of the foot, resulting in ulcerations. The same can be said when the first ray has been amputated, as discussed earlier in this chapter. Although Charcot's joint disease is discussed in detail elsewhere, a brief review is warranted as a prelude to any discussion on surgical intervention.

Harris and Brand[61] outlined five patterns of destruction. Recognition of these patterns is important when surgical intervention is being considered for the neuropathic foot with ulceration. The most common site of involvement is the medial column (patterns 3 and 5). When signifi-

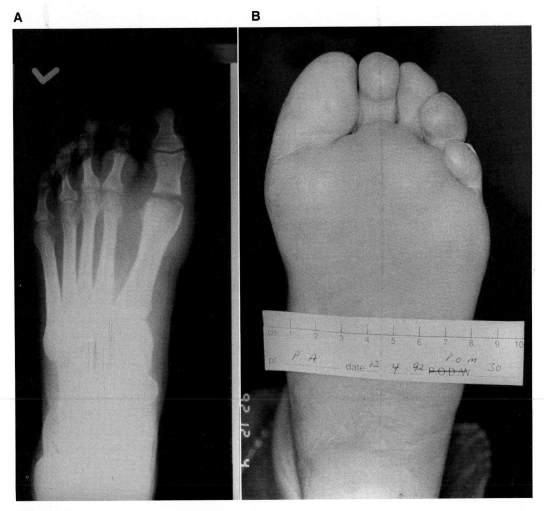

FIG 22–10.
Two and one-half years after Keller-Mayo arthroplasty using a plantar approach. Note second metatarsal osteotomy was performed at same time.

cant loss of bone substance occurs in the midfoot, severe instability may occur even in the presence of appropriate therapy. Further instability can result from complete disruption of the intermetatarsal and cuneometatarsal ligaments. The first metatarsal base and medial cuneiform will plantarflex as a unit, creating a plantarmedial prominence. When more proximal destruction occurs, collapse of the navicular and talus is likely to occur, creating the typical rockerbottom deformity often described as the hallmark of Charcot's joint disease. Pattern 4 disruptions result in loss of ligamentous integrity between the fourth and fifth metatarsals and the cuboid bone. The ligamentous connection between these three bones is more variable so that loss of this ligament may result in partial or complete plantar extrusion of the cuboid. The cuboid will often be clinically palpable on the plantar aspect of the foot, leading to plantar ulceration. Harris and Brand[61] state this pattern of destruction does poorly with conservative care and often requires surgical intervention.

Based on our experience with this pattern of destruction, we are in complete agreement with them. A thorough preoperative evaluation includes assessment of foot mechanics, including all structures affecting foot mechanics. With destruction of the midfoot and resulting structural abnormalities, joint axes are changed, as is the normal relationship between agonist and antagonist muscle function. The posterior tibial muscle, which functions to invert and adduct the foot, is weakened on collapse of the medial arch, resulting in a relative lengthening of its origin to insertion. This allows the peroneus brevis muscle and the extensor digitorum longus to evert and abduct the forefoot, creating the classic rockerbottom appearance to the foot. The Achilles tendon is likewise affected by this change in joint axis. Normally the Achilles tendon plantarflexes and supinates the foot. When the midfoot is destroyed by the Charcot process and collapses, the axis of action of the Achilles tendon changes such that the Achilles tendon will pronate the foot and plantarflex the rearfoot with the fulcrum at Lisfranc's joint. It is important to realize this preoperatively because failure to address this surgically may lead to failure of the procedure.

Surgical Procedures

First Metatarsal-Medial Cuneiform Exostectomy

Plantar medial ulcerations in the region of the midfoot may result from previous surgical intervention on the distal first metatarsal, such as hallux or first ray amputation or first metatarsal head resection. Loss of this important weight-bearing structure leads to transfer of weight and pressure more proximally. In the presence of an enlarged first metatarsal base, this focal pressure may lead to ulceration. In addition, loss of the first ray leads to medial column instability and increased pronation functional loss of the extensor hallucis longus.

Exostectomy of the plantar surface of the first metatarsal base is a simple and highly successful procedure for medial column ulcerations. A list of the indications for this procedure follows. Lack of attention to these indications can result in surgical failure and recurrent ulceration:

1. Plantar or plantar-medial ulceration directly underlying first metatarsal base.
2. Plantarly prominent, enlarged first metatarsal base, or both.
3. Stable first metatarsal-medial cuneiform joint.
4. No equinus deformity unless addressed by a second procedure.

Procedure.—The presence of an open ulceration does not preclude surgical intervention. Precautions, however, must

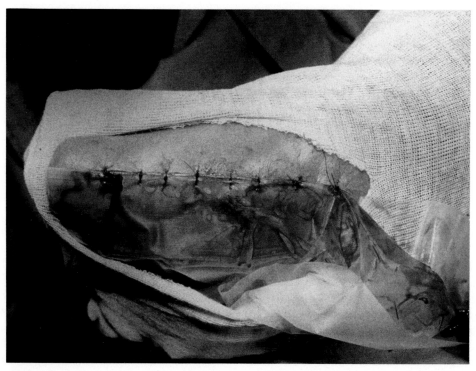

FIG 22–11.
Cross-contamination between ulcer and surgical incision can be prevented by use of an impermeable drape sewn in place.

be taken to avoid contamination of the surgical site. The use of a sterile adhesive drape sutured over the ulceration reduces the risk of cross-contamination by the surgeon and assistant (Fig 22–11). The surgical approach is dictated by the depth of the ulcer. When the ulceration is superficial and does not directly communicate with bone, a medial incision at the juncture of the dorsal and plantar skin is preferred. This avoids a plantar incision and prolonged periods of non-weight-bearing. This also allows for excellent exposure of the first metatarsal medial cuneiform articulation. This articulation should be visualized because it is often necessary to plane both the plantar surface of the first metatarsal base and the plantar surface of the medial cuneiform. Once the periosteum is elevated from the underlying bone, an osteotome or sagittal saw can be used to resect the bony prominence. Care

must be taken to avoid creating a bony prominence. Therefore, it is important that all bony spicules are removed and all rough surfaces are smoothed. The surgical wound is closed in layers with suture material of the surgeon's choice. The use of drains is rarely necessary in this procedure. However, when large amounts of bone are resected, it may be advisable to use closed-suction drainage because a hematoma can lead to wound problems (e.g., dehiscence or infection). The immediate postoperative management of these patients must include total non-weight-bearing and elevation of the extremity. In the presence of an open ulceration, the dressing is changed on the first postoperative day. When no ulcer is present, it is best to leave the dressing alone until the third postoperative day. Sutures are left in place a minimum of 2 weeks. Weight-bearing begins only when sutures are removed and the ulcer is completely healed.

Open ulcerations with direct communication to the underlying bone are often best approached with an exostectomy and excision of the ulcer. The ulcer is then closed primarily. The advantages of this technique are:

1. Complete removal of ulcer and surrounding necrotic and infected tissue.
2. Direct exposure of involved bone.
3. Primary healing of ulceration.

Although several advantages exist, there certainly are several disadvantages with this approach. The main disadvantage is the possibility of inadequate debridement, thus leaving behind infected tissue. This may serve as a focus of residual infection and potential wound problems. A second disadvantage is the presence of a plantar incision. This has not been a major disadvantage in our experience, provided certain guidelines are followed. Total non-weight-bearing must be adhered to for a minimum of 3 weeks. Earlier ambulation may lead to wound dehiscence and infection. However, in the presence of a chronically recurrent ulceration with clinical osteomyelitis, this technique may reduce healing to 3 to 4 weeks when healing by secondary intention would have taken much longer. In addition, primary closure of wounds is desirable in ischemic or marginally ischemic patients because their ability to granulate large wounds is extremely poor.

The surgical approach is to perform a double elliptical incision, fully excising the ulceration (Fig 22–12). The critical factor in operative planning is to make the incision long enough such that wound closure can be achieved with as little tension on the wound as possible. It is recommended that the length of the incision be at least three to four times the width. The incision is carried down to the level of the

dermis, removing the ulcer and all necrotic and infected tissue surrounding the ulceration. Once the ulcer is fully excised, the underlying bony prominence should be clearly visible. All soft tissue attachments are released such that the bony prominence can be easily dissected from the surrounding tissue. The bony prominence is then resected using either an osteotome or sagittal saw. Sufficient bone is removed so as to create a "valley" in the region of the ulceration. All bone that is soft and necrotic is removed until firm, bleeding bone is encountered. Once again, care must be taken not to leave prominent bony spicules or edges. These edges are smoothed and beveled using a double-action rongeur or bone rasp. Wound closure is achieved by using 3-0 nylon sutures in the form of full-thickness retention sutures. This allows for reapproximation of deeper layers without the introduction of deep sutures, which may act as a focus of infection. In addition, these retention sutures will reduce tension along the incision line. The remainder of the incision is reapproximated with 4-0 nylon suture. It is often advisable to pack the proximal aspect of the incision to allow for dependent drainage. However, in the ischemic diabetic patient, complete closure of the wound is recommended because these patients lack the ability to granulate wounds. The postoperative management of these patients requires a minimum of 3 weeks of non-weight-bearing. It is advisable that sutures remain in place for 3 weeks. Once sutures are removed, the patient is returned to shoes gradually.

As with all surgical procedures, complications may occur. The most common complications seen include postoperative infection, wound dehiscence, or recurrent ulceration. Surgery performed in the presence of an open ulceration increases the risk of an infection. The use of perioperative antibiotics, along with intraoperative draping of the ulcer, helps reduce the incidence of infection. Wound dehiscence is more likely to occur after excision of the ulceration and primary closure as a result of either wound closure under tension or possible hematoma formation. The use of retention sutures and meticulous dissec-tion will aid in reducing wound tension and dead space and subsequent hematoma collection. In addition, the judicious use of closed-suction drainage can reduce hematoma collection. As previously dis-

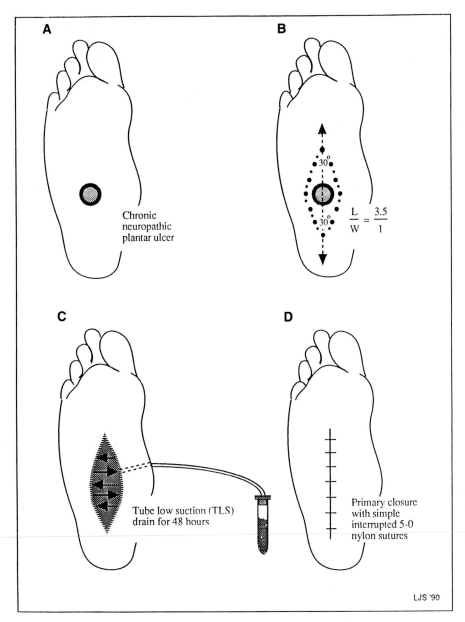

FIG 22–12.
A–D, technique for the surgical management of chronic plantar ulceration associated with diabetic neuropathic osteoarthropathy. (From Sanders LJ, Frykberg RG: Diabetic neuropathic osteoarthropathy: The Charcot foot. In Frykberg RG, editor: *The high risk foot in diabetes mellitus,* New York, 1991, Churchill Livingstone. Used by permission.)

cussed, it is important to evaluate the Achilles tendon for possible contracture. This is critical with either of these procedures. Very often these procedures are performed in the presence of either a first ray amputation or first metatarsal head resection. These procedures lead to loss of medial column stability and excessive pronation. This pronatory action is further accentuated by the presence of a gastrocsoleus equinus. Not recognizing this preoperatively may lead to failure of surgery and recurrence of the ulceration.

Surgical resection of the bony prominence will allow for successful management of the majority of these medial column ulcerations. However, if preoperative evaluation suggests hypermobility at the first metatarsal medial cuneiform joint as a result of severe Charcot's joint destruction, consideration should be given to primary fusion of this joint. Clinical examination of this foot may not reveal a significant bony prominence underlying the ulceration. Further, no obvious exostosis will be noted on radiographs. When the foot is allowed to bear weight, however, the collapse of the medial column becomes obvious. This instability can be further demonstrated when the first metatarsal-medial cuneiform joint is put through a range of motion. The joint can be subluxated manually in a plantar direction. There may be crepitus in the joint with range of motion, suggesting loss of joint congruity with significant loss of articular cartilage. These may be seen on plain radiographs. In addition to involvement of the first metatarsal medial cuneiform joint, radiographs may show involvement of other joints in the midfoot. The degree of destruction and instability dictates the extent of surgical reconstruction required.

Operative Technique.—A dorsomedial incision is made of sufficient length to allow adequate exposure of the joint and surrounding soft tissue. This is deepened in a standard fashion until the articulation between the first metatarsal and medial cuneiform is identified. This can be performed by putting this joint through a range of motion and noting buckling in the joint capsule or inserting a 25-gauge needle into what appears to be the joint. Once the joint is identified, a longitudinal incision is made through the joint capsule, and the capsule is freed from the underlying bone using a periosteal elevator. Once this maneuver is completed, the articular surfaces should be readily visible. The articular surfaces are next resected from the base of the first metatarsal and the distal surface of the medial cuneiform. All cartilage should be removed to improve the likelihood of joint fusion. If a sagittal plane deformity (e.g., dorsiflexion or plantarflexion) exists in the first ray, it may be corrected by resecting the articular surface in a wedge fashion. For example, if the first ray is plantarflexed and dorsiflexion is desired, the cartilage should be resected such that the base is directed dorsally and the apex is directed plantarly. Remodeling of the bony surfaces should be performed until the osteotomy site is closed without gapping. It is also important to avoid any interposition of soft tissue within the osteotomy because this could lead to delayed union.

Fixation of the osteotomy can be achieved by a variety of techniques. Use of two crossed 0.062 Kirschner wires across the osteotomy will provide stability in all three planes. However, this mode of fixation does not provide compression. A second means of fixation involves the use of two staples inserted with the 3M Stapilizer (Fig 22–13). One 10 by 13 mm staple should be inserted on the dorsal surface of the joint, and a second 10 by 13 mm staple should be inserted on the medial surface of the joint. Once again, this fixation device will allow for good approximation of the bony surfaces with stability in all three planes but does not provide compression. Most recently, plates and screws have been used for internal fixa-

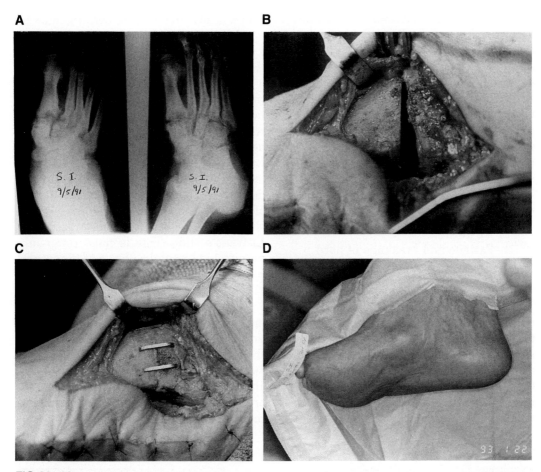

FIG 22–13.
A, loss of bone substance can lead to significant in-stability at the first metacarpophalangeal joint–medial cuneiform articulation such that fusion should be con-sidered. **B,** the articular cartilage is removed from the base of the first metatarsal and the distal surface of the medial cuneiform. **C,** the joint is stabilized with two staples medially and one staple dorsally. **D,** patient 9 months after first metacarpophalangeal joint–medial cuneiform fusion with staples.

tion. A five-hole dynamic compression T plate with 3.5-mm cortical screws and a 4.0-mm interfragmentary screw is well suited for this type of osteotomy (Fig 22–14). Although this technique is techni-cally more difficult, this form of fixation provides excellent compression and will allow for primary bone healing and earlier ambulation. The wound is then closed in a layered fashion starting with the joint capsule. Regardless of type of fixation used, all patients are maintained on a to-tally non-weight-bearing regimen for a minimum of 3 months. The decision of when to begin ambulation is dictated by clinical, as well as radiographic, findings. If rigid internal fixation is used in the form of screws and plates, ambulation can usually begin at this point in a well-pad-ded walking cast. If K wires or staples are used, patients usually do not begin weight-bearing for at least 4 to 5 months. The surgeon must be cautious when al-lowing these patients to begin weight-bearing. Because of peripheral sensory neuropathy, patients' activity will not be limited by pain. Strict instructions and parameters must be outlined for the patient to avoid potential complications such as cast irritations or disruption of the osteotomy site. The surgeon would be well served to extend the period of non-weight-bearing one and one-half to two times the normal non-weight-bearing period in non-neuropathic patients.

In addition to the complications already listed for the previous procedures, other possible complications include:

1. Delayed or nonunion of fusion site.
2. Skin irritation from underlying hardware.
3. Fatigue and breakage of hardware.
4. Cast abrasion or irritation.

The patient must be well informed not only of the prolonged rehabilitation from this procedure but also of the potential complications and risks. The patient must also be made aware of the possibility of further surgery in the future either to manage these complications or to deal with a recurrent ulceration. The impor-

tance of total non-weight-bearing must be emphasized to the patient.

Lesser Metatarsal-Cuneiform Fusion

It has been our experience that primary fusion of Lisfranc's joint is often unnecessary and that patients do quite well with prolonged non-weight-bearing or with isolated first metatarsal-medial cuneiform fusion. If, however, Lisfranc's joint (tarsometatarsal articulation) is deemed unstable laterally and the degree of destruction is severe, consideration should be given to primary fusion of Lisfranc's joint. This is most commonly manifested by total collapse of the lateral column of the foot.

Operative Technique.—The first metatarsal-medial cuneiform articulation is fused as described previously and should be performed as the initial procedure. This will allow for correction of any abductory deformity by removing the appropriate wedge of bone. Once this procedure is completed, the midfoot is eval-

A

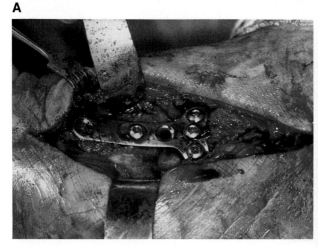

B

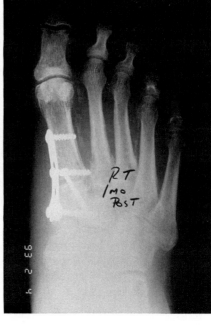

FIG 22–14.
Primary fusion may also be achieved using a T plate and interfragmentary screw.

uated for further instability. If necessary, the second metatarsal-intermediate cuneiform joint is next fused. A dorsal longitudinal incision is made over the involved joint. If fusion of the third metatarsal-lateral cuneiform joint is necessary, the dorsal longitudinal incision can be centered between the second and third metatarsals. The incision is then deepened to the joint level. The joint capsule is incised longitudinally, exposing the articular surfaces of the involved joints. Any loose bony debris should be removed at this time. The articular cartilage is resected in a dorsal to plantar direction, care being taken to avoid the intermetatarsal artery. Once the cartilage is resected, the bones are temporarily fixated with a 0.062 K wire. Fixation of the arthrodesis can be achieved using the 3M Stapilizer, because this will provide adequate stability. An identical procedure can be performed for the remaining articulations.

Lateral Column Procedures

Cuboid Exostectomy.—Ulcerations underlying the cuboid bone are the most problematic ulcers to treat for the podiatric physician. These are the pattern five lesions described by Harris and Brand.[61] Although medial collapse rockerbottom deformity is the most common pattern, plantar extrusion of the cuboid with adduction of the forefoot is not unusual. In this pattern there is disruption of the lateral tarsal-metatarsal ligaments, causing the cuboid to become dislocated in a plantar direction. This results in the cuboid not only becoming plantarly prominent but also rotated such that the peroneal groove is directed plantarly. This can lead to callus formation and ulceration. All conservative measures (e.g., shoe and orthoses) should be exhausted before surgical intervention. When conservative care fails to maintain ulcer healing, surgical intervention is appropriate. The surgical approach is dependent on the degree of ulcer healing and ulcer depth.

The ulcer that is healed at the time of surgery or is superficial without bone involvement is best approached by a plantar longitudinal incision. When the ulcer probes to bone with definite bone involvement, surgical excision of the ulceration and underlying bony prominence is recommended. Occasionally when the ulceration is extensive, making primary closure tenuous, consideration may be given to bony resection with fasciocutaneous flap and split-thickness skin graft. All three procedures will be described.

Procedure.—When no ulcer is present at the time of surgery or the ulcer is superficial, a plantar longitudinal incision is made over the bony prominence (in the presence of an open ulceration, this incision is placed just lateral to the ulceration). The wound is deepened in standard fashion until the cuboid is visualized. It is crucial that the surrounding soft tissue structures are freed so that adequate cuboid is exposed. Once this is completed, an osteotome and mallet are used to resect the prominent bony eminence. The surgeon should be aggressive in the exostectomy because the most common cause of failure is inadequate resection. In addition, the wound should be carefully explored for any bony spicules, which are then remodeled with a double-action rongeur. Once the surgeon is comfortable with the degree of bony resection, the wound is closed in a layered fashion. Because the amount of bone resected can sometimes be considerable, the development of postoperative hematoma can be a complicating factor. It is often beneficial to use closed-suction drainage for the first 24 to 48 hours. This should be inserted before closure of the deep layers.

The postoperative management of these wounds is the same as with any plantar incision, in other words, total non-weight-bearing for 3 to 4 weeks and gradual advancement to shoe gear. The use of a posterior splint is often recommended to reduce shear forces across the incision, as well as to protect the incision in case of accidental weight-bearing. Elevation and gentle compression may likewise be beneficial.

When the ulceration is more extensive and, in fact, communicates with the underlying bone, surgical excision of the ulceration is often indicated. This excision and bony resection may be accomplished in one of two ways: primary closure or with muscle and fasciocutaneous flap and skin graft. The decision as to which procedure to perform is based on the overall size of the ulceration. In the cases of relatively small ulcerations, primary closure can be achieved with little tension on the wound. In the case of larger ulcerations, however, primary closure would result in excessive tension on the wound. These wounds are best managed with a rotational fasciocutaneous skin flap and skin grafting of the resulting defect.

Operative Technique.—When the ulceration is excised, the same basic rule applies as previously stated: the length of the incision should be three to four times the width. This usually allows for primary closure of the wound with little tension. The initial skin incision is made to the level of the dermis, excising all necrotic and infected tissue along the way. Very often an adventitious bursa exists at the base of these ulcerations. It is important to excise this bursa as completely as possible because this may serve as a constant source of infection and drainage. Once this is completed, the surgeon should be at the level of the bony prominence. The soft tissues surrounding this prominence should be dissected from the underlying bone. As before, once the bone is adequately exposed, an osteotome and mallet is used to resect the prominence. A double-action rongeur is used to further remodel the cuboid. The use of closed-suction drainage may be indicated because hematoma formation is the most common complication.

Wound closure is achieved by applying full-thickness retention sutures of 3-0 nylon suture. This is reinforced with 4-0 or 5-0 nylon suture for full wound closure. We do not recommend the use of any deep absorbable sutures in a recently infected wound. This adds an additional risk of deep wound infection. Should a postoperative infection develop, the nylon sutures can be removed without having to worry about deep sutures acting as a focus of infection. The postoperative management includes daily dressing changes until the wound is completely free of any drainage. Once again, total non-weight-bearing is required for 3 to 4 weeks (Fig 22–15).

When ulcerations are larger than 2.0 cm in diameter, primary closure of the wound may result in excessive tension that may lead to wound dehiscence. These cases are best managed by wound closure involving some type of rotational skin flap. Over the past 5 years we have gained increasing experience using a rotational fasciocutaneous skin flap with interposing muscle flap over the bony prominence. This flap is based on the medial plantar artery as its main blood supply. This has provided primary closure of the wound with additional soft tissue coverage over the resected bone. This procedure is best performed with the patient in the prone position. The ulcer and all underlying bursal tissue is excised in a circumferential manner. All necrotic and infected tissue must be excised. Care must be taken to avoid the lateral plantar artery and nerve, which usually course directly over this area from medial to lateral. Care must also be taken to spare any intrinsic musculature because this will be needed for interposition over the resected bone. This then allows for exposure of the bony prominence, which is once again freed from the surrounding soft tissue as in previous procedures. The bone is resected, and attention must be taken not to leave any prominent bony spicules behind. Once this is completed, intrinsic musculature is ro-

A

B

C

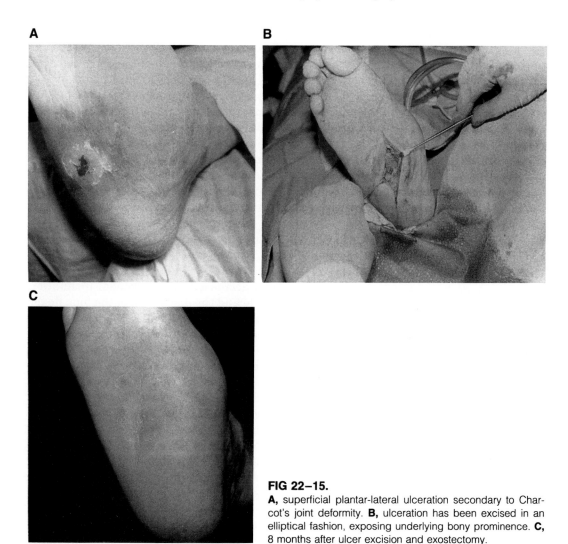

FIG 22–15.
A, superficial plantar-lateral ulceration secondary to Charcot's joint deformity. **B,** ulceration has been excised in an elliptical fashion, exposing underlying bony prominence. **C,** 8 months after ulcer excision and exostectomy.

tated from medial to lateral over this area. Because of the location of these ulcerations, the most common muscle used is the flexor digitorum brevis. The muscle belly is dissected free distally and centrally, allowing it to be rotated on its proximal attachment. The distal end and the lateral side of the muscle belly are then reattached to the surrounding soft tissue. A flap composed of skin and fascia is fashioned that can be rotated distally and medially and is based proximally on the medial plantar artery. The flap is gradually dissected until it can be rotated freely and without vascular compromise. Once this is completed, the distal and lateral edges of the flap are sutured to the adjacent skin. The donor site from the medial arch is then covered with a split-thickness skin graft taken from the lateral thigh. Closed-suction drainage and a gentle compression dressing are critical to the success of the skin graft. The postoperative management of this procedure requires not disturbing the graft site for at least 72 hours. Therefore, the dressing is not changed for 3 days. Once it is determined that the skin graft has taken, dressings can be changed more regularly. Once again, the use of a posterior splint is helpful in reducing shear across incision lines. The major complication (aside from infections) is hematoma formation either under the flap or skin graft. This may result in loss of the flap or skin graft. If a hematoma is detected under the skin graft, these should be evacuated with small superficial incisions in the graft itself to facilitate drainage. Daily dressing changes are then performed. Total non-weight-bearing must be maintained for 4 to 6 weeks if the flap is to be fully incorporated (Fig 22–16).

The advantages of this procedure are that (1) it allows for primary closure of large defects on the plantar surface; (2) it rotates thicker, healthier skin over a previously ulcerated area; (3) it adds additional soft tissue cushioning over a previously prominent area; (4) the fasciocutaneous flap is a vascularized flap with a higher chance of success; and (5) it provides a flat surface for ambulation that is more resistant to further ulceration.

TENDO-ACHILLES LENGTHENING AFTER TRANSMETATARSAL AMPUTATION

It has been stated by Dr. Paul Brand that if a neuropathic patient's stride length could be restricted to 14 in., one might expect the chronically recurrent ulceration to remain closed. This is especially true if the ulcer is occurring on a transmetatarsal amputation in which the surface area has diminished but the forces remain the same. Excess vertical and shear forces become concentrated at the distal plantar aspect of the transmetatarsal amputation and can lead to skin breakdown. Heterotopic bone formation at the distal aspects of the metatarsal stumps will also contribute to skin breakdown. When these dynamic and structural changes occur, recurrent ulceration leading to osteomyelitis can threaten the limb.

A short shoe with a functional rocker sole and molded Plastazote insert will have the effect of causing the affected limb to buckle at the knee at midstance, thereby causing a shortened stride. This nonsurgical method of shortening stride should be attempted first. The lack of a toe box on the shoe will prevent a lever effect against the end of the foot. If a toe box is desired, it should be scooped at the end so it does not impact the distal end of the transmetatarsal amputation. Plans for surgery should ensue if the foot continues to ulcerate.

Equinovarus deformity is common after transmetatarsal amputation because of a decrease of the calcaneal inclination angle and the disruption of the long flexor and extensor tendons. The tendo-Achilles lengthening is successful because it shortens the stride length during gait. The gastrocsoleus acts to slow down the forward progression of the tibia especially at midstance and beyond. If the gastrocsoleus complex is weakened by the tendo-Achilles lengthening, a short step must be taken for the knee not to buckle on the affected side. Patients learn very quickly that they will feel very unsteady in gait if too long a step is taken.

The tendo-Achilles lengthening is usually done at the same time as a transmetatarsal amputation revision. Acute infection must be absent. Because it is a clean procedure, the tendo-Achilles lengthening should be done first. Transmetatarsal amputation revision may then proceed using the same instruments.

Procedure

Lengthening may be achieved by a slide or Z lengthening. Removal of a section of the Achilles tendon is not necessary. A lateral posterior approach is preferred. The paratenon is punctured, and a dissecting scissor is used to incise it along the full length of the 8-cm incision. The tendon is exposed and lengthened. The plantaris tendon is tenotomized. Hemostasis is imperative before closure. The paratenon is closed, followed by the skin in the desired fashion. Postoperatively the foot is placed in a posterior splint with abundant padding to protect the heel from pressure to avoid a decubitus ulcer. The patient is kept off the foot until the transmetatarsal amputation revision has healed, usually 1 month. If tendo-Achilles lengthening was done without transmetatarsal amputation revision, ambulation

may ensue within 1 week. An ankle foot orthosis is usually not necessary.

The thought of weakening the gastrocsoleus complex with tendo-Achilles lengthening goes against the very principles of maintaining biomechanical balance of the lower extremity. Limb-threatening problems, however, will alter what may be expected as the future use of the affected limb. If tendo-Achilles lengthening will help prevent the patient from needing a prosthesis and preserve a living structure for him or her to step on, the

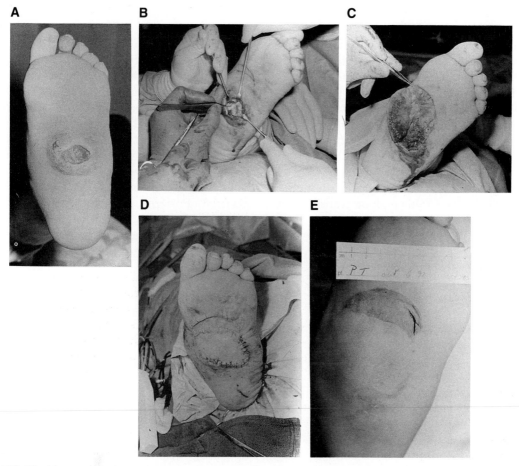

FIG 22–16.
A, deep plantar-lateral ulceration secondary to Charcot's joint deformity. **B,** ulceration has been saucerized, exposing plantarly prominent cuboid bone, which can now be resected. **C,** fasciocutaneous flap is rotated over ulcer site, which has been filled by flexor digitorum brevis muscle flap. **D,** flap is sutured in place and donor site is covered with split-thickness skin graft. **E,** 2 years after fasciocutaneous flap with split-thickness skin graft.

appropriate use of this procedure can be justified. This has been our experience, and we believe it has helped many neuropathic patients avoid major amputation.

ARTHRODESIS PROCEDURES

There are many situations in which the clinician is faced with offering a diabetic patient with severe neuropathic complications the choice of amputation or reconstructive procedure. Amputation is many times looked on by the diabetic patient as the last chapter in a lifetime of continual upset caused by diabetes. Because of this, an option other than amputation will in most cases be preferred by the patient. The clinician must take pains to ensure that the expectations of the patient are clearly defined and the expected outcome of the procedure is realistic in the framework of the patient's medical, financial, and social condition. All of these procedures require extended periods of non-weight-bearing. The home situation must be conducive to this end, or placement in

an extended care facility must be sought. Other services such as intravenous therapy, visiting nurses, physical therapy, occupational therapy, and homemaker all must be planned in advance. Meetings must be held with the immediate family so all involved will understand what is expected of them and the patient.

Arthrodesis procedures in neuropathic patients are usually selected as an alternative to major amputation. Deep sepsis must be controlled and be progressing toward healing before consideration of reconstruction. Osteomyelitis is commonly a complicating factor and is ideally removed before the definitive procedure is performed. We do not advocate reconstructive surgery merely to straighten a deformed foot. We prefer to accommodate a deformity with appropriate shoeing and follow up as long as possible. Structural stability is the goal of reconstructive surgery in the foot that cannot remain healed otherwise. We do not try to restore longitudinal or transverse arch structure to the operated foot but seek a plantigrade position. Patients are kept non-weight-

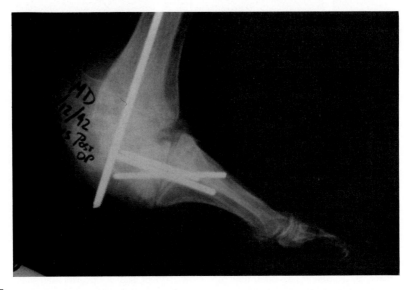

FIG 22–17.
Pantalar fusion. Patient with Charcot's midfoot, subtalar, and ankle. Chronic, nonhealing ulcer developed over dislocated talar head. Steinmann's pins were re-moved at 17 weeks. Patient is now ambulating in molded shoe and rigid, padded ankle foot orthosis.

A   B   C

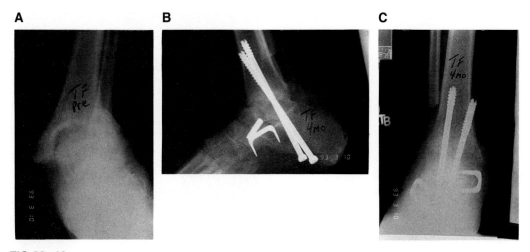

FIG 22–18.
A, preoperative anteroposterior radiograph of destroyed Charcot ankle with osteomyelitis of the fibula in a patient with 20-year history of type I diabetes mellitus. **B,** 4 months' postoperative pantalar arthrodesis. Two 6.5-mm cannulated screws were used to fuse subtalar and ankle joints. Staples fixate the talonavicular and calcaneocuboid joints. Note the medial calcification of the posterior tibial artery. **C,** anteroposterior radiograph at 4 months, indicating bony union at ankle arthrodesis site.

bearing for 3 to 4 months after surgery. This is adjusted according to the postoperative clinical and radiographic findings.

Procedure Selection

The procedure is selected by the location of the instability. Whatever is unstable is to be stabilized by arthrodesis. Procedures will occur at single or multiple locations at the tarsometatarsal, midtarsal, subtalar, and ankle joints. The decision to fuse one or more of the locations must be individually considered. Tarsometatarsal joint instability is usually done alone. Subtalar and midtarsal joint involvement will usually translate to triple arthrodesis. An unstable ankle with talar or calcaneal collapse will usually require pantalar arthrodesis (Fig 22–17). Fractured malleoli without tarsal involvement is usually an acute event and should be treated early with open reduction and internal fixation.

Whenever possible, internal fixation with compression is desired. Cannulated 6.5-mm cancellous screws have worked quite nicely in fusion of the ankle and subtalar joint (Fig 22–18). The guide K wires may be drilled from above or below for placement of at least two screws. Intraoperative x-ray films are useful to determine screw placement. Vitallium epiphyseal staples with predrilled eccentrically placed entry points are preferred for the midtarsal joint (Fig 22–19). Compression can be expected if they are placed in this fashion. When bone density is less than desirable for large internal fixation screws, threaded Steinmann pins may be used liberally. They do not cause compression but afford adequate stability. When osteomyelitis is a predominant feature around the ankle joint, external fixation devices will be of use (Fig 22–20). We have not used external fixators for midtarsal or tarsometatarsal fusions.

Successful fusion is dependent on absence of infection, adequate vascular supply, non-weight-bearing, and meticulous removal of all cartilage surfaces along with subchondral bone. Careful attention to these factors will lead to an acceptable result. Ankle foot orthoses lined with soft material is commonly used after such procedures (Fig 22–21). We prefer the use of

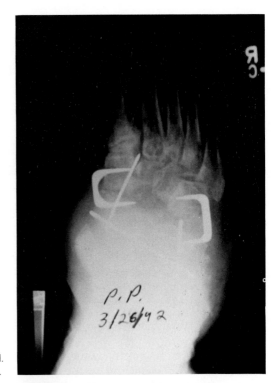

FIG 22–19.
Triple arthrodesis. Complete talonavicular dislocation with chronic ulcer medial and plantar to the talar head. Fixation with epiphyseal staples and Steinmann's pins.

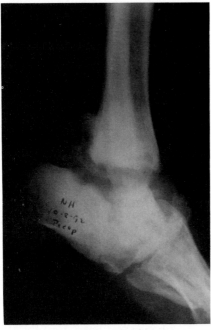 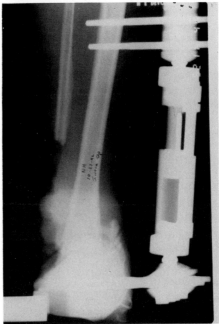

FIG 22–20.
A, Charcot's rearfoot and ankle. Complete destruction of the rearfoot with medial deviation of the foot. The medial malleolus is fractured. **B,** ankle-subtalar joint fusion with external fixator in place. Fibula was re-moved because of osteomyelitis. External fixator re-mained in place for 16 weeks. Patient is now walking with rigid, padded ankle foot orthosis.

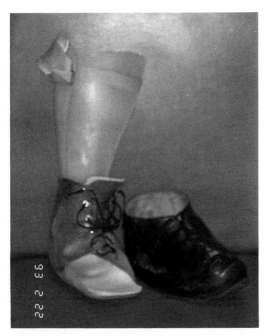

FIG 22–21.
Rigid, padded ankle foot orthosis and molded shoe. These are most commonly used in post–rearfoot and ankle reconstruction patients.

molded shoes if significant deformity persists. Finally, protection of the contralateral side must be employed because of the possibility of neuropathic fracture on that side.

CONCLUSION

The diabetic foot is not one to be feared but respected and treated appropriately. With an ultimate goal toward limb preservation, structural and mechanical alterations in the feet of persons with diabetes must be dealt with cautiously, as well as deliberately. When conservative efforts fail, reconstructive procedures are advisable to eliminate underlying bony prominences that directly contribute to ulcer causation. It is much preferable to select an opportune time to correct structural deformities than to wait until amputation becomes necessary as a result of progressive infection and gangrene.

With proper attention to detail and the principles herein outlined, no one should be denied the opportunity for reconstructive foot surgery simply because of the presence of diabetes mellitus.

REFERENCES

1. Borssen B, Bergenheim T, Lithner F: The epidemiology of foot lesions in diabetic patients aged 15–50 years, *Diabetic Med* 7:438–444, 1990.
2. Holewski JJ et al: Prevalence of foot pathology and lower extremity complications in a diabetic outpatient clinic, *J Rehabil Res Dev* 26:35–44, 1989.
3. Cavanagh PR, Sims DS, Sanders LJ: Body mass is a poor predictor of peak plantar pressure in diabetic men, *Diabetes Care* 15:750–755, 1991.
4. Delbridge L et al: The aetiology of diabetic neuropathic ulceration of the foot, *Br J Surg* 72:1–6, 1985.
5. Ctercteko GC et al: Vertical forces acting on the feet of diabetic patients with neuropathic ulceration, *Br J Surg* 68:608–614, 1981.
6. Delbridge L, Appleberg M, Reeve TS: Factors associated with development of foot lesions in the diabetic, *Surgery* 93:78–82, 1983.
7. Frykberg RG: Diabetic foot ulcerations. In Frykberg RG, editor: *The high risk foot in diabetes mellitus,* New York, 1991, Churchill Livingstone.
8. Lang-Stevenson AI et al: Neuropathic ulcers of the foot, *J Bone Joint Surg [Br]* 67:438–442, 1985.
9. Boulton AJM et al: Dynamic foot pressure and other studies as diagnostic and management aids in diabetic neuropathy, *Diabetes Care* 6:26–33, 1983.
10. Duckworth T et al: Plantar pressure measurements and the prevention of ulceration in the diabetic foot, *J Bone Joint Surg* 67:79–85, 1985.
11. Delbridge L et al: Limited joint mobility in the diabetic foot: relationship to neuropathic ulceration, *Diabetic Med* 5:333–337, 1988.
12. Fernando DJS et al: Relationship of limited joint mobility to abnormal foot pres-

sures and diabetic foot ulceration, *Diabetes Care* 14:8–11, 1991.

13. Mueller MJ et al: Insensitivity, limited joint mobility, and plantar ulcers in patients with diabetes mellitus, *Phys Ther* 69:453–462, 1989.

14. Masson EA et al: Abnormal foot pressures alone may not cause ulceration, *Diabetic Med* 6:426–428, 1989.

15. Pirart J: Diabetes mellitus and its complications: a prospective study of 4,400 patients observed between 1947 and 1973, *Diabetes Care* 1:168–188, 1978.

16. Davidson MB: An overview of diabetes mellitus. In Frykberg RG, editor: *The high risk foot in diabetes mellitus,* New York, 1991, Churchill Livingstone.

17. Niklas BJ: Prophylactic surgery in the diabetic foot. In Frykberg RG, editor: *The high risk foot in diabetes mellitus,* New York, 1991, Churchill Livingstone.

18. Dannels E: Neuropathic foot ulcer prevention in diabetic American Indians with hallux limitus, *J Am Podiatr Med Assoc* 79:447–450, 1989.

19. Dannels E: A preventive metatarsal osteotomy for healing pre-ulcers in American Indian diabetics, *J Am Podiatr Med Assoc* 76:33–37, 1986.

20. Downs DM, Jacobs RL: Treatment of resistant ulcers on the plantar surface of the great toe in diabetics, *J Bone Joint Surg [Am]* 64:930–933, 1982.

21. Diabetic foot ulcers [editorial]. *Lancet* 1:232–233, 1977.

22. Frykberg RG: Podiatric problems in diabetes. In Kozak GP et al, editors: *Management of diabetic foot problems,* Philadelphia, 1984, WB Saunders.

23. Giurini JM, Habershaw GM, Chrzan JS: Panmetatarsal head resection in chronic neuropathic ulceration, *J Foot Surg* 26:249–252, 1987.

24. Gudas CJ: Prophylactic surgery in the diabetic foot, *Clin Podiatr Med Surg* 4:445–458, 1987.

25. Harkless LB, Dennis KJ: The role of the podiatrist. In Levin ME, O'Neal LW, editors: *The diabetic foot,* St Louis, 1988, Mosby–Year Book.

26. Jacobs RL: Hoffman procedure in the ulcerated diabetic neuropathic foot, *Foot and Ankle* 3:142–149, 1982.

27. Kelly PJ, Coventry MB: Neurotrophic ulcers of the feet, *JAMA* 168:388–393, 1958.

28. Martin JD et al: Radical treatment of mal perforans in diabetic patients with arterial insufficiency, *J Vasc Surg* 12:264–268, 1990.

29. McCook J et al: Surgical treatment of the perforating ulcer of the foot, *J Cardiovasc Surg* 7:101–107, 1966.

30. Singer A: Surgical treatment of mal perforans, *Arch Surg* 111:964–968, 1976.

31. Tillo TH et al: Review of metatarsal osteotomies for the treatment of neuropathic ulcerations, *J Am Podiatr Med Assoc* 80:211–217, 1990.

32. Goldenberg S et al: Nonatheromatous peripheral vascular disease of the lower extremity in diabetes mellitus, *Diabetes* 8:261–273, 1959.

33. Logerfo FW, Coffman JD: Vascular and microvascular disease of the foot in diabetes, *N Engl J Med* 311:1615–1619, 1984.

34. Wagner FW: The dysvascular foot: a system for diagnosis and treatment, *Foot Ankle* 2:64–122, 1981.

35. Classen JN: Neuropathic arthropathy with ulceration, *Ann Surg* 159:891–894, 1964.

36. Coventry MB: Resection of the metatarsal heads to relieve pain and deformity, *Mayo Clin Proc* 40:240–247, 1965.

37. Griffiths GD, Wieman TJ: Metatarsal head resection for diabetic foot ulcers, *Arch Surg* 125:832–835, 1990.

38. Cohen M, Roman A, Malcolm WG: Panmetatarsal head resection and transmetatarsal amputation versus solitary partial ray resection in the neuropathic foot, *J Foot Surg* 30:29–33, 1991.

39. Giurini JM et al: Sesamoidectomy for the treatment of chronic neuropathic ulcerations, *J Am Podiatr Med Assoc* 81:167–173, 1991.

40. Rossini AA, Hare JW: How to control the blood glucose level in the surgical diabetic patient, *Arch Surg* 111:945–949, 1976.

41. Skyler JS: Complications of diabetes mellitus: Relationship to metabolic dysfunction, *Diabetes Care* 2:499–509, 1979.

42. Bagdade JH, Root RK, Bulger RG: Impaired leukocyte function in patients with poorly controlled diabetes, *Diabetes* 23:9–15, 1974.

43. Gibbons GW, Eliopoulos GM: Infection of the diabetic foot. In Kozak GP et al, editors: *Management of diabetic foot problems,* Philadelphia, 1984, WB Saunders.

44. Sapico FL, Bessman AN: Diabetic foot infections. In Frykberg RG, editor: *The high risk foot in diabetes mellitus,* New York, 1991, Churchill Livingstone.

45. Kaneshige H: Nonenzymatic glycosylation of serum IgG and its effect on antibody activity in patients with diabetes mellitus, *Diabetes* 36:822–828, 1987.

46. US Department of Health and Human Services: Healthy people 2000—National health promotion and disease prevention objectives, DHHS publication no 91-50213, Washington, DC, 1991, US Government Printing Office.

47. Kosinski EJ, Pippin JJ, Kozak GP: Preoperative evaluation of the diabetic patient. In Kozak GP et al, editors: *Management of diabetic foot problems,* Philadelphia, 1984, WB Saunders.

48. Campbell D: Diabetic vascular disease. In Frykberg RG, editor: *The high risk foot in diabetes mellitus,* New York, 1991, Churchill Livingstone.

49. Griffiths GD, Wieman TJ: The influence of renal function on diabetic foot ulceration, *Arch Surg* 125:1567–1569, 1990.

50. Bacharach JM et al: Predictive value of transcutaneous oxygen pressure and amputation success by use of supine and elevation measurements, *J Vasc Surg* 15:558–563, 1992.

51. Carter SA: Role of pressure measurements in vascular disease. In Bernstein EF, editor: *Noninvasive diagnostic techniques in vascular disease,* St Louis, 1985, Mosby–Year Book.

52. Gibbons GW et al: Noninvasive prediction of amputation level in diabetic patients, *Arch Surg* 114:1253–1257, 1979.

53. Hoffman AF: Evaluation of arterial blood flow in the lower extremity, *Clin Podiatr Med Surg* 9:19–56, 1992.

54. Bone GE, Pomajzl MJ: Toe blood pressure by plethysmography: an index of healing in forefoot amputation, *Surgery* 89:569–574, 1981.

55. Kirby KA, Arkin DB, Laine W: Digital systolic pressure determination in the foot, *J Am Podiatr Med Assoc* 77:340–342, 1987.

56. Niehaus LP, Kallibjian A: Application of transcutaneous oxygen measurement in podiatric surgery, *J Foot Surg* 28:124–126, 1989.

57. Masson EA, Boulton AJM: Pressure assessment methods in the foot. In Frykberg RG, editor: *The high risk foot in diabetes mellitus,* New York, 1991, Churchill Livingstone.

58. Silvino NA, Evanski PM, Waugh TR: The Harris and Beath footprinting mat: diagnostic validity and clinical use, *Clin Orthop* 151:265–269, 1980.

59. Rose NE, Felwell LA, Cracchiolo A: A method for measuring foot pressures using a high resolution computerized insole sensor: the effect of heel wedges on plantar pressure distribution and center of force, *Foot Ankle* 13:263–270, 1992.

60. Kaufman JL et al: Local anesthesia for surgery on the foot: efficacy in the ischemic or diabetic extremity, *Ann Vasc Surg* 5:354–358, 1991.

61. Harris JR, Brand PW: Patterns of disintegration of the tarsus in the anesthetic foot, *J Bone Joint Surg [Br]* 48:4–16, 1966.

23 _____ Controversies in Footwear for the Diabetic Foot at Risk

Jan S. Ulbrecht, M.D.

Julie Perry, M.S.

F. G. Hewitt, Jr., M.S.

Peter R. Cavanagh, Ph.D.

Patients who develop significant lower extremity diabetic sensory neuropathy— "loss of protective sensation"[1-4] (see Chapter 4)—are at risk for skin ulceration on their feet because they cannot feel injury occurring. Much of the rest of this book deals with the morbidity and even mortality resulting from such skin breakdown. Skin ulceration in the neuropathic diabetic foot occurs most frequently as a consequence of significant mechanical contact between the foot and a shoe, contact that is not felt by the patient.[5] It is, therefore, not surprising that the foot-shoe interface has been the subject of much interest in this field. Footwear can both cause injury and help prevent it, and various footwear modifications have been proposed over the years to prevent causation and enhance prevention.

Despite this long-standing interest in footwear for the diabetic patient with loss of protective sensation, the footwear options now available do not predictably prevent problems. This is because developments in the field of therapeutic footwear have, until recently, been largely empirical. (There are some notable exceptions to this statement.[6-9])

The empirical approach flourished because the usual end points for success or failure were maintained skin integrity or skin ulceration, respectively. Experts in the field have tended, therefore, to introduce footwear "improvements" into practice rather than testing them rigorously in randomized studies. Much has been achieved, but the process of prescribing a particular shoe for a particular patient remains largely an art.[10]

Plantar pressure distribution measurement has the potential to become a new end point for the measurement of footwear success for the diabetic patient at risk of foot injury. Because the association between plantar ulceration and areas of high plantar pressure has now been clearly established, and because the methodology for measuring pressure at the foot-shoe interface (including dorsum of the foot and the shoe upper) is now available, assessment of pressure in shoes should provide a surrogate and anticipatory measure of footwear "success" or "failure." We are therefore in a position to learn what the currently available footwear modifications do to relieve pressure. This should lead to a streamlining of the options used and to a more rational selection of the particular design appropriate to a given situation. It is logical to assume that completely new footwear improvements would follow. Practitioners would no longer have to modify footwear and risk trying it out on patients to see if tissue integrity is maintained.

Several excellent articles and book chapters have been written dealing with the principles and practice of footwear design and manufacture for the neuropathic foot as they stand now.[11-16] In this chapter we plan to point to some of the areas that must be considered controversial. In each case we will attempt to define the controversy, suggest methods to resolve it, and speculate about the outcome. The aim of this chapter is to identify rather than resolve problems and to stimulate research.

SURGERY VERSUS FOOTWEAR

Perhaps the most basic controversy in the field is the choice of altering the architecture of the foot or the design of the shoe to prevent the recurrence of plantar lesions. Because the topic of prophylactic surgery is dealt with elsewhere in this volume (see Chapter 22), we have chosen not to address this particular controversy directly. However, it should be pointed out that there have been no randomized, controlled studies to demonstrate the superiority of either approach as far as complications, patient satisfaction, cost, and ulcer recurrence are concerned. This is certainly an issue that needs some resolution in the future.

SHOE UPPERS

Many injuries occur on the toes.[5] The toebox of a shoe must therefore have adequate depth, length, and width. Dorsal foot lesions are also commonly caused by poor fit. "Fit" is a word which is uniformly used with reference to the shoe upper, but it is very difficult to define. Measures of fit have, to date, been in the hands of the "shoe fitter" and are completely subjective.

It may be helpful to consider the concept of "fit" in the context of the possible functions of the upper. At the simple mechanical level, that function is to attach the sole of the shoe to the foot. Forces generated between a foot and the shoe upper during standing are simply a matter of how tight or loose the shoe upper is. However, propulsive forces during toe-off and deceleration forces during heel strike in walking can be transmitted to the ground only as either shear between the plantar surface of the foot and the insole or as forces acting between the shoe upper and the foot. Consider the bare foot landing on a surface consisting of roller bearings (Fig 23–1,A). No shear stress can be developed between the tissue and support surface because the rollers will simply rotate. The result is that the foot will slide off the front edge of the surface.

Next, consider a shoe that has the same roller bearing as the interface between the plantar aspect of the foot and a shoe that also has an upper attached (Fig 23–1,B). On landing, the forward movement of the foot will be restrained by the upper, which results in a shear stress between the upper and the dorsum of the foot. In reality, there is friction between the sole of the foot and the insole in a typical shoe, but the upper still plays the same role in restricting forward movement of the foot. Shear stress on the dorsum can relieve shear stress on the plantar surface of the foot, which many authors believe (without proof so far) to be important in the pathogenesis of plantar ulceration. The relationship between plantar shear stress and the stresses acting through the shoe upper are therefore worth exploring further.

To our knowledge the stresses between shoe upper and foot have never been measured, but such measurement is now possible using one of the flexible pressure-measuring insole devices. It is probable that these stresses are largest over the dorsum of the foot during heel strike when

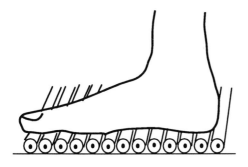

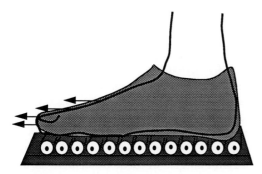

FIG 23–1.
Schematic demonstration of the role of the shoe upper. Consider the bare foot landing on a surface consisting of roller bearings **(A)**. No shear stress can be developed between the tissue and support surface because the rollers will simply rotate. The result is that the foot will slide off the front edge of the surface. Next consider a shoe that has the similar roller bearings as the interface between the plantar aspect of the foot and a shoe that also has an upper attached **(B)**. On landing, the forward movement of the foot will be restrained by the upper, resulting in a shear stress between the upper and the dorsum of the foot. In a typical shoe, there is friction between the sole of the foot and the insole, but the upper still plays the same role in restricting forward movement of the foot.

walking downhill and largest over the posterior aspect of the heel at toe-off walking uphill, but these theoretical predictions must be confirmed. We do not know how much stress the dorsal surface of the foot can withstand, and the only way to approach this would be to measure pressure between the shoe upper and the foot in situations where ulceration had occurred (compare with the discussion of

thresholds for ulceration in Chapter 5, which deals with the ulceration threshold for the plantar surface). However, with this knowledge, with actual data about the relationship between plantar shear stress and stress over the dorsum of the foot and with some additional knowledge about the relevance of shear to the injury of the plantar surface, the mechanical goals of design of shoe uppers could be established. (Note that the possibility of altering the frictional properties of the foot-insole interface and of the shear properties of the insole also exists; see later discussion.)

It is apparent on theoretical grounds that a full shoe should be better than a sandal in distributing dorsal stresses. We would, however, propose that it might be most advantageous to design the upper so that the part of the upper covering the toes and bunion areas does not participate in force transmission (because these are the areas that often ulcerate dorsally). How much this approach would increase loading of the dorsum of the midfoot would need to be measured.

INSOLES

Let us now turn to the plantar surface of the foot and to prevention of plantar foot ulcers. Plantar ulcers are, in fact, more common than dorsal lesions[5] and more difficult to deal with because they are caused by the large forces generated between the feet and the ground during standing and walking. Because of this mechanical cause, we believe that the term "healing shoes" is somewhat of an oxymoron. Plantar ulcers will not heal, or at least will heal much more slowly, if subjected to continued mechanical insult that occurs during walking in most types of footwear. The pressure threshold needed to prevent healing is likely to be much lower than the pressure required to cause the initial tissue breakdown, although little is known about this threshold at present.

It is appropriate at this point to address the methods of treatment for plantar neuropathic ulcers and, specifically, total contact casting and the principle on which it is based because the same principle is likely to be useful in the design of footwear for prevention of ulceration. Because neuropathic plantar ulcers occur as a consequence of mechanical trauma at sites of high plantar pressure,[17] it should come as no surprise that total non-weight-bearing or bed rest can heal neuropathic plantar lesions.[18] Conversely, the nonhealing plantar ulcer in the neuropathic foot must be thought of as a "poorly unloaded" ulcer; it is probable that just a few steps of full weight-bearing on an ulcer will undo a day's healing.

However, total non-weight-bearing is difficult to achieve. The walking total contact cast has now been repeatedly shown to heal neuropathic plantar ulcers, which may have existed for many months, in an average of 6 to 10 weeks.[19–25] The total contact cast is made by intimately molding the plaster up against the plantar surface. In theory, such molding should cause a more even distribution of load on the plantar aspect of the foot. This has been confirmed in practice by preliminary studies using an in-shoe pressure device.[26] Earlier studies with single shear transducers also suggested that shear stress may be dramatically reduced.[27]

Thus, using techniques such as total contact casting, healing a neuropathic plantar ulcer is not difficult. The ease with which neuropathic ulcers can be healed supports the notion that a nonhealing neuropathic ulcer is a poorly treated ulcer. However, keeping such feet healed is difficult, in part because we have not yet developed the techniques to devise the perfect footwear for a given foot and in part because patients do not always choose to wear the footwear we prescribe. How might shoes protect the plantar surface

from injury? Because pressure is a measure of force applied to a given area, and because skin injury presumably occurs when the pressure to which soft tissues are exposed exceeds the threshold for injury for that tissue, reduction of high plantar pressure must be accomplished.

Large-impact forces can be reduced by spreading the force out over time (e.g., by dropping an egg on foam rather than on a hard surface). The pressure under the object is also reduced by this approach, but this can happen only in a dynamic situation and probably applies only to the heel at the time of heel strike.[28] This might be best described as shock absorption. A focal concentration of pressure can also be reduced by spreading the applied force over a greater area through increasing the area of contact (based on the same principle on which the total contact cast operates). This is probably what happens in the forefoot during middle and late support and might be best described as accommodation. Thus a reasonable principle for the design of insoles in footwear for the neuropathic diabetic foot should be that insoles should accommodate the plantar surface and thereby distribute plantar forces over a greater area, thereby lowering focal pressure.

What do different insole shoe modifications actually do? The research addressing this question in terms of in-shoe pressure measurement has only just started, and so far we have found in our own work more questions than answers. Clinical observation has suggested that even simple sports shoes may be of value in protecting the plantar surface of the patient at risk,[29] so that a good place to start might be to look at what off-the-shelf shoes do in terms of distributing plantar pressure. After all, any sophisticated footwear we design must be better than standard shoes to justify the expense to the patient. This question must be answered in a systematic fashion, and Figure 23–2 is an example of what happens to plantar pres-

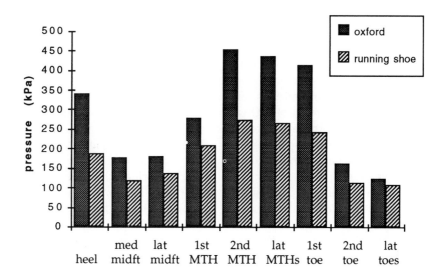

region of the foot

FIG 23–2.

The effect of two different over-the-counter shoes on in-shoe plantar pressures in a 60-year-old diabetic man with significant peripheral neuropathy. Data were measured using a Micro EMED device. When averaged over all regions, the running shoe resulted in a 32% decrease in pressure relative to the leather-soled Oxford. The greatest decrease occurred in the heel (44%), followed by the hallux (41%), metatarsal heads (34%), midfoot (29%) and second through fifth toes (21%). (From Perry JE: The effect of running shoes and Oxfords on plantar pressures in diabetic patients. Unpublished master's thesis. University Park, Pa, 1992, Pennsylvania State University. Used by permission.)

sure in a single neuropathic patient in a standard leather-soled Oxford shoe and in a midpriced running shoe. As is apparent in this particular case the running shoe reduced plantar pressure by an average of 34% in the metatarsal head region and 41% in the hallux compared to the oxford shoe. This is a substantial reduction that may, in a given case, take the plantar pressure below the threshold for tissue damage. There are also indications that the higher the initial pressure, the greater the reduction achieved.[30]

What about custom design of insoles for the patient at risk? If accommodation is the goal, the ideal insole would be relatively soft to allow perfect molding of the insole to the foot during compression. It would then need to be very thick so that it did not bottom out during compression. In addition, the insole could already be molded to match the shape of the foot, so that only fine molding would need to take place during compression. These are the principles that have most often been used in the design of insoles for diabetic patients at risk of foot injury. However, it is unclear, on theoretical grounds, what the best combination of characteristics might be. Thick insoles are difficult to fit into shoes, and soft insoles bottom out (reach maximum compression and therefore afford no protection). Molded insoles cannot be made from a very soft material, or they will lose their shape. It is therefore not surprising that combinations of materials have also been used to combine material properties. The other important issue in insole design is durability of the insole because all the materials used in insole design wear out eventually, and some can wear out in just a few weeks.

Many materials exist; some are softer and some are harder; some can be molded and some cannot; some deform to the shape of the foot sooner than others; some deteriorate sooner than others; some are open cell foams, some are closed cell foams, and some are liquids or gels (see Chapter 19).[11] The effects of softness (or modulus in engineering terms) of either single materials or of laminated materials, of thickness, and of molding on pressure reduction can and should now be investigated in a systematic manner. For example, the effect of molding a particular insole in two different patients is shown in Figure 23–3. As can be seen in both patients, pressure was significantly reduced in the heel by the molded insole. Forefoot pressure was, on the other hand, increased in one patient and decreased in the other. It must be remembered that these results are from only two patients

and for a single combination of materials at a single thickness. Therefore, these results cannot be interpreted as telling us anything about the general effectiveness of molded insoles. However, the possibility that the same intervention may actually have opposite effects in different people is intriguing and worrisome in the clinical setting, and therefore these results further underscore the importance of systematic research in this field.

It would be overwhelming to test in this way all variations of materials, thicknesses, and molding, and this is where modeling can help. Modeling in this case refers to computer prediction of outcome in terms of pressure because these various attributes (modulus, molding, and thickness) of an insole are varied. Key to any such modeling is knowledge of the mod-

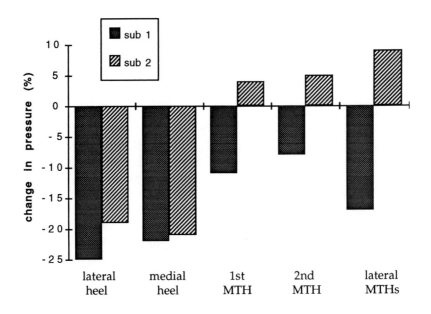

region of the foot

FIG 23–3.
In-shoe plantar pressure changes when two patients used molded rather than nonmolding insoles made from the same materials inside a rigid rocker shoe (negative numbers indicate a reduction when using the molded insole). Note that although pressure in the heel was reduced by the molded insole in both patients, the metatarsal head pressures were increased in one patient and decreased in the other. This example illustrates the importance of quantitative measurement in the prescription of in-shoe devices. (From Hewitt FG Jr: The effect of molded insoles on inshoe plantar pressures in rockered footwear. Unpublished master's thesis, University Park, Pa, 1993, Pennsylvania State University. Used by permission.)

ulus of the given material, and this value must first be measured because the physical characteristics of the various insole materials are not usually provided by the manufacturer. This is somewhat like trying to sell a car without bothering to test what the power output of the engine is (it could be too low to even move the car), and it is to be hoped that the manufacturers of the many insole materials available will recognize this point and address the problem. We have begun to use an engineering technique called finite element modeling to ask questions about insoles.[28,31] Once development is complete, modeling can be used to answer the general questions about insole properties, allowing the key predictions of the models to be confirmed by in-shoe pressure testing. This should be a cost-effective approach to answering questions that would otherwise need a long series of experiments on patients.

We have discussed the concept of accommodation and have argued in favor of full-length soft insoles as having the best likelihood of perfectly molding to the plantar surface. However, the total contact cast effectively heals ulcers, and it is obviously not soft. Would perfectly molded "hard" insoles work in shoes? This is an intriguing and important question that as yet has no answer. It is a relevant question because of the frequent need to fit a neuropathic patient with a molded ankle-foot orthosis that cannot be provided with the same kind of accommodative padding as an insole.

Hard insoles would have the advantage of not needing to be particularly thick. It is our belief at this time that hard molded insoles do not prevent plantar ulceration as effectively as accommodative insoles do. However, it is unclear if this is because the hard insoles we have encountered have not been well molded, have been designed to correct foot function, or have been molded in weight-bearing rather than non-weight-bearing. The total

contact cast is molded to the non-weight-bearing foot and is likely to unload the plantar surface much better than an insole molded during weight-bearing. This is because an insole molded to the weight-bearing foot will allow compression of the soft tissues at the points of high pressure to occur before it makes contact over the whole surface. Also maintenance of the perfect apposition of the foot and insole in a shoe is not likely to be achieved as well as it is in a cast where movement of the foot with respect to the cast is very limited.

The issue of insoles designed to correct structural deformities or function problems is also worth exploring. There are many experts who believe that it is important, even in the insensitive foot, to correct significant functional deformities such as uncompensated forefoot varus or valgus. However, it must be recognized that to change the dynamic alignment of the bony structures of the foot, focal forces must be applied, and these will tend to lead to focal pressure elevations. Furthermore, relatively hard insoles must be used to achieve any correction. All of these questions can and must be answered in the future by modeling and finally by measurement.

Another aspect of insole construction that has not yet been discussed is that of pressure reliefs in an area of frequent tissue breakdown. Opinions favoring the use of reliefs have been expressed, but so have concerns about the possibility of increasing pressure at the edge of such areas. We have not yet studied this question systematically, but Figure 23–4 represents a single example of what one can expect to learn from the application of in-shoe pressure measurement in an attempt to answer this question. This particular case was very illustrative because the first modification of the patient's footwear in the region of ulceration actually led to a slight worsening of pressure in the region of the relief. However, the difference was not statistically significant. We believe

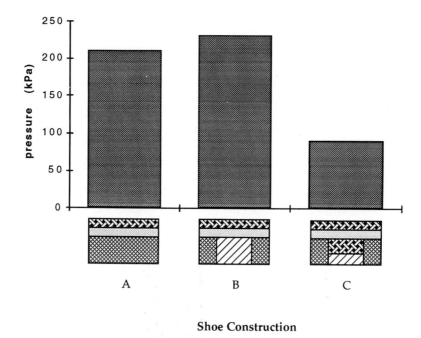

Shoe Construction

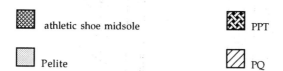

athletic shoe midsole   PPT

Pelite   PQ

FIG 23-4.
Peak plantar pressure at the site of previous forefoot ulceration inside three different shoes of a neuropathic patient. Condition *A* represents the first prescription, which was a running shoe with a flat closed-cell polyethylene (Pelite) and open-cell urethane foam (PPT) insole. When the patient ulcerated in this shoe, an attempt was made to provide a pressure relief "plug" of a poured silicone material (PQ). Pressure measurement showed *(B)* that the pressure was actually slightly increased in the new shoe, which was, therefore, not given to the patient. The third approach using a PPT "plug" on top of the PQ *(C)* was remarkably successful in reducing the plantar pressure by more than 50%, and the patient has remained ulcer free in this shoe for 6 months.

that the increase occurred because the material used was a silicone gel (PQ). This material is noncompressible and behaves like a liquid and not like a spring.[28] Liquids offer intriguing possibilities as insole materials, but in this case we believe confining the gel to the limited space of a relief allowed no room for displacement of the gel. Fortunately, pressure measurement before dispensing the shoes resulted in the footwear not being given to the patient, and it is likely that another round of ulceration and healing was thereby prevented. An open cell urethane foam (PPT) relief in the same area reduced pressure without apparently increasing pressure markedly around the relief, and the patient has done well in the shoes with the relief for more than 6 months.

Socks are another important component of the interface between foot and shoe, and recent studies have shown that special socks also lower plantar pressure, probably in a manner identical to that of insoles. Padded socks can lower plantar pressure by up to 30%,[32] and in some preliminary studies in our laboratory we have found reductions of up to 10% with regular thin socks. Padded socks may therefore play a role in the treatment of patients at risk of neuropathic ulceration. It is unlikely that the effects of different interventions (i.e., socks, insoles, and outsoles) will be directly additive, although this prediction must also be confirmed by direct measurement.

OUTSOLES

The outsole of a shoe can be modified, and the rigid rocker or roller bottom modification of footwear[8] has been frequently used to treat the neuropathic foot. As with many of the innovations in this field, including total contact casting, much of the pioneering work with the rocker bottom shoe has come from Dr. Paul Brand and his group working with patients who have Hansen's disease. The techniques were then transferred by that group to patients with diabetic neuropathy.[7,33] The rocker bottom shoe is designed to shift loading posteriorly away from the toes and metatarsal heads. Walking can occur without extension of the metatarsophalangeal joints, and this is believed to reduce metatarsal head pressures during a critical time in the gait cycle.

As with all the other modifications we have discussed, the rocker bottom shoe was originally developed and used completely on an empirical basis. In the last decade some measurements have been accomplished, and these have largely confirmed the effects that the design was intended to achieve. For example, Coleman,[9] using small individual capacitance pressure transducers, noted significant reduction of pressure underneath the second and fourth metatarsal heads using a number of rocker bottom shoe configurations. Using a similar experimental arrangement, Sims and Birke[34] found a progressive decrease in metatarsal head pressure as the apex of a rocker was moved posteriorly. However, Schaff and Cavanagh,[35] using a pressure-measuring insole, found that although a particular rocker bottom shoe resulted in a reduction of more than 30% in pressure over the medial forefoot during walking, peak pressures over the lateral margin of the forefoot were increased. Thus, measurement again discovered an opposite effect to that expected, at least under some circumstances, a finding which we have emphasized elsewhere in this chapter.

It is therefore probable that different feet will need different designs of the rocker shoes. The possible design variations include the position of the rocker along the long axis of the shoe relative to the metatarsophalangeal joints, the angle of the rocker with respect to the long axis of the shoe, the height of the rocker, and whether a rocker or a roller design is used. As with the insole modifications previously discussed, the effects of these different modifications to the rocker shoe must be investigated in a systematic fashion. This could also prove to be an extremely long and cumbersome process, and mathematical modeling of rocker shoes should again prove useful as a starting point.

SHEAR

Many authors believe that shear stress and not vertical stress is the quantity which injures plantar tissues. This is certainly a reasonable hypothesis, and it is quite possible that both types of stress are injurious because compression of soft tissues (from vertical stress) causes intermittent ischemia[36] and shear forces tend to tear tissues. On theoretical grounds, it is also likely that shear stresses are highest at sites of the highest vertical stress.[27] Not all neuropathic patients with very high vertical plantar pressure ulcerate;

the difference between patients who do and do not ulcerate may be in the amount of shear stress present.

To resolve these questions, ways of measuring shear must be developed. This work is in progress,[37] but few results are as yet available. A notable exception is the study of Pollard et al.[27] who measured longitudinal shear stress in a variety of footwear options using single shear transducers. They found significant reductions in shear in rocker bottom shoes and in a total contact cast. They did not attempt to measure shear stress at sites of ulceration, however, and there are as yet no quantitative data linking shear stress to ulceration. As the results of this early study suggest, reduction of shear stress by footwear is possible, and the theoretical role of the shoe upper in limiting plantar shear was already discussed. The total contact cast probably limits plantar shear by providing a very rigid "upper."

When shear forces exceed the available frictional force, sliding occurs and heat is generated. Whether sliding on the insole (e.g., of the tips of clawed toes during walking) plays any role in tissue injury or callus formation is unknown, but the strong possibility exists that this is the case. Shear stress on the plantar surface could be decreased by lowering the coefficient of friction of the insole and allowing sliding to occur. However, the possible negative consequences of sliding both to the plantar and dorsal surfaces of the foot and to the toes would need to be understood and considered.

FOOTWEAR PRESCRIPTION

So what shoe is right for a given patient? One might expect diagnosis and treatment to follow a similar paradigm to that used in other branches of medicine. The oncologist, for example, will diagnose a particular type of cancer and treat it with a specific chemotherapy program. The pulmonologist will diagnose a form of pneumonia, identify the particular bacteria involved, and use a specific antibiotic for treatment. A similar approach simply does not exist in the area of preventing ulceration or reulceration in the diabetic neuropathic foot. We can diagnose loss of protective sensation, we can identify foot deformity, and we can identify areas of high pressure under the foot, but we cannot yet prescribe a specific footwear option to treat each patient. Theoretically the best shoe for a given patient would be that shoe that would lower the focal pressures on the plantar and dorsal surfaces below the ulceration threshold of the tissue at that site. But, as we have discussed in this chapter, at this point neither the pressure threshold for ulceration nor the relative roles of normal or shear stress in ulceration are known. Neither are the effects of different types of footwear modifications on the mechanical conditions at the foot-shoe interface accurately known.

We can expect, however, that in the next decade these questions will be answered. We can reasonably anticipate the day when the risk profile for ulceration of a given foot will be developed in terms of sensory loss, vertical stress, shear stress, blood supply, patient activity level, and probably other as yet not apparent factors. The correct, esthetically attractive footwear solution will then be prescribed, and in-shoe pressure (vertical and shear) measurement will be used to make sure that the footwear is indeed lowering all relevant forces below the known ulceration threshold.

In the meantime we, among other physicians, continue to practice the art of footwear design for the patient at risk. We measure barefoot pressure routinely in all patients with loss of protective sensation and tend to prescribe sports shoes or their equivalent to patients with barefoot plantar pressures less than 500 kPa on an EMED SF platform (see Chapter 3). We use extra-depth shoes with ¼-in. accommodative insoles for patients with forefoot pressures of 500 kPa, sometimes incorporating a rigid rocker bottom design as well. Custom-molded shoes with custom-molded ½-in. accommodative insoles and rocker bottom modifications are given to patients with forefoot pressures close to or greater than 1,000 kPa. This scheme, as all such schemes, is based only on our clinical experience and remains to be validated by the appropriate studies.

CONCLUSION

In this chapter we have tried to provide an overview of some of the controversies that underlie footwear design for the diabetic patient with neuropathy. Design of such footwear still remains basically an art, although there is the potential for it to become much more scientifically based within the next decade. We must learn about thresholds for injury, and we must learn what the different footwear modifications do in terms of reducing the injurious forces that act on feet during gait. The importance of shear must be determined.

The goal will be to prescribe the right footwear for a particular patient. In-shoe pressure measurement is one of the technologic advances that will allow this progress to occur. Even the few preliminary results using this methodology that we have presented in this chapter serve to illustrate the importance of measurement in this field. Quite often in the experiments described, footwear modification did not do what it was supposed or intended to do according to conventional wisdom. Sometimes even the opposite effects were observed.

Given the rather primitive state of footwear science at the present time, clinicians and their patients have much to look forward to.

REFERENCES

1. Cavanagh PR, Ulbrecht JS: Biomechanics of the diabetic foot: A quantitative approach to the assessment of neuropathy, deformity, and plantar pressure. In Jahss MH, editor: *Disorders of the foot and ankle,* ed 2, Philadelphia, 1991, WB Saunders.
2. Birke JA, Sims DS: The insensitive foot. In Hunt GC, editor: *Physical therapy of the foot and ankle,* New York, 1988, Churchill Livingstone.
3. Holewski JJ, Stess RM, Graf PM, et al: Aesthesiometry: Quantification of cutaneous pressure sensation in diabetic peripheral neuropathy, *J Rehabil Res Dev* 25:1–10, 1988.
4. Sosenko JM, Kato M, Soto R, et al: Comparison of quantitative sensory-threshold measures for their association with foot ulceration in diabetic patients, *Diabetes Care* 13:1057–1061, 1990.
5. Apelqvist J, Larsson J, Agardh CD: The influence of external precipitating factors and peripheral neuropathy on the development and outcome of diabetic foot ulcers, *J Diabetic Complications* 4:21–25, 1990.
6. Bauman J, Girling E, Brand PW: Plantar pressures and trophic ulceration. An evaluation of footwear, *J Bone Joint Surg* 45B-4:652–673, 1963.
7. Brand PW, Coleman WC: The diabetic foot. In Rifkin H, Porte D Jr, editors: *Ellenberg and Rifkin's diabetes mellitus: theory and practice,* ed 4, New York, 1990, Elsevier Science.
8. Nawoczenski DA, Birke JA, Coleman WC: Effect of rocker sole designs on plantar forefoot pressures, *J Am Podiatr Med Assoc* 78:455–460, 1988.
9. Coleman WC: The relief of forefoot pressures using outer shoe sole modifications. In MothiramiPatil K, Srinivasa H, editors: *Proceedings of the International Conference on Biomechanics and Clinical Kinesiology of Hand and Foot.* Madras, India, 1985, Indian Institute of Technology.
10. Milgram JE, Jacobson MA: Footgear: Therapeutic modifications of sole and heel, *Orthop Rev* VII:57–62, 1978.

11. Coleman WC: Footwear in a management program of injury prevention. In Levin ME, O'Neal LW, editors: *The diabetic foot,* St Louis, 1988, Mosby–Year Book.

12. Coleman WC: Footwear considerations. In Frykberg RG, editor: *The high risk foot in diabetes mellitus,* New York, 1991, Churchill Livingstone.

13. Coleman WC: Shoe gear for the insensitive foot. In Harkless LB, Dennis KJ, editors: *Clinics in podiatric medicine and surgery: the diabetic foot,* Philadelphia, 1987, WB Saunders.

14. Tovey FI: The manufacture of diabetic footwear, *Diabetic Med* 1:69–71, 1984.

15. Tovey FI, Guy R, Platt H, et al: Surgical footwear, *BMJ* 299:1216, 1989.

16. Tovey FI, Moss MJ: Specialist shoes for the diabetic foot. In Boulton AJM, Ward JD, editors: *The foot in diabetes,* New York, 1987, John Wiley & Sons.

17. Boulton AJM, Hardisty CA, Betts RP, et al: Dynamic foot pressure and other studies as diagnostic and management aids in diabetic neuropathy, *Diabetes Care* 6:26–33, 1983.

18. Steed DL, Moosa HH, Webster MW: The importance of randomized prospective trials in evaluating therapy for wound healing, *Wounds* 3:111–115, 1991.

19. Birke JA, Sims DS Jr, Buford WL: Walking casts: Effect on plantar foot pressures, *J Rehabil Res Dev* 22:18–22, 1985.

20. Boulton AJM, et al: Use of plaster casts in the management of diabetic neuropathic foot ulcers, *Diabetes Care* 9:149–153, 1986.

21. Coleman WC, Brand PW, Birke JA: The total contact cast: A therapy for plantar ulceration on insensitive feet, *J Am Podiatr Assoc* 74:548–552, 1984.

22. Kominsky SJ: The ambulatory total contact cast. In Frykberg RG, editor: *The high risk foot in diabetes mellitus,* New York, 1991, Churchill Livingstone.

23. Myerson M, Wilson K: Management of neuropathic ulceration with total contact cast. In Sammarco GJ, editor: *The foot in diabetes,* Philadelphia, 1991, Lea & Febiger.

24. Sinacore DR: Total-contact casting in the treatment of diabetic neuropathic ulcers. In Levin ME, O'Neal LW, editors: *The diabetic foot,* ed 4, St Louis, 1988, Mosby–Year Book.

25. Mueller MJ, Diamond JE, Sinacore DR, et al: Total contact casting in treatment of diabetic plantar ulcers, *Diabetes Care* 12:384–388, 1989.

26. Masson EA: What causes high foot pressures in diabetes: How can they be relieved? (Proceedings of the IDF Satellite Symposium on the Diabetic Foot, Washington 1991), *Foot* 2:212–217, 1992.

27. Pollard JP, Le Quesne LP, Tappin JW: Forces under the foot, *J Biomed Eng* 5:37–40, 1983.

28. Cavanagh PR, Ulbrecht JS: Biomechanics of the foot in diabetes. In Levin ME, O'Neal LW, Bowker JH, editors: *The diabetic foot,* ed 5, St Louis, 1993, Mosby–Year Book, pp 199–232.

29. Soulier SM: The use of running shoes in the prevention of plantar diabetic ulcers, *J Am Podiatr Med Assoc* 76:395–400, 1986.

30. Perry JE: The effect of running shoes and Oxfords on plantar pressures in diabetic patients. Master's thesis, University Park, Pa, Pennsylvania State University, 1992.

31. Shiang TY, Cavanagh PR: Finite element analysis of the foot-shoe interface in diabetic patients. Paper presented at the 1992 International Symposium, Biomedical Engineering in the 21st Century, Taipei, Republic Of China, Sept 23–26, 1992.

32. Veves A, Masson EA, Fernando DJS, et al: Use of experimental padded hosiery to reduce abnormal foot pressures in diabetic neuropathy, *Diabetes Care* 12:653–655, 1989.

33. Brand PW: Repetitive stress in the development of diabetic foot ulcers. In Levin ME, O'Neal LW, editors: *The diabetic foot,* ed 4, St Louis, 1988, Mosby–Year Book.

34. Sims DS, Birke JA: Effect of rocker sole placement on plantar pressures [abstract]. In *Proceedings of the 20th Annual Meeting of the USPHS Professional Association,* Atlanta, 1985.

35. Schaff PS, Cavanagh PR: Shoes for the insensitive foot: The effect of a "rocker bottom" shoe modification on plantar pressure distribution, *Foot Ankle* 11:129–140, 1990.
36. Levin ME: The diabetic foot: Pathophysiology, evaluation, and treatment. In

O'Neal LW, et al, editors: *The diabetic foot,* ed 4, St Louis, 1988, Mosby–Year Book.
37. Laing P, Cogley D, Crerand S, et al: The Liverpool Shear Transducer [abstract]. In *The diabetic foot.* The Netherlands, p 49, 1991.

24   Pedorthics and the Diabetic Foot

Herb S. Steb, C. Ped., M.B.A.

Statistics show that up to 15% of all diabetic patients bear significant risk of lower limb amputation at some point during their affliction. Of these patients, the contralateral limb usually develops some high-risk pathology within 18 months. Assuming these patients survive,[1] half of these patients will experience contralateral amputation within 3 to 5 years. It is also noteworthy that more than half of all nontraumatic amputations are performed on diabetic patients. The big question is why?

It is peripheral vascular disease, sensory neuropathy, and infection that are the primary causitive factors of lower level and foot trauma afflicted with diabetes mellitus.

The resulting loss of a protective threshold of sensation increases incidence of foot lesions and resulting ulcerations, especially in areas of overlying bony prominences vulnerable to pressure. The lack of protective pain sensation thus predisposes these diabetic feet to the risk of undetected injuries and repetitive stress factors.

Development of neuropathic limb ulcerations were first shown in 1959 by Kosiak[2] and later defined by Paul Brand[3] to be pressure and time related. High pressure, applied for a short duration, or low pressure, applied repetitively over an area for long periods, are likely to result in ulcerations.

It is pressures in the environment of improper, ill fitting footwear or unprotected bare feet that become the primary concern. With insensate feet any dorsal, medial, lateral, or plantar pressures, in either short or long duration, caused by motor neuropathy or otherwise, can cause ulceration. These include:

1. Buildup of plantar keratoses
2. Digital instability characterized by plantarflexed metatarsals, hammer, claw, and mallet toe deformities
3. Hallux rigidus
4. Hallux valgus, bunions
5. Sesamoiditis
6. Overlapping toes

Dynamic factors of hyperpronation and supination as a result of biomechanical abnormalities also predispose the foot to high-pressure areas that can cause trauma and resulting ulceration.

It is the neuropathic patient's unawareness of pain, the complete antitheses of the non-neuropathic patient's awareness of pain, as well as the potential resultant disfigurement, ulceration, infection, and complications, that exacerbates the problems of the diabetic foot.

Among the essential components in the prevention, treatment, and therapy of diabetic foot problems is a diabetic patient's pedorthic* foot management.

---

*The art of design, fabrication, fit, and modification of footwear prosthetics and foot orthoses applied from the ankle and below.

PEDORTHIC MANAGEMENT

Pedorthic management commences after a physician's diagnosis and description of specific presenting pathology. The intended treatment plan, objective, and prognosis are then communicated to the pedorthist by the physician. This serves as the basis on which pedorthic determination of intrinsic accommodative or functional orthoses, footwear, and extrinsic biomechanical footwear modifications can be recommended. The physician is then able to write an appropriate prescription to achieve the desired goal.

PEDORTHIC PRACTITIONER

The paramedical expert qualified to make these recommendations is a clinician known as a pedorthist, certified by the American Board for Certification in Pedorthics (C. Ped). Pedorthists are trained in basic functional anatomy and biomechanics of the lower limb and foot. Further training and experience qualify him or her as an authority in the design, fabrication, and fitting of accommodative and functional foot orthoses, therapeutic stock and custom foot gear, and intrinsic and extrinsic biomechanical shoe modifications.

The pedorthist's further responsibility is to contribute to the education of the patient as pertains to pedorthic foot management. This includes:

1. Information on footwear options
2. Needed orthotic requirements
3. Initial and ongoing use of orthotics
4. Frequency of change, renewal, and longevity
5. Therapeutic expectations
6. Monitoring visual self-inspection of the feet
7. Proper shoe tread pattern
8. Hygienic foot care practice

The certified pedorthist is a paramedical member of the health team and is the primary contributor in advising which orthotic devices, materials, and types of footgear are best suited to the treatment of the presenting condition.

PEDORTHIC EVALUATION TECHNIQUES

With knowledge of a physician's diagnosis, the pedorthist performs a systematic pedorthic prefitting assessment and analysis of the presenting pathology (Table 24–1). The first criterium is the gathering of subjective historical data from the patient. This provides a comprehensive picture of how the patient views his or her problems. This is followed by a static, non-weight-bearing examination, when careful visual examination is made.[8] It is critical to look for anatomic areas of keratosis or hypertrophy, which in itself is evidence of pressure. The origin or cause of this pressure must be determined. Also to be observed is foot shape, longitudinal and metatarsal arch contour, heel and toe relationships, toe deformities, and any other tuberosities such as Charcot's joints.

After visual examination, palpation and a range of motion of each anatomic component of the foot should be performed. The objective is to determine either motional laxity, rigidity, or normalcy of the foot in a non-weight-bearing position. Foot tonicity and tolerance are thus

TABLE 24–1.

Pedorthic Techniques Evaluating Diabetic Patient's Presenting Pathology

1. Comprehension and interpretation of physician's diagnosis
2. Comprehensive pedorthic foot examination
3. Evaluation of foot-floor reactive forces by recorded imprint
4. Examination and analysis of fit, tread pattern, and upper distortions of patient's worn footwear
5. Classification of patient according to foot risk

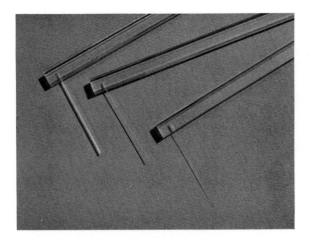

FIG 24–1.
Sensory testing nylon filaments. *Top left,* 6.10; *middle,* 5.07; *bottom right,* 4.17. (Grams of force) (Semmes-Weinstein monofilaments-S.W)

assessed for later determination of required orthotic elevations. Particular attention must be given to dorsiflexion and plantarflexion of the hallux because of the tremendous pressure exerted on this area at toe off, during the final stage of stance phase of gait. Careful evaluation must also be made of passive foot plantarflexion, dorsiflexion, supination, and pronation. Either limited or excessive motion can cause pressure areas and would indicate need for functional control within the limits of the patients tolerance levels.

One of the most important elements of this static examination is to ascertain or evaluate sensation. This information may have been provided with the physician's diagnosis. However, in the absence of this information, it is easily measured by using the Semms Weinstein (SW) monofilament quantification method (Fig 24–1). This is the use of three different nylon sensory filaments, which measures pressure per square inch, calibrated as 4.17 (1 G), 5.07 (10 G), and 6.10 (75 G) of pressure, prodded vertically against the epidermal surface of skin. This is done at various anatomic locations of the foot and lower leg and the patient's reaction recorded. Normal sensation is measured as 4.17, diminished sensation as 5.07, and the anesthesized insensate foot at 6.10. One must be careful not to confuse a foot that does not feel sensation from one that

is aware of and feels pressure. There is a difference!

The remaining considerations of the static examination are observation of diminished hair growth and dryness of skin, indicative of circulatory problems, and foot temperature, indicative of inflammation or internal subluxation. Hot anatomic areas are often indicative of the need for pedorthic stabilization. Determination of foot temperature is helpful.

The pedorthist next performs a standing and dynamic examination to compare the observations made during the static phase of the examination with obvious deviations, both weight-bearing and kinetically. Changes in foot shape, excessive calcaneal varus or valgus, forefoot abductive or adductive gait patterns, or loss of the subtalar neutral position all must be noted and evaluated for potential pathologic anomalies.

FLOOR REACTION IMPRINTS

The next phase of pedorthic analysis and an equally cogent aspect, is recording by imprint, floor reactive forces. It is a mechanical technique to ascertain floor-foot reactive forces to which the plantar area of the foot is subjected.[6]

This technique is based on the newtonian principle "for every action there is

A

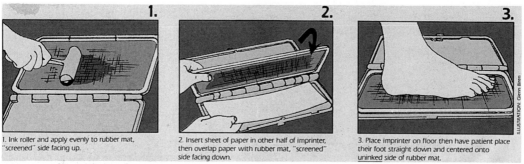

1. Ink roller and apply evenly to rubber mat, "screened" side facing up.

2. Insert sheet of paper in other half of imprinter, then overlap paper with rubber mat, "screened" side facing down.

3. Place imprinter on floor then have patient place their foot straight down and centered onto uninked side of rubber mat.

B

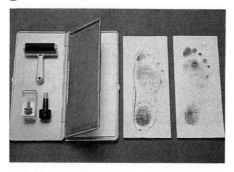

FIG 24–2.
A, floor reaction imprinter above shows *(1)* inking, *(2)* placing paper under inked screen, and *(3)* placement of foot on uninked screen. **B,** floor reaction imprinter, roller, ink, static print left, dynamic print right. (Courtesy of Langer Biomechanics Group, Inc., Deer Park, NY.)

an equal and opposite reaction." The forces identified by these imprints are generally the repetitive, disruptive forces that damage feet with impaired sensation, as well as non-neuropathic feet.

The floor reaction imprint graphically depicts the component-reacting forces during the stance phase of the gait cycle. These component forces are fore and aft, medial and lateral, vertical, torque, and sheer. They are exerted throughout the foot but principally on the plantar surface of the foot. The print pictorially reveals the weight-loading pattern and anatomic location of excessive pressure, indicated by high-density to low-density colorations. The imprint also identifies foot shape, heel-toe relationship, arch definition and type, foot-body balance, and pressure variables.

Floor reaction testing should be re-corded in both static and dynamic phases. This is done to compare the intensity differential between static and dynamic stance phases of gait.

A static print is done by placing the non-weight-bearing foot gently on an imprint and then having the patient stand, bearing full body weight (Fig 24–2, A). This is repeated on the other foot.

A dynamic print is achieved by having a patient place the foot on the imprinter as he or she walks through stance phase of the gait cycle (Fig 24–2, B). However, this is occasionally difficult for some people, especially geriatric patients. If this situation arises, an alternate method of testing can be offered. This is a semidynamic imprint achieved by having a patient place one foot on the imprinter while bending the knee, bringing the opposite foot forward and then back. This somewhat simulates the stance phase of gait and gives an acceptable semidy-namic imprint, revealing high-pressure areas.

INTERPRETATION OF IMPRINT

To interpret a floor reaction imprint, one must first define the foot type. A normal pescavus foot would display a well-defined arch expected to reveal somewhat more pressure at both the heel, first and fifth metatarsal head areas, with little or no contact at midfoot. The print would be moderately dark at the heel and the first and fifth metatarsal phalangeal head areas. Conversely, the imprint of an abnormal pes cavus foot exposed to excessive plantar pressure would reveal high-intensity coloration not only on the first and fifth metatarsal heads but possibly on the second, third, and fourth as well. This high-intensity coloration would be suggestive of plantar pressure resulting from plantarflexed metatarsals, plantar callus, scar tissue, and a convex depressed metatarsal arch, each pressure point presenting potential sites for ulceration. Medial

or lateral heel imbalance may also be indicated (Fig 24–3).

Definition of a pes planus foot would display a foot with little or no arch definition. However, the lack of arch definition does not necessarily constitute an abnormal foot. A congenital low arch in a subtalar neutral position that is asymptomatic and free of excessive pressure points might not reveal an imprint with any high-density discoloration areas. The medial border outline of this normal foot would be fairly straight. An abnormal pes valgus, hyperpronated foot would be indicated by a convex medial border outline (Fig 24–4, A). The line of weight-bearing would reveal high-intensity coloration at the medial heel and longitudinal arch. It would then continue anteriorly to the first metatarsal phalangeal sesamoid area on to the distal end of the hallux. The entire forefoot being malbalanced may reveal several high-intensity metatarsal pressure areas.

There are other more sophisticated means of measuring floor reactive forces as just described. The most advanced are electronic with computer refinement.

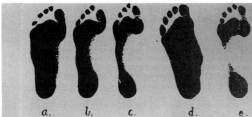

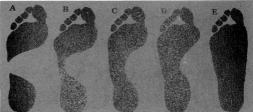

FIG 24–3.

A, an excessively high arch *(e)*, pes cavus footprint, normal only if asymptomatic with neutral calcaneus. Abnormal pes planus with convex medial arch *(d)*, normal prints of arches low *(a)*, medium *(b)*, and high *(c)*, with neutral calcaneus. **B,** all footprints reveal differences in normal arch prints. *A,* high pes cavus; *B,* medium-high; *C,* medium; *D,* low; *E,* normal pes planus. (**A** and **B** adapted from Rossi WA, Tennant R: *Professional shoe fitting,* New York, 1984, National Shoe Retailers Assoc. Used by permission.) **C,** floor reaction imprint of an insensate 61-year-old man with ulceration on distal end of second and third toes of

right foot. Foot type is pes cavus. Note typical high plantar pressure shown by darkened coloration at the heel, fifth and first metatarsal head areas. Also indicated and shown by darkened areas is pressure on the entire metatarsal arch and cuboid areas. **D,** pes cavus feet with pressure on medial aspect of varus calcaneus. Also note pressure on fifth and first metatarsal heads and on second and third metatarsal heads. Note entire metatarsal arch and heel with fat pad atrophy. Feet are outlined to show perimeter of plantar surface.

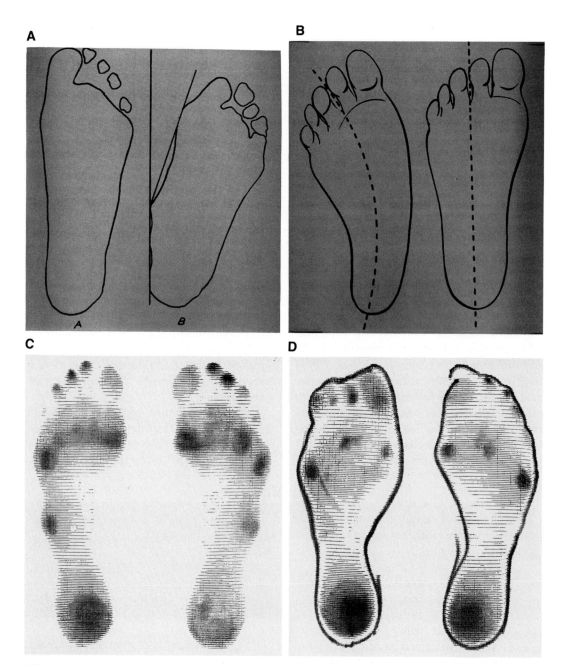

FIG 24–4.
A, Normal congenital low arch *(A).* Abnormal pes planno valgus *(B).* **B,** *left,* normal foot with axis through center. *Right,* curved axis on pronated foot. (Adapted from Rossi WA, Tennant R: *Professional shoe fitters,* New York, 1984, National Shoe Retailers. Used by permission.)

These systems are force plate or pedo-barographic in principle, record relative forces, and interpret and produce quantitative data in televisual and printed form. The negative aspect of electronic computerized systems is not only the excessive cost but also problems of calibration and standardization of data.

Experience has proved that to date the floor reaction imprinter is the most cost-effective means for a pedorthist to record floor-foot reactive forces. The most common names to describe these imprinters are the Harris Mat System and Pedograph System.

WORN FOOTWEAR PRESSURE ANALYSIS

Diabetic patients with insensate feet most often purchase improperly fitting footwear. Unknowingly, they truly believe shoe fit must be snug, which actually translates to tight, to create an awareness of the shoes on their feet. What they actually feel is pressure, because an insensate foot may be aware of dynamic pressure in the absence of sensation.[10]

The trained experienced pedorthist can visually analyze malbalance and actual as well as potential pressure areas by "reading" or inspecting footwear.

SOLE WEAR

Tread pattern on the heels and soles indicates foot deformities, body imbalance, and pathologic gait. It could also indicate incompatible selection of shoe shape (last),[9] with foot shape, improper fit, and construction. In addition, outsole wear indicates the following:

1. Wear concentrated under the head of the first metatarsal points to potential callus under the first metatarsal head.
2. Wear concentrated in center of the ball is a sign of a depressed metatarsal arch.
3. Worn toe tips indicate insufficient toe spring or a short shoe.
4. Excessive wear on the medial or lateral borders of the heels indicates a calcaneal valgus or varus heel rotation.
5. Excessive wear on the medial or lateral borders of the sole indi-

cates possible pronation or supination.

The clinician should investigate all unusual unilateral or bilateral tread patterns for causative biomechanical gait deficiencies with the potential of creating pressure areas and ultimately ulcerations. Normal tread pattern on a shoe should simulate the normal line of weight-bearing during stance phase of the gait cycle. Treading moves from posterior to anterior as follows:

1. Heel strike occurs just off the center to the lateral aspects of the heel.
2. Proceeds forward along the outer longitudinal arch to the approximate head of the fifth metatarsal.
3. Moves medially and forward across the metatarsal arch to the head of the first metatarsal phalangeal articulation.
4. Continues its forward motional pattern from the head of the first metatarsal to the distal end of the hallux to toe off. The final tread will be just medial of center to the tip of the shoe.

Any deviation of this tread pattern is an indication of a potential problem of malbalance or existing pathology and should be further explored.

UPPER DISTORTIONS

The upper portion of a shoe both externally and internally reveals pressure problems such as:

1. Distorted heel counters, indicating calcaneo varus or valgus upper bulges over sole on medial side and away from the foot on the lateral side.
2. Upper overriding the insole, suggesting incompatibility of shoe

shape with foot shape, poor fit, pronation, or supination.

3. Excessive vamp break, toe wrinkling, indicating fit too long or incorrect last.
4. Insufficient toe flex, vamp break, indicating fit too short.

OTHER DIAGNOSTIC SIGNS

1. Discoloration of the interior because of excessive perspiration caused by lack of porosity. This results in a hot humid environment and increased disruptive friction.
2. Curled uneven insoles causing plantar pressures.
3. Pressure points because of overstretching at the hallux or fifth phalanx. A hammer or claw toe show distortion over the vamp or toe box.
4. Examination of the footprint on the insole visually, indicating plantar pressure areas, as well as shoe fit.

The vulnerability of the diabetic foot to fundamental pressures and problems have been delineated. The role, expertise, and function of the pedorthist as a member of the foot management team have been detailed.

Equipped with this information, the pedorthist can synergize all of the data in determining patients' footwear and accommodative or functional orthotic requirements to prevent trauma or achieve and maintain therapeutic goals.

However, what still remains is classification of patients according to degree of "foot risk." It is the final basis on which management recommendations are made.

Wagner[4] has published foot risk classifications by the "ulcer classification system," which the pedorthist uses as a guide (Table 24–2). The SW monofilament quantification system further provides grading of sensitivity, calibrated in grams of force. A series of filaments are vertically applied against the skin until the filament bends.

Persons able to identify the various grams of force are classified in risk categories as follows:

TABLE 24–2.

Foot Risk Chart

	Nylon Filament Sensory Test*			
	Sensate	Insensate		
	4.17	5.07	6.10	6.10
	Category			
Patient Criteria Determinations	0	1	2	3
Newly diagnosed as diabetic	X			
Potential of insensitivity	X			
With protective threshold of sensitivity	X			
Partial or total loss of protective level of sensitivity		X		
Total loss of protective level of sensitivity			X	X
No ulceration history	X	X		X
With ulceration history and recurrence potential			X	X
Without foot deformity	X or with			
With foot deformity and high ulceration potential				X

*Foot risk calibrated in grams of force.

Risk category 0 (SW 4.17)

1. Positive diagnosis as diabetic
2. Has protective sensation
3. With or without foot deformity
4. Potential of insensitivity

Risk category 1 (SW 5.07)

1. Partial or total loss of protective level of sensation
2. No history of ulceration
3. Without foot deformity

Risk category 2 (SW 6.10)

1. Total loss of protective level of sensation
2. Has history of ulceration
3. Has no foot deformity

Risk category 3 (SW 6.10)

1. Total loss of protective level of sensation
2. Has history of previous foot ulceration more likely to reoccur
3. Has foot deformity

The one basic problem with this classification system is that patients with significant peripheral vascular disease may have a limb-threatening situation even though they are in one of the lesser categories.

DETERMINATION OF FOOTWEAR OPTIONS

With a thorough understanding of diabetics' foot pathology, an understanding of proper shoe fitting and accommodation of these feet are extremely critical.

The proper fitting of a non-neuropathic foot is difficult enough, because it is an art rather than a pure science. However, patients with sensation have the ability to verbalize feeling pressure, pain, or discomfort. An insensate patient cannot!

Knowledge of compatibility of foot shape with shoe shape, (last*), variability of lengths, widths and girth according to last, toe spring, and shoe construction and patterns must be understood by the clinician responsible for the fitting (Fig 24–5).

There are three principal types of footwear made on a variety of lasts and constructions[7] that are recommended according to diabetic foot risk classifications:

*A last is the form over which a shoe is fabricated, the shape of which determines the fitting characteristics of a shoe.

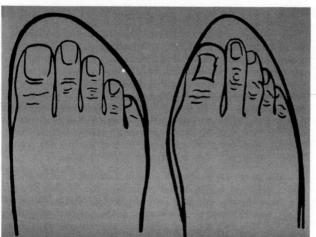

FIG 24–5.
Left, shoe shape similar in contour to the foot. *Right,* improper last, creating forefoot pressure. (Adapted from Rossi WA, Tennant R: *Professional shoe fitter,* New York, 1984, National Shoe Retailers Assoc. Used by permission.)

Extra Girth Footwear

This type of footwear is made on a variety of lasts that have added girth and depth, varying from ⅛ to ⅝ in., depending on last, in both welt and cement constructions. Available in this category are shoes anatomically shaped according to foot contour (Fig 24–6). They provide significant wiggle room for the forepart of the foot with secure hindfoot control. All of this type of footwear is made with removable insoles that can be optionally replaced with accommodative or functional custom-molded, multidensity soft tissue supplemental inlay orthotics.

Also available in extra girth construction are heat-moldable, polyethylene foam–lined, deerskin shoes (Thermold, P.W. Minor Co., Batavia, N.Y.). These are excellent on feet with pronounced deformities, providing a protective inert surface for vulnerable foot areas.

Custom Footwear

Both conventional construction and custom-molded footwear are made over actual models of patients' feet, which are called "lasts" (Fig 24–7).

A last is created by first taking a negative mold of the foot. The most common technique is to take a "bivalve", dorsumplantar cast or, at the clinician's option, a plaster bandage, wrap cast.

The negative thus created is subsequently converted to a positive plaster model of the patient's foot, in reality a plaster last (Fig 24–8). Modification necessary to provide balance and accommodation are then made to this positive mold or last.

The shoes are made of soft lightweight materials and leathers. One of the most desirable leather used is kangaroo kid for its softness and durability. The insole mold and upper fit is an exact replica of a patient's foot. They are now made with removable molded insoles, which provide the added option of any subsequent ad-

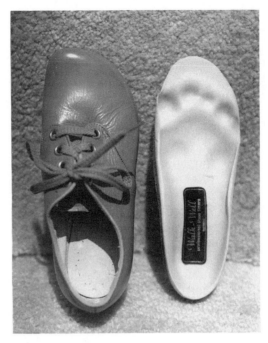

FIG 24–6.
Shoe anatomically shaped according to foot contour with depth to accept custom-molded inlay on right.

justments. Critical to the success of this type of footwear is the detailing the clinician provides to the fabricator to assure accommodation of pathology and proper biomechanical function. Close scrutiny to specific details must be made on the completed shoes. For the insensate foot with some deformity, I almost always use the custom-mold construction rather than conventional.

Selective Athletic Footwear With Extra Girth Capability

Though footwear cosmetics should not be a consideration in determining the choice of footwear to use on the diabetic foot, it nevertheless occasionally is a factor. Fortunately, certain manufacturers now provide athletic footwear in a variety of lasts in widths from extra narrow to extra wide (EEEE) (Fig 24–9). They come with removable insoles providing extra girth capability for custom-molded accommoda-

A

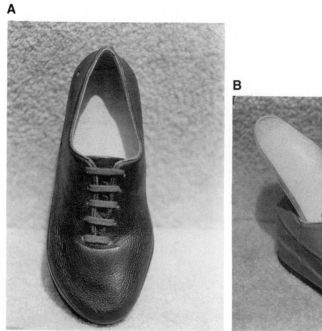

B

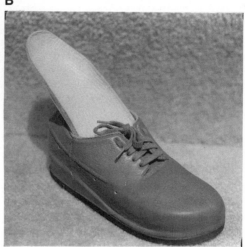

FIG 24–7.
A, custom-molded shoe of patient with hallux valgus. Note outflare shape of shoe. **B,** custom-molded shoe with replaceable total contact accommodative inlay.

tive and functional orthotics. They are available in varying degrees of firmness and flexibility with significant advantageous shock-absorbing qualities. When the specific type of athletic shoe to use is selected, a patient's requirements must be carefully considered because the stress points of a running shoe, for example, differ from those of a shoe for tennis, fitness,

aerobics, and so forth. When athletic footwear is used, consideration of extrinsic modification is also a factor.

Healing, or Temporary, Footwear

Patients with insensate feet should never walk on their bare feet. The foot must always be protected! After total contact cast-

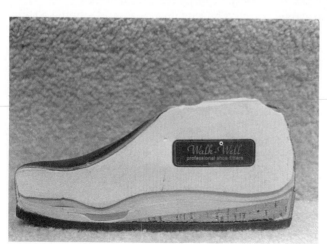

FIG 24–8.
Cross-section of custom-molded shoe with pressure relief excavation under first metatarsal phalangeal joint.

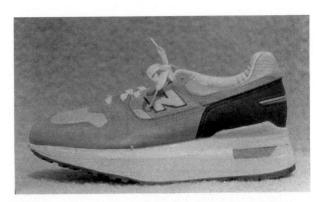

FIG 24–9.
Extra girth athletic shoe that will accept custom-molded multidensity inlay. The sole is converted to a steel-braced rigid rocker bottom, men's size 12 EEEE.

ing or at any time immediately after closure of an ulcer, temporary, or healing, footwear is required (Fig 24–10). When the patient is waiting for the fabrication of a custom-molded shoe, which takes 3 to 6 weeks, temporary footwear, sometimes referred to as "healing sandals," are required. The critical factor is that the patient cannot wait, because time is of the essence.

The shoe must be protective, accommodative, and as close to foot shape as possible during this interim period. One of the preferred materials to be used for this purpose is polyethylene foam such as Plastazote (available from APEX Foot Health Industries, South Hackensack, N.J.) (Fig 24–11). It is nontoxic, is resilient, and easily molds to the contour of the foot.

A commercially made total Plastazote shoe, is available with extra girth capa-

bility that will accept a custom-molded inlay (see Fig 24–11). When there is difficulty in fitting an edematous or disfigured foot, a custom-molded Plastazote sandal should be fabricated by the clinician (Fig 24–12). This would consist of a soft density ½-in. Plastazote insole molded to the plantar surface of the foot. This insole should extend about ½ in. on all sides of the foot for protection. A layer of firm Plastazote is then glued to this insole. Straps of cotton webbing should be fitted to the patient's foot and then glued to the firm Plastazote bottom. A strip of firm ¼-in. Plastazote is then heated and glued around the perimeter to secure it together, adding a degree of rigidity to the sandal.

For added rigidity, a leather midsole and spring steel shank piece may be added. A final outsole of ⅜-in. neoprene crepe completes construction.

The sole design should employ a roller

FIG 24–10.
A temporary healing sandal custom-molded to a patient's foot.

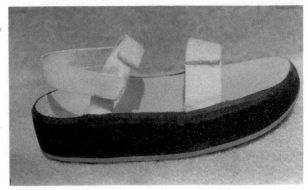

A

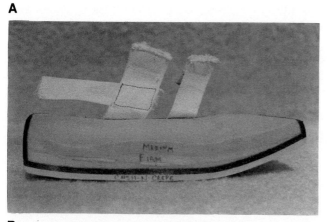

B

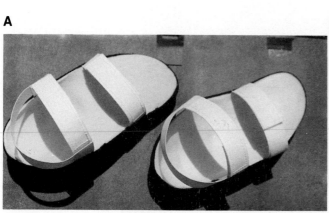

FIG 24–11.
A, cross-section of healing sandal. Note cush-N-crepe bottom sole, black rigid Plastazote above, followed by firm Plastazote, all serving as a base for medium-density, custom-molded Plastazote insole. Cotton webbing serves as straps with Velcro closure. Black rigid Plastazote sidewalls on perimeter of sandal adds rigidity for rocker bottom. Note toe spring. **B,** commercial Plastazote temporary healing shoe with replaceable inlays. (Manufactured by APEX Foot Health Industries, South Hackensack, NJ.) Figure 24-12c courtesy of APEX Foot Health Industries.

B

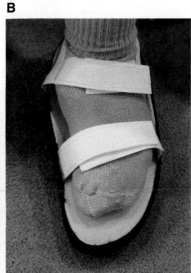

A

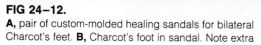

FIG 24–12.
A, pair of custom-molded healing sandals for bilateral Charcot's feet. **B,** Charcot's foot in sandal. Note extra space on perimeter on sandal for extra protection.

or rocker concept. This is accomplished by grinding down the forepart of the firm Plastazote, and outsole layers.

On delivery of permanent footwear, healing footwear may be used as alternate house shoes.

CUSTOM-MOLDED INSTRINSIC FOOT ORTHOSES

Two ways of spreading stress is by softness and molding.

Softness spreads stress in space and time by reducing the speed of the foot's impact shock with the ground.

Molding to the exact contour of the foot distributes weight to the total plantar surface of the foot, eliminating high-pressure areas. Equalized weight distribution is achieved through the use of softness and molding by using total contact inlays made of various space-age materials, depending on accommodative and functional goals (Fig 24–13).

These inlays are referred to as "total

A

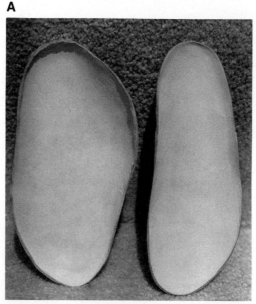

B

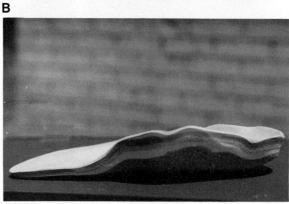

FIG 24–13.
A, custom-molded multidensity inlay. **B,** in lay for unilateral Charcot's foot.

contact multi-density thermo-formable inlays," which in reality are removable custom-molded inlays. They are used for both potential or recurrent pressure areas or ulcerations and are extremely cogent in diabetic foot management.

There is a moment of high pressure under the metatarsal heads during the stance phase of gait at heel off while the other foot is in swing phase. This peak pressure is the cause of most initial and recurrent ulcers in the distal third of the foot. A total contact multi-density thermo-formable inlay directly molded to the foot or over a positive plaster cast of the plantar surface of the foot dramatically decreases or eliminates this peak pressure.[10]

These custom inlays are best fabricated from various types of closed-cell polyethylene foams, open-cell polyurethane foams, thermoplastic cork, open-cell sponge rubber, and expanded closed-cell rubber.

Polyethylene foam materials are heat moldable, vacuum formable, and easily ground for sculpting and adjusting. Most important, they are inert and do not react with human tissue. They are available in variable densities (durometers) from soft to semirigid. Selection is dependent on the desired accommodative or functional goals or requirements. These materials have variable compression settings from 5% to 30%, according to thickness and density.[11] They are used individually or in multidensity dual, tri or quad systems, each contributing their own positive characteristics, compensating for negative reactive forces that cause pressure.

Other determinant factors as to which materials to use depend on their properties such as weight, tensile strength and durability. Some of the cross-linked, closed-cell polyethylene foams are better known by their commerical names of Plastazote, Pelite, Aliplast, Dermaplast, and XPE.

Polyurethane foam, open-cell materials are commercially known as P.P.T. and Poron. These materials maintain 90% of thickness under excessive load and are excellent in absorbing shock and shear forces. However, because polyurethane is not heat moldable, it is often used in combination with polyethylene foams.

Expanded closed-cell rubber is more commonly known as Spenco or Ribatex. It is often combined with multistretch fabric acting as an interface between the foot and the rubber. This combination absorbs both shock and shear forces in a firm durometer material and maintains 90% of its thickness when used as a component of a foot orthosis.

Open-cell sponge rubber is commercially known as Pedic Sponge, Lynco, and Kemblo. It is soft and porous, permitting ventilation and rapid recovery, maintaining up to 90% of its thickness. It also can be combined with a multistretch fabric interfacing between the foot and rubber surface. It is used in both firm and soft densities, combining well with other materials.

Thermoplastic cork is commercially known as Thermocork and Burko-Cork. When heated, it becomes tacky, molds beautifully to a positive cast, and bonds exceptionally well with other materials. The cooled device creates a firm orthosis, maintaining greater than 90% of its thickness.

Visco elastic polymers are better known as Sorbothane, P.Q., and Viscolas. It is a rubberlike material that, when compressed, tends to flow, dissipating shock and sheer forces. A major disadvantage to its use is its element of weight. It is difficult to cut, sand, or grind, making fabrication and adjustments difficult.

EXTRINSIC FOOTWEAR MODIFICATIONS

The third method of spreading stress in conjunction with softness and molding is "rocking."

A totally rigid spring steel reinforced rocker bottom can significantly reduce plantar pressure and shear stresses on the forefoot. This results from the knee flexing early, thus accelerating the gait cycle, reducing the stride length and forefoot plantar pressure. To assure uninhibited toe-off phase of gait, a critical component in the rocker function, the integrity of toe spring must be maintained. The distal end of the sole must eliminate any ground contact (Fig 24–14). The peak of the rocker apex becomes the fulcrum, is generally a minimum of ¾ in. high, and is often higher to assure toe clearance. Precise angulation of toe spring is difficult to specify but ranges from an average of 10% to 40%. An excellent starting point in determining curvature of rocker angle is to create a radius the length of 75% of the shoe. This radius should be placed perpendicular to the sole of the shoe at a point 55% to 60% from the posterior tip of the heel and an arc drawn to the toe. The curve and angle thus created are an excellent starting point. Added elevation, however, if needed for tolerance, may create a stability problem, especially with geriatric patients. For the sake of stability and a smoother gait cycle, the use of a roller bottom, though a degree of compromise, may be advisable. The roller bottom has a less radical angle at the apex, assuring a mollified, safer gait pattern. The methodology of determining the exact location of the apex may vary with some clinicians, but the preceding has proved successful.

In addition to reduction of metatarsal pressure, the rocker concept at both sole and heel are effective in relieving strain on a Charcot ankle or fused ankle.

There is often a need to broaden the base of support at both midfoot and hindfoot to stabilize Charcot's joints, rigid pes valgus, and severely pronated feet. The heel, referred to as an "offset heel" and "flared heel," is extended medially, laterally, or both to a linear extension, meeting the deviated vertical line of body weight. An imaginary plumb line from the knee to the floor gives the approximate degree of heel extension.

However, a pragmatic determination must be made when the degree of extension becomes too cumbersome. When a custom-molded shoe is detailed, the offset heel concept can become an integral part of the detailing of the shoe. The basic difference between the simple flared heel and an offset heel is the filling of the cavity between the heel extension and the upper counter.

FOOTWEAR RECOMMENDATIONS BASED ON FOOT RISK

With the physician's diagnoses and pedorthic assessment and perceived classification of foot risk, appropriate footwear, orthoses, and biomechanical footwear modifications can be recommended (Table 24–3).

FIG 24–14.
Men's extra girth shoe with rigid steel-braced (heel to toe) rocker bottom. Note 20° toe spring.

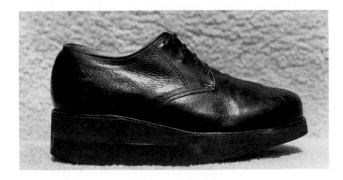

TABLE 24–3.

Footwear Chart

	Foot Risk Category			
	Sensate	Insensate		
Footwear Recommendations*	4.17 (0)	5.02 (1)	6.10 (2)	6.10 (3)
Conventional Footwear	X	X		
Last similar to contour of foot, soft porous leather, no abrasive seams, fitting with extreme caution (not tight)	X	X	X	X
Extra girth footwear	X	X	X	X
Cushioned inlays (dual density)		X		
Custom multidensity inlays		X	X	X
Rocker or roller bottoms (rigid)			X	X
Heat-moldable shoe (Thermold)			X	X
Athletic footwear (replaceable inlays)	X	X	X	
Cushioned inlays (dual density)		X		
Custom multidensity inlays		X	X	
Rocker or roller bottoms (rigid)			X	
Custom-molded footwear				X
Custom tridensity inlays				
Precise detailing to deformities			X	X
Steel-braced rigid rocker or roller bottoms			X	X

*Select shoe manufacturers include Classic Custom Shoe, Acor Custom Shoe, Jerry Miller I.D. Shoe, Abernathy Inc., Birkenstock, Trumold Shoes, P.W. Minor Co., Drew Shoe Corp., Footsaver, Alden Shoe Co., Foot-So-Port, Markell Shoe Co., Rockport Shoe Corp., S.A.S. Shoe Co., New Balance Athletics, Spiess Shoe Co., Munro & Co., Etonic Athletics, and Pendas.

Foot Risk Category 0 (SW 4.17)

For all purposes, this foot can be considered as any normal foot. It has all protective levels of sensation, but the sensory systems within the foot is always at risk. It is for this reason that a posture of preventive care should be assumed.

Most conventional footwear may be used with special attention to selection of a last compatible with the contour of the foot. Soft porous leather free of abrasive seams should be preferred. Care to keep the forepart of the foot free to articulate with secure heel and arch control is the goal of proper fit.

Foot Risk Category 1 (SW 5.07)

These patients have lost protective levels of sensation partially or totally in different anatomic sectors of their feet and therefore are at a high risk of injury. They do not have any history of ulceration and are without any significant foot deformity. However, they would be unaware of any repetitive stress that could cause tissue breakdown. For that reason, footwear with extra girth able to accept cushioned or custom multidensity inlays would be recommended.

Athletic footwear with extra girth capability able to receive inserts may also be considered.

A custom-molded shoe could also be considered but usually is not a necessity.

Foot Risk Category 2 (SW 6.10)

Not only do these patients have a lost protective threshold of sensation, but they have a history of foot ulceration. Human tissue once ulcerated is extremely vulnerable to recurrent ulceration; therefore, these patients' feet present a high risk factor. Because this patient is without foot deformity, an extra girth shoe is a favored footwear option with a tridensity total contact multi-density thermo-formable inlay. A rigid rocker or roller bottom would be advisable. Other options would be a well-fitted athletic shoe with appropriate total contact multi-density thermo-formable inlays and rocker or roller bottoms. Consideration of a custom-molded shoe is also advisable with total contact multi-density thermo-formable inlays and appropriate biomechanical modifications.

Foot Risk Category 3 (SW 6.10)

The major problem with the feet of these patients is their deformities. Deformities cause high-pressure stress in concentrated areas, causing tissue breakdown and ulceration on insensate feet. These patients may or may not have a history of ulceration, which adds an additional dimension of risk.

Recommended footwear is almost always a custom-molded shoe with uppers of kangaroo kid for durability and softness, a custom total contact multi-density thermo-formable inlay and rigid rocker or roller bottoms. Special relief techniques such as excavations under high-pressure areas are also advisable.

Another consideration for patients in category 3 is use of an extra girth shoe, providing there is fit capability. Heat-moldable footwear that can be customized to foot deformities may possibly be used, with appropriate multidensity inlays, rigid rocker bottoms, and offset heels if required.

There is no substitution for a clinician's pragmatism and creativity when recommending footwear, orthoses, and modifications according to risk classifications in the therapeutic management of diabetic feet.

CHARCOT CONDITIONS

Changes in the osseous structure of the neuropathic foot resulting in Charcot's joint, sometimes referred to as Charcot's foot because it includes changes in the metatarsal bones, leading to severe foot deformation (Fig 24–15,A-B). With deformed configuration, a pathologic gait pattern develops, creating high-pressure points and usually ulceration because of the absence of a protective threshold of pain.

Also, Charcot's feet with an impaired vascular system often leads to gangrene and eventual amputation.

With patients who have Charcot's feet, it is critical that a precise biomechanical assessment be made of the line of body weight. This must be done to plan how to compensate for the pathologic gait pattern responsible for causing pressure points. Compensation is achieved by re-aligning body weight to whatever degree is possible through the design and detail of a custom-molded shoe. Stabilization is required to prevent further disfigurement, and a total contact multi-density thermo-formable inlay with compensating excavations must be made to assure equalized weight distribution on the plantar weight-bearing surfaces.

The custom shoe must also accommodate pressure on the dorsal areas of the foot with appropriate compensation (Fig 24–16). A rigid rocker or roller sole should be used to assure stabilization and assure some normalization of a gait pattern. Care must be exercised in the placement of the rocker apex to assure transfer of any possible pressure from vulnerable anatomical areas.

Because of the deformed configurations and impaired gait pattern of the Charcot foot, along with foot stabilizing and accommodation, additional ankle leg bracing is often required. When the joints are found to be mechanically unstable, plastic or metal ankle-foot support may be required. It is here that the expertise of a certified orthotist should be sought to work in concert with the pedorthist and physician.

At the time of delivery of this special footwear, complete instructions as to how to commence their use, along with how to

A

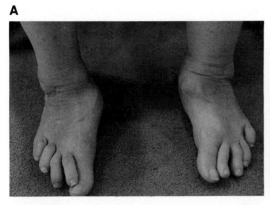

B

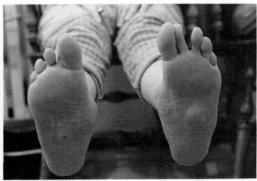

FIG 24–15.
A, superior view of bilateral Charcot's feet. Note medial tuberosities, curled, hammered, and overlapping toes. **B,** plantar view of bilateral Charcot's feet. Note almost

healed ulcer right pressure area and midfoot pressure area on left foot.

self-inspect the foot, must be given to the patient. Initial short periods of wear progressing to full time, taking shorter steps and employing a slower cadence, should not be taken for granted. Instructions should be given to a patient both verbally and in written form. Working in concert with a diabetic nurse educator is advised.

AMPUTATIONS

Transmetatarsal, Chopart, Lisfranc, unilateral or multilateral phalanx amputa-

tions each present special considerations.

Weight-bearing distribution and gait patterns should be the primary concern of the clinician (Fig 24–17). Cosmesis, though a psychologic concern of the patient, should be secondary. Patients with a transmetatarsal or more advanced amputation ideally should have a custom-molded shoe. The shoe accommodating the amputation should be made shorter than the normal foot. Often in an effort to match the footwear in size, problems result with an undesirable flex point and a cumbersome gait. A custom-molded shoe

A

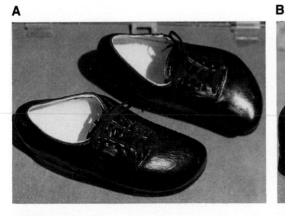

B

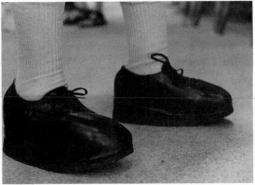

FIG 24–16.
A, custom-molded shoes for bilateral Charcot's feet with total contact multi-density thermo-formable inlays. Upper leather in kangaroo kid for softness and

durability. **B,** Side view of custom-molded shoe with rigid steel-braced rocker bottom. Note 25° toe spring on right foot.

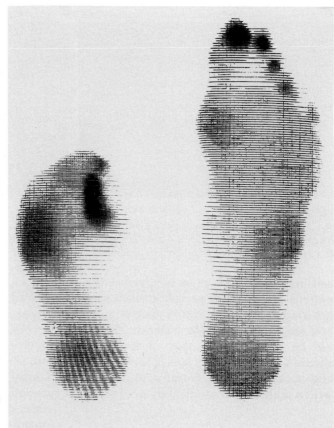

FIG 24–17.
Insensate diabetic patient with trans-metatarsal amputation. Scar tissue on plantar area of balance of first metatarsal shaft, resulting in excessive lateral weight-bearing. Right foot still intact shows pressure for potential ulceration on distal end of hallux and second toe. Medial bulging convex arch indicates pes planus and calcaneus valgus. Also note some potential pressure at right cuboid area.

FIG 24–18.
Athletic shoe with extra depth feature. Has total contact multi-density thermo-formable inlay. Bottoms are rigid rocker steel braced with good toe spring.

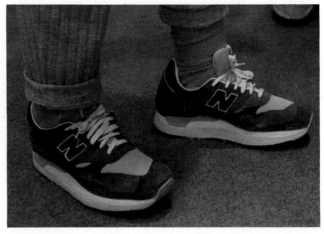

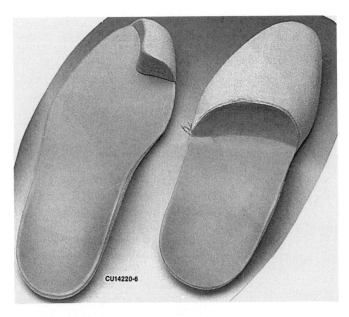

FIG 24–19.
Left, prostheses with toe filler accommodation in conjunction with total contact soft tissue supplement (TCSTS) inlay. *Right,* prostheses with transmetatarsal amputation toe filler in conjunction with TCSTS inlay. *(Courtesy of APEX Foot Health Industries, Inc., South Hackensack, N.J.).*

fit as close to the stump as practical, with a roller bottom, is our preference.

An extra girth shoe or appropriate athletic shoe with extra girth capability can also be used (Fig 24–18). With either of these options, total contact multidensity soft tissue inserts with prosthetic forepart accommodation should be used (Fig 24–19). The shoes should have rigid steel-braced rocker or roller soles and may require mismating.

In the cases of Chopart and Lisfranc amputations, it is most desirable to use an above ankle custom shoe. However, a Chopart filler boot or leather ankle foot lacer in conjunction with an extra girth stock shoe may be considered. The same shoe details as previously described should be used.

ONGOING PEDORTHIC-PATIENT RELATIONSHIP

Noncompliance is always a problem with many diabetic patients. It is therefore essential that the clinician put himself or herself in a strong control posture with the patient. This commences with the initial prefitting analysis by educating the patient through explanation as to what you are assessing. The negative aspects of neuropathic and ischemic foot disorders, the ramifications of neglect, and potential of amputation should be made clear. The patient must be made to understand that the very nature of the disease requires compromise in life-style, activities, and extra foot care. The patient, physician, nurse educator, and pedorthist must work as a team to protect the feet against any trauma. With this team effort diabetic patients can avoid the resulting tragedies experienced by so many diabetic patients. Above all, patients must realize that the care of the diabetic foot is a lifelong, ongoing responsibility.

CONCLUSION

Ultimate pedorthic judgment is dependent on comprehension of patient pathology in relationship to therapeutical goals and management. The pedorthist is responsible for:

1. Determining need for an accommodative or functional orthoses or combination of both.
2. Determining types of materials to be used and their influence on the dissipation of disruptive forces.
3. Determining the biomechanics of modifications and their effect on restoration of an acceptable gait pattern.
4. Recommending proper types of footgear.
5. Providing patients' pedorthic education.
6. Periodically reevaluating orthoses and footwear.

With all of these responsibilities, systematic pedorthic management of the diabetic foot can contribute to the prevention of millions of foot amputations and the enhancement of the lives of the millions of diabetic patients.

REFERENCES

1. Levin ME, O'Neal LW, editors: *The diabetic foot,* ed 4, St Louis, 1988, Mosby–Year Book.
2. Kosiak M: Etiology and pathology of ischemic ulcers, *Arch Phys Med Rehabil* 40:62–69, 1959.
3. Brand PW: *Repetitive stress on insensitive feet,* US Public Health Service, Carville, La, 1975.
4. Wagner FW Jr: *A classification and treatment program for diabetic, neuropathic, and dysvascular foot problems,* AAOS Instructional Course Lectures, Vol. 28, St Louis, 1979, Mosby–Year Book.
5. Rossi WA, Tennant R: *Professional shoe fitting,* New York, 1984, National Shoe Retailers Assoc.
6. Wu KK: *Foot orthoses: principals of clinical practice,* Baltimore, 1990, Williams & Wilkins.
7. Steb HS: Footwear and the diabetic foot [lecture], Carville, La, 1988, US Department of Health and Human Services, National Hansens Disease Center.
8. Steb HS: Pedorthic pre-fitting analysis, [lecture], New York, 1989–1991, New York University Post Graduate Medical School, Orthotic Prosthetic Division.
9. Steb HS: The anatomy of a shoe, professional shoe fitting, and pedorthic assessment of the foot, [lectures], Chicago, 1991–1992, Northwestern University Medical School, Prosthetic-Orthotic Center.
10. Steb HS: Pedorthic and the diabetic foot [lecture]. Grand Rapids, Mich, 1991, Michigan Podiatric Medical Assoc.
11. Schwartz RS, Schwartz RB: *Material selection for foot orthoses.* South Hackensack, NJ and New York, 1990, Eneslow Classic Mold Shoes–Apex Foot Health Industries.

25   Comprehensive Foot Care

Jeffrey Cohen, D.P.M.

As podiatric physicians, we frequently treat diabetic patients. In many of these instances the patient has an infected foot, cellulitis, deep abscess (or abscesses), fever, and possible septicemia. These patients must be treated swiftly and aggressively with appropriate antibiotics, consultations, surgical procedures (both emergency and reconstructive), and follow-up (Fig 25–1). This form of therapy has been well covered in other chapters in this book; therfore, this chapter will concentrate on the conservative treatment of the diabetic patient from both a preventive and a therapeutic approach. In many cases this conservative care will preempt the necessity for the previously mentioned scenario to be played out.

No part of the human body is as vulnerable as the foot. The foot is often subjected to ill-fitting, poorly ventilated shoes, which are stressful even to the nondiabetic foot. Add to all this the fact that the foot is at the end of the vascular tree, subjected to gravity like no other part of the human anatomy. All these are vector factors that challenge the podiatric physician in the management of the diabetic foot.

EXAMINATION

Before any patient is treated, it is necessary to first examine the patient and assess what is problematic and what requires attention. A complete lower-extremity examination should be done as described in Chapter 2. The diabetic patient is approached the same way as the nondiabetic patient, taking into account the patient's chief complaint, unless this is a routine examination. The physicain should also listen carefully to the patient's history, specifically for activities that may lend themselves to foot problems.

The 30-year old type I diabetic of 15 years' duration who is standing for long hours at his or her occupation must be considered in a different light than the 62-year-old type II diabetic who has been on an oral hypoglycemic agent for the past 5 years and who works in a sedentary occupation wearing sneakers all day. Both patients will require special care, however, and each will need individualized education, instruction for home care, treatment, and preventive maintenance.

Once a complete history is acquired, the examination of the diabetic patient should include assessment of both the vascular and neurologic status of the patient. Particular attention should be given but not limited to the lower extremity. The patient can then be classified according to the level of pathophysiology associated with his or her diabetes. By doing so, one can readily ascertain whether a presenting or potential foot lesion is caused by vascular complications, neuropathic complications, or a combination of both. This, in turn, allows us to use the most efficacious form of therapy for each individual patient according to the patient's specific needs.

In the remainder of this chapter, we

A

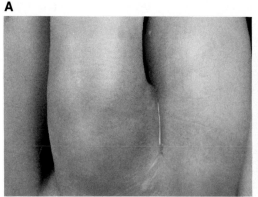

B

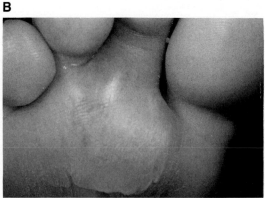

FIG 25–1.
A, dorsal view of diabetic patient with second inter-space abscess. **B,** plantar view of same patient. This patient required hospital admission, incision and drainage, intravenous antibiotics, and appropriate follow-up.

will explore various diabetic lesions, briefly discuss their pathophysiology and methods of diagnosis, and elaborate on many ways to conservatively treat and prevent these conditions.

VASCULAR LESIONS

Medical Management

Diabetes is a disease process that affects multiple organ systems. Of concern to the podiatrist is its effect on the lower extremity and especially the most distal aspect of the body and vascular tree, the foot.[1–3] The triad of sequelae associated with diabetes is nephropathy, neuropathy, and angiopathy. Let us concern ourselves with the latter two complications, and at this juncture, the angiopathy, or as it is often referred to, the vascular disease. The terminology refers to the effects of the changes that take place in the arteries, both large and small, in the body. However, this is not the only area of the vascular tree that is affected by this disease.

The vascular lesions associated with the diabetic foot are generally caused by ischemia. The lack of circulation to the limb is a result of large-vessel disease in the leg and thigh as a result of athero-sclerosis of these vessels.[4] So when we examine a patient with a vascular lesion, we are seeing the end result of occlusive arterial disease, and the symptoms will include pain, absence of pulses, possibly intermittent claudication, tissue necrosis with or without erythema surrounding the lesion, and possibly gangrene. If the patient has concomitant peripheral neuropathy, it is possible to have a vascular lesion that is nonpainful or less painful than would otherwise be expected.[1]

Patients who have vascular lesions should be evaluated for the severity of their ischemia because this will determine how the patient should be treated. For example, the patient may be a candidate for conservative medical care, may be treated surgically by debridement or amputation, or may be referred to a vascular surgeon for revascularization. "The features which suggest that local treatment is unlikely to succeed are the presence of ischaemic rest pain and extensive necrosis."[5] For the purpose of this chapter, we shall consider those vascular lesions that are associated with an ankle brachial index (ABI) of greater than 0.6. We will also consider those lesions in which the index is less than 0.6 but are not candidates for surgical intervention because of their medical status or other reasons why they cannot be revascularized.[2]

If we could successfully increase the flow of blood to the area of ischemia, theoretically the lesion should heal more quickly and more successfully. There are several possible approaches to accomplish this task. The first would be to inject local anesthetic to block a nerve, in effect creating a local sympathectomy. By blocking the sympathetic nerves, vasodilation occurs distal to the block. This can be accomplished at the level of the ankle, the knee, or through a referral to an anesthesiologist for injection at the spinal level. If successful, a permanent sympathectomy could be performed surgically by the vascular surgeon. This procedure is not performed very often any more. Some practitioners have found success by performing ankle blocks several times in a period of a few weeks with some ischemic lesions. However, if the ischemia is caused by a blockage proximal to the ankle, dilating the distal vessels should have very little effect on increasing the blood flow to the foot.

A second methodology that has shown some promise is the use of pentoxifylline (Trental; Hoechst Ag) which has a mode of action different from the vasodilating effect of local anesthetics.[6,7] In this scenario, the medication causes the red blood cells to become more flexible, allowing them to circulate through blood vessels that were previously impassable to them in part or whole. The net effect of this medication, therefore, is to increase the amount of hemoglobin reaching the area of ulceration, thereby increasing the healing capacity of the tissues. We have used this treatment regime in conjunction with topical medications and local debridement. The result was an improvement in those patients who took the drug, with the remainder of care being relatively equal.

A third method of increasing the flow to the ischemic ulcer or creating the same effect, in other words, increased oxygenation at the level of necrosis, is through the use of hyperbaric oxygen.[2] The theory behind the use of hyperbaric oxygen is that by placing oxygen under the proper amount of pressure, the oxygen tension (Po_2) level in the affected tissue is increased through external sources, and therefore healing can proceed.

Topical applications of medication have shown to have positive effects in many cases. These topical formulations range from antibiotics to antibacterial agents to debriding agents. In many instances more than one medication can be used at the same time.

The first group of medications are the antibacterial or antiseptic agents. The most common of these used today is povidone-iodine (Betadine), which can be applied as a solution (full strength or dilute), an ointment, or as a soak. As a solution applied directly to the lesion, it decreases the bacterial flora and dries the lesion. As an ointment, it causes less drying of the tissues while still having the remaining positive effects. As a soak, it may help to promote drainage if there is purulence present within the wound. In many instances, especially in a nursing home setting where the patient is sedentary or bedridden, the use of a dressing with povidone-iodine solution and dry sterile gauze can change an infected, wet ischemic lesion to a clean, dry eschar-type of lesion that may heal slowly deep to the eschar, or may continue unchanged without causing serious harm to the patient. Unfortunately, povidone-iodine in all of its forms retards the development of granulation tissue; therefore, it has limited use in this patient population.

The next class of topical agents that may be used for these wounds are the antibiotics. These are especially useful in those lesions that have identifiable organisms that can be neutralized or destroyed by antibiotics. Most of these diabetic ulcers will culture out multimicrobial flora that are superficial. These agents will deter many of the topical organisms from becoming more deeply seated pathogens. There are many common topical antibiotics to choose from, most having a wide spectrum of effectiveness. A few physicians favor using polysporin powder or spray, which some physicians believe helps to dry many of the lesions. At the same time, a decreased microbial flora is maintained in the area, which, in turn, helps create a healing wound. Other commonly used antibiotics are polymyxin B–bacitracin–neomycin (Neosporin) cream or ointment, bacitracin, and mupirocin (Bactroban) ointment.

The last class of topical medications worthy of mention are the debriding agents. These generally work through the use of enzymes that break down the necrotic tissues, thereby allowing the healthy tissues to heal more quickly. We believe the best of these formulations is collagenase (Santyl), which has a mode of action that "has the ability to digest native and denatured collagen and to contribute toward the formation of viable granulation tissue and subsequent epithelization of wounds."[8] The ointment may be applied along with a topical antibiotic such as polysporin powder to

have the added effect of the topical antibiotic.

As part of treating any infected or suspected infected diabetic lesion, we must use appropriate antibiotic therapy. Oral antibiotics should be administered as determined by culture and sensitivity studies or, when there is no significant drainage, by empiric evaluation of the patient. It is best to initiate antibiotic treatment in a diabetic patient if there is any suspicion of infection. As the degree of ischemia increases, the ability of the patient to mount a classic response to infection decreases (see Chapter 15 for more detailed discussion of the use of antibiotics in the care of the diabetic patient).

Although most vascular lesions in diabetics are ischemic, there are diabetic patients who have concomitant venous disease that will cause them to have ulcerations because of stasis (Fig 25–2). These patients must be treated with elevation and compression in addition to the local care of the wounds. They should also be instructed to keep their legs elevated, preferably higher than the level of their heart, whenever sitting and not to stand for extended periods of time (½ hour at most). In addition to elevation, there are several forms of therapy to help compress the fluid out of the limbs.

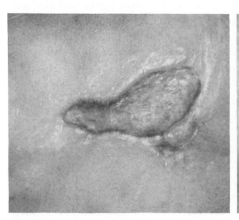 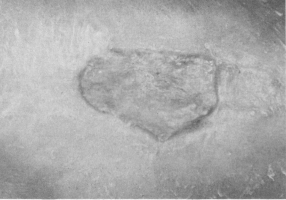

FIG 25–2.
Long-standing venous ulcerations on medical malleolus bilaterally.

The use of Ace bandages wrapped concentrically and evenly up the foot and leg from the toes to just below the knee or to the midthigh is effective. However, this is difficult to accomplish in the home-care patient, who may not reapply the bandages correctly on a daily basis. These patients should have either over-the-counter or custom-fit support to improve the return flow of blood to the deep venous system and on to the heart. On a more acute level, when there is one or more venous stasis ulcers on the leg, using Unna boot dressings has proved to be effective. These are applied directly onto the skin from the toes to below the knee with sterile dressings applied first to the open wounds that have been cleansed appropriately. Care should be taken when the dressings are applied to create even compression or graduated compression up the leg. The dressing should be changed every 3 to 7 days, depending on the patient. A noticeable improvement can be seen at each such change of the bandage.

The last form of medical management that is used on patients with venous stasis ulcers is actually considered surgical. The need for the wound to be kept clean and free of necrotic tissue requires debridement of the wound. This applies especially to wounds that are wet, as opposd to those that appear to be a dry eschar, as referred to earlier, which may best be left alone. In ischemic lesions, it may be too painful to debride the necrotic tissue, and many times the enzymatic debriding agents referred to earlier may best be used. Hydrogen peroxide acts well as a mechanical debriding agent and may be used by both the patient and the physician at each dressing change. When the podiatric or vascular physician sees the patient, he or she may wish to further remove loose or thickened necrotic tissue to let granulation tissue invade the wound and create a new base of epithelization to take place.

Biomechanical Management

External pressure on living tissue decreases the blood flow to that tissue while the pressure is applied.[2,9–11] In the ischemic foot, the effect of even mildly increased pressure on the skin may be the difference between minimal blood flow and no blood flow to the particular area.

The human foot normally bears weight evenly distributed across specific areas of the foot's plantar surface designed to tolerate increased pressures. These weight-bearing areas are the heel, lateral side of the sole, metatarsal heads, and plantar tuft of the toes.[12] When there is an irregularity in the mechanics of the foot, one or more of these areas or other areas unintended for weight-bearing become the target of unacceptable high pressure, loss of circulation to the tissue, and in the ischemic foot, the site of necrosis (Fig 25–3).[13]

Therefore, in the foot with a biomechanical dysfunction or in the ischemic foot with or without biomechanical dysfunction, it is clear that there is a logical cause for the development of ulcers. It should therefore be just as logical that many of these lesions can and should be prevented or once developed, controlled by maintaining the foot in a proper biomechanical alignment. This can be accomplished in many different ways. Simple dispersion dressings to prevent pressure areas, various accommodative appliances or orthotics, and a multitude of custom-made and semicustom-made shoes are the ways to accomplish this task. Many of these techniques will be discussed in detail later in this chapter.

If a patient whose foot has one or more lesions is suitable for conservative treatment, his or her treatment regime should involve both a medical approach and a biomechanical approach. This regime would provide the best possible chance of healing and prevent the need for more aggressive procedures.

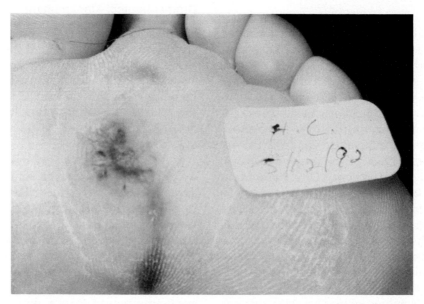

FIG 25–3.
Patient with insulin-dependent diabetes mellitus with cavus-type foot and pressure area submetatarsal 2 left foot. Note eccymotic areas within the keratosis indicative of necrotic changes deep to the callous.

NEUROTROPHIC LESIONS

Medical Management

The effect that the nervous system has on the lower extremity is so diverse and important to normal function that with malfunction of the system we see a broad range of symptoms develop, such as peripheral neuropathy. "Diabetic neuropathy is a common name for what probably constitutes several conditions involving the lower extremities, including: (1) progressive symmetrical distal polyneuropathy; (2) ischemic mononeuropathy multiplex; (3) neurogenic arthropathy; (4) diabetic anhidrosis; (5) diabetic amyotrophy; and (6) diabetic cold feet."[3] The most common of these is the first, which causes the stocking and glove distribution to first the hands and then the feet; this condition is seen frequently in podiatric practice. These patients have symptoms ranging from mild tingling or fleeting sensations down to their feet to complete sense of numbness, stiffness, and heaviness with loss of proprioception, muscle atrophy, and changes of the joints that can develop into Charcot joints. The remaining effects are seen in conjunction with the first and tend to complicate their treatment with symptoms such as drop foot, wasting of the large muscles, joint destruction, and dryness of the skin of the lower extremity.

A common complaint of diabetic patients to their podiatrist or physician is that of pain in their legs, especially at night. On examination, there is often no visual or palpable signs of an abnormality, and many times these patients suffer from early neuropathy despite the ability to feel relatively normal sensations. In time, most of these patients develop all or most of the symptoms of typical diabetic neuropathy. Those patients who do suffer from painful peripheral neuropathy can be helped some of the time with medications. In a study demonstrating the effectiveness of 0.075% capsaicin, most of the patients tested found that they had good relief of their symptoms. The medication is a cream that is applied topically to the painful areas four times daily and rubbed in. The most common side effect was burning at the site of application.[14]

In patients who already have diabetic neuropathy, the development of foot ulcerations is not uncommon and poses a challenge to the treating podiatrist and a threat to the patient. Lesions develop on the insensate foot from improperly fitted shoes, abnormal weight-bearing patterns, trauma, foreign bodies, or thermal injuries or exposures. In many cases, the patient may not be aware of the occurrence of such a lesion. There may also be a long delay in recognizing its presence or seeking attention, especially with the first such incident, because there is no pain. It is not uncommon for patients to respond, when asked by the physician, that the lesion developed only 1 or 2 days before their visit. In fact, they may have realized what was occurring only during that time, although the incident developed much earlier. Regular examinations by the patient or family member on a daily basis can prevent or reduce some of the more severe sequelae of neuropathic lesions. It is therefore important to educate these patients about the signs and symptoms of neuropathic lesions of the foot.

The treating physician must be able to assess which patients are in danger of developing neuropathic lesions. It is often a difficult task to assess objectively how severe the patient's neuropathy has become and when he or she will be prone to dangerous skin lesions because of decreased sensitivity.

Two methods have been used to identify diabetics who are prone to foot ulcerations. These methods are known as vibration perception threshold and pressure perception. The former uses a biothesiometer, which is an electronic device that senses, through various degrees of vibration, the point at which an individual can perceive the sensations and records these thresholds. This device "has the disadvantages of being expensive, needing calibration and a power source, and . . . may vary widely between tests and sites for the same patient."[15] The pressure perception

technique uses a device known as a Semmes-Weinstein monofilament aesthesiometer.[17] This device "consists of a series of graded, pressure sensitive nylon filaments of increasing calibre that buckle at a reproducible stress, and can measure the patients' cutaneous pressure perception threshold."[15] This device is an inexpensive method of determining which patients are susceptible to neuropathic ulcers and should be used as a screening device when practical.

In the diabetic with a peripheral neuropathy and ischemia, the lesions will develop and must be treated in the same manner as those with ischemia alone. These patients are in more danger, however, because they lack sensation in their feet. Therefore, they generally seek help later, and their ischemia has usually worsened. If these patients do develop pain, it is usually caused by the presence of abscess formation. Immediate hospitalization and surgical intervention are required to effectively heal these abscesses. These patients are discussed in detail in other portions of this book.

Diabetics who have peripheral neuropathy without the ischemic component will benefit most from comprehensive conservative foot care. These patients have the ability to heal from a vascular standpoint, and this can be well visualized when surgery is performed and primary wound healing occurs normally. The difficulty in healing these patients' wounds occurs generally with secondary and tertiary healing, which can be seen when one is dealing with ulcer formations.

The absence or diminution of sensation causes patients with diabetic neuropathy to develop increased pressures on the foot. This pressure usually occurs in the sole, although any area of the foot can be affected by shoe pressure. The foot's skin responds to increased pressure by thickening or forming callus. These hyperkeratotic areas in the nonneuropathic patient will cause pain, and the patient will usu-

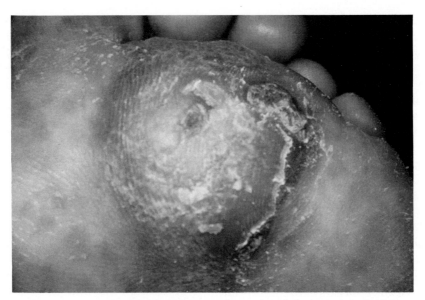

FIG 25–4.
Patient with insulin-dependent diabetes mellitus with large area of necrosis under keratotic tissue.

ally seek help to alleviate the source of pain. In the neuropathic foot, the hyperkeratotic tissue is often left to cause more pressure until local pressure necrosis develops and an ulceration ensues deep to the callus (Fig 25–4). The callus itself, therefore, is causing further increased pressure and thus causes the formation of neuropathic diabetic foot ulcers.[16] Primary podiatric care should involve inspection of the feet for signs of increased pressure and debriding calluses that may be present. These inspections deter the formation of ulcers and therefore vital in the regular care of the diabetic patient.

Much of the medical management of neuropathic lesions of diabetics is the same as for the vascular lesions. The removal of necrotic tissue by debridement, whether mechanical, surgical, or medical, is required (Fig 25–5). The use of topical antibiotics or antiseptics in conjunction

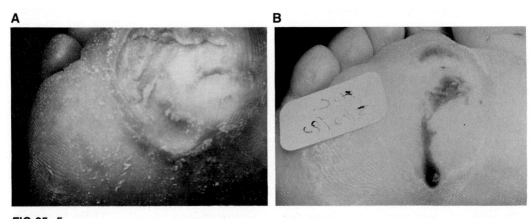

FIG 25–5.
A, Neuropathic ulcer present under keratosis in same patient as in Figure 25–3. **B,** large neuropathic ulcer present after debriding keratosis on same patient as in Figure 25–4.

with this treatment is essential to maintain a clean environment and to promote healing. The use of silver nitrate whether in 10% ointment form or by applicator sticks in 75% concentration can be an important adjunct to promote epithelization, especially in a lesion with a clean granulation tissue base.

In addition, even though these patients have good large vessel flow and patent pulses, there is still a lack of healing capacity at the dermal level, which is believed to be caused by arteriosclerosis, soft tissue swelling, or nutritional deficiencies, which cause microangiopathy to take place. With the decreased blood flow, those nutrients required for proper healing, including oxygen, cannot reach the proper tissue level. With the use of a hemorheologic agent such as pentoxifylline (Trental), which "acts by decreasing blood viscosity and serum fibrinogen levels and increasing red blood cell flexibility, . . . tissue perfusion is enhanced."[17] In a study performed on diabetic neurotrophic ulcers, the use of pentoxifylline appeared to have accelerated the healing process in 9 of 12 patients studied.[17,18]

Biomechanical Management

The relationship of abnormal pressures on the tissues of the diabetic foot was discussed in the section on vascular lesions. Those lesions, which are generally painful, become more painful when the increased pressure causes additional ischemia. The ischemia, in turn, causes the necrosis of the tissues to spread. In the neuropathic diabetic foot or the combined vascular and neuropathic foot with its associated lesions, the biomechanical dysfunction cannot be assessed by an increase in the amount of pain felt by the patient. With the neuropathic lesions, this abnormal weight distribution is manifested by new, unchanged, or worsening lesions developing on the feet of these patients. It therefore becomes essential that the physician be aware of the forces transmitted through any particular areas of the foot and how to control these forces to minimize the amount of pressure necrosis that may occur.[12]

Biomechanical management of the neuropathic foot may be accomplished by both weight-bearing techniques and non-weight-bearing techniques. Weight-bearing devices that accommodate the lesions or redistribute the weight-bearing forces can be as simple as felt padding or dressings applied directly on the foot with dressing changes as described earlier for vascular lesions. These are intended for short-term use, generally until the lesions are healed, and usually are best suited for cases where the cause of the wound is a temporary imbalance caused by a poor-fitting shoe or improper activity and either the offending shoe or activity has been discarded or discontinued. In the more common scenario of a pressure imbalance in the foot, weight-bearing devices of an accommodative or functional nature can be fabricated to redistribute the forces either away from the affected area completely or to more evenly distribute those forces, thereby lessening the affect on the particular area of ulceration. Also within the category of weight-bearing devices would be the use of a casting technique known as a total contact cast, which allows the patient to continue ambulating with the forces of pressure almost bypassing the foot.[10,11]

Non-weight-bearing techniques include either the use of crutches or a specially designed shoe where a portion of the foot is left unaffected by the forces of gravity. There are at least two such shoes on the market where the forefoot is held off the ground, hanging over a short sole that is inclined at the heel (Figs 25–6 and 25–7). This can be very effective in treating ulcers of the forefoot and toes.

All of these devices will be discussed in more detail in the section describing orthotic devices later in this chapter.

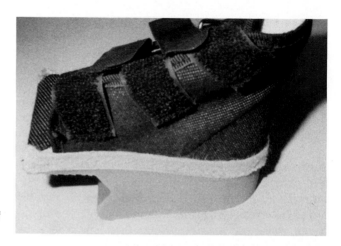

FIG 25–6.
Ipos shoe with entire forefoot elevated off ground and with no underlying pressure.

COMMON SKIN PROBLEMS OF THE DIABETIC FOOT

Anhidrosis

Because of the vascular and neurotrophic changes associated with most, though not all, diabetics, the skin of these patients often becomes dry. The dryness can lead to itching and therefore scratching. A simple excoriation because of scratching can lead to infection if left untreated. In addition, the dryness of the skin may, and often does, lead to cracking of the epidermis. This is especially prevalent around the heels, which have an inherently poor vascular supply.

Treatment for the anhidrosis is best accomplished with an array of topical skin creams and emollients. Most of these are available over the counter and supply moisture and softeners that can increase the suppleness of the tissues. Some of the more commonly used items are Lacticare lotion, Keri lotion, and Hydrisonal lotion or cream. Some of the urea-based products, such as Ureacin-10 and Ureacin-20, can also assist in lessening the keratoses around the heels. Vitamin E, aloe vera, cocoa butter lotions, and Crisco are other emollients that work well.

Fissures

When the skin is dry for a long enough period, the cracks that may develop can become quite deep, especially around the heel and in pinch-type calluses that develop on the medial aspect of the first

FIG 25–7.
Darby shoe with elevated and angulated heel reducing forefoot pressure but maintaining support under the forefoot.

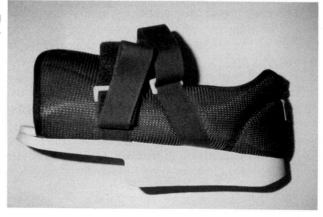

metatarsophalangeal joint. Once this occurs, in addition to using emollients, the keratotic tissue surrounding the fissure needs to be debrided in the office. This is a simple procedure and does not require anesthesia. The crater that forms the fissure should be made as flat as possible to allow epithelization across the gap in the skin. By immobilization of the skin after the debridement, the healing may take place sooner. One can apply a topical antibiotic cream or ointment with a small piece of sterile gauze and moleskin to dissipate forces of friction and prevent the skin from pinching. On the heel, the application of topical antibiotic and sterile gauze and creation of a box heel using Elastoplast tape will accomplish the same goal. If the fissures become necrotic, they must be treated in the same fashion as any other ulcer, as outlined previously.

Tinea Pedis

Although not specific to the diabetic population, tinea pedis, or Athlete's foot, is more prevalent in diabetics and can have more disastrous consequences in these patients. As such, it is incumbent on the podiatrist or diabetologist to inspect the feet closely for signs of dermatophytosis, which may include any or all of the following (Fig 25–8).

1. Small punctate vesicular rash
2. Dry scaling rash
3. Cracking under toes at junction with ball of foot
4. Mild erythema, usually with dry, scaling skin
5. Maceration between the toes, often with foul odor
6. Pruritus

In the diabetic population, it is essential to treat this condition early in its observance to prevent a secondary bacterial infection that will develop more readily than in the general population. To assist in the diagnosis, a fungal culture should be taken before therapy is initiated.

Therapy will usually consist of topical antifungal medications, all of which are applied to the affected areas twice daily to be effective. In mild cases, an over-the-counter product may be all that is required to alleviate the condition. Sometimes it is important to give patients a prescription for a cream to demonstrate the importance of their treating the condition. In severe cases, oral medication may be indicated. Two medications are used for this purpose. The first is griseofulvin, which is produced under many different trade names, and the other is ketoconazole (Nizoral). Both can have significant side effects causing blood dys-

A

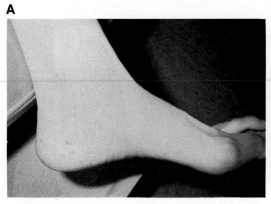

B

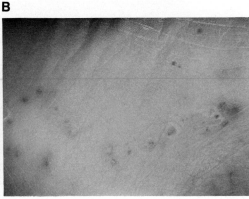

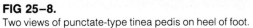

FIG 25–8.
Two views of punctate-type tinea pedis on heel of foot.

crasias and liver damage and should be used with caution. If long-term use is required, blood tests should be taken at the beginning of therapy and every 2 months thereafter as long as the treatment continues because most changes are reversible if found early enough.

NAIL PROBLEMS

Onychogryphosis

Just as the pressure of a tight shoe or abnormal weight-bearing forces can cause damage to the underlying tissues in the form of pressure necrosis, a thickened and deformed nail (onychogryphosis) will cause necrosis to occur in the nail bed, which is often deformed from the misshapen nail (Fig 25–9). It is not uncommon to find fluid accumulation under a thickened nail of a diabetic patient. Once it is detected, the nail must be debrided to allow whatever accumulation of fluid or necrotized tissue present to drain out. In addition, for the nail bed to heal, enough nail must be removed so that the area of

breakdown has no pressure from any remaining nail. If necessary, the patient should be advised to wear open-toed shoes or sandals or may be placed in a surgical shoe until healing occurs.

Onychocryptosis

Onychocryptosis, or ingrown nail, is not a condition which diabetics are naturally prone to encounter. As with most other conditions, however, the diabetic patient may quickly develop complications from such a condition with devastating sequelae, including amputation. The ingrown nail that becomes infected must be immediately treated to prevent infection from spreading rapidly. The offending section of nail must be removed, using local anesthetic if required, and the abscess drained and debrided (Fig 25–10). The nondiabetic patient rarely requires antibiosis once the nail is removed and the infection is drained. However, the diabetic patient should always be placed on oral antibiotic therapy when there has been purulent drainage, even without evidence

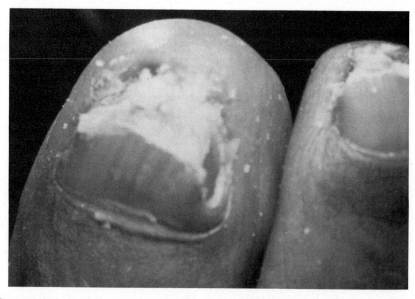

FIG 25–9.
Typical thickened, discolored, deformed, crumbling nail involved with mycotic infection, causing underlying pressure on nail bed. Note reddened area under distal aspect of nail.

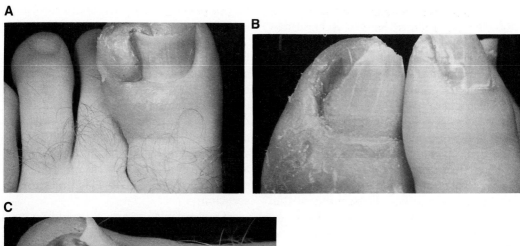

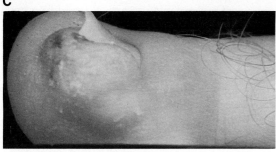

FIG 25–10.
A, dorsal view of severe infected ingrown nail right hallux. **B,** lateral view of same toe as in **A. C,** a different toe after removal of offending ingrown nail. Note clean granulation tissue.

of spreading cellulitis. Empiric oral therapy should be initiated, with the drug selection broad enough to cover gram-positive and gram-negative organisms. Once the culture results are available, appropriate antibiotic changes should be made.

Many limbs are amputated in the diabetic population as a result of a pathologic condition that begins as a simple ingrown toenail. Proper attention to this area could reduce morbidity, disability, and significant hospitalization. Periodic podiatric care of the patient with incurvated nails or nails with a tendency to ingrow by debridement of the nails, debridement of calloused nail grooves if present, and packing of the nail grooves when required can prevent these patients from developing infected onychocryptosis and associated sequelae. If the ingrowing condition is chronic or severe enough and the patient is not ischemic, it is often wise to perform a surgical correction by partial or total matriectomy so that the condition will not recur. In these instances, we pre-

fer to perform incisional techniques such as a Frost or Winograd procedure as opposed to using chemical agents such as phenol and alcohol or sodium hydroxide to eradicate the nail matrix. As discussed earlier, the diabetic patient heals better by primary intention than secondary intention healing.

Onychomycosis

One of the most common maladies of the toenails is fungus infection. When a nail is infected with the fungus, it becomes thickened, discolored, sometimes macerated, sometimes brittle, and often deformed. There are two modes by which the mycotic or fungal nail can precipitate difficulties for the diabetic patient.

The first is because of the increase in the thickness of the nail, which will cause it to function much the same as the gryphotic nail discussed previously. Therefore, the sequelae of this phenomenon would be the same.

Second, with the chronic fungal infection present, the patient is likely to develop a fungal skin infection and, therefore, as elucidated earlier, may form secondary bacterial infections, having serious consequences.

Once again, periodic podiatric care of patients with these conditions can preempt many of these negative effects. With mycotic nails, keeping them cut or burred down as thin as possible will usually prevent necrosis or secondary bacterial infection to the nail bed. With many of the topical medications available such as Loprox, Nizoral, or Spectazole, some improvement or in some cases eradication of the infection is possible with regular treatment over a 6 to 12-month period. Even after that period it is usually necessary to treat prophylactically to prevent recurrences. Oral medications, either griseofulvin or ketoconazole, can be used, but they require 9 to 12 months of continuous use and should be used with caution, as discussed earlier. One must weigh the benefits vs. the risks of such therapy on a patient-by-patient basis.

SHIELDING AND PADDING

Preventive

Just as many of the nail problems are controlled or prevented by reduction of the pressure associated with those nails, it is also important to reduce the areas of pressure on the skin of the diabetic's foot. Areas of increased pressure are calloused areas and are referred to depending on their configuration and location. A calloused area over a prominence on a toe is generally referred to as a heloma durum or hard corn; a calloused area between two toes is referred to as a heloma molle. Calloused areas on the bottom or plantar surface of the foot are referred to as superficial shearing calluses if they are diffuse or intractable plantar keratosis if they are discrete areas with a dense central core

corresponding to the area of greatest pressure.

The location of the calluses determine the type of padding needed to protect that area. There are two general principles in treating these areas of pressure. One is to divert pressure away from the affected area of tissue, and this is termed weight dispersion. The other is to diminish the amount of pressure to a particular area by absorbing that pressure into another medium, and this can be termed pressure absorption.

On a toe with a corn, the padding used is generally made of felt or foam and ranges from $\frac{1}{16}$ to $\frac{1}{8}$ in. thick. The pad surrounds the corn so that the pressure applied to the toe by the shoe is dispersed over a wider area more evenly (Fig 25–11). The result is a decrease in pressure to the area of the corn. These are generally applied with adhesive-backed felt and should not be left on the skin more than 2 days if they get wet or 4 to 7 days if kept dry. The pad should be covered with tape to keep the pad in place. These work very well after palliative care to prevent the rapid recurrence of these lesions. As a method of permanent or long-term protection, the use of a nonadhesive, removable pad is more desirable. One item that works very well, especially for the soft corns (Fig 25–12) is foam in the form of a tube that is applied over the affected toe or the adjacent toe to cushion the pressure and can also be used with an aperture to disperse the pressure (Fig 25–13).

Another way to prevent corns to known areas of pressure is to use a Silipos pad, which is removable and reusable and has the properties of weight dispersion because of an aperture and pressure absorption by the nature of its gel-like consistency.

On the plantar of the foot, weight dispersion is accomplished by once again using $\frac{1}{16}$- to $\frac{1}{4}$-in. felt, either adhesive or nonadhesive, cut in the form of a U or double U to avoid the areas of pressure,

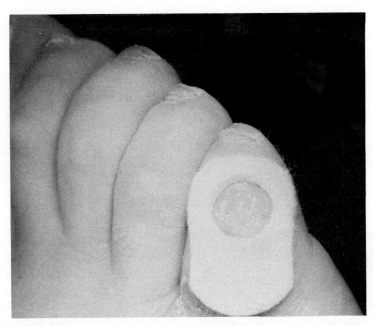

FIG 25–11.
Aperture pad made of ⅛-in. thick felt to disperse pressure from keratosis (corn) overlying bony prominence.

as illustrated in Figure 25–14. To keep the pad in place, apply tape far enough past the area of padding so as to adhere to the surrounding skin. Elastoplast conforms well to the contours of the foot with one piece of 3-in. tape. In patients with sensitive skin or who are allergic to tape, nonadhesive felt may be used with paper tape to hold the padding in position.

Another form of padding that is well used with corns either between the toes or at the ends of the toes is a molded pad formed between the toes. There are several of this type on the market. Two types of molded pads that provide the best and most consistent results are called MPC (Moldable Podiatric Compound; North Health Care, Rockford, Ill.) and

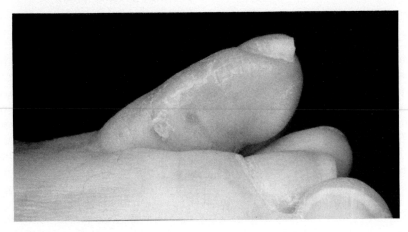

FIG 25–12.
Soft corn (heloma molle) that has begun to form ulceration found between toes.

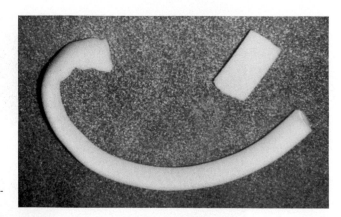

FIG 25–13.
Rolled foam padding available in long strip, which can be cut to length of toe and placed over toe to protect for interdigital pressure.

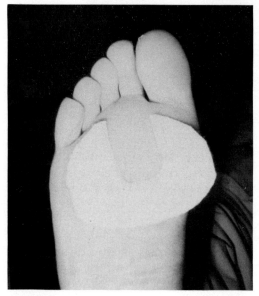

FIG 25–14.
Demonstration of a U-shaped dispersion padding fabricated from ⅛-in. adhesive felt.

Berkoplast (Berkeman Podiatry Products, Mount Kisco, N.Y.). The basic material is premeasured with the MPC, and comes with accompanying catalyst and a plastic bag for mixing the two components. This material forms a latex rubber shield to protect the toe. It is the most expensive and comes in only one size, so often there is some waste involved, but the final product is the most reproducible and lasts the longest (Fig 25–15, A and B). The Berkoplast comes in different sizes and can be mixed to size (Fig 25–15, C).

There are other materials that can be used for the distal toe lesions that are fabricated into pads that fit under the toes and cause the toes to be lifted off the ground, thereby reducing the pressure. One such device was termed by the late Leonard Hymes, D.P.M., as a cotton roll toe crest. It was originally made from a section of dental cotton roll that was cut to the size of the width of one or more toes. The roll was then covered with Elastoplast tape to make a ring from the tape. This ring would then be pulled over the toes to allow the cotton roll covered with the tape to sit under the toes (Fig 25–16). This can be used for short-term treatment of distal calluses or small ulcers. Today, however, instead of cotton dental roll, we use high-density foam.

Therapeutic

The same areas of concern that were treated with preventive padding can, despite the best of care, develop areas of tissue breakdown or sublesional inflammation. There are also areas that can develop early pressure or blisters as a result of abnormal friction caused by unusual activity or improperly fitted shoes, which need to be treated with padding or shielding on a therapeutic basis.

The corn or callus that breaks down on a mild level can be treated with balance padding in much the same way as just

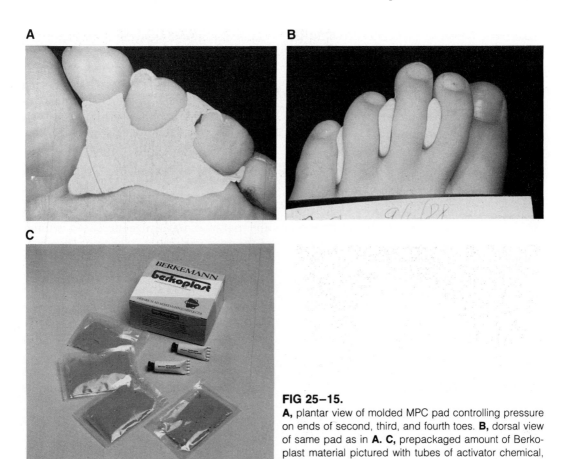

FIG 25–15.
A, plantar view of molded MPC pad controlling pressure on ends of second, third, and fourth toes. **B,** dorsal view of same pad as in **A. C,** prepackaged amount of Berko-plast material pictured with tubes of activator chemical, which, when mixed with the puttylike material, causes the mold to set in the desired shape after several minutes.

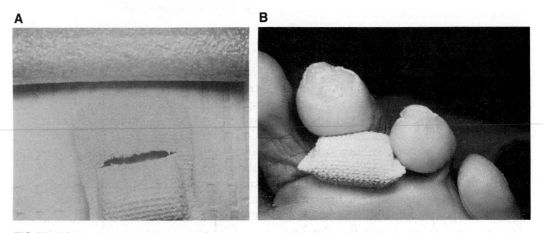

FIG 25–16.
A, appearance of foam tubing and completed cotton rolled toe crest (CRTC). **B,** appearance of CRTC on third toe, which has a distal keratosis present.

described; however, a sterile dressing is incorporated into the padding with whatever medicament is appropriate, and the dressing should be changed regularly until healing has occurred.

Blisters or areas of early friction can be treated with padding that will absorb excess pressure and minimize the forces of friction. If an area is not blistered and the skin is not sensitive to adhesive, moleskin can buffer the effects of friction. If there is mild blistering and the physician does not want to open the blister, Spenco 2nd skin (Spenco Medical Corp., Waco, TX) with the accompanying cover material provides proper absorptive and friction-reducing properties in these situations. The material is placed directly over the affected tissue and held in place with the lightweight cover material.

ORTHOTIC DEVICES

This section will deal with those devices or appliances that have some effect on the entire foot, although they are often used for controlling or accommodating a specific area of the foot.

Functional Orthotics

Using an orthotic device that is rigid or semirigid when one is dealing with the diabetic foot is limited to patients who are being treated prophylactically. If we can prevent the occurrence of deformities that may later cause pressure areas leading to breakdown, this modality may be quite important. The patient who has early hallux valgus, hammertoes, or any biomechanical dysfunction that lends itself to the formation of pressure areas on the plantar aspect of the foot can be preempted from developing diabetic ulcers by balancing their foot at an early stage of their illness. One has to be very careful, however, to weigh the advantages of orthotic therapy against the possible consequences of such treatment. The addition of any material to the shoes of a diabetic can be fraught with a myriad of complications. The edges of the orthotic device can create blistering, which can lead to ulcer formation or can create callus, which is exactly what you are trying to prevent. If you are dealing with a neuropathic foot that is insensate, the patient will not be able to realize the areas of increased pressure associated with such devices. In addition, the mere filling of the shoe with any material may cause increased friction of the toes within the toebox of the shoe, causing corns or blisters, which may lead to the formation of ulcers. Therefore, if the patient is to be fitted with an orthotic device of any kind, there must be sufficient room in their shoes.

Diabetics can develop other conditions associated with strain and fatigue, as can any other individual. Many times these problems, such as plantar fasciitis or tendinitis, will be treated with a functional orthotic with excellent results. Diabetic patients should not preclude the physician from using the devices as long as the precautions previously mentioned are considered and accounted for when fitting the support.

Accommodative Devices

Once the patient has developed pressure areas or areas of prominence that may become irritated, especially in the insensate foot, the best protection would be an accommodative appliance fabricated from a material that can protect the foot. The optimum device should be moldable, supportive, protective, easily shaped and modified, easily fit into shoes, and have shock-absorption capacity. Many different materials are available for this purpose, and several will be mentioned here.

The first is a thermoplastic material manufactured under the name of Sports Molds (Stein's Foot Specialities, Hackensack, NJ). These are used for sports but

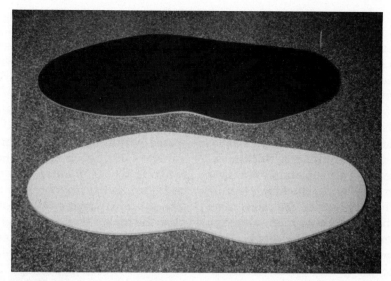

FIG 25–17.
Top and bottom view of Sports Mold before heating and molding to shape of foot.

are particularly useful for diabetic patients. The Sports Molds are thin, easily molded, and provide soft, even support to the foot (Fig 25–17). They can be used presized in men's and women's sizes small through large or by cutting out of a large sheet of material. Once fitted to the patient's shoe, they are heated with a hot air gun (Fig 25–18); when warmed and very soft, they are placed into the patient's shoes, and the patient walks with the device to mold the material to the shape of the patient's foot and his or her weight-bearing pattern. Within several minutes the Sports Molds can be removed from the shoes and will be shaped to the contour of the foot. Because of the thermoplastic qualities of the material, as the patient walks, the heat of the foot constantly reshapes and remolds the device according to changes in pressure. Often the thickness of the material is enough to allow

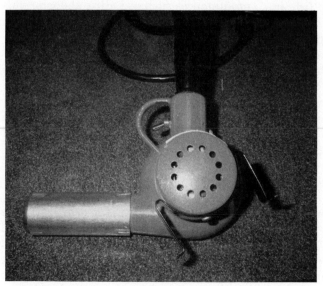

FIG 25–18.
Heat blower used to heat up the sports molds or other orthotic materials for shaping or adjusting. This unit creates enough heat to melt plastic without using open flame.

differences in pressure areas, but when it is not enough, additional material (taken from a sheet without naugahyde covering) can be added as a balance pad, metatarsal support, arch support, or any other pattern so desired or found to be necessary according to the patient's wear pattern, weight distribution, or complaints. These work particularly well in women's shoes that cannot accommodate a thicker device. If necessary, a complete second layer of mold can be added to the first, creating a double-thickness device that adds more stability and shock absorption, although requiring more space in the shoes.

Plastazote is a material that works similarly to the Sports Molds because it also can be shaped and molded to the patient's feet. It is generally thicker than the Sports Molds and firmer, therefore providing more support in addition to the molding capability. It does not change as readily without specific adjustment by the physician or orthotist. It is commonly used in many molded shoes and requires increased space in the shoes.[19]

Wood flour is made from a combination of ground cork, a grade of very fine sawdust and latex, which is known as rubber butter. The wood flour is applied over a positive plaster impression of the foot in semi-weight-bearing. It is applied in thicknesses of about ¼ in., and when dry, it is removed from the cast, shaped, and covered with naugahyde, leather or other suitable covering and fit into a shoe deep and wide enough to accommodate the support. This is a good mold and an exact replica of the foot with all its prominences and unusual contours. It was very popular in the 1960s and 1970s and is still used today. However, with the advent of thinner, more easily created materials its popularity has waned.

Another device that provides accommodative protection and support is what is termed dynamic molds.[8] The rationale behind this material is that it provides weight distribution by using hydraulic techniques to reduce vector forces and redistribution from excessive weight-bearing points. The dynamic molds are similar to the rubber butter molds because they are fabricated from a combination of finely ground cork, wood flour, a small amount of plaster, and a latex composition. The difference is that these molds are produced within the patient's shoes over 30 minutes, during which time the patient is walking for 10 minutes, standing for 10 minutes, and sitting for 10 minutes (Fig 25–19). The purpose of this procedure is that the mold takes on a shape that more realistically reproduces the actual functional position of the foot with its abnormal weight-bearing distribution and prominences. By the foot being pressed into the mixture of ingredients that takes on the consistency of mud, the weight-bearing is equalized so that all the plantar surfaces bear weight equally all closer to equal than before molding.[8] Once the device is fabricated and completely cured (about 1–2 weeks), additional corrections may be added to the bottom of the mold as needed. This could further remove pressure from an area of ulceration and preulceration. This can be used with a Charcot foot and a cavus-type foot. It is possible to even form part of the mold around lateral prominences such as hallux abductor valgus or tailor's bunion. This mold has been used successfully on a patient with neuropathy, secondary to spina bifida, which caused the patient's foot type to be in a calcaneus position, thus developing recurrent ulcerations at the posteroplantar junction. In this case, the mold was formed high up onto the posterior of the feet and is still very successful.

Total Contact Casting

By removing the weight-bearing forces entirely, most neuropathic ulcers will heal quickly. Placing patients on complete bed rest or keeping them non-weight-bearing with the use of crutches will usually be

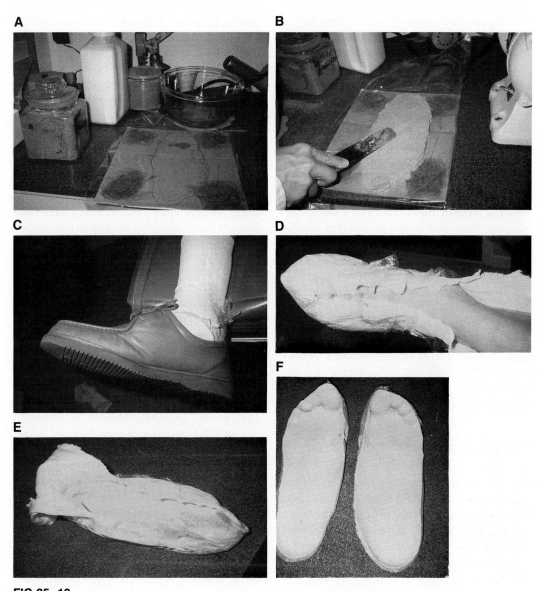

FIG 25–19.
A, materials and setup required for fabricating dynamic molds, including mixing bowl, spatula, finely ground cork, wood flour, latex, plaster, and cardboard with plastic printed with outline of patient's foot. **B,** after the ingredients are mixed, the batter consistency material is spread over the plastic to the shape of the patient's foot. **C,** after the patient rests his or her leg on the mixture, the plastic is glued to the sock, and the entire foot and mold are placed into the patient's shoe, which was sized large enough to accommodate all the materials. **D,** after 30 minutes, the shoe is removed and the sock cut down the middle. **E,** the mold is removed and, **F,** trimmed of excess material. These are now covered with plastic and placed in the patient's shoes for 1 week, after which time they are adjusted as needed and covered. Once covered, they may be moved from shoe to shoe, and further adjustments or additions are made to the bottom surface of the mold.

effective. However, this is often not practical or possible because of patient compliance or other problems they may have. Brand in 1982 introduced the total contact cast technique, which is still used.[11] This consists of a below-knee plaster cast "applied with minimal to no padding and is designed to fit the lower leg like a glove. The vertical forces are evenly distributed over the sole of the foot, shear forces are reduced and the ulcer heals while the patient continues to walk."[11] Laing et al.[11] in January 1991 published an article in which they demonstrated an average healing time of approximately 6 weeks for neuropathic ulcers on the bottom of the foot when total contact casts were used. They also found that if there were no follow-up with appropriate shoe wear or appliances, these patients experienced a recurrence rate of approximately 50%. In another study of the recurrence rates after healing of diabetic ulcers with total contact casting, Helm et al.[10] found a recurrence rate of 20% for various reasons, including poor follow-up with appropriate shoes or appliances.

SHOE THERAPY

The role of properly fitting shoes in treating diabetic ulcers is a function of removing the source of pressure or imbalance on a particular area of the foot. An ulcer on the top of a toe is often best treated by eliminating shoe pressure. This may be accomplished with a healing sandal, followed by extra-depth shoes. A pressure area on the plantar of the foot can be relieved by placing a rocker sole on the outside of the shoe. This allows the pressure to be transferred from proximal to the area of concern to distal and past the area of ulceration on the foot.

In addition to various molds being introduced into the shoe as mentioned previously, padding can be placed strategically within the shoes the same way that padding is placed directly on the foot. This can be easily done by the physician in the office without elaborate equipment or planning. Again, special attention to the fit of the shoe is critical.

As opposed to adjusting or correcting the patient's existing shoe, a special shoe can be manufactured or ordered for the patient. There are many different types of footwear that have been used for this purpose, and they have all worked well for different individuals on different occasions. There is a Plastazote shoe termed a healing shoe (Apex) that has a Velcro® strap, simple rounded toe, and Plastazote construction of both the insole and upper material that conforms to the patient's foot.

A perfect long-term solution to a problem foot is having a shoe custom molded to the patient's specific size and shape, allowing for deformities of the toes or other prominences. The molded shoes usually have a Plastazote insole that has been heat molded to a cast of the patient's foot and can be further adjusted or replaced with another accommodative appliance such as the Dynamic Molds.

Similar to the molded shoe is an atraumatic boot, which is a molded boot used by Singleton et al.[20] The boot is described as a device that reduces shear stress and its ensuing damage to the neurotrophic foot by providing a large medium in which the forces of gravity and reactive force of gravity may interact, with minimal consequences to the overlying foot.

SUMMARY

It is readily apparent that the diabetic foot can occur at any time. Its occurrence can be slowed or even extinguished with a diverse armamentarium that comprises comprehensive care of the diabetic foot. A complete program of primary podiatric care, functional or accommodative appliances, protective or therapeutic shoewear, and a keen awareness of treating the diabetic foot will help prevent prolonged hospitalization or absenteeism from work and improve the patient's quality of life.

Acknowledgment

A good deal of the research and knowledge that is incorporated in this chapter was provided by Raymond K. Locke, D.P.M., whose dedication as a leader to the podiatry profession for more than 50 years, teacher to the students of podiatric medicine, and advisor, teacher, and partner to me shall never be forgotten.

REFERENCES

1. Edmonds ME: The diabetic foot: Pathophysiology and treatment, *Clin Endocrinol Metab* 15:889–916, 1986.
2. Harkless LB, Dennis KJ, editors: *Clinics in podiatric medicine and surgery: vol 4. The diabetic foot,* Philadelphia, 1987, WB Saunders.
3. Levin ME, O'Neal LW, editors: *The diabetic foot,* ed 2, St Louis, 1977, Mosby–Year Book.
4. Logerfo FW, Coffman JD: Vascular and microvascular disease of the foot in diabetes, *N Engl J Med* 311:1615–1619, 1984.
5. Faris I: Foot lesions in diabetic patients: Pathogenesis and management, *Med J Aust* 1:632, 1977.
6. Brenman SA: Pentoxifylline as adjunctive therapy in leg ulcer management, *J Am Osteopath Assoc* 91:677–686, 1991.
7. Young MJ, et al: The effect of callus removal on dynamic plantar foot pressures in diabetic patients, *Diabetic Med* 9:55–57, 1992.
8. Locke RK, Heifitz NM: Collagenase as an aid in healing. *J Am Podiatr Assoc* 65:242–247, 1975.
9. Balkin SW, Kaplan L: Silicone injection management of diabetic foot ulcers: a possible model for prevention of pressure ulcers, *Decubitus* 4(4):38–40, 1991.
10. Helm PA, et al: Recurrence of neuropathic ulceration following healing in a total contact cast, *Arch Phys Med Rehabil* 72:967–970, 1991.
11. Laing PW, et al: Neuropathic foot ulceration treated by total contact casts, *J Bone Joint Surg* 74B:133–136, 1992.
12. Scheffler NM, et al: Treatment of painful diabetic neuropathy with capsaicin 0.075%, *J Am Podiatr Med Assoc* 81:288–293, 1991.
13. Stevens MJ, et al: Paradoxical blood flow responses in the diabetic neuropathic foot: An assessment of the contribution of vascular denervation and microangiopathy, *Diabetic Med* 9:49–54, 1992.
14. Mueller MJ, et al: Relationship of foot deformity to ulcer location in patients with diabetes mellitus, *Phys Ther* 70:356–362, 1990.
15. Kumar S, et al: Semmes-Weinstein monofilaments: A simple, effective and inexpensive screening device for identifying diabetic patients at risk of foot ulceration, *Diabetes Res Clin Pract* 13:63–68, 1991.
16. Thurston R, Beattie C: Foot lesions in diabetics: Predisposing factors, *Nurs Times* 80(34):44–46, 1984.
17. Adler PF: Assessing the effects of pentoxifylline (Trental) on diabetic neurotrophic foot ulcers, *J Foot Surg* 30:300–303, 1991.
18. Weitgasser H: The use of pentoxifylline ('Trental' 400) in the treatment of leg ulcers: results of a double-blind trial, *Pharmatherapeutica* 3(suppl 1):143–151, 1983.
19. Block P: The diabetic foot ulcer: A complex problem with a simple treatment approach, *Milit Med* 146:644–666, 1981.
20. Singleton EE, et al: Another approach to the long-term management of the diabetic neurotrophic foot ulcer, *J Am Podiatr Assoc* 68:242, 1978.

26 _____ Nutrition

Maureen Smith Plombon,
M.S., R.D.

Nutritional concerns are similar for patients with diabetes whether they have type I or type II. Educational programs, dietary guidelines, and eating plans must be designed and followed by the individual to maintain blood glucose balance and minimize complications.

Although the focus of this book is on the type I diabetic with complications of the foot, the nutritional recommendations are applicable to all diabetics.

RATIONALE

Nutritional intervention has been a key component of the management of diabetes since the earliest forms of treatment. Although a balanced diet is essential for optimal health for all individuals, it has special significance for the diabetic. The goals of dietary management of the diabetic patient are achieving and maintaining desirable body weight, ensuring adequate intake for all essential nutrients, achieving healthy lipid levels, maintaining optimal blood glucose levels, preventing acidosis and shock, and meeting the special needs of certain medical complications.

Before a nutritional plan of therapy is designed for the diabetic, a number of factors must be taken into consideration. These include their diabetic therapy (insulin injections, pills, or dietary management), level of physical activity, daily caloric needs, and the individual's life-style. To be effective, any dietary management plan must complement the diabetic's life-style and be followed easily, without a large degree of inconvenience.[1]

If the diabetic is not at a desirable weight range or is not achieving the proper nutritional intake, steps must be taken. Approximately 80% of those who develop type II diabetes are overweight. The caloric balance between intake and expenditure must be manipulated to achieve the desirable or goal weight, and the food chosen should supply the necessary nutrition. In most cases, this involves a balanced plan for weight loss, the monitoring of caloric intake, and the increase in physical activity whenever possible.

For the type I diabetic, consistency in the timing and amount of food eaten each day is important. Matching food intake and physical activity to the amount of insulin is essential for maintaining blood glucose levels.

Eating habits and food preferences are behaviors that are difficult to change. Even health concerns that are directly related to diet are not always strong motivators for change. Therefore, both the content of nutritional programming and the process by which it is delivered must be addressed for an effective diabetes education program.

CALORIES AND ENERGY BALANCE

The typical American diet provides sufficient calories to meet our energy needs for growth, body metabolism, and physical activity. Excess calories are stored in the body as fat or adipose tissue, which is related to increased risk for diabetes and other chronic disease such as heart disease and cancer.

Height-weight tables can be used to determine goal weight ranges for the patient, but they provide only a value that represents total body weight. The fat weight/lean body weight ratio is not considered in these tables. Therefore, an individual may be considered overweight when a high percentage of that weight comes from lean body tissue, but this does not translate into a health risk concern.

The same is also true of a method that estimates body weight based only on height. The following formula is used:

	Women	Men
For first 5 ft start with:	105 lbs	106 lbs
For each additional inch add:	5 lbs	6 lbs
Small frame:		Subtract 10%
Large frame:		Add 10%

Body fat assessment provides additional information, more specifically, what the total percentage of body fat weight is when compared with its lean body weight. Normative value ranges for men and women are 10% to 18% and 18% to 24%, respectively. A goal body weight can then be calculated knowing the current percent body fat and body weight and choosing a goal percentage body fat.

Once a goal or desirable body weight is determined, a daily caloric intake required to achieve that weight can be calculated. Total energy needs can be estimated by a variety of ways. The most accurate method would be by measuring the basal metabolic rate and then converting the oxygen consumption to kilocalories required at rest. Extra calories are then added to meet the needs of daily and physical activities. This would tell you how many calories are necessary to maintain the current body weight with specific additional daily activities.

A more simplified method for estimating energy needs may be made by multiplying the goal body weight by a factor of 10, 12, or 14 for women or 12, 14, or 16 for men based on a relative activity level: inactive, moderately active (two to three exercise sessions per week), or highly active (more than three exercise sessions per week), respectively (Table 26-1).

The difference between the current caloric intake and the newly calculated caloric intake will represent the daily deficit of calories. Multiplied by 7 and then divided by 3,500 (3,500 calories per 1 lb), you will have a value for pounds lost per week. It is recommended that weight loss should be on average no more than 1½ to 2 lb per week.

Weight loss plans for adults should provide a minimum of 1,200 calories for women and 1,500 calories for men. If a

TABLE 26-1.

Estimation of Energy Needs

	120-lb Woman		190-lb Man	
	Female Factor	Calories	Male Factor	Calories
Inactive	10	1,200	12	2,280
Moderately active	12	1,440	14	2,660
Highly active	14	1,680	16	3,040

greater deficit of calories is desired, additional calories expended in physical activity should account for the difference. It is quite difficult to maintain optimal nutritional quality with fewer daily calories.

PHYSICAL ACTIVITY

The benefits of physical activity are numerous. With regard to weight management, the decreased percentage of body fat and increased lean body mass will typically result in an increased metabolic rate, therefore more calories expended per day. Obesity has been shown to decrease the body's ability to use insulin; a reduction in body fat will reverse this trend. Independently, exercise has been shown to result in more efficient use of insulin as the cells become more sensitive to insulin. This beneficial effect is on a short-term basis only, so exercise must be scheduled regularly to be effective. Regular physical activity has also shown to reduce coronary heart disease risk factors and blood pressure, which are two important considerations for the diabetic.

Guidelines for the development of an exercise program are provided in other resources.[2,3] Precautions must be taken to ensure that blood glucose levels are maintained before, during, and after the exercise session. It is recommended that 10 to 15 g of carbohydrate be eaten 1 hour before moderate exercise and repeated for each additional hour of activity for those with controlled blood glucose values. Exercise is contraindicated when the blood glucose level is greater than 300 mg/dl. Additional guidelines are available for adjusting food intake and insulin dosage for various types of exercise.

For consideration at this time, the two key features are caloric expenditure for weight management and safety for the diabetic with foot complications. The timing and management of the insulin administration are also important considerations

when a program of physical activity is planned but will not be covered in the scope of this chapter.[4]

When the daily caloric needs for the individual are planned, the type of activity, intensity, and duration must be considered. Resources provide caloric expenditure per minute for various athletic and everyday life activity to assist in calculating caloric expenditure.[5] Once calculated, this figure should be added to the basal metabolic rate to determine daily caloric needs.

For the diabetic with foot complications, special attention should be taken in wearing high-quality athletic shoes and socks. It is important that the footwear fit properly and that blisters are minimized. Activities that may involve physical trauma, especially when neuropathy or nerve damage is present, should be avoided.

NUTRIENT NEEDS

Once the total caloric intake is determined on a daily basis, the distribution of those calories should be addressed. The typical American diet today derives approximately 12% to 15% of total calories from protein, 48% from carbohydrate, and 38% to 40% from fat. National nutritional goals are aimed at lowering the total fat intake to 30% of total calories and increasing the complex carbohydrate intake to at least 55% to 58%. This heart-healthy diet is also appropriate for the diabetic. It may be especially important for the diabetic who runs the increased risk of developing cardiovascular disease.

The allowance for protein intake is determined first, calculated as a percentage of total calories or by using the recommended daily allowance of 0.8 g/kg of body weight. The result of your calculations will be expressed as either protein calories or as grams of protein. Dividing protein calories by 4 (4 calories/g of protein) will provide you with the allowance in grams. At the start of treatment a poorly regulated diabetic may be in negative nitrogen balance, so the protein intake may need to be increased until this comes under control.

The carbohydrate allowance is established next, with approximately 55% of total calories comprised of carbohydrate. As with protein, the carbohydrate calories can be divided by 4 (4 calories/g of carbohydrate) to provide you with total grams of carbohydrate in the allowance.

The fat allowance is calculated last and typically represents the balance of calories remaining (no greater than 30% of total). The fat calorie balance is then divided by 9 (9 calories/g of fat) to determine the fat allowance in grams (Table 26–2).

Dietary research regarding obese type II diabetics indicate that a low-fat weight reduction plan should be initiated. If the patient is resistant to weight loss, the composition of the diet should be adapted to increase the fat content at the expense of carbohydrates. Maintaining a high-carbohydrate, low-fat diet for these individuals can result in increased hyperglycemia, increased plasma triglycerides levels and lowered high-density lipoprotein (HDL)–cholesterol levels. It does not appear to reflect a heart healthy diet for this group of individuals. It is recommended, however, that the fat be unsaturated, preferably monounsaturated, and that cholesterol intake be monitored, so that low-density lipoprotein (LDL)–cholesterol levels are not affected.

Diabetic management of the diet covers a broad spectrum of individuals and medical conditions. Therefore, the optimal plan must be designed based on the specific medical conditions of the individual patient, his or her type of diabetes, if obesity is present, the patient's response to weight reduction diets, and other risk factors for coronary heart disease.

DIABETIC EXCHANGE LISTS

Translating dietary goals into actual food choices is often a difficult task. The "basic four food groups" have been a long-standing model that classifies foods into four groups based on similar nutrient content. The four groups, meat, milk, fruits and vegetables, and breads and cereals, have recommended servings for children and adults.

The Diabetic Exchange Lists are based on a similar model. Specific daily analysis of food choices proved to be time consuming and confusing. The Diabetic Exchange Lists were developed in 1950 by the American Diabetes Association, the American Dietetic Association, and the U.S. Public Health Service to provide a simple, universal system by which meals may be planned in a wide variety of circumstances in accordance with individual preferences.[6] The Diabetic Exchange Lists were updated in 1976 and 1986, and the current system emphasizes a high-carbohydrate, low-fat dietary plan.

Foods are classified as equivalent units or exchanges within one of six ex-

TABLE 26–2.

Calculation of Nutrient Needs

Nutrient	2,000 Calories		
	% of Total Calories	Calories	G
Protein	12–15%	240–300	60–75
Carbohydrate	55–58%	1,100–1,160	275–290
Fat	30%	600	67

change lists or categories. Exchanges have approximately equivalent amounts of carbohydrates, proteins, and fats and contain similar kinds and types of foods. The six exchange groups are starch, bread, and meat, vegetable, fruit, milk, and fat.

Once a caloric intake level is established, the exchange distribution is outlined as a daily eating plan, typically by a registered dietitian. Exchanges are distributed throughout the day in meals and snacks. Most plans provide three meals and between one and three daily snacks. The diabetic is then able to choose any food within the exchange list or one that is a combination of exchanges.[7,8]

The timing of the meals and snacks is based on the timing of the insulin injections and the type of insulin taken. Home blood glucose monitoring allows the diabetic to assess if the meal plan is working and make adjustments accordingly. Blood glucose levels should return to preprandial readings within 4 to 5 hours.

Historically, it was recommended that diabetics avoid simple sugars because of the immediate sharp increase in blood glucose levels. Research has shown, however, that different carbohydrates elicit different glucose responses. This variation has resulted in the development of the Glycemic Index, which ranks different carbohydrate glucose response rates relative to a standard of 100 for white bread.[9] Those foods that produce a slower release of blood glucose have a low glycemic index. Examples are yogurt, ice cream, or pasta. Foods that produce an excessive release of blood glucose, representing a high Glycemic Index, include baked potatoes, corn flakes, sugar, and honey. The actual form that the food is eaten in can also result in variant glycemic responses. Foods identified with a high Glycemic Index may still be included in the dietary plan in moderation, but their response should be monitored by the individual with a home blood glucose test.

VITAMINS AND MINERALS

Vitamin and mineral requirements are not significantly different for the well-controlled diabetic than for the general population. In many ways, the diabetic may actually eat a more balanced diet. When a greater quantity of fruits and vegetables are consumed and complex carbohydrates are emphasized, the diet becomes lower in fat and higher in fiber and carbohydrates. Eating a wide variety of foods will typically ensure adequate intake of essential nutrients, therefore, vitamin and mineral supplementation is not warranted.

FIBER

Fiber requirements do not differ from the general population either. Typical fiber intakes range from 12 to 18 g daily, although recommendations are for between 20 to 35 g daily. Fiber, both soluble and insoluble, helps in lowering blood cholesterol levels and helps in blunting the rise of blood glucose levels after meals. It is also related to lowered insulin requirements. Increasing the fiber content of the diet should be done gradually to avoid any gastrointestinal distress. Adequate water intake (at least eight 8-oz glasses daily) should also be monitored.

ALCOHOL

It is recommended that alcohol be avoided. Alcohol can boost the affects of insulin, resulting in a lowered blood sugar level, which can be further exacerbated if food intake is then forgotten. If consumed, it should be accounted for in the daily Diabetic Exchange Plan. Sweet mixers, sweet liquors, or wines should also be avoided. Type I diabetics should consume alcohol only when they are in glucose control, and then only in moderation and accompanied by food.

SUGAR ALTERNATIVES

Sugar alternatives on the market either contain calories or are calorie free. Those with calories, known as nutritive sweeteners, are found as mannitol, fructose or high-fructose corn syrups, sorbitol, invert sugars, molasses, or brown sugar on food labels. These sweeteners are not calorie free, so they need to be watched for excess calories and may cause cramping or diarrhea when used in large quantities. Fructose is typically not recommended for diabetics with poor control because fructose is readily converted to glucose.

Those alternatives without calories, nonnutritive sweeteners, are found as the diet food additive Nutrasweet or the tabletop sweetener Equal (both are aspartame), saccharin, acesulfame-K, and sucralose. All should be used in moderation.

ALTERNATIVE MEAL PLANS

The diabetic exchange lists method outlined previously is the most popular method for diabetic meal planning, but it is not the only existing system. A number of alternatives offer a variety of approaches to meal planning.

Total Available Glucose, or TAG, a complicated system requiring a high degree of motivation, knowledge, and skill is at one end of the difficulty scale, whereas a Month of Menus, which provides 28 days of interchangeable menus for breakfast, lunch, and dinner (1,500 calories) is at the simplistic end. A high-carbohydrate, high-fiber plan designed by Dr. James Anderson in 1974 uses eight exchanges for a primarily vegetarian diet. The great quantity of food required to meet the caloric needs, the complexity of the plan, and the acceptability of the food choices make this a difficult plan to follow. But it does appear helpful for the obese type II diabetic. A Calorie-Fat Counting System is very simple to learn, but it does not consider the nutrient content or the glycemic reaction of foods that may be consumed. A Point System provides a listing of food with accompanying point values, and the patient may choose foods up to their daily point allotment; 1 point is equivalent to 75 calories. Again, the overall nutritional quality of the diet is not accounted for with this system. Individualized sample menus are designed in a one-on-one approach that is time intensive but may be suited for certain individuals who wish a very customized eating plan. A more in-depth review of these alternatives is available.[10]

VERY LOW-CALORIE DIETS

Quick weight-loss plans and very low-calorie diets (VLCDs) designed to maximize weight loss in a minimum of time are usually not effective in the long term and may be especially dangerous to the diabetic. With such a dietary plan, the body enters a state of semistarvation, depleting glycogen stores from the muscle and incompletely oxidizing fats for energy. This results in a buildup of ketones in the blood or ketoacidosis. Left unchecked, ketoacidosis can result in coma or death for the diabetic.

With minimal caloric intake (< 800 calories), the body is not able to maintain normal glucose levels and receives an inadequate supply of nutrients. Any weight loss experienced is due to a loss of water that is released when the glycogen is released from its storage in the muscle. Each gram of glycogen released from the muscle is accompanied by approximately 3 g of water. This does not represent any loss of fat or lean body mass.

When even a moderate increase of calories is reinstituted, the body replenishes its glycogen stores, which is again stored with water. Weight loss is short lived. Research has shown that the long-term effects of VLCD, or yo-yo dieting as it is known, can actually be more detrimental to health status than carrying the additional body weight. True, healthy weight loss should not exceed 1 to 2 lb/week. The most effective method for achieving and maintaining weight loss is a combined program of caloric management and regular physical activity, which is also recommended for optimal diabetic control.

A medically supervised VLCD plan, which supplies high-quality protein and carbohydrate and fortified with vitamins and minerals, has been used for some patients. Although its use is controversial, particularly regarding its safety, a medical decision may be made that the risks involved are outweighed by the benefits of a more immediate, if short-termed, weight loss. It should only be considered with close medical supervision.

BEHAVIOR MODIFICATION

Eating is a behavior influenced by our habits, food preferences, social interactions, and life-style. Knowing what to eat for optimal health and actually doing it may be two different issues. Too often nutrition information is provided to patients and they are left to struggle with the integration of this knowledge into a working plan of action. Diets are perceived as being restrictive and a temporary situation. It is important to present the diabetic's eating plan as a guide for a new set of habits in establishing a positive way of life.

In approaching these changes, a comprehensive plan must be devised that is simple, practical, well organized, and supervised. Structure is important to help establish the routine of the new habits. If the plan is too complicated or does not have relevance to the patient's life-style, it will not be followed. Supervision helps to provide immediate positive reinforcement for the patient's accomplishments.

Counseling may be conducted individually or in a group setting. Often, the di-

abetic patient will participate in a combination of counseling options. These options include one-on-one sessions with a diabetic educator for developing a specific treatment plan, as well as group classes for more general education and support sessions. The number and content of these sessions depend on the patient's needs and the format of the program in your geographic area.

The diabetic educator must serve as a facilitator who will venture into the counseling project with a patient as a partner. Patients must feel ownership in this project and play an active role in designing their own eating plans. If the patient is not satisfied with the quality of the interaction with the counselor, adherence tends to suffer. Actions that initially may appear unrelated to the specifics of counseling, such as waiting time before the appointment, have been shown to have a negative affect on adherence.

Counseling has been defined as a two-part process; the first is the development of a rapport or a trusting relationship with the client, and the second is the implementation of the behavior change strategies.[11] The implementation is dependent on successfully establishing this relationship. A well-qualified, compassionate, and understanding facilitator will have a direct impact on the success rate for adherence.

In addition to a technical knowledge base, the diabetic counselor must be well trained in effective communication skills. Such skills include the techniques of active listening, demonstrating understanding with reflective statements, asking questions to gather information, and becoming aware of the client's concerns, expectations, and perceived obstacles for success. Although it is not within the scope of this chapter to delve into this arena, there are numerous sources that delineate communication skills for effective counseling.[12]

Changing how you eat involves making changes in a variety of interrelated activities. This may include how you shop for food, how you prepare foods, whether you take time to keep fresh fruits and vegetables available for snacks rather than a candy bar, your typical pattern for eating or skipping certain meals, and the social interaction that may occcur at that meal, It may also entail learning new skills for meal preparation or time management skills to provide the time for advanced planning of meals or even time for breakfast during a hectic, early morning schedule.

As with any behavior change, modifying the diet takes a number of clearly defined steps. The diabetic health care team should help the patient progress through these steps to successfully achieve a more healthful eating plan:

1. Awareness,
2. Education,
3. Behavioral changes,
4. Reinforcement.

AWARENESS

The first step in behavior change is creating awareness. It is difficult to change a behavior if you are not fully aware of the actual content in which you perform that behavior. What you eat, how it is prepared, when you eat, and for what reason are all important aspects of the awareness component. Keeping a dietary record or log is the most effective way to collect these data. A log should include a time, location/activity, food description, quantity of food consumed and description of the patient's mood. Where available, reviewing itemized grocery receipts will also help identify positive food choices purchased and increase awareness of shopping patterns.

Analyzing the food diary will allow the diabetic educator to see eating patterns emerge, as well as food preferences.

In addition, methods of food preparation will become apparent and may highlight the need for learning new skills or modifying recipes. Matching the new eating plan as closely as possible to current practices will help increase the success rate.

Often, foods are forgotten or dismissed as unimportant nibbles or snacks and are not written down. Initiating the habit of recording food intake will provide a more accurate snapshot of eating behaviors and will help patients self-monitor their success in following a new eating pattern.

A second component of awareness involves recognition of cues or triggers that lead to the initiation of a behavior that is to be changed. Cues may be certain social situations that lead to a certain eating pattern or a television commercial that places the thought in your head for having a sweet treat:

Cues → Behavior → Consequences

In keeping a food diary, it helps to include notes regarding your thoughts and emotions when eating and concomitant activities. Such information may show that feeling lonely and watching television by yourself is a strong stimulus for overeating snack foods unconsciously. Once the actual pattern is known, with as much detailed information as possible, an action plan for change can begin. This technique is known as stimulus control, where cues that may stimulate the undesirable behavior are limited.

The path between the cue and the behavior is usually not one single step; it is a series of activities that leads you to the main event or behavior. Sitting in front of the television does not automatically produce a snack that is eaten. A cue triggers the thought of a snack, which then must be acted on. This might entail standing up, walking out of the room into the kitchen, searching the refrigerator, finding a suitable snack, and then returning to the television:

T.V. → Cue → Thought → Stand up → Walk out of Room → Go to Kitchen → Open Refrigerator → Find Snack → Return to T.V. → Eat Snack

Each step in this scenario has the potential for breaking the chain of events that subconsciously leads from televison viewing to eating a snack. If awareness of these habit chains is increased, alternative activities that will disconnect the chain can be designed and implemented. The new path can lead to a new behavior or event. For example, having only low-fat, nutritious snacks in the refrigerator, or you walk into a different room and pick up a crossword puzzle or other task that will take your mind off the snack. The new behaviors that can be learned to break the chain are as varied as the individuals who perform these new behaviors. The key to success is awareness and planning ahead for the event.

EDUCATION

Education is the second step in behavior change. It is important for diabetics to understand the interrelationship between glucose, insulin, food, and physical activity. What factors may affect glucose maintenance, symptoms of serious side effects, and precautions that should be taken must also be understood. They should understand that diabetes is controllable and they are personally responsible for maintaining control over their health status. What they do and do not do can have long-term and serious impact on their health.

The diabetic should immediately take actions to be proactive in the maintenance of his or her health. These are the basic survival skills that must be learned. Medication dosage, timing, meal plans and the Diabetic Exchange Lists, self-monitoring blood glucose test, as well as the signs and symptoms of side effects all must be incorporated into their lives. The assimilation of this knowledge and these tasks into their daily routine is the first stage of the learning process. Knowledge is empowerment, and with the accomplishment of these skills, the diabetic will gain self-confidence. For those diabetics who have been diagnosed for a long time but are not remaining in control of their disease, this initial learning stage may need to be reinforced.

Once these basic survival skills are learned, a more in-depth educational program may be offered. The format for these programs may vary across the country, from 1-week camps to weekend getaways or evening meetings at the local hospital. The goal of these programs is to provide the next level of information and support that will help diabetics manage their disease in all situations, from holiday parties or vacation to engaging in highly competitive athletic events. This continuity of care is an important aspect for establishing the groundwork for long-term success.

An ongoing program of education would involve updates on new forms of treatments and continuing support for the behavior changes. Local support groups and programs can be found by contacting the local chapter of the American Diabetes Association.

BEHAVIORAL CHANGES

Taking the cognitive knowledge base and incorporating this information and the accompanying skills into daily activities is the source for most difficulties in learning new habits. Influencing factors in this process are physiological (e.g., blood glucose levels and symptoms from loss of control), psychologic (attitudes regarding health status and need for change), and environmental (the degree of support from family and friends).

Behavioral research has classified four distinct stages in the process of self-change. Although the original research dealt with a different health life-style change—smoking—the concept can be adapted for other health-related behavioral changes.[13]

The four stages include precontemplators, contemplators, recruits, and adherers. As the awareness and decision process proceeds, the individual will progress from one level to the next as a level of comfort is obtained.

Diabetics have already been recruited by their health care team, possibly before they have had the opportunity to contemplate the life-style changes that will be necessary. Those who do not adhere to their therapy may be the ones who have not accepted the facts of their situation and deny that there is a problem that needs to be addressed. Those with diabetic complications, regardless of the cause, may need to readdress the components of their therapy and develop a new action plan.

The characteristics of those recruits who become adherers are not easily isolated. Because there are confounding influences, it is difficult to single out any specific behavior or attitude that will definitively identify those who will succeed. Again, behavioral research shows that a good sense of self-esteem, self-efficacy, and self-motivation, as well as an internal locus of control, are all factors that positively influence success.

Self-efficacy reflects the individual's perception that they are able to develop a mastery of the skill necessary to complete any given task. Their perceived competency and ability to succeed will directly affect how they respond to challenges. A positive mental attitude may be an important component. Therefore, it is important that their health care providers be supportive and helpful in their comments if there is difficulty in maintaining control of blood glucose levels. Negative remarks will be taken as failures by those with feelings of low self-efficacy and may promulgate more failures.

The concept of locus of control is also an ingredient for helping those accept personal responsibility for health. Those with a sense of an internal locus believe that they can control the outcome of their lives. External controllers believe that their destinies are controlled by chance or some powerful other. External controllers with diabetes may have a difficult time adopting new health behaviors meant to impact such a serious health matter.

Setting goals, both short- and long-term goals, will direct the path of change. The goals should be written and follow the standards for any goal setting activity. The acronym SMART goals reflects the characteristics for effective goal setting. Goals should be:

S Specific
M Measurable
A Attainable
R Realistic
T Timetable

A global goal of eating a healthier diet is too unwieldy to manage. It cannot be easily measured, and it may not be realistically attained within a reasonable time frame. A more effective goal would be to state that "I plan to eat three meals and two snacks per day for at least 5 out of the next 7 days."

Goals should be stated in a positive manner, what you *will* do rather than what you *will not*, and reinforce positive behaviors.

Setting specific positive short-term goals will reassess what are considered the parameters for success. Perfect glucose control may not be a realistic parameter for success initially. Perhaps maintaining modest control while incorporating new eating patterns is more attainable for the patient. Success breeds success. As the patient achieves these goals and experiences the positive feelings for this success, he or she will be motivated and have the self-confidence to achieve the next level of success.

In establishing goals, it is important to determine any obstacles, real or perceived, that may need to be overcome to achieve success. These obstacles may be behavioral, such as an attitude of inability to cope; physical, such as cooking skills that must be obtained; financial, the misconception that healthy eating is more expensive; or a lack of social support systems.

Most successful patients have a network for support: friends, family, or other diabetics. Support provides a source of positive feelings and an opportunity to share concerns and fears. Support systems have been shown to increase adherence to the new eating plan. Attention should be given to negative support where good intentions may sabotage efforts.

Supportive environments at home involve incorporating as many new habits for the diabetic family member into the life-style of the entire family. This includes the family all eating the same meals so the diabetic does not feel isolated or different, including physical activity into the family's typical recreational activities, or providing free time for the diabetic to engage in his or her own form of exercise or physical activity. Integrating as many diabetic activities into the family's life-style so that they are not special but just a way of life will reinforce long-term adherence.

REINFORCEMENT

As stated previously, achieving small goals is a path that can lead to the overall objective of diabetic control, and a healthy diet provides ample opportunity for positive reinforcement and rewards. Depending on the individual patient, a system of rewards may be established that is received on the attainment of specific goals. Rewards should be nonfood oriented, pos-

itive, healthy, and chosen by the patient. Nagging is an example of a negative reinforcer, and as well intentioned as it may be, it is simply not effective. In a similar manner, punishment has a strong negative effect on compliance.

COPING STRATEGIES

During times of stress or change, it is human nature to return to long-standing habits. For anyone who has recently made a life-style change, either dietary or even quitting smoking, it is important to develop coping strategies for these difficult times. A short-term lapse can easily become a way of life again if a relapse strategy is not planned.

A relapse is always a negative experience for individuals who feel they have failed in their attempt to make a life-style change. When counseling, it is important to be nonjudgmental with the patient and discuss what can be done in the future to prevent such an occurrence. Rehearsing "what if?" scenarios can help the patient role-play specific situations that they consider risky for relapse. Practice brings familiarity and will better prepare the diabetic client when faced with the real-life situation.

For diabetics, role playing includes how they may respond to certain stressors and what they must consider regarding their dietary and insulin plan. If the situation results in an unpredictable eating schedule, they must take steps to ensure that they will maintain their diabetes treatment plan. Their immediate health status must remain a priority.

SPECIAL CONSIDERATIONS

Treatment plans for diabetics can vary as widely as the individual patient who presents themselves to you. Special considerations must be made for women through menstruation, pregnancy, and menopause; children and teenagers; and athletes. In addition, those with other complications, such as retinopathy or kidney disease, will require additional treatment and care. The flexibility of treatment plans allows each set of conditions to be dealt with individually. Although it is not within the scope of this chapter, additional information and resources are available through the references provided.

Wound healing and infection control are issues of concern for the diabetic with complications such as foot lesions. Unfortunately, research into the cause of delayed healing often does not control for the type of diabetes, the level of glucose control, or the overall nutritional status. Each of these variables must be considered when researching treatment strategies.

For the physician, it now appears that blood glucose should be controlled to levels less than 200 mg/dL and between 120 and 160 mg/dL if possible to optimize wound healing and minimize the spread of infection. Often diabetes is dealt with as a separate condition from the immediate medical concern, and blood glucose levels of 200 to 300 mg/dL are tolerated. The mechanism resulting in these recommendations has only recently been analyzed, and it is not apparent if it is directly associated with the diabetes or is a secondary result of the degree of blood glucose control.

Ischemia associated with foot ulcers may be directly affected by blood glucose levels. Hyperglycemia increases the viscosity of the blood and causes an increased concentration of glycosylated hemoglobin, which has an increased affinity for oxygen. This shifting of the O_2 dissociation curve results in a diminished delivery of O_2 to the capillary and a decreased tissue oxygen tension (Po_2) level. This response has been shown to be reversible when blood glucose levels are returned to normal.[14]

It has also been observed that there is a high incidence of staphylococcal infection in diabetics, which varies depending on the blood glucose level. When the blood glucose level is greater than 130 mg/dL, there is an increased growth in gram-positive organisms and an inhibition in gram-negative organisms. When the blood glucose level is less than 100 mg/dL, gram-negative organisms proliferate.[14]

A study of the inflammatory stage of wound healing showed impairment of polymorphonuclear leukocytes (PMN) action in poorly controlled diabetics (blood glucose level > 200 mg/dL). Overall, there is delayed cellular response to injury when blood glucose levels are out of control, which may affect collagen synthesis. It appears that this condition is associated with diabetes mellitus and can be improved with blood glucose control.[15]

The diabetic's hyperglycemia may also be exacerbated by their stress reaction to their condition. The stress hormones—epinephrine, glucagon, cortisol, and growth hormone—act to increase blood glucose levels. As the body's metabolic system responds to the challenge of infection, these hormones may counteract the available insulin, resulting in an increased need for insulin.

These are just a few examples of how blood glucose levels may directly affect wound healing in the diabetic. Blood glucose levels should be monitored preoperatively and postoperatively to maintain optimal levels, which will promote wound healing and limit the impact on the immune system.

The typical type II diabetic is older and overweight and may have a tendency for impaired wound healing that is independent of the diabetic condition. A diabetic out of control is often malnourished and in a catabolic state, deriving energy from fat and protein stores. He or she may be in negative nitrogen balance and have decreased albumin and total lymphocyte levels. Lowered albumin levels may be correlated with infection and delayed wound healing.

Protein status should be monitored; the goal is to achieve nitrogen balance. Protein intakes are usually sufficient in most patients to maintain balance. Care must be taken because these patients with complications may also be at risk for renal complications of diabetes; the complications are exacerbated by excessive protein intakes. Diet plans should include foods that have high-quality, complimentary protein in sufficient amounts, as previously discussed.

It is currently recommended that before any surgical procedure blood glucose levels should be maintained as close to normal as possible (< 200 mg/dL). The effects of even this short-term control has been demonstrated to be quite beneficial to the patient. Additional research should help identify the factors related to the diabetic condition and those that are independent to improve surgical outcomes.[15]

Interest in improving wound and absess healing has motivated research into the use of vitamins and minerals both supplementation and topical applications. Studies of the efficacy of supplementation have not provided any evidence for increased needs in these circumstances. The overall nutritional status of the patient should be assessed and managed to achieve optimal nutritional status. Supplementation is only recommended in cases of nutritional deficiency.

Topical application of zinc is currently being used in experimental circumstances with promising results. Further study in allied areas such as treatment for burn patients should help provide new options in the treatment of the complications of the diabetic foot.

RESOURCES

Access to nutrition counseling and diabetes education programs are available through most hospitals and medical centers. Treatment is typically delivered through a health care team approach. Diabetes educators represent a variety of professionals, from nurses to dietitians, health educators, and exercise physiologists. Certified diabetes educators are those professionals who have passed a Certification Examination provided through the American Association of Diabetes Educators (AADEs).

The initials CDE identify these professionals. The AADE provides a directory of diabetes education programs and will also provide a listing of certified diabetic educators within your geographic area.

Registered dietitians are nutrition professionals trained in the areas of diabetes, foods, and counseling skills who qualify through educational requirements, an internship experience, and the successful completion of a registration examination through the American Dietetic Association (ADA). Qualified dietitians are identified with the initials RD. A specialty practice group with the ADA, the Diabetes Care and Education Dietetic Practice Group, is composed of dietitians who specialize in the care of diabetes.

Additional information and resources are available through the American Diabetes Association, the American Dietetic Association, and the American Association of Diabetic Educators.

REFERENCES

1. American Diabetes Association: Nutritional recommendations and principles for individuals with Diabetes Mellitus: 1986. [position statement], *Diabetes Care* 10:126–132, 1987.
2. American College of Sports Medicine: *Guidelines for exercise testing and prescription*, ed 4. Philadelphia, 1991, Lea & Febiger.
3. American Diabetes Association: Diabetes mellitus and exercise, [position statement], *Diabetes Care* 13:804–805, 1990.

4. Franz MJ, Norstrom MA: *Diabetes actively staying healthy (DASH): your game plan for diabetes and exercise,* International Diabetes Center, 1990, Minneapolis.

5. Katch FI, McArdle WD: *Nutrition, weight control and exercise,* ed 2. Philadelphia, 1983, Lea & Febiger, pp 308–315.

6. Franz MJ, Barr P, Holler H et al: Exchange lists: Revised 1986, *J Am Diet Assoc* 87:28–36, 1987.

7. American Diabetes Association and American Dietetic Association: *Nutrition guidelines for professionals—diabetes education and meal planning,* Alexandria, Va, 1988, American Diabetes Association.

8. Holler HJ: Understanding the use of exchanges lists for meal planning in diabetes management, *The Diabetes Educator* 1991, 17:474–484.

9. American Diabetes Association: Glycemic effects of carbohydrate [policy statement], *Diabetes Care* 1984, 7:607–608, 1984.

10. Pastors JG: Alternatives to the exchange system for teaching menu planning for persons with Diabetes, *The Diabetes Educator* 18:57–62, 1992.

11. Danish SJ: Developing helping relationships in dietetic counseling, *J Am Diet Assoc* 67:107–110, 1975.

12. Danish SJ, D'Augelli AR, Hauer AL: *Helping skills: a basic training program,* ed 2, New York, 1980, Human Sciences Press.

13. Prochaska JO, DiClemente CC: Stages and processes of self-change of smoking: Toward an integrative model of change, *J Consult Clin Psychol* 51:390–395, 1983.

14. Morain WD, Colen LB: Wound healing in Diabetes Mellitus, *Clin Plast Surg* 17:493–501, 1990.

15. Rosenberg CS: Wound healing in the patient with Diabetes Mellitus, *Nurs Clin North Am* 25:274–361, 1990.

APPENDIX: RESOURCES

American Diabetes Association
1600 Duke St.
Alexandria, VA 22314
1-800-232-3472

American Dietetic Association
216 W. Jackson
Suite 800
Chicago, IL 60606-6995
1-800-877-1600

American Association of Diabetes
  Educators
500 N. Michigan Ave.
Suite 1400
Chicago, IL 60611

27 _____ The Importance of Patient Education

Sandra Frankenheim, R.N., C.D.E.

Linda Selemba, C.D.E.

Education has become one of the accepted cornerstones in the edifice of diabetic care. The increase in publications addressing self-care behaviors, the increase in numbers of health care providers certified as diabetes educators, the assumptions regarding the ideas surrounding the access to information leading to behavior change, and the increasing consumerism of health care are some of the indicators of the strong rationale for the role of education in diabetic foot care. When the effectiveness of educational efforts aimed at a largely adult population is measured, compliance with a prescribed treatment regimen is often used as the criterion of success. It is frequently assumed that patient access to the correct information regarding his or her condition will generate appropriate behavior change. Perhaps a better way to evaluate successful educational endeavors is a dialog between the educator and the learner and significant others regarding their perceptions of the usefulness and accessibility of the material presented. It is our contention that especially where diabetic foot care is concerned, a collaborative relationship will prove to be most effective in enabling patients to participate in the care of their feet. This collaborative relationship will be discussed from the perspective of the client and the educator, and some principles, characteristics, and content relative to diabetic foot care will be suggested. We believe that with attention to the individualism of the client and the educator, the treatment and preventive modalities presented in the rest of this book will become more accessible to the client and successful care more attainable for the practitioner.

ROADBLOCKS TO LEARNING

A multitude of factors can and do provide hindrances to the ability of our clients to hear and use foot care information and specific regimens for situational care. Basically these factors can be condensed into three parts: the client, the learning environment, and the instructor. We will look at each of these in turn and offer specific suggestions for the amelioration of problems in educational success.

Our clients have personalities, needs, knowledge, both correct and incorrect, and fears. They also bring past learning experiences and relationships with physicians and other health care providers that will absolutely influence their relationships with us and that will usually not be obvious to us initially. Clients will need to develop trust before they will let us in on some of their past health experiences, to which we should listen very carefully. Once a level of trust is developed, clients will often let us know their own roadblocks, problems, and biases in learning and modifying their behavior. It will then be possible to work together in eradicating these problems. It is important for the practitioner to consider the level of complicity they may have in the behavior of the client. How the practitioner presents himself or herself to the client can make a decisive impact on the ability of the client to retain and apply information. With diabetic foot care we are usually working with adult clients; therefore, it is important to uncover the knowledge base each client has acquired. We will not be working with a blank slate; each person will bring to our relationship many past learning experiences, some erroneous pieces of information, and many interpretations of accurate information. These interpretations will include the filtering of the client's own experiences and those of others. Of course, the experiences of others usually are not analogous to the situation of our client, but we must be sure to examine these interpretations because they have an enormous bearing on whether or not our clients will perceive a need or ability to alter their own behavior. In addition to providing us with much needed information, the conversations in which we explore these topics will give us the chance to solidify the personal relationship with our client that will enable effective learning to occur.

Probably the single greatest roadblock to effective learning is fear. Clients with diabetes are always aware that their feet will require some level of care. They also believe that if they have developed some problem with their feet, it is only a matter of time before their feet will be amputated. It is perhaps difficult for those of us who work daily with the success stories possible with these clients to understand the depth of this fear. Every one of them has expressed to us the existence of a relative or friend who had to undergo an amputation, and all clients expressed this event as an immediate prelude to death. This belief in the inevitability of amputation usually leads to some degree of fatalism and depression, which must be acknowledged by the educator and the

client. To take a Pollyanna approach is to negate clients' very real feelings and prevent the realism that must be an important part of an effective learning situation. Asking client's about others they know or their own experiences with the possibility of amputation and then truly listening to the answers, are frequently all that is needed. Potentially false reassurances must not be given, but a realistic discussion of the options and of clients' ability to impact on their own health, along with an acceptance of fear, instead of belittling it, will lead to the formulation of a level of trust necessary for clients to learn and to make effective behavior change.

There are several other roadblocks to learning for adults with diabetes, especially once foot problems have begun to occur. These include other physical problems, such as retinopathy and neuropathy, cardiac problems, and, frequently, excessive weight. All these may make it difficult, if not impossible, for our clients to participate in some aspect of their foot care needs. The person with an insensate foot may overlook the importance of compliance not out of willfulness but truly because the lack of pain feedback undermines the need for attention to real or potential problems. Such clients need individualized problem solving and frequently several potential solutions may need to be tried before the client and the practitioner hit on a workable one. The client must be the significant problem solver, because only then will he or she have the motivation to try.

Visual disturbances may contribute to a client's inability to learn. Persons who cannot see their feet will not look at them, with mirrors or otherwise. It is very useful to ask clients about their vision and, if it is a problem, to explore possible solutions with them. Usually there is someone in that person's life who can make visual examinations of the feet, but it might not be possible for this to be done daily. While not losing track of the optimum, it would be wise to discuss with the client the reasons for daily foot examination and then to accept the schedule that the client can attempt to adhere to. To insist that only daily examinations will accomplish the task is to ensure that no examinations or only erratic ones will be done. It is also appropriate to mention that health care practitioners should practice what they preach. When 85% of visits to a practitioner by people with diabetes take place with the shoes still on, we are sending a strong message about the real importance of foot care.

Another significant and often unconsidered roadblock concerns whether our clients believe they are able to comply with their health care requirements. Because we are so concerned with foot care, we often forget to consider that our clients may be, in fact, very ill. Foot care may not be a priority for them. Unless adults see a benefit to themselves, learning will not take place. The benefit of enhanced foot care for these clients is not just a reduction in amputation rates but an increased sense of control and success, which frequently eludes them regarding the rest of the disease process. Just an acknowledgement, on our part of the complex picture with which the client and his or her family deal every day lets our clients know that we view them as complete human beings, not just as feet.

Asking clients to tell us what they know about their feet and their disease process and what they think they need to learn will tell us about their priorities and give us the opportunity to correct any inaccurate information. It would be well for us to remember that clients may not easily relinquish incorrect information and may need a trial and error period while they test out what we are telling them. There may be many repetitive questions, which might frustrate us. Frequently clients will need to achieve some level of success, then relapse, before they can really begin to accept that a particular behavior change, such as always wearing a particular shoe,

does impact on what happens with their feet. We will need to be patient while our clients try out both compliance and noncompliance on their way to recognizing their behavioral responsibilities.

The learning environment for adult clients should be as pleasant as possible. In an individual experience, privacy should be provided if at all feasible. Privacy enhances the establishment of trust necessary to individual revelation and problem solving. There should be no distractions, such as magazines, traffic through the room, or interruptions. If a television or radio is on, it should be turned off for the duration of the learning situation. Family members should be included whenever possible, and the experience should be interactive, with information being exchanged among all participants. Group situations should be arranged with seating to facilitate sharing. Visual aids, such as charts, pictures, blackboards, and handouts, should be used if indicated (Table 27–1). However, it is a good idea to avoid a schoolroom effect, which may foster performance anxieties.

The personality of the educator may be used as an educational tool. To the extent that the educator is able to form personal bonds with the client will be the extent of real effectiveness. It is extremely helpful if the educator is warm and nonjudgmental while at the same time conveying to clients that they are responsible for their foot-care decisions. The educator is most useful to the client as a resource person and facilitator. Of course, to develop these roles, time and energy must be spent sounding each other out.

ASSESSMENT

A comprehensive and accurate assessment lays the foundation for delivery of an individualized and effective educational intervention. Studies have suggested that the assessment process con-

TABLE 27–1.

Principles of Diabetes Foot Care*

1. Discontinue tobacco use.
2. Inspect feet daily; incorporate in activities of daily living (e.g., after bathing).
3. Check entire foot and between toes for calluses, blisters, abrasions, tenderness, discoloration, dryness, redness, and areas of friction.
4. Use a hand mirror to see bottom of feet or enlist the help of another person to look at feet.
5. Wash feet daily with mild soap.
6. Test water with thermometer or elbow first; water should feel comfortable. Avoid temperature extremes.
7. Do not soak feet unless instructed to do so by health care provider.
8. Dry feet carefully; pat with towel gently, especially between toes.
9. Apply a thin layer of nonperfumed moisturizer to feet after bathing. Do not apply between toes.
10. Avoid use of powder between toes. A light dusting of nonperfumed talc may be used on the rest of the foot if desired.
11. Wear socks to bed at night if feet are cold. Do not use heating pads, hot water bottles, or hot water to warm feet.
12. Cut nails in contour with the toes. Do not trim down the sides or corners.
13. Do not perform "bathroom surgery" by scraping or cutting corns, calluses, or blisters. Do not use corn removers or plasters because these products may damage healthy tissue. Consult with your podiatrist or health care provider.
14. Break in new shoes gradually; wear them for only a few hours at a time the first 2 weeks. On purchase of shoes, feet should be measured and shoes carefully fitted.
15. Avoid tight-fitting shoes, high-heeled shoes, open-toed shoes, and sandals, especially thongs.
16. Wear shoes made of breathable material, such as leather.
17. Before wearing shoes each time, inspect and feel interior of shoes for foreign objects, nail heads, pebbles, or rough surfaces.
18. Specialized shoes may be prescribed by podiatrist for specific foot problems such as hammertoes or Charcot foot.
19. Wear appropriate shoes or stockings at all times. Avoid darned or mended socks.
20. Avoid constricting stockings, socks, or garters.
21. Know early signs of inflammation and infection, such as increased warmth, pain, swelling, or discharge, and report to health care provider immediately.
22. Be sure to have health care provider inspect feet at each appointment.

*From American Diabetes Association: *Diabetic foot Care.* Alexandria, Va, 1990, American Diabetes Association. Used by permission.

stitutes up to 55% of a client interaction.[1] An assessment should comprise input from each member of the health care team. A collaborative effort may reduce the amount of time spent by each team member on the assessment stage.

When a patient first seeks treatment, an initial assessment should be undertaken. Ongoing assessment during the health care delivery process is of equal importance. Communication of assessment findings to other team members may occur through the use of charting, care plans, and multidisciplinary client care conferences.

Numerous variables must be assessed to determine learning needs. Information can be obtained from a thorough health history and physical examination. Additional assessment methods include the use of observation, interviews, questionnaires, records, and skill inventories. Generally a combination of these methods is used to obtain a comprehensive database.

Demographic variables such as age, gender, and level of formal education must be taken into consideration. For example, specific educational strategies may need to be undertaken to accommodate the presence of cognitive or functional disabilities and the lack of financial resources and support systems in the elderly client. Level of formal education, according to Billie,[2] may impact on clients orientation to learning and suggests that "as the number of years of formal education increases, the amount of structure needed decreases" in the format of the learning experience.

Cultural variables must be addressed. Members of a particular culture may differ in their views on values, roles, and responsibilities. Environmental factors such as physical limitations of the home in the newly disabled client or lack of a safe neighborhood in the client beginning a walking program must be examined. Employment status and type of health insurance can affect the ability of the client to carry out a desired skill such as self-monitoring of blood glucose levels.

Information about concurrent illnesses, chronic complications from diabetes such as retinopathy or neuropathy, sensory-perceptual deficits, medications, participation in health promotional activities (e.g., diet and exercise), and use of alcohol, tobacco, or illicit drugs should be obtained.

A psychologic assessment should incorporate identification of support systems, coping mechanisms, and level of acceptance of diabetes.

Billie[2] states that "people decide to learn, they cannot be made to learn." Therefore, readiness to learn must also be assessed, and it may be influenced by any of the aforementioned variables.

The assessment of a potential learner must recognize principles of teaching and learning. Effective delivery of education must delineate the differences between the teaching of an adult to that of a child.

Knowles[3] describes four principles that set the basis for approaching the prospective adult learner. According to Knowles,[3] the adult incorporates his or her own past experiences into the learning process. Therefore, examination of the client's current diabetes management and foot care knowledge base, prior educational experiences, and previous attempts

at life-style change must be undertaken. For example, a client may have previously attempted a walking program on his or her own without success but was able to comply with an exercise regimen as a member of a walking group.

Second, as adult learners mature, their self-concept moves from dependency to self-direction. Undoubtedly, learners with newly diagnosed diabetes will rely on family members or the health care team for assistance with skills such as administration of insulin and treatment of hypoglycemia. However, as clients become more at ease with these skills, they will assume responsibilities for these tasks. The health care team should encourage clients to participate in the learning process by performing return demonstrations of skills and problem solving exercises.

Third, adults are problem-oriented learners rather than subject-oriented learners. The acquisition of knowledge may be desired by the client; however, if the potential knowledge gain could be applied to an immediate problem, learning will ensue more readily. For example, the client who is being treated for a first-time foot infection that resulted from the manipulation of a blister would be willing to learn foot care first aid and proper shoe selection.

Unfortunately, this characteristic of the adult learner may contribute to difficulty in teaching preventive foot care. The educator must then rely on the other attributes of the adult learner to ensure that application of knowledge gained will take place. The educator may encourage the client to incorporate foot assessment into an established routine such as the bathing ritual. Continued assessment and reinforcement is mandatory.

Finally, adults have to see the need for learning to participate in the educational interaction. Clients' readiness to learn is affected by the perceived impact of diabetes care on their current life-styles. Clients see a need to incorporate changes without significant compromise to their existing life-styles. Moreover, readiness to learn is dependent on clients' acceptance of the diagnosis of diabetes mellitus and the degree of treatment needed.

DIAGNOSIS, GOAL SETTING, AND DETERMINATION OF PLAN

Using the assessment data, members of the health care team are now able to construct diagnoses and formulate plans. Clear objectives must be developed and described in behavioral terms that are quantifiable. Evaluation of the educational process will reflect on these objectives. If possible, the goals should be mutually set with the client. The formulation of a contract with the client may be useful.

The client educational plan should be outlined in stages. Haire-Joshu and Houston[1] describe three distinct stages: survival, ongoing, and in-depth. At the survival stage, clients should receive only the critical information necessary to live on their own outside of the health care environment. For example, the client with newly diagnosed type I diabetes, on discharge from the health care setting, needs to be able to perform insulin preparation and injection, management of hypoglycemia, and possibly self-monitoring of blood glucose. The client may be unable to assimilate large amounts of information and therefore should not be expected to learn how to manage sick day, travel, or exercise guidelines.

Similarly, hospitalized clients with established diabetes who are undergoing stress secondary to an acute illness may not be able to advance to more in-depth education despite having mastered basic skills in diabetes management through actual life experiences with diabetes. However, clients with established diabetes who are not undergoing an acute illness may be able to move to a more advanced stage of education if they verbalize a readiness to do this.

The ongoing educational stage transpires when the client is comfortable with survival skills and verbalizes a readiness to learn additional information and skills. A significant amount of foot care education may take place during this stage, as well as education in sick day management, insulin adjustments, and exercise.

The in-depth education stage may involve instruction in more specialized skills, for instance, use of an insulin pump. Also, it may include any review of skills or information, update on new technologies or treatments, or whatever knowledge the client desires.

Members of the health care team may contribute much input during the survival skill stage. As the client moves into the more advanced stages, he or she will bring more experience to the educational interaction. It is important to recognize and acknowledge the client's experiences and problem solving skills.

TEAM MANAGEMENT

The multidisciplinary team approach is the most effective vehicle for delivery of a quality foot care and diabetes management program. The treatment team may consist of a diabetologist, podiatric physician, diabetes nurse educator, foot care nurse specialist, orthopedist, vascular surgeon, pedorthist, nutritionist, physical therapist, exercise specialist, and social worker. Ideally, the principle members of the team are based in one centralized location such as a diabetes management or foot care center. Alternatively, team members may be based in one institution or community, whereby one of the team members assumes the role of client care coordinator and the remaining team members consult and provide input to the client's treatment plans.

Regardless of the setting, the main objective is the provision of an individualized and effective treatment plan to the client. Effective communication is critical to the accomplishment of this objective. The client should have access to each member of the team, and accordingly each team member must maintain open lines of communication with the client. Then all of the team members must communicate with each other. This form of communication has been described as the each to all model of health care team communication.[4]

Team client care conferences provide the ideal setting for communication to take place. Conferences of this nature should incorporate goal setting, problem solving, and clarification of the management plan. Clients should be assured of congruent recommendations from all team members. Documentation of the behaviorally stated goals and management plan is essential to maintain the communication link between the team members. In addition, documentation provides the basis for ongoing evaluation of both client progress and the educational-management program, as well as demonstration of medicolegal accountability.

The benefit to the physician or podiatric provider in having a team-based practice is that valuable time may be freed up if he or she can spend less time on in-depth education and more time in clinical practice. This is not to say that the practitioner should not provide education. The physician may have more time to teach, which should be taken advantage of. Anderson and Funnell[5] describe the moment of diagnosis as a teachable moment because the client does not comprehend the meaning of diabetes. In addition, the time of the onset of complications may provide an opportunity for teaching because the client feels that he or she is more suscep-

tible to the complications of diabetes. Similarly, abnormal findings such as calluses or improperly cut nails during a foot examination may prompt immediate attention by the client to visualize the findings and learn proper actions to take to prevent these occurrences. This is a particularly important teaching moment for the client with insensate feet who may not realize that such insults have taken place.

ROLE OF THE CERTIFIED DIABETES EDUCATOR

A certified diabetes educator (CDE) assumes an invaluable role on the health care team. The CDE is knowledgeable in all aspects of diabetes care, particularly in the area of teaching and learning theories. This content provides the framework for carrying out an educational plan; however, it is most often lacking in health care professionals' curriculum. The CDE may assist in protocol development along with the physician provider. Establishment of protocols may expand the educator's role to include adjustment of insulin and sick day management.

The expanding role of a CDE implies certain medicolegal responsibilities such as the nonphysician members of the team practicing medicine without appropriate licensure. According to Ratner,[6] in 1991 there had not yet been any legal challenges to the expanding role of the CDE. The most formidable defense against litigation is maintenance of the highest standards of diabetes care and education, which includes certification of diabetes educators by the National Certification Board for Diabetes Educators and recognition of the educational program by the American Diabetes Association (ADA).[7,8] Written protocols directing the practices of the diabetes educator should be developed and implemented. Furthermore, practitioners should comply with

Standards of Medical Care set forth by the ADA.[7]

EFFECTIVENESS OF EDUCATION

How has the effectiveness of client education been demonstrated in the literature? One can assess effectiveness from the perspectives of the chronic disease, diabetes education, comprehensive foot care, and diabetes foot care education models.

Many studies have been conducted using the model of chronic disease. A metaanalysis conducted by Mazzuca[9] reported that education was successful in improving compliance, physiologic progress, and health outcomes. In addition, behaviorally oriented programs were more effective than programs that addressed only knowledge building. For example, education would be more effective when clients learn how to incorporate management of the disease into their current lifestyles rather just learning the pathophysiology of the disease.

There are few randomized, controlled, long-term studies with regard to the effectiveness of diabetes education on physiologic outcome, compliance, and acquisition of knowledge. Much of the references to effectiveness are disseminated through anecdotal reports.

In a randomized, controlled diabetes education study only clients with type II diabetes by Mazzuca et al.,[10] the experimental group showed a sustained statistically significant difference in self-care skills and compliance behaviors when compared with the control group 14 months after participating in a group education program. However, a rare difference was seen between the two groups in diabetes knowledge. The experimental group also showed modest but statistically significant improvement in fasting blood glucose levels, hemoglobin A_{1C} values, blood pressure, and creatinine levels at 6

to 12 months and greater weight loss at 6 months. Numerous studies have been conducted relating diabetes education to cost effectiveness. Reduction in diabetes-related hospital admissions and reduction in days spent hospitalized have been documented in the literature.[11–13]

Studies do suggest that a comprehensive foot care program, which includes the prescription of therapeutic shoes, foot inspection, and patient education, decreases lower-extremity amputations by approximately 50% and decreases hospital admissions.[14–16]

Unfortunately, no studies demonstrate the effectiveness of foot care education alone. Kruger and Guthrie[17] examined the effects of a prospective hands-on foot care education program on the subjects' foot care knowledge, self-care practices, and the actual condition of the feet. The results of the study were inconclusive, and the high attrition rate contributed to the study's limitations.

We recognize the need for longitudinal studies that will demonstrate the effects of client education in both diabetes management and foot care with regard to cost effectiveness, application of knowledge, compliance, and reduction in morbidity. Timely application of relevant educational principles and commitment to a team approach will enable health care practitioners to provide quality and efficacious education to their clients.

REFERENCES

1. Haire-Joshu D, Houston C: Promoting behavior change: Teaching/learning strategies. In Haire-Joshu D, editor: *Management of diabetes mellitus: Perspectives of care across the life span,* St Louis, 1992, Mosby–Year Book.
2. Billie D: *Module #1: An approach to individualizing instruction: Assessing patient readiness and activities of daily living,* Pitman, NJ, American Association of Diabetes Educators, 1984.

3. Knowles M: *The adult learner: a neglected species,* Houston, 1980, Gulf Publishing.
4. Lorber D, Lagana D: The health care team in diabetes: A model for communication, *Pract Diabetol* 10:16, 1991.
5. Anderson R, Funnell M: The role of the physician in patient education, *Pract Diabetol* 9:10–12, 1990.
6. Ratner R: Overview of diabetes mellitus. In Haire-Joshu D, editor: *Management of diabetes mellitus: Perspectives across the life span,* St Louis, 1992, Mosby–Year Book.
7. American Diabetes Association: Clinical practice recommendations, *Diabetes Care* 14(suppl):10–13, 18–19, 76–81, 1991.
8. National Certification Board for Diabetes Educators: Certification: Progress and prospects for diabetes educators, *Diabetes Educator* 13:206–208, 1987.
9. Mazzuca S: Does patient education in chronic disease have therapeutic value? *J Chronic Dis* 35:524–529, 1982.
10. Mazzuca S et al: The diabetes education study: A controlled trial of the effects of diabetes patient education, *Diabetes Care* 9:1–10, 1986.
11. Alogna M: CDC diabetes control programs: Overview of diabetes patient education, *Diabetes Educator* 10:32–36, 1985.
12. Impact of diabetes outpatient education programs: Maine, *MMWR* 31:307–308, 1982.
13. Runyan J: The Memphis chronic disease program, *JAMA* 231:264–267, 1975.
14. Davidson JK et al: Assessment of program effectiveness at Grady Memorial Hospital-Atlanta. In Steiner G, Lawrence PA, editors: *Educating diabetic patients,* New York, 1981, Springer-Verlag.
15. Edmonds ME et al: Improved survival of the diabetic foot: The role of a specialized foot clinic, *Q J Med* 60:763–771, 1986.
16. Miller LV: Evaluation of patient education: LA County Hospital experience, Report of National Commission on diabetes to the Congress of the United States. Washington, DC, Department of Health, Education, and Welfare, 1975, Publication no (NIH) 76-1021, vol 3, part V.
17. Kruger S, Guthrie D: Foot care: Knowledge retention and foot care practices, *Diabetes Educator* 18:487–490, 1992.

28

From Hospital to Home: Role of Home Care in Management of Foot Problems

Sharon Wollman, R.N.

Mark S. Lenes, R.Ph., P.D.

There is no place like home for providing a familiar and supportive environment for healing. This concept is frequently being embraced today by the medical community, as well as the patient. Home health care services are provided by a variety of health care professionals. The level of involvement of each professional is tailored to the specific needs of the patient. The family also plays a major role in the caregiving of the patient. The broadest definition of the term home health care consists of medical, nursing, pharmaceutical, and social services to patients in their places of residence. For the purpose of this chapter, home care and home health care will be one in the same. Also, all services described in this chapter will be classified as "skilled" services, in other words, services provided by health professionals, including pharmacists, nurses, and medical social workers.

Home care is a very diverse system of services provided for patients. These services are not provided by any single entity but are instead multidisciplined in scope.

The ultimate goal of home care should be that it provides a less intimidating, less costly, and more humane approach to care than the old conventional care models.

BRIEF HISTORY OF HOME CARE

Home care is not a new concept. Nursing care to the sick poor, as home care was originally designed, is nearly 200 years old. Before 1980, the home health care market represented just less than 1 billion dollars per year; by 1980, the market had grown to 2.5 billion dollars per year and, by 1990, had reached between 8 and 9 billion dollars per year. The Health Care Financing Administration (HCFA) estimates that home health care will grow at approximately 20% per year. Medical technology has been adapted from the hospital to the home setting, and new home-specific technologies, with an emphasis on safety, simplicity, and reliability, are being developed. The growth is also attributed to an expanded array of professional services now available in the home. All aspects of health care that can be administered in the hospital setting, from physical therapy, and social work to all laboratory tests, can be done in the home setting.

A major factor in the rapid growth of home care is cost containment to both the patient and the health insurer. A growing number of acute and chronic health problems can be managed entirely in the home or have management completed in the home after a brief stabilizing hospitalization at a significant savings to the health insurer payor. One example of the cost savings of home care is through the use of home intravenous antibiotic therapy. It has been shown that the cost of home antibiotic therapy on the average is approximately one half the cost of treating the patient in the hospital. A wide variety of infections have been shown to be treatable with parenteral antibiotics on an outpatient basis, the most common being osteomyelitis and associated skin and soft tissue infections. Of course, many of the patients who have such infections have diabetes or vascular insufficiency, and often a prolonged course of up to 6 weeks of intravenous antibiotic administration is necessary. Occasionally patients will have to visit the office setting or clinic for debridement of wounds, removal of sequestra, or other surgical manipulations.

HOME HEALTH CARE TEAM

The physician prescribes a specialized program of treatment, certifies the need for home care, approves any changes to the patients plan of care, and must be available for any changes in the medical treatment to the patient.

The home care nurse provides skilled nursing care to implement the medical and nursing care plans. It is the responsibility of the home care nurse to provide a vital link between the patient, the physician, and the pharmacist, keeping all informed by telephone, consultation, and progress notes.

The pharmacist dispenses the prescribed medications, checking for dosage, indications, adverse reactions, drug-drug interactions, and drug-food interactions. It is also the responsibility of the clinical pharmacist to develop a pharmaceutical plan of care, keeping all laboratory values (blood urea nitrogen values, creatinine clearance, etc.) in focus and monitoring

any changes that may take place with the patient.

The hospital social worker or discharge planner work with the patient and the family to coordinate personal, family, physician and home health nursing needs before the patient is discharged to home. The dietitian makes a nutrition assessment of the patient and assists with special dietary needs, nutrition education, and meal planning.

EVALUATION OF THE PATIENT FOR HOME CARE

Home health care begins with an evaluation of the patient's medical and other health care needs, available resources, family support, and treatment preferences. The physician decides whether home care is safe and medically appropriate. Consideration is given not only to the patient's medical condition and continued health care support needs but also to family dynamics, physical aspects of the home environment, and the availability of quality home care services.

CRITERIA FOR PATIENT ADMISSION TO HOME CARE

Patients referred for home health care from a hospital setting have to meet certain criteria:

1. *Medical stability:* Before a diabetic patient is discharged from the hospital the patient's medical condition should be stable. Initially the patient should be afebrile. If a wound is present, the wound should be properly evaluated and guidelines established for treatment by either the patient, family members, or a health care provider.

2. *Manageable infection:* The diabetic patient should have an infection process that can be treated effectively in the home

with appropriate family and health care support.

3. *Compliance:* The diabetic patient must be willing to be compliant with all aspects of the home health care plan. The patient or family should express a willingness to actively participate in the medical treatment program.

4. *Education:* The diabetic patient or significant other must have the ability to comprehend a training program for home care. Patients will find greater flexibility in their home care treatment and play a greater role in their home health care decision-making process.

4. *Environmental factors:* It must be determined if the patient's home has availability of a telephone for medical emergencies, a refrigerator for prescribed medications, electricity, running water, and clean surroundings.

6. *Reimbursement:* Home health care services are either reimbursed by the patient or through third-party payors. Confirmation of reimbursement must be established at the onset of acceptance of the patient for home care. Currently Medicare has limited home infusion benefits. New DMERC coverage is expected to be broader.

PREPARING THE PATIENT, THE FAMILY, AND CAREGIVERS

When home care is prescribed for the diabetic patient, the patient and family are prepared for the transition of hospital to home through predischarge teaching. A key element of the discharge preparation process is the education of the patient and the caregiver. This education begins with the patient's present medical condition, how it is expected to progress, the treatment regimen, and how the patient or caregiver can effectively participate in treatment decisions and make informed choices. It is important to realize that the training and preparation of the diabetic patient for home care must be an individual approach. However, a comprehensive teaching plan is necessary to ensure all components of home care are thoroughly presented to the patient and family.

Hospital social workers, discharge planners and home health care professionals are the logical personnel to begin this training. The physician plays an important role in this educational process by participating in the discharge planning, supporting the discharge teaching, and gaining a deeper understanding of the patient's expectations about the home care experience. Unity between the physician, social work or discharge planner, the home health care professional regarding home care training and education clarifies expectations and increases the success of the outcome.

DEVELOPING A CARE PLAN

The course of treatment for the home health care patient is prepared in a written care plan. Most of the elements of the initial care plan are based on information gathered from the physician, the initial patient evaluation, the patient's medical records, and the nurses and other health care professionals who cared for the patient in the hospital. This plan of care is developed with interdisciplinary input as appropriate to address the needs of the patient and in conjunction with the patient or caregiver.

The care plan is finalized after the home health care nurse has made an initial visit to the patient in the home and has completed a comprehensive home health assessment. This evaluation includes a medical history and physician assessment, a psychosocial assessment, an environmental assessment, and a family-caregiver assessment. The home health care nurse consults with the physician and any additional health care providers, and an adjusted care plan is completed.

The plan of treatment for the diabetic patient includes:

1. A primary diagnosis, a secondary diagnosis, and all underlying medical conditions if applicable.
2. Prognosis, rehabilitation potential, functional limitations, and permitted activities.
3. Nutritional requirements, maintenance, and compliance.
4. Medications, including dosage, frequency, route, compliance, side effects, and complications.
5. Wound care, including monitoring (presence of drainage, color, odor, appearance), dressing changes, and complications.
6. Signs, symptoms, potential complications, monitoring requirements, and physical or behaviorial parameters that signal the need for the home health care nurse to notify the physician of a change in the patient's medical status.
7. Contingency plan for emergencies, such as telephone numbers in an acute emergency (to include the physician, local emergency room and ambulance, home health care nurse, and pharmacist).

The information in the plan of treatment provides the basis for home health care. The care plan is revised and updated frequently throughout the home care experience. There are written and verbal changes made by the physician, changes in the responsibility and discipline of the patient, and changes the home health care nurse may decide on with support from the multidisciplinary medical team.

MULTIDISCIPLINARY MEDICAL TEAM FOR HOME CARE

During the course of home care for the diabetic patient, the physician will be called on to update, review, and recertify the care plan. Frequent physician monitoring may become necessary, depending on the patient's condition and progress. Physician involvement with the home health care nurse, pharmacist, family members, and any other home care providers are imperative for efficiency and quality of the home care treatment. The home health nurse should be trained and knowledgeable in all areas of home care. The nurse needs to be responsible for regulatory requirements related to the practice of home care, home care agency policy and procedures, disease processes, psychosocial aspects related to illness and home care, infection control and universal precautions, and pharmacology (specifically those drugs that will be administered or that the patient is already taking).

PATIENT COMPLIANCE AND MONITORING

The emotional adjustment to diabetes by the patient and the family can be a crucial element in the success of patient healing. When the patient returns home after hospitalization, fear and anxiety may be quite overwhelming. With medical support, education, and reassurance by the physician, family, and home care nurse, the patient does not feel abandoned or isolated and is apt to become very respectful and involved in his or her disease process. As the patient and the family become educated about the disease, expectations about the diabetes disease process becomes more realistic. It is difficult for persons with diabetes to fully appreciate the demands of a diabetic regimen (e.g., insulin injections, blood glucose level monitoring, dietary restrictions, treatment of hypoglycemia, and the constant need to monitor and make decisions regarding these concerns).

A major source of concern for the diabetic patient is the diabetic foot. When the patient is discharged from the hospital with a diabetic foot ulcer, wound care is routinely instituted in the home. With detailed instructions from the physician, the home health nurse treats the diabetic wound daily, or as prescribed, always assessing the wound for signs of infection that include fever, erythema, purulent drainage, and fluctuant swelling. The home care nurse will immediately contact the physician for additional treatment or a change in therapy.

HOME INFUSION THERAPY

The diabetic patient is frequently discharged from the hospital to the home with home infusion therapy. As a result of osteomyelitis, cellulitis, wound infections, and postoperative pain, the patient receives antibiotic therapy or pain management in the home. The purpose of home intravenous therapy for the diabetic patient is to administer medications, especially those needed to take effect immediately. Again, the physician, the home care nurse, and the pharmacist work together to create a safe discipline for the patient.

Home infusion therapy is administered in many ways. The traditional practice of intravenous therapy is peripheral venipuncture. This is the most common technique. It involves less trauma to the patient, is less likely to create problems for the patient, and is more convenient. Most patients find the peripheral catheter easy to work with when administering their medication. The home care nurse changes the catheter every 72 hours to prevent infection. This type of catheter is good for short-term therapy.

Often diabetic patients, however, have poor veins. An alternate method of catheterization is the midline catheter for patients requiring several weeks of intravenous therapy or those with poor venous access. The midline catheter provides a stable midline access within the peripheral circulatory system. These catheters

are generally placed in the basilic, median cubital, or cephalic veins of the anticubital region. The home care nurse is certified to insert this catheter in the home care setting.

An alternative to the peripheral catheter and the midline catheter is the central line catheter. Patients requiring long-term therapy or who have no venous access will require the insertion of a central line catheter:

PICC Line Catheter

This catheter is a peripherally inserted central line catheter generally inserted by a physician or specially trained registered nurse. PICC lines are inserted in the hospital or in the physician's office. They are usually placed in the basilis, median cubital, or cephalic vein of the antecubital region of the patient's arm.

Hickman/Broviac Catheter

This catheter is an open-end tunneled catheter, a long-term indwelling catheter inserted into the superior vena cava via the subclavian vein. These catheters are inserted by a physician in an operating room of a hospital. This can be done on an outpatient basis.

Groshong Catheter

This catheter is a close-end tunneled catheter, a long-term indwelling catheter, inserted into the superior vena cava via the subclavian vein. These catheters are generally inserted by a physician in an operating room of a hospital. This can be done on an outpatient basis.

Plain Central Line Catheter

This catheter is generally inserted in the subclavian or jugular vein with the tip located in the superior vena cava. These catheters are generally inserted in the emergency room, the patient's hospital room, or the hospital operating room by the physician. They may be inserted on an outpatient basis. The home care nurse is educated in line maintenance, infection control, and universal precautions. It is the responsibility of the home care nurse to monitor the patient's medical progress. The intensity of the monitoring process depends on the severity of the patient's condition and the patient or caregiver's ability. Written reports and orders, interdisciplinary conferences with the physician and pharmacist, and verbal reports keep communication and coordination of the disciplines involved with patient care.

ROLE OF THE PHARMACIST

The decision to dispense medications for intravenous infusion outside the hospital setting places the community pharmacist in a situation whereby the safety and efficacy of such therapy must be ensured. Policies and procedures must be written, and all documentation must be similar to that of the institutional pharmacy before medications are dispensed for home intravenous administration.

Continuity of care from the hospital setting to the home must be ensured. Multiple surveys have demonstrated that the community pharmacist is a well-respected source of health care information, particularly in the area of self-treatment. Therefore, the areas of instruction on drug administration, common side effects, and expected outcome with therapy represent a common extension of the role of the pharmacist in patient care. All clinical and microbiologic data must be shared with the pharmacist to ensure the continuity of care for the patient.

The community-based pharmacist (in a home infusion company situation, with the proper equipment and materials) must have the knowledge of available parenteral products, as well as knowledge of drug stability and storage. The pharma-

cist should be aware of proper dilution volumes, reconstitution techniques, available infusion devices, and the most effective device to use for each particular patient. Dispensing of sufficient quantities of each product should be dictated by length of therapy and product stability.

Constant communication with the prescriber, home care nurse, and patient is imperative in the home care setting. The pharmacist is a key player in this loop, maintaining the proper documentation and communication with each care giver and patient. Proper charting of information in a timely and coherent manner is a must. Because patient laboratory data are accessible, interpreting these data and determining appropriate laboratory tests for the duration of therapy are essential. Evaluation of the proposed therapy, awareness of common adverse effects and expected outcomes, and the ability to troubleshoot explanations for unexpected responses are skills that must be had by the pharmacist in the home care setting. The community pharmacist in this setting must also have the skills to provide therapeutic assessments and provide or suggest viable alternatives to apparently ineffective therapy. As an example, the referring physician and the pharmacist must work together to pick the best possible antibiotic for each individual patient. The choice of antibiotic must meet certain criteria:

1. Active against the infecting organism
2. Minimal side effects
3. Minimal venous irritation
4. Prolonged half-life
5. Cost effective

The physician and pharmacist must also communicate to monitor the many parameters that home intravenous therapy provides. In the instance of osteomyelitis, where intravenous antibiotic therapy is usually necessary for 4 to 6 weeks (in some cases of chronic osteomyelitis up to 4 months), the pharmacist must consider monitoring the following parameters for the infected osteomyelitis patient*:

1. Serum creatinine levels
2. Blood urea nitrogen levels
3. Minimal inhibitory and bactericidal concentrations
4. Erythrocyte sedimentation rate
5. White blood cell count
6. Peaks and troughs of amikacin, ciprofloxacin, gentamicin, tobramycin, and vancomycin
7. Changes in hearing or balance
8. Patient-specific parameters
   a. Temperature
   b. Night sweats
   c. New or increased wound drainage
   d. Erythema of skin over infected bone
   e. Doses adjusted for patient body weight
   f. Increased level of pain medication used by patient

One of the most important areas for the pharmacist to monitor is the toxicity level of the drugs involved. Because of the prolonged treatment course with the increased risk of adverse effects, the home care pharmacist must carefully monitor patients. Toxicity, relapse, and treatment failure are principal concerns in the management of acute and chronic osteomyelitis.

*These parameters are indicated for patients infected with Staphylococcus and methicillin-resistant Staphylococcus.

CONCLUSION

The future of home care will be characterized by managed care, tighter financial constraints, increased technologies, and a greater impetus to avoid long and costly institutionalization. Physicians will become an even greater force to drive the home health care industry, with more reliance on the home health care team to help them take care of the patient from hospital to home.

BIBLIOGRAPHY

Ackerman BH, Wolfe JJ: Monitoring chronic outpatient infections: Providing comprehensive home health care pharmacy services. *Drug Intell Clin Pharm* 25:840, 1991.

American Medical Association: *Physician guide to home health care,* Washington D.C., 1989, American Medical Association.

Bernstein LH: An update on home intravenous antibiotic therapy, *Geriatrics* 46:47, 1991.

Cummings JE, Weaver FM: Cost-effectiveness of home care, *Clin Geriatr Med* 7:865, 1991.

Poretz DM: Home intravenous antibiotic therapy, *Clin Geriatr Med* 7:749, 1991.

Scott WC, et al: Educating physicians in home health care, *JAMA* 265:769, 1991.

INDEX